Metal Ions in Life Sciences

Volume 24

Targeted Metallo-Drugs: *Design, Development, and Modes of Action*

Guest Editors
Etelka Farkas
University of Debrecen
Faculty of Science and Technology
Department of Inorganic and
Analytical Chemistry
H-4010 Debrecen
Hungary
efarkas@science.unideb.hu

Celine J. Marmion
RCSI University of Medicine and
Health Sciences
Department of Chemistry
123 St. Stephen's Green
Dublin 2
Ireland
cmarmion@rcsi.com

Series Editors
Astrid Sigel, Helmut Sigel
Department of Chemistry
Inorganic Chemistry
University of Basel
St. Johannsring 19
CH-4056 Basel
Switzerland
astrid.sigel@unibas.ch
helmut.sigel@unibas.ch

Eva Freisinger, Roland K. O. Sigel
Department of Chemistry
University of Zürich
Winterthurerstrasse 190
CH-8057 Zürich
Switzerland
freisinger@chem.uzh.ch
roland.sigel@chem.uzh.ch

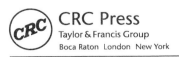

CRC Press is an imprint of the
Taylor & Francis Group, an **informa** business

Cover illustration : The figure on the dust cover represents bacterial cell resistance mechanisms and was taken from Chapter 6 by permission of Andres Evans and Professor Kevin Kavanagh.

First edition published 2023
by CRC Press
6000 Broken Sound Parkway NW, Suite 300, Boca Raton, FL 33487-2742

and by CRC Press
4 Park Square, Milton Park, Abingdon, Oxon, OX14 4RN

CRC Press is an imprint of Taylor & Francis Group, LLC

© 2023 selection and editorial matter, Etelka Farkas and Celine J. Marmion, individual chapters, the contributors

Reasonable efforts have been made to publish reliable data and information, but the author and publisher cannot assume responsibility for the validity of all materials or the consequences of their use. The authors and publishers have attempted to trace the copyright holders of all material reproduced in this publication and apologize to copyright holders if permission to publish in this form has not been obtained. If any copyright material has not been acknowledged please write and let us know so we may rectify in any future reprint.

Except as permitted under U.S. Copyright Law, no part of this book may be reprinted, reproduced, transmitted, or utilized in any form by any electronic, mechanical, or other means, now known or hereafter invented, including photocopying, microfilming, and recording, or in any information storage or retrieval system, without written permission from the publishers.

For permission to photocopy or use material electronically from this work, access www.copyright. com or contact the Copyright Clearance Center, Inc. (CCC), 222 Rosewood Drive, Danvers, MA 01923, 978-750-8400. For works that are not available on CCC please contact mpkbookspermissions@tandf. co.uk

Trademark notice: Product or corporate names may be trademarks or registered trademarks and are used only for identification and explanation without intent to infringe.

Library of Congress Cataloging-in-Publication Data
Names: Farkas, Etelka, editor. | Marmion, Celine J., editor.
Title: Targeted metallo-drugs : design, development, and mode of action / guest editors
Celine J. Marmion (RCSI University of Medicine and Health Sciences, Department of Chemistry,
Dublin, Ireland), Etelka Farkas (University of Debrecen, Faculty of Science, Department of Inorganic
and Analytical Chemistry, Debrecen, Hungary).
Description: First edition. | Boca Raton : CRC Press, 2023. |
Series: Metal ions in life sciences, 1559-0836 ; volume 24 |
Includes bibliographical references and index.
Identifiers: LCCN 2022043783 (print) | LCCN 2022043784 (ebook) |
ISBN 9781032223308 (hardback) | ISBN 9781032223537 (paperback) |
ISBN 9781003272250 (ebook)
Subjects: LCSH: Metals–Therapeutic use. | Metals in medicine. |
Drugs–Design. | Pharmaceutical chemistry.
Classification: LCC RM666.M513 T37 2023 (print) | LCC RM666.M513 (ebook) |
DDC 615.9/253–dc23/eng/20230228
LC record available at https://lccn.loc.gov/2022043783
LC ebook record available at https://lccn.loc.gov/2022043784

ISBN: 9781032223308 (hbk)
ISBN: 9781032223537 (pbk)
ISBN: 9781003272250 (ebk)

ISSN: 1559-0836   e-ISSN: 1868-0402

DOI: 10.1201/9781003272250

Typeset in Times New Roman
by codeMantra

About the Editors

Etelka Farkas is Emeritus Professor (2016) at the Faculty of Science and Technology, Department of Inorganic and Analytical Chemistry at the University of Debrecen, Hungary. After receiving her scientific degree (D.Sc.) from the Hungarian Academy of Sciences (HAS) in 1998, she has worked as elected member in some HAS Committees, e.g., the Committee on Physical Chemistry and Inorganic Chemistry (2011–) and the Doctoral Council of Chemical Sciences (2018–2021), and she chaired the Working Committee of Coordination Chemistry (2011–2017). From 2006 to 2019, she was also Chair of the International Relations of the Hungarian Chemical Society. Her research has been focused, first of all, on the bio-induced solution study of metal complexes with a large variety of ligands, e.g., amino acid-, peptide-, and hydroxamic acid-based ligands, and the results have been presented in ca. 180 publications. Professor Farkas was Editor of the RSC Specialist Periodical Reports (Vols. 37–39) on Amino Acids, Peptides, and Proteins for the years 2012, 2013, and 2015. Furthermore, she was Guest Editor of the Special Issue 472 (2018) of *Inorganica Chimica Acta* and of the issue 206 (2020) of the *Journal of Inorganic Biochemistry*. She received many awards; to mention just three of them: (2005) Gold Cross of Merit of the Hungarian Republic; (2012) Albert Szent-Györgyi Award; and (2022) Academy Prize, Awarded by the HAS.

Celine J. Marmion is Professor of Bioinorganic Chemistry (since 2018) and Deputy Dean for Student Engagement (2018–2024) in RCSI, University of Medicine and Health Sciences, Dublin, Ireland. Her current research focuses on the rational design and development of innovative, multi-targeted metallo-drug candidates as anticancer or antimicrobial drugs. She has a track record in commercializing her research with the patient at the heart of all that she does. In this regard, she, together with colleagues, executed a pharma license agreement on a metallo-drug technology in 2010 and, more recently, entered into an industry-funded collaboration and option agreement with another pharma in 2016. Professor Marmion has undertaken many senior leadership roles within and outside her university. She is currently an active Council member of the Society of Biological Inorganic Chemistry (SBIC). She was President of the Institute of Chemistry of Ireland, the national body representing all chemists in Ireland from 2019 to 2022, the third female only to be elected as President since its establishment in 1922. She also co-founded the Irish Biological Inorganic Chemistry Society in 2017 and served as its President from 2018 to 2020. Professor Marmion is a strong and vocal advocate for young scientists. In this regard, she played a key role in the establishment of the Institute of Chemistry of Ireland Young Chemists' Network. She is also deeply committed to nurturing excellence in the education of students. She was the recipient of national "Teaching Hero" awards in 2021 and 2016 (as nominated by students) and numerous RCSI President's Teaching Awards.

About the Editors

Astrid Sigel has studied languages; she was an Editor of the *Metal Ions in Biological Systems* (*MIBS*) series (until Volume 44) and also of the *Handbook on Toxicity of Inorganic Compounds* (1988), the *Handbook on Metals in Clinical and Analytical Chemistry* (1994; both with H. G. Seiler and H.S.), and on the *Handbook on Metalloproteins* (2001; with Ivano Bertini and H.S.). She is also an Editor of the *MILS* series from Volume 1 on, and she co-authored more than 50 papers on topics in Bioinorganic Chemistry.

Helmut Sigel is Emeritus Professor (2003) of Inorganic Chemistry at the University of Basel, Switzerland. He is a Co-editor of the series *Metal Ions in Biological Systems* (1973–2005; 44 volumes) as well as of the Sigels' new series *Metal Ions in Life Sciences* (since 2006). He also co-edited three handbooks and published over 350 articles on metal ion complexes of nucleotides, amino acids, coenzymes, and other bio-ligands. Together with Ivano Bertini, Harry B. Gray, and Bo G. Malmström, he founded (1983) the International Conferences on Biological Inorganic Chemistry (ICBICs). He lectured worldwide and was named *Protagonist in Chemistry* (2002) by *Inorganica Chimica Acta* (issue 339). Among Endowed Lectureships, appointments as Visiting Professor (e.g., Austria, China, Japan, Kuwait, UK), and further honors, he received the P. Ray Award (Indian Chemical Society, of which he is also a Honorary Fellow), the Alfred Werner Award (Swiss Chemical Society), and a Doctor of Science honoris causa degree (Kalyani University, India). He is also an Honorary Member of SBIC (Society of Biological Inorganic Chemistry).

Eva Freisinger is Associate Professor of Bioinorganic Chemistry and Chemical Biology (2018) at the Department of Chemistry at the University of Zürich, Switzerland. She obtained her doctoral degree (2000) from the University of Dortmund, Germany, working with Bernhard Lippert, and spent three years as a postdoc at SUNY Stony Brook, USA, with Caroline Kisker. Since 2003, she has performed independent research at the University of Zürich where she held a Förderungsprofessur of the Swiss National Science Foundation from 2008 to 2014. In 2014, she received her *Habilitation* in Bioinorganic Chemistry. Her research is focused on the study of plant metallothioneins with an additional interest in the sequence-specific modification of nucleic acids. Together with Roland Sigel, she chaired the 12th European Biological Inorganic Chemistry Conference (2014 in Zürich, Switzerland) as well as the 19th International Conference on Biological Inorganic Chemistry (2019 in Interlaken, Switzerland). She also serves on a number of Advisory Boards for international conference series; since 2014, she has been the Secretary of the European Biological Inorganic Chemistry Conferences (EuroBICs), and is currently co-Director of the Department of Chemistry. She joined the group of Editors of the *MILS* series from Volume 18 on.

Roland K. O. Sigel is Full Professor (2016) of Chemistry at the University of Zürich, Switzerland. In the same year, he became Vice Dean of Studies (BSc/MSc), and in 2017, he was elected Dean of the Faculty of Science. From 2003 to 2008, he was endowed with a Förderungsprofessur of the Swiss National Science Foundation, and he is the recipient of an ERC Starting Grant 2010. He received his doctoral degree summa cum laude (1999) from the University of Dortmund, Germany, working with Bernhard Lippert. Thereafter he spent nearly three years at Columbia University (now Yale University), New York, USA, with Anna Marie Pyle. During the six years abroad, he received several prestigious fellowships from various sources, and he was awarded the EuroBIC Medal in 2008 and the Alfred Werner Prize (SCS) in 2009. Between 2015 and 2019, he was the Secretary of the Society of Biological Inorganic Chemistry (SBIC), and since 2018, he has been the Secretary of the International Conferences on Biological Inorganic Chemistry (ICBICs). His research focuses on the structural and functional role of metal ions in ribozymes, especially group II introns, regulatory RNAs, and on related topics. He is also an Editor of Volumes 43 and 44 of the *MIBS* series and of the *MILS* series from Volume 1 on.

Historical Development and Perspectives of the Series
*Metal Ions in Life Sciences**

It is an old wisdom that metals are indispensable for life. Indeed, several of them, like sodium, potassium, and calcium, are easily discovered in living matter. However, the role of metals and their impact on life remained largely hidden until inorganic chemistry and coordination chemistry experienced a pronounced revival in the 1950s. The experimental and theoretical tools created in this period and their application to biochemical problems led to the development of the field or discipline now known as *Bioinorganic Chemistry*, *Inorganic Biochemistry*, or more recently also often addressed as *Biological Inorganic Chemistry*.

By 1970, *Bioinorganic Chemistry* was established and further promoted by the book series *Metal Ions in Biological Systems* founded in 1973 (edited by H.S., who was soon joined by A.S.) and published by Marcel Dekker, Inc., New York, for more than 30 years. After this company ceased to be a family endeavor and its acquisition by another company, we decided, after having edited 44 volumes of the *MIBS* series (the last two together with R.K.O.S.) to launch a new and broader minded series to cover today's needs in the *Life Sciences*. Therefore, the Sigels' new series is entitled

"Metal Ions in Life Sciences".

After publication of 22 volumes (since 2006), we are happy to join forces from Volume 23 on in this still growing endeavor with Taylor & Francis, London, UK, a most experienced Publisher in the *Sciences*.

The development of *Biological Inorganic Chemistry* during the past 40 years was and still is driven by several factors; among these are (i) attempts to reveal the interplay between metal ions and hormones or vitamins, etc.; (ii) efforts regarding the understanding of accumulation, transport, metabolism, and toxicity of metal ions; (iii) the development and application of metal-based drugs; (iv) biomimetic syntheses with the aim to understand biological processes as well as to create efficient catalysts; (v) the determination of high-resolution structures of proteins, nucleic acids, and other biomolecules; (vi) the utilization of powerful spectroscopic tools allowing studies of structures and dynamics; and (vii) more recently, the widespread use of macromolecular engineering to create new

---

* Reproduced with some alterations by permission of John Wiley & Sons, Ltd., Chichester, UK (copyright 2006) from pages v and vi of Volume 1 of the series *Metal Ions in Life Sciences* (MILS-1).

biologically relevant structures at will. All this and more is reflected in the volumes of the series *Metal Ions in Life Sciences*.

The importance of metal ions to the vital functions of living organisms, hence, to their health and well-being, is nowadays well accepted. However, in spite of all the progress made, we are still only at the brink of understanding these processes. Therefore, the series *Metal Ions in Life Sciences* links coordination chemistry and biochemistry in their widest sense. Despite the evident expectation that a great deal of future outstanding discoveries will be made in the interdisciplinary areas of science, there are still "language" barriers between the historically separate spheres of chemistry, biology, medicine, and physics. Thus, it is one of the aims of this series to catalyze mutual "understanding."

It is our hope that *Metal Ions in Life Sciences* continues to prove a stimulus for new activities in the fascinating "field" of *Biological Inorganic Chemistry*. If so, it will well serve its purpose and be a rewarding result for the efforts spent by the authors.

Astrid Sigel and Helmut Sigel
Department of Chemistry, Inorganic Chemistry
University of Basel, CH-4056 Basel, Switzerland

Eva Freisinger and Roland K. O. Sigel
Department of Chemistry
University of Zürich, CH-8057 Zürich, Switzerland

October 2005 and March 2022

Preface to Volume 24

Targeted Metallo-Drugs:
Design, Development, and Modes of Action

The *Metal Ions in Life Sciences* (*MILS*) series has occupied a pivotal role in fostering and stimulating interdisciplinary research in the vibrant field of Biological Inorganic Chemistry since the publication of its first volume in 2006. This 24th volume entitled "Targeted Metallo-Drugs: Design, Development, and Modes of Action" is no exception.

Inspired by the clinical success of cisplatin as a leading anticancer drug but mindful of the shortcomings associated with its use including dose-limiting toxic side effects and acquired or intrinsic drug resistance, scientists across the globe have been endeavoring to identify new metallo-drugs beyond cisplatin for therapeutic exploitation.

While the biological properties of cisplatin, like numerous drugs, were serendipitously discovered, advances in science, technology, and medicine have resulted in a paradigm shift in recent years, moving from a single-target to a more streamlined and multi-targeted approach in metallo-drug development. While the primary target of cisplatin is cancer cell DNA, the identification of numerous biological targets beyond DNA has led to a plethora of innovative, multi-targeted metallo-drug candidates, rationally designed to (i) enhance cancer cell selectivity, thus reducing toxic side effects and/or (ii) possess new modes of action to improve efficacy and also target resistance pathways. Developing drugs incorporating metals other than Pt, with a mechanism of action and toxicity profile distinct to Pt drugs, is also being pursued not only as anticancer agents but as antimicrobial, antiviral, and other agents such as those targeting neglected tropical diseases and cyanide poisoning. This is very timely given the surge in antimicrobial resistance to current organic-based antibiotic treatments and the recent COVID-19 global pandemic. The development of nanoclusters as diagnostic and therapeutic agents and radiometal-based medical imaging and therapeutic entities are also prominent areas of active research in the biological inorganic chemistry field. Understanding the mode of action of these targeted drug entities at a molecular level is critical if we are to progress drugs from the bench, to pre-clinical evaluations and ultimately to the clinic. We are seeing wonderful progress in this regard with the advancement of new spectroscopic methods as well as the emergence of metalloproteomics, a discipline used to elucidate the expression, quantity, and function of metalloproteins in the human body. This MILS-24 volume captures all of the above in 12 comprehensive, well-illustrated and up-to-date chapters spanning 370 pages with over 1,600 citations and 100 figures, with key contributions from 32 international experts from Europe, Asia, and North and South America.

Chapters 1–3 focus on metallo-drugs as anticancer agents. The first chapter provides an eloquent overview of metal-based prodrugs and their nanoformulations that employ intrinsic tumor-specific triggers (redox, hypoxia, and pH) to selectively promote drug activation in the unique environment found in tumor cells. Chapter 2, in contrast, focuses on light as an external activation source. A comprehensive overview of light-activated metallo-drugs for photodynamic and photoactivated therapies is provided. A particular feature of Chapter 2 is a comparison of inorganic- versus organic-based photo-active systems, and the development of new guidelines that embody the requisite features of light-activated metal-based systems, thus promoting a more rational approach to drug design in this area.

In recent years, exploiting signaling pathways and cellular stressors other than DNA damage have come to the fore as alternative drug targets. Chapter 3 offers a unique insight into the mitochondria as one such target. Complexes incorporating different metal ions and metal-based mitochondria-targeting photosensitizers, designed to disrupt mitochondrial bioenergetics and redox homeostasis and, in so doing, bypass resistance mechanisms and (re-)activate tumor cell death programs, are comprehensively described.

Given the recent COVID-19 pandemic and its enormous global impact, the onset of new viruses, the emergence of resistance to current antiviral drugs, and the fact that many antiviral agents have a narrow spectrum of action, we are witnessing a surge in interest in research into the development of novel antiviral agents, including those targeting the SARS-COV-2 virus. Chapters 4 and 5 eloquently review the role of metallo-drug candidates as innovative antiviral agents. Chapter 4 provides a state-of-the-art summary related to metal-based antiviral agents derived from metals from periods 4 to 7 of the Periodic Table, while Chapter 5 highlights the potential of not only repurposing clinically-approved drugs as antiviral agents but also tapping into the chemical diversity of metal complexes as a source of novel drug treatments for COVID-19.

The emergence of antimicrobial resistance is posing an enormous threat to humanity. Chapter 6 provides us with hope by presenting an up-to-date overview of the safety and toxicity profiles and modes of action of a range of metal-based complexes as representative examples, which have been developed as potential alternatives to conventional antibiotics. A section on Zn chelators is also included as they directly interact with Zn to re-sensitize some bacteria resistant to β-lactam antibiotics.

Chapter 7 showcases how fine-tuning metal complexes by incorporating bioactive ligands or co-ligands that modulate the physicochemical and biological properties of the resulting complexes can lead to new and exciting multi-functional metallo-drugs targeting neglected tropical diseases.

Chapter 8 builds on the content covered in Chapter 14 of the 19th volume of MILS, providing an up-to-date account of the challenges in targeting cyanide poisoning and how these may be overcome by exploiting metal-based agents or indeed by activating biological metal-containing proteins such as hemoglobin to treat cyanide toxicity in humans.

Preface to Volume 24

Understanding the mode of action of these targeted drug entities at a molecular level is critical if these new drug entities are to progress from the bench, to pre-clinical evaluations, and ultimately to the clinic. Chapter 9 provides a state-of-the-art account of spectroscopic tools (X-ray fluorescence, luminescence lifetime imaging, and two-photon excitation microscopies) that can be employed to elucidate the localization of metal-based complexes in tumor cells. Chapter 10 comprehensively showcases the field of metalloproteomics, paying particular attention to how metalloproteomics can be utilized to unveil the modes of action of anticancer and antimicrobial metal-based drugs. It also highlights how a metalloproteomics approach could be equally applied to other areas of research including neurological disorders given that there is increasing evidence that deregulation of metals can contribute to numerous neurodegenerative diseases.

The penultimate Chapter 11 provides an eloquent account of metal-based nanoclusters with a particular emphasis on their ability to detect metal ions and inorganic anions, small molecules, proteins, and nucleic acids. Their application as promising fluorescence probes for biological imaging and labeling and their capacity to act as potential drug delivery nano-objects and as diagnostic and therapeutic agents are also covered in detail.

The final chapter, Chapter 12, provides a comprehensive overview of the enormous potential and applications of radiometals in nuclear medicine, their chemical and radiation characteristics, as well as the synthetic protocols and strategies facilitating their incorporation into radiopharmaceuticals as well as future trends in the development of radiometals into medically useful tracers.

In summary, we have endeavored to showcase the far-reaching potential of metal-based agents as therapeutic and diagnostic agents as well as highlighting key developments in spectroscopic techniques and metalloproteomics to further advance our understanding of the modes of actions of metallo-drugs. We are enormously grateful to our colleagues who have contributed their extensive expertise to MILS-24, enabling us to keep our scientific community abreast of the latest developments in this vibrant field of research. We hope also that MILS-24 will serve as an invaluable resource to stimulate further cutting-edge research in these important areas and that it will also inspire our next generation of young scientists who are interested in pursuing research in metallo-drug design and development.

Celine J. Marmion

Etelka Farkas

Contents

About the Editors iii
Historical Development and Perspectives of the Series vii
Preface to Volume 24 ix
Contributors to Volume 24 xv
Handbooks and Book Series Published and (Co-)edited by the SIGELs xix

Chapter 1   Metal-Based Prodrugs Activated by Cancer-Specific Stimuli 1

Martijn Dijkstra, Hemma Schueffl, Isabella Poetsch, Petra Heffeter, and Christian R. Kowol

Chapter 2   Light-Activated Drugs for Photodynamic and Photoactivated Therapy 39

Dmytro Havrylyuk, Austin Hachey, and Edith Glazer

Chapter 3   Mitochondria as a Metallo-Drug Target for Therapeutic Purposes 67

Andrea Erxleben

Chapter 4   Transition Metal-Based Antiviral Agents Against SARS-CoV-2 and Other Pathogenic Viruses 105

Maria Gil-Moles and Ingo Ott

Chapter 5   Exploiting the Chemical Diversity of Metal Compounds as a Source of Novel Anti-COVID-19 Drugs 139

Damiano Cirri, Carlo Marotta, Alessandro Pratesi, Tiziano Marzo, and Luigi Messori

Chapter 6   Evaluating the Potential of Novel Metal-Based Drugs for Treating Drug-Resistant Bacteria 163

Andris Evans and Kevin Kavanagh

Chapter 7   Prospective Metallo-Drugs Including Bioactive Compounds: Selection of Co-Ligands to Tune Biological Activity Against Neglected Tropical Diseases 193

Dinorah Gambino and Lucía Otero

xiii

xiv Contents

Chapter 8 Challenges in Targeting Cyanide Poisoning: Advantages in Exploiting Metal Complexes in Its Treatment..............................215

Sigridur G. Suman

Chapter 9 Advanced Microscopy Methods for Elucidating the Localization of Metal Complexes in Cancer Cells 239

Johannes Karges and Nils Metzler-Nolte

Chapter 10 Metalloproteomics: A Powerful Technique for Metals in Medicine...265

Tiffany Ka-Yan Ip, Ying Zhou, Hongyan Li, and Hongzhe Sun

Chapter 11 Metal-Based Nanoclusters for Biomedical Applications 289

Edit Csapó

Chapter 12 Radiometals in Molecular Imaging and Therapy 319

Izabela Cieszykowska, Wioletta Wojdowska, Dariusz Pawlak, and Renata Mikołajczak

Index...347

Contributors to Volume 24

Izabela Cieszykowska
National Centre for Nuclear Research
Radioisotope Centre POLATOM
Andrzej Sołtan 7
PL-05–400 Otwock, Poland

Damiano Cirri
Department of Chemistry and
Industrial Chemistry
Via Giuseppe Moruzzi 13
I-56124 Pisa, Italy

Edit Csapó
MTA-SZTE Lendület "Momentum"
Noble Metal Nanostructures Research
Group, Interdisciplinary Excellence
Center
Department of Physical Chemistry
and Materials Science
University of Szeged
Rerrich B. square 1
H-6720 Szeged, Hungary

Martijn Dijkstra
Institute of Inorganic Chemistry
Faculty of Chemistry
University of Vienna
Waehringer Strasse 42
A-1090 Vienna, Austria

Andrea Erxleben
School of Biological and
Chemical Sciences
University of Galway
University Road
Galway, H91TK33, Ireland

Andris Evans
Department of Microbiology and
Immunology
The University of Western Ontario
London
Ontario N6A 3K7, Canada

Dinorah Gambino
Área Química Inorgánica
Departamento Estrella Campos
Facultad de Química
Universidad de la República
Montevideo, Uruguay

Maria Gil-Moles
Institute of Medicinal and
Pharmaceutical Chemistry
Technische Universität Braunschweig
Beethovenstr. 55
D-38106 Braunschweig
Germany
and
Departamento de Química
Universidad de La Rioja
Centro de Investigación de Síntesis
Química (CISQ)
Complejo Científico Tecnológico
ES-26004 Logroño, Spain

Edith Glazer
Department of Chemistry
North Carolina State University
Raleigh, NC, USA

Austin Hachey
Department of Chemistry
University of Kentucky
Lexington, KY 40506, USA

Dmytro Havrylyuk
Department of Chemistry
University of Kentucky
Lexington, KY 40506, USA

Petra Heffeter
Center for Cancer Research
Medical University of Vienna
Borschkegasse 8a
A-1090 Vienna
and
Research Cluster "Translational
Cancer Therapy Research"
Vienna, Austria

Tiffany Ka-Yan Ip
Department of Chemistry
The University of Hong Kong
Hong Kong SAR, China

Johannes Karges
Faculty for Chemistry and
Biochemistry
Ruhr University Bochum
Universitätsstrasse 150
D-44801 Bochum, Germany

Kevin Kavanagh
SSPC Pharma Research Centre
Department of Biology
Maynooth University
Co. Kildare, Ireland

Christian R. Kowol
Institute of Inorganic Chemistry
Faculty of Chemistry
University of Vienna
Waehringer Strasse 42
A-1090 Vienna, Austria
and
Research Cluster "Translational
Cancer Therapy Research"
Vienna, Austria

Hongyan Li
Department of Chemistry
The University of Hong Kong
Hong Kong SAR, China

Carlo Marotta
Department of Chemistry and
Industrial Chemistry
Via Giuseppe Moruzzi 13
I-56124 Pisa, Italy

Tiziano Marzo
Department of Pharmacy
University of Pisa
Via Bonanno Pisano 6
I-56126 Pisa, Italy

Luigi Messori
Department of Chemistry
'Ugo Schiff'
University of Florence
Via della Lastruccia 3–13
I-50019 Sesto Fiorentino, Italy

Nils Metzler-Nolte
Chair of Inorganic Chemistry I –
Bioinorganic Chemistry
Faculty for Chemistry and
Biochemistry
Ruhr University Bochum
Universitätsstrasse 150
D-44801 Bochum, Germany

Renata Mikołajczak
National Centre for Nuclear Research
Radioisotope Centre POLATOM
Andrzej Sołtan 7
PL-05–400 Otwock, Poland

Contributors to Volume 24

Lucía Otero
Área Química Inorgánica
Departamento Estrella Campos
Facultad de Química
Universidad de la República
Montevideo, Uruguay

Ingo Ott
Institute of Medicinal and
Pharmaceutical Chemistry
Technische Universität Braunschweig
Beethovenstr. 55
D-38106 Braunschweig, Germany

Dariusz Pawlak
National Centre for Nuclear Research
Radioisotope Centre POLATOM
Andrzej Sołtan 7
PL-05–400 Otwock, Poland

Isabella Poetsch
Institute of Inorganic Chemistry
Faculty of Chemistry
University of Vienna
Waehringer Strasse 42
A-1090 Vienna, Austria
and
Center for Cancer Research
Medical University of Vienna
Borschkegasse 8a
A-1090 Vienna, Austria

Alessandro Pratesi
Department of Chemistry and
Industrial Chemistry
Via Giuseppe Moruzzi 13
I-56124 Pisa, Italy

Hemma Schueffl
Center for Cancer Research
Medical University of Vienna
Borschkegasse 8a
A-1090 Vienna, Austria

Sigridur G. Suman
Science Institute
University of Iceland
Dunhagi 3
IS-107 Reykjavik, Iceland

Hongzhe Sun
Department of Chemistry
The University of Hong Kong
Hong Kong SAR, China

Wioletta Wojdowska
National Centre for Nuclear Research
Radioisotope Centre POLATOM
Andrzej Sołtan 7
PL-05–400 Otwock, Poland

Ying Zhou
Department of Chemistry
The University of Hong Kong
Hong Kong SAR, China

Handbooks and Book Series Published and (Co-)edited by the SIGELs

"Handbook on Toxicity of Inorganic Compounds" (ISBN: 0–8247-7727-1) Eds H. G. Seiler, H. Sigel, A. Sigel; Dekker, Inc.; New York; 1988; 1069 pp

"Handbook on Metals in Clinical and Analytical Chemistry" (ISBN: 0–8247–9094-4) Eds Hans G. Seiler, Astrid Sigel, Helmut Sigel; Dekker, Inc.; New York, Basel, Hong Kong; 1994; 753 pp

"Handbook on Metalloproteins" (ISBN: 0–8247–0520–3) Eds I. Bertini, A. Sigel, H. Sigel; Marcel Dekker, Inc.; New York, Basel; 2001; 1182 pp

Metal Ions in Biological Systems
Volumes 1–44
https://www.routledge.com/Metal-Ions-in-Biological-Systems/book-series/
IHCMEIOBISY
(see also the website given below)

Metal Ions in Life Sciences
Volumes 1–23
Details about all books (series) edited by the SIGELs, including the Guest Editors, can be found at
http://www.bioinorganic-chemistry.org/mils

1 Metal-Based Prodrugs Activated by Cancer-Specific Stimuli

Martijn Dijkstra[#]
Institute of Inorganic Chemistry, Faculty of Chemistry
University of Vienna, Waehringer Strasse 42,
A-1090 Vienna, Austria

Hemma Schueffl[#]
Center for Cancer Research
Medical University of Vienna, Borschkegasse 8a,
A-1090 Vienna, Austria

Isabella Poetsch
Institute of Inorganic Chemistry, Faculty of Chemistry
University of Vienna, Waehringer Strasse 42,
A-1090 Vienna, Austria
and Center for Cancer Research
Medical University of Vienna, Borschkegasse 8a,
A-1090 Vienna, Austria

Petra Heffeter*
Center for Cancer Research
Medical University of Vienna, Borschkegasse 8a,
A-1090 Vienna, Austria
and Research Cluster "Translational Cancer
Therapy Research", Vienna, Austria
petra.heffeter@meduniwien.ac.at

Christian R. Kowol*
Institute of Inorganic Chemistry, Faculty of Chemistry
University of Vienna, Waehringer Strasse 42,
A-1090 Vienna, Austria
christian.kowol@univie.ac.at

[#] These authors contributed equally to this work.
[*] Corresponding authors

DOI: 10.1201/9781003272250-1

and Research Cluster "Translational Cancer Therapy Research", Vienna, Austria
christian.kowol@univie.ac.at

CONTENTS

1 Introduction 3
   1.1 Anticancer Metal Complexes: Clinical Situation 3
   1.2 Intrinsic Parameters of the Malignant Tumor Suitable for Drug
       Activation 4
      1.2.1 Activation by Reduction Based on the Changed Redox
            Environment of the Tumor 5
      1.2.2 Physicochemical Triggers: Hypoxia and Reduced pH 5
      1.2.3 Biological Characteristics: Tumor-Specific Upregulation
            of Enzymes 7
2 Redox-Responsive Metal-Based Prodrugs 7
   2.1 Redox-Responsive Pt Complexes 8
   2.2 Nanomaterials Releasing Redox-Responsive Pt Drugs 12
   2.3 Redox-Responsive Ru Complexes 13
   2.4 Redox-Responsive Nanomaterials of Ru Compounds 17
   2.5 Redox-Responsive Cu Complexes and Their Nanoformulations 17
3 Hypoxia-Responsive Metal-Based Prodrugs 18
   3.1 Hypoxia-Responsive Co Complexes 19
   3.2 Hypoxia-Responsive Cu, Fe, and Au Complexes 21
   3.3 Hypoxia-Responsive Nanosystems Releasing Metal Drugs 22
4 pH-Responsive Metal-Based Prodrugs 23
   4.1 pH-Responsive Pt Complexes 23
   4.2 pH-Responsive Pt Nanomaterials 24
   4.3 pH-Responsive Ru Drugs and Nanomaterials 26
5 Enzyme-Activatable Metal-Based Drugs and Nanomaterials 28
   5.1 Enzyme-Activatable Prodrugs 28
   5.2 Enzyme-Activatable Nanomaterials Releasing Metal Drugs 30
6 General Conclusion 30
Acknowledgments 31
Abbreviations 31
References 32

Abstract

Malignant tissue is characterized by several very specific traits, which offer the opportunity for the development of drugs with increased tumor specificity and tolerability. Here especially a changed redox homeostasis, altered blood supply, the occurrence of low oxygenated areas (hypoxia), decreased pH values, and specific enzyme expression need to be considered. Since several decades, metal compounds (especially Pt drugs) are key players in the daily therapy of cancer patients. The chemistry of diverse metal drugs has several characteristics, which allow the design of tumor-specific activated prodrugs. Of particular note is the activation by reduction principle, which is based on chemical changes induced by reduction of the central metal ion, representing a very

Prodrugs Activated by Cancer-Specific Stimuli

elegant and powerful strategy for, e.g., Pt, Ru, Cu, and Co (pro)drugs. This chapter aims to give an overview of metal-based prodrugs and their nanoformulations, which have been designed to be activated by tumor-specific stimuli.

KEYWORDS

Metal Complex; Stimuli-Responsive; Activation by Reduction; Hypoxia; pH; Platinum; Ruthenium

1 INTRODUCTION

1.1 ANTICANCER METAL COMPLEXES: CLINICAL SITUATION

Numerous transition metals are essential elements that, due to their versatility, regulate some of the most basic physiologic aspects of human bodies. They act, for example, as the catalytic center in enzymes, transport oxygen and electrons, or generally support structural cellular functions [1]. Their multi-faceted nature also makes them resourceful pharmacologic tools for the treatment of various diseases. Since the fortuitous discovery of the anticancer properties of cisplatin over 50 years ago, this drug and its derivatives still play a significant role in today's clinical routine [2]. Pt drugs have revolutionized anticancer therapy by their unanticipated high therapeutic efficacy and, consequently, the marked increase in the life span of cancer patients with previously poor prognoses. Currently, there are three Pt(II) drugs with worldwide clinical approval: cisplatin (1978), carboplatin (1989), and oxaliplatin (2002). In addition, the Pt(II) complexes nedaplatin, lobaplatin, and heptaplatin are approved regionally (Figure 1).

It can be estimated that more than every second, an anticancer patients receive a Pt drug as part of their therapy [3]. Moreover, Pt drugs (especially carboplatin) have shown to exert potent synergistic activity with immune checkpoint inhibitors, which further consolidates their important role in modern cancer therapy [4]. Their overwhelming success induced a surge of interest in the anticancer potential of not

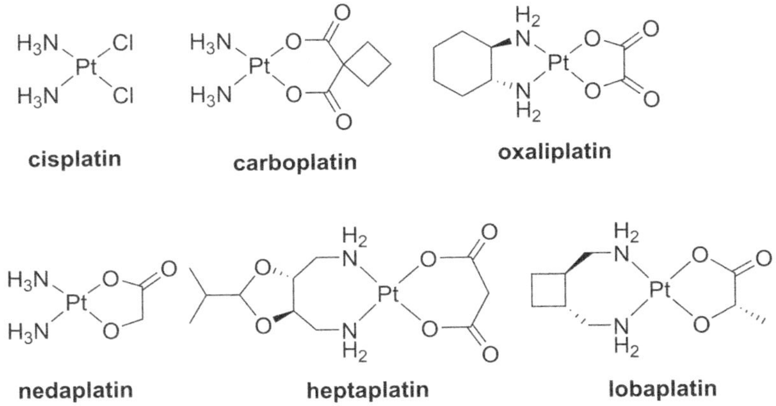

FIGURE 1 Globally and regionally approved Pt(II) anticancer drugs.

only novel Pt-based complexes but also of other transition metals. However, even though a plethora of novel compounds have been developed and investigated, only a small fraction has actually entered clinical investigations. Thus, despite these intense efforts, apart from Pt, arsenic trioxide is the only other metal (metalloid) drug that has been approved for cancer therapy so far [5]. Reasons for the failure of these metal-based drugs are far-reaching, frequently discussed in the literature, and range from toxic side effects and insufficient activity (compared to the already approved therapeutics) to unfavorable activation dynamics and kinetics [6]. As metal drugs are, by nature, highly reactive, they may react with many intra- or extracellular targets [7]. Although this is the basis for their significant activities, these undirected mechanisms are also the main cause of severe side effects [8]. As a consequence, metal drugs often have a rather narrow therapeutic window [8]. Therefore, one of the most active research fields of modern metal-based anticancer drug development is the design of compounds with a more controlled drug activation and/or release in tumor tissue. The applied strategies range from passive drug accumulation in the malignant tissue (with, e.g., nanocarriers) to strategies where the drug is released based on a tumor-specific trigger event. Stimuli-dependent drug activation has the potential to circumvent off-target toxicity in healthy tissue, while maintaining the full power of the highly reactive metal drugs in the malignant tumor. Although there have been several physical triggers (e.g., temperature, electrical and magnetic fields as well as mechanical forces) utilized for drug activation, these types of stimuli typically require an external activation source [9–11]. In fact, one of the most extensively investigated fields of metal drug activation is photodynamic therapy (PDT), in which photosensitive prodrugs are activated by light. As PDT involves an external light source such as lasers or light-emitting diodes, this approach will not be discussed in this chapter. However, as these strategies frequently suffer from difficulties such as an insufficient penetration of the light, e.g., through the skin, there are also many attempts to design PDT compounds with tumor-specific drug release.

This book chapter aims to give an overview of the main chemical and biological concepts and strategies used for the design of metal-based drugs, which can be activated by the specific (intrinsic) conditions in the solid cancer tissue.

1.2 INTRINSIC PARAMETERS OF THE MALIGNANT TUMOR SUITABLE FOR DRUG ACTIVATION

A solid and reliable starting point to find tumor-specific properties is to closely examine the physiological and biological properties of cancer cells and tumors, which are summarized in the hallmarks of cancer [12–14]. Many reviews describe certain aspects of the tumor microenvironment [15, 16] or metabolic and physiologic alterations [17] in tumor tissue that may be suitable for drug activation. However, even though there are a lot of possible intrinsic triggers, certain aspects need to be considered. For example, triggers not only need to be specific but should also display a sufficient signal intensity/magnitude to efficiently activate drugs in a tumor-specific manner. However, probably most limiting is the availability of a specific "chemical moiety", which can be activated by the trigger

Prodrugs Activated by Cancer-Specific Stimuli

for drug release. This moiety has to be stable under "normal conditions" and activated in a confirmed tumor-specific manner. We classify the intrinsic stimuli relevant for metal-based drugs into three broad areas: activation by reduction, physicochemical triggers (e.g., hypoxia, pH), and biological (enzymatic) triggers.

1.2.1 Activation by Reduction Based on the Changed Redox Environment of the Tumor

In mammalian cells, reactive oxygen species (ROS) are produced regularly as a part of mitochondrial oxygen consumption [18]. However, these molecules harbor a great risk for the cell, as they may react with and potentially destroy intracellular proteins or lipids, which in the worst case, can lead to cell death. Therefore, in healthy cells, these reactive molecules are constantly controlled by reducing agents as well as specific enzymes (catalase, superoxide dismutase) that keep up a reducing intracellular milieu of approximately −200 and −240 mV [19]. This steady-state is maintained by complementary levels of reduction/oxidation (redox) couples such as for glutathione (GSH) and glutathione disulfide (GSSG). In malignant cells, the situation is much more complex, as several fail-safe key regulators such as damage sensors have been frequently lost or overridden [20]. Nevertheless, cancer cells prevent ROS-mediated cell death by disassembling further fail-safe mechanisms and strongly increasing the expression of reducing agents such as ascorbic acid, GSH, or other thiol-containing molecules [21]. In addition, intracellular thiols play an important role in the resistance of cancer cells against, e.g., Pt drugs. For example, the GSH-S-transferase mediates conjugation of the thiol residue from cysteine in GSH to metal-based drugs, with particularly high affinity for Pt [22]. Such GSH-conjugates can be recognized by efflux transporters, eliminating the drug from the cell [23]. Consequently, cisplatin-resistant tumors frequently display elevated levels of GSH, which inactivate the drug and thereby efficiently suppress the therapeutic effect [24]. In addition to GSH, in malignant cells, the whole cellular machinery responsible for maintaining the redox balance is often significantly altered. As a result, the development of redox-active metal-based prodrugs, exploiting the reductive environment of cancer cells as an internal stimulus for drug activation, has become one of the most extensive and successful research areas [25].

1.2.2 Physicochemical Triggers: Hypoxia and Reduced pH

One of the earliest and perhaps most obvious differences between solid tumors and healthy tissue is a misbalance between apoptosis and proliferation, which results in a large population of rapidly dividing cells. This newly establishing tumor tissue is in constant high need of nutrients and oxygen. However, the supplying vasculature is typically not able to keep up with the growth rate of the malignant cells and has often an atypical, chaotic, not fully functional structure. This results in areas of (at least transiently) under-supplied cells or even necrosis. In these areas of the tumor, several characteristic traits arise, which can be exploited as triggers for stimuli-responsive drugs (Figure 2).

In more detail, the lack of a stable blood supply leads to (sometimes only transient) insufficient oxygenation (hypoxia) together with starvation of the

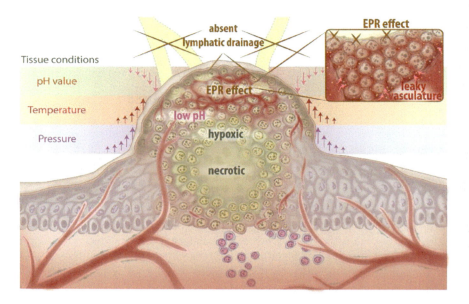

FIGURE 2 Overview on the physical chemical parameters of the malignant tumor tissue, underlying the EPR effect.

cells, while waste products (including carbon dioxide) are retained. On the one hand, this aberrant vasculature and the lack of lymphatic drainage in the tumor results in the so-called enhanced permeability and retention (EPR) effect, which describes the enhanced retention of larger particles such as serum proteins (albumin) and nanocarriers [26]. On the other hand, these areas are also typically characterized by a drop in the pH value. The latter is also supported by a metabolic switch, the so-called Warburg effect [27]. To cope with the changing unstable environmental conditions in the solid tumor, cancer cells often have certain metabolic flexibility to produce energy either by anaerobic or aerobic glycolysis, independent from their oxygen supply. This altered metabolism offers these malignant cells several advantages including (1) an enhanced survival probability in haemal-poor regions with low oxygen supply, (2) increased chances to evade the immune system, and (3) utilization of metabolic products to build essential biomolecules that are required for their accelerated cell growth [28, 29]. Accordingly, this leads to lactate production which further supports the acidification of the tumor tissue [30]. Chemically, both the hypoxic conditions as well as the characteristic pH gradient from healthy to malignant tissue can be exploited to trigger drug activation (see the sections below). Interestingly, even though tumor tissues and cancer cells differ distinctively from healthy cells in various other physical aspects such as temperature [31], elasticity and interstitial pressure [32], or the permeability of the extracellular matrix [33, 34], to our knowledge there have not yet been reports on metal drugs, which can be activated by such physical stimuli.

1.2.3 Biological Characteristics: Tumor-Specific Upregulation of Enzymes

Enzymes play a crucial role in all stages of cancer development. Alterations in enzyme expression or activity enable malignant cells to take the reins of essential cell signaling pathways, thereby ensuring their survival and proliferation [12–14, 35]. The majority of these pathways involving redox homeostasis, xenobiotic biotransformation, or remodeling of the extracellular matrix ultimately lead to drug resistance [36]. However, this divergent enzymatic behavior of malignant cells can also be efficiently exploited as an activation trigger for anticancer drugs. Therefore, the low number of enzyme-activatable metal drugs reported so far is rather surprising [25].

2 REDOX-RESPONSIVE METAL-BASED PRODRUGS

The most prevalent group of redox-responsive anticancer metal drugs is based on the "activation by reduction" concept, which is rooted in the chemical observation that metals in certain oxidation states have strongly different reactivities and ligand release kinetics (Figure 3). One well-known example is Pt, a metal that predominantly exists in the oxidation states +2 and +4. All clinically approved Pt drugs are based on a Pt(II) core, which readily forms crosslinks with DNA nucleobases. In contrast, Pt(IV) complexes are usually several magnitudes less

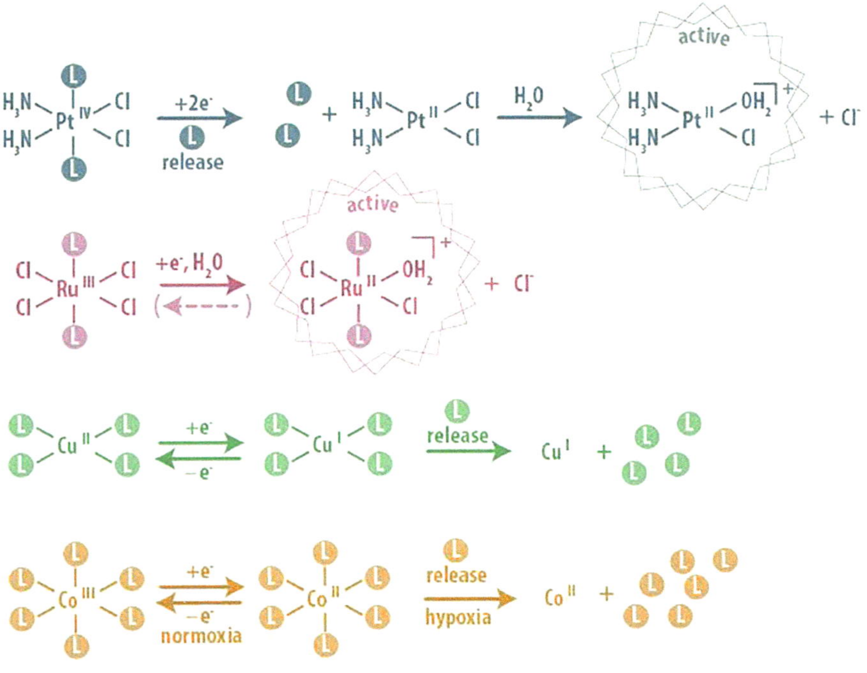

FIGURE 3 Types of "activation by reduction" for different metal ions (L=ligand).

reactive than their Pt(II) counterparts. Due to these advantageous properties, Pt(IV) complexes are ideal prodrug candidates and present the earliest attempts to generate metal-based reduction-activatable drugs [37]. In recent years, the development of several other reducible metal complexes has gained increasing attention. Particularly, Ru(III)/(II) and Cu(II)/(I) complexes have been investigated, due to their easily accessible intrinsic redox activity and a high degree of functionality. A special subclass (mainly for Co and Cu complexes) are hypoxia-activatable drugs, which are specifically activated by reduction under hypoxic conditions and will be discussed in Section 3.

2.1 REDOX-RESPONSIVE Pt COMPLEXES

The generally accepted mode of action of Pt(II) drugs is that they are activated by aquation in the cytoplasm of cancerous cells and, subsequently, form bis-adducts with double-stranded DNA, preferably on guanine N^7 positions. This binding results in DNA damage during DNA synthesis, which in turn activates several damage-responsive signaling pathways, cell cycle arrest, and apoptosis [38]. Noteworthy, the reactivity of Pt drugs also leads to the interaction with plasma molecules/proteins limiting their stability and transport efficiency to the malignant tumor. Thus, only a small fraction of the administered drug eventually reaches its target in the nucleus of the cancer cell. To reduce side effects and improve tumor delivery of the drugs, the majority of Pt-based drug development shifted to Pt(IV) prodrugs in the past decade [37]. Pt(IV) complexes have an octahedral geometry and are coordinatively saturated. Furthermore, they are chemically inert to substitution reactions with biological nucleophiles, increasing the stability compared to Pt(II) analogs (although hydrolysis can occur, e.g., in case of oxaliplatin(IV) complexes [39]). In addition, the axial positions of Pt(IV) complexes can be functionalized with, e.g., biomolecules [40], tumor-targeting moieties [41], or other auxiliary ligands [42] to improve efficacy, selectivity, and stability. To activate the Pt(IV) prodrugs, they have to be reduced to the respective active Pt(II) complexes. For a long time, it was believed that GSH, ascorbate, and other low-molecular-weight reducing agents are responsible for this "activation by reduction". Yet, there is strong evidence that the high-molecular-weight fraction of cells, e.g., metalloproteins like cytochrome c or hemoglobin, are far more efficient in the reduction of Pt(IV) drugs [43, 44]. Nevertheless, there is little knowledge about where and how the reduction and thus activation of Pt drugs exactly happens *in vivo*.

One of the most important parameters for the efficacy of a Pt(IV) prodrug is its reduction potential, which dictates both the stability in the bloodstream and the efficacy of activation in cancerous tissue. When the reduction potential is too high, the Pt(IV) complex will be mainly reduced in the bloodstream and will thus lose its prodrug properties. In contrast, a too low reduction potential will result in excretion of the drug before it can be activated. Therefore, the reduction potential has to be fine-tuned to obtain the optimum compromise between activity and stability. The redox potential of a Pt(IV) complex is strongly

Prodrugs Activated by Cancer-Specific Stimuli

influenced by the nature of the axial ligands. Choi et al. discovered that for [Pt(en)Cl$_2$(X$_2$)] (en=ethylenediamine), the reduction potential increases in the order X=OH<OCOCH$_3$<Cl<OCOCF$_3$ [45]. This trend shows that Pt(IV) complexes bearing electron-withdrawing axial ligands are destabilized and more easily reduced. However, there is no correlation between the reduction potential and the actual reduction kinetics [46]. Gibson et al. could show that oxaliplatin(IV) complexes with the lowest reduction potential (X=OH) have the highest reduction rate in the presence of ascorbic acid and *vice versa* in the case of X=OAc [47]. Thus, these parameters have to be investigated and judged very carefully.

The redox activity of a Pt(IV) drug can be deliberately exploited to develop redox-responsive compounds that should selectively be reduced in cancer tissue. In general, redox-active Pt(IV) complexes can be divided into three main categories: complexes bearing (i) non-bioactive ligands, (ii) bioactive ligands, or (iii) active/passive targeting carriers.

The most important and famous examples of redox-responsive Pt(IV) complexes bearing non-bioactive ligands are tetraplatin, iproplatin, satraplatin, and LA-12, which all entered clinical trials (Figure 4) [48]. Investigations on tetraplatin were abandoned because the compound was reduced too fast causing severe neurotoxicity [49]. In contrast, iproplatin proved to be more stable than cisplatin and carboplatin but failed to show superior anticancer activity in clinical trials [50]. Satraplatin finished a phase III clinical trial, where it revealed superior antitumor activity in pretreated metastatic castrate-resistant prostate cancer patients over cisplatin but no significantly improved overall survival [51]. Notably, satraplatin revealed very fast reduction kinetics in the bloodstream ($t_{1/2}$~6min) *via* activation by red blood cells [52, 53]. LA-12 has a very similar structure to satraplatin but with the cyclohexylamine ligand replaced by a bulkier adamantylamino moiety. LA-12 finished clinical phase I trials [54], but no phase II studies have been reported so far.

The early successes of these drugs triggered the development of new types of Pt(IV) complexes. In particular, the functionalization of the axial ligand(s) with (synergistic) bioactive molecules to give bifunctional compounds was strongly investigated (Figure 4). For example, Pt(IV) derivatives with well-known anticancer drugs like paclitaxel (**1**), gemcitabine (**2**), or aspirin (**3**) as their axial ligands have been reported [40, 55, 56]. Two other examples will be discussed in more detail: (1) Dichloroacetate is a potent inhibitor of pyruvate dehydrogenase kinase and has been examined for its potential application in cancer therapies. Cisplatin(IV) (**4**), also known as mitaplatin, and oxaliplatin(IV) (**5**) prodrug derivatives containing two axial dichloroacetate moieties have been investigated for their anticancer activity (Figure 4) [57, 58]. Although the cytotoxicity of **4** was very similar to cisplatin in the tested cell lines, *in vitro* assays demonstrated that the released dichloroacetate was able to restore the hyperpolarized mitochondrial membrane potential, which promoted apoptosis and activity also against cisplatin-resistant A2780 ovarian carcinoma sublines. Surprisingly, the oxaliplatin equivalent **5** was more cytotoxic than oxaliplatin, particularly in cisplatin-resistant cell models. In addition, it was discovered that the anticancer activity of

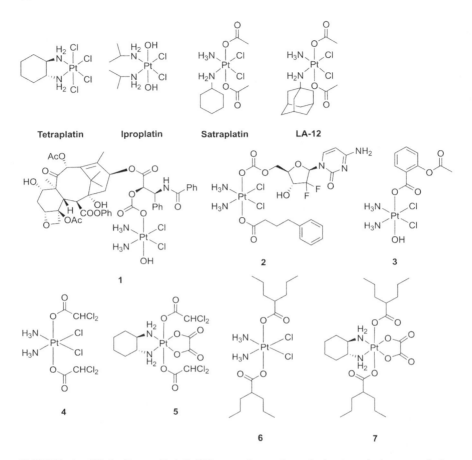

FIGURE 4 Clinically studied Pt(IV) complexes (tetraplatin; iproplatin; satraplatin; LA-12) and examples of investigational drugs bearing an additional anticancer drug as axial ligand(s).

5 against colorectal carcinoma could be enhanced by combination with 5-fluorouracil. (2) Valproic acid is a well-known histone deacetylase inhibitor with promising antitumor activity *via* a variety of functionalities including cell cycle arrest and differentiation [59]. A cisplatin derivative with valproic acid as axial ligands (6) was reported as a dual-action prodrug with improved anticancer activity [60]. The cytotoxicity of 6 was 50- to 100-fold higher compared to [Pt(NH$_3$)$_2$(OH)$_2$Cl$_2$] (oxoplatin) against several cancer cell lines (at least partially due to distinctly increased lipophilicity). Notably, *in vitro* cell culture assays showed that complex 6 exhibited histone deacetylase inhibition comparable to free valproic acid. *In vivo* anticancer activity was investigated in an A549 lung cancer xenograft mouse model and showed that a dispersion of 6 in tween-80 or loaded in PEG-PCL nanoparticles not only exerted higher tumor regression compared to oxoplatin,

Prodrugs Activated by Cancer-Specific Stimuli

but also significantly reduced nephrotoxicity. Cytotoxicity of the bis-valproic acid-oxaliplatin complex **7** was evaluated in cisplatin-sensitive and -resistant A2780 cells demonstrating that although the IC_{50} values were due to the prodrug nature consistently higher than oxaliplatin, the cytotoxicity of **7** increased significantly compared to dihydroxido oxaliplatin(IV) and the mono-valproic acid reference complex [61]. In addition, **7** was 1,000-fold more cytotoxic than free valproic acid. Histone deacetylase inhibition was investigated by Western blotting in A2780 cells, showing that **7** had remarkable histone deacetylase-inhibitory activity, while the inhibition by free valproic acid or a 1:2 mixture of valproic acid and oxaliplatin was negligible even at higher doses.

Besides bioactive ligands, targeting/carrier molecules can also be attached to the axial positions of Pt(IV) complexes. Here, we have to distinguish between active and passive tumor-targeting strategies. To achieve active tumor targeting, functional moieties such as, e.g., peptides, vitamins, sugars, or lipids, which bind to overexpressed receptors on cancer cells, are attached to the Pt core. The increased cell uptake of these targeted drugs (often *via* endocytosis) enables accumulation at the tumor site. For purely organic drugs, several of these active targeting approaches have already been studied in clinical phase III trials [62]. For Pt-based drugs, the attachment of different active tumor-targeting moieties (e.g., biotin, different sugars) has already been reported [40]. For example, glycosylated Pt(IV) compounds were developed by Ma et al. [63]. In this study, oxaliplatin-releasing derivatives functionalized by a sugar moiety (glucose, mannose, or rhamnose) were tested. They showed that the cellular uptake was dependent on the glucose uptake transporter in the breast cancer cell model MCF-7. Additionally, these complexes were (at least in part) able to overcome the oxaliplatin resistance of A549R cells compared to corresponding A549 wt cells. However, as the glucose uptake transporter levels of the two different cell models were not evaluated, it is not known whether the enhanced activity is due to higher cellular uptake. To exploit the enhanced expression of the biotin (vitamin H) receptor at the cancer cells, Muhammad et al. developed cisplatin-releasing Pt(IV) complexes that harbored one or two biotin molecules in the axial position(s) [64]. The biotinylation of the complexes resulted in enhanced drug accumulation in breast cancer cells compared to healthy breast epithelial cells. The mono-biotinylated compound showed pronounced anticancer activity against the breast cancer cell models MCF-7 and MDA-MB-231 compared to the corresponding bis-biotinylated complex. The difference between the two complexes in their activity could be explained by the impact of the hydroxido ligand of the mono-biotinylated drug on the reduction properties, resulting in changed activation and/or cellular uptake.

Passive tumor targeting is based on the EPR effect (already mentioned in the Introduction section), which leads to the accumulation of macromolecules (nanoparticles, proteins) in tumor tissue. A very elegant nanocarrier is albumin, the most abundant protein in blood serum, which has a long half-life time of ~19 days in the human body [65]. Noteworthy, this large molecule (~66 kDa) is not only tumor-accumulating due to the EPR effect but, as an important nutrient carrier of the body, it is also preferentially taken up (and even degraded) by cancer cells to satisfy their requirement for building blocks. For organic drugs, albumin targeting has already been successfully translated into the clinical routine by the development of the albumin/paclitaxel nanoformulation Abraxane® (approved for several cancer types) as well as the albumin-binding pH-sensitive Aldoxorubicin (finished phase III against soft-tissue sarcoma) [66, 67]. Albumin-targeting Pt(IV) complexes were developed by axial addition of a maleimide moiety that allows the drug to bind the free thiol group of the cysteine 34 residue of the endogenous albumin [41, 68]. Promising examples are Pt(IV) complexes harboring one or two axial maleimide moieties. These drugs show fast and stable binding to albumin *ex vivo* as well as *in vivo*, resulting in a prolonged plasma half-life, tumor accumulation, and finally distinctly improved anticancer activity *in vivo* [41, 68, 69]. One maleimide-bearing Pt(IV) drug recently entered clinical phase I trials (NCT02950064).

2.2 NANOMATERIALS RELEASING REDOX-RESPONSIVE Pt DRUGS

Based on the observation that several Pt(IV) complexes have limited *in vivo* activity due to unfavorable pharmacological properties like fast excretion and/or premature reduction, diverse strategies to encapsulate these drugs into nanocarriers were investigated [70–72]. In particular, stimuli-responsive Pt(IV) nanomaterials, commonly referred to as "smart" drugs, gained scientific interest in the last years [73, 74]. Encapsulation can be achieved by a variety of carrier agents like peptides, micelles, synthetic or biopolymers, and many others [75]. In general, Pt-containing nanoparticles are designed by either direct conjugation of the desired drug molecule to a macromolecular moiety or by coupling the anticancer agent to ligands that are driven into supramolecular assemblies *via* non-covalent interactions (e.g., hydrophobic interactions of polyethylene glycol) or cross-linking (*via*, e.g., disulfides or diazides). In the following section, two selected examples will be discussed. Recently, Wang et al. reported a cisplatin(IV) indolamine-2,3-dioxygenase inhibitor (IDOi) hybrid nanosystem for effective chemotherapy against cervical cancer [76]. Small molecule IDOi received significant attention in the past decades for their ability to revive T cells for cancer immunotherapy [77]. Disuccinatocisplatin ($[Pt(NH_3)_2Cl_2(O_2CCH_2CH_2COOH)_2]$) and a potent IDOi (4-{[2-(4-bromophenyl)hydrazinyl]sulfonyl}benzoic acid) were loaded into biocompatible layered double hydroxide (LDH) nanoparticles *via* an anion exchange process. The authors suggested that the nanohybrid enters tumor tissue *via* endocytic pathways and, subsequently, collapses due to the reduction of the respective Pt(IV) complex. Different loading ratios (10:1; 1:2; 1:10 and 1:40) of Pt(IV) complex to IDOi were tested. The IC_{50} values of Pt(IV)-IDOi/LDH decreased substantially with increasing IDOi content (up to 0.3 µM) in IDO high-expressing cancer cells (HeLa and A549). *In vivo* antitumor activity of bovine serum albumin-coated Pt(IV)-IDOi(1:40)/LDH was investigated in nude mice bearing HeLa cervix carcinoma xenografts. To ensure adequate immune response, the animals were pretreated with injection of stimulated peripheral

Prodrugs Activated by Cancer-Specific Stimuli

blood mononuclear cells (PBMCs) 24 h before the first administration of the nanohybrid. Notably, the mice that were treated with PBMCs and albumin-coated Pt(IV)-IDOi(1:40)/LDH showed the strongest anticancer response and no body weight loss, confirming the immunochemotherapeutic potential and tolerability of the treatment with this nanomaterial.

Another example, published by Lin et al., incorporated Pt(IV) complexes into polysilsesquioxane nanoparticles. In addition, $\alpha_v\beta_3$ integrin-binding cyclic RGD (cRGD) peptides or anisamides were attached on the nanoparticle surface, combining passive and active-targeting strategies [78]. Anisamides are believed to interact with sigma receptors, which are overexpressed in many cancers [79]. The authors demonstrated the controlled redox responsiveness by showing that 80% of the Pt cargo was released after 48 h incubation with 10 eq. of cysteine. Cytotoxicity studies in human colon and pancreatic cancer lines revealed that the RGD-nanoparticle was up to 10-fold more cytotoxic than oxaliplatin in $\alpha_v\beta_3$ integrin-overexpressing cancer cells. The anisamide-loaded nanoparticles were up to 3-fold more active than oxaliplatin in sigma receptor-positive AsPC-1 pancreas carcinoma cells. *In vivo* antitumor efficacy of the anisamide-loaded nanoparticle was investigated against pancreatic cancer in mice and showed superior tumor growth inhibition compared to oxaliplatin.

2.3 REDOX-RESPONSIVE Ru COMPLEXES

Ru complexes are the most intensively studied "non-Pt" metal-based anticancer drugs, developed with the aim to overcome resistance against Pt drugs and reduce adverse effects. Ru is a suitable candidate, due to its rather similar chemical and coordinative properties to Pt [80]. Although Ru can have oxidation states between -2 and $+8$, only Ru(II) and Ru(III) are relevant under physiological conditions. Similar to Pt(IV), the octahedral Ru(III) complexes are considered as prodrugs, which are activated by reduction [81]. However, in case of these Ru(III) complexes, reduction does not change the octahedral geometry, but distinctly accelerates ligand release *via* aquation (Figure 3). The formed Ru(II) species is highly reactive and considered to interact with biomolecules. In contrast to Pt(IV) complexes, also re-oxidation and redox cycling can occur for Ru complexes. However, this strongly depends on the exact coordination sphere and, furthermore, not even all Ru(III) complexes are reducible under physiological conditions. To the best of our knowledge, Ru(III) complexes have not been used to release bioactive ligands after reduction. To stabilize the reactive Ru(II) species, usually arene complexes are prepared, which have a very characteristic "piano stool" structure and are normally not able to change their +2 oxidation state.

Until now, two Ru(III) and one Ru(II) complexes have been clinically evaluated (Figure 5) [82]. Phase II trials of NAMI-A were performed in combination with gemcitabine, yet investigations were discontinued due to a lack of superior antitumor activity compared to gemcitabine alone [83]. After an initial phase I clinical trial with KP1019, the sodium salt analog NKP1339 (BOLD-100) was

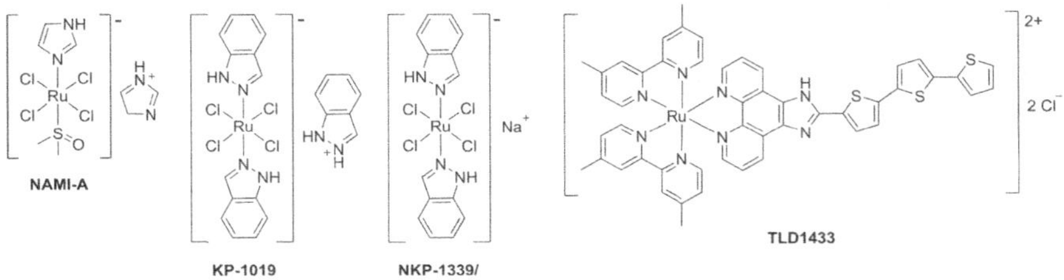

FIGURE 5 Clinically studied Ru complexes (NAMI-A; KP-1019; BOLD-100; TLD1433).

further investigated due to distinctly increased water solubility. BOLD-100 is currently subjected to phase II clinical trials in combination with the FOLFOX regimen for the treatment of advanced gastric, pancreatic, colon, and bile duct cancers (NCT04421820). BOLD-100 has orphan drug designations in gastric and pancreatic cancer from the food and drug administration. The Ru(II) complex TLD1433 is a photo-active polypyridyl-complex that entered phase II as PDT agent against bladder cancer [84].

With regard to their modes of action, originally Ru complexes have been assumed to target DNA comparable to Pt drugs. However, although Ru has been detected in the nuclei of treated cells, there is increasing evidence that the anticancer activity of, e.g., KP1019/BOLD-100 or NAMI-A is not based on direct DNA damage [81]. Ru(III) complexes have a high affinity for sulfur and readily react with (serum) proteins [85, 86]. In particular, albumin has been suggested to be crucial for drug transport into the tumor tissue and to be responsible for the only mild adverse effects observed in clinical trials with KP1019/BOLD-100 [87, 88]. The reduction of Ru(III) compounds by GSH and other biological reductants such as ascorbic acid has been extensively investigated, however, mainly in cell-free settings. Notably, due to the tight binding of Ru(III) complexes to serum proteins, the extracellular reduction of the Ru center seems improbable [89, 90]. Consequently, it is assumed that reduction of Ru compounds is an intracellular process, after release of the Ru moiety from its biological carrier, which makes the complex accessible for reduction. Inside the cell, several biological targets are discussed. For BOLD-100, the drug shows a unique multimodal activity spectrum (Figure 6). Briefly, after reduction to Ru(II), the main mode of action is the induction of endoplasmic reticulum stress due to the inhibition of GRP78, which leads to activation of the unfolded protein response and apoptotic cell death. Additionally, the interplay of ROS induction, autophagy regulation, epigenetic modification, activation of immunogenic cell death, and altered metabolic pathways contribute to the promising activity of BOLD-100 [6].

Notably, in comparison to the enormous efforts in the development of Pt(IV) prodrugs, the search for novel Ru(III) therapeutics is extremely under-investigated. This might also be linked to the paramagnetic properties of Ru(III) complexes which prevent convenient characterization by NMR spectroscopy.

Prodrugs Activated by Cancer-Specific Stimuli   15

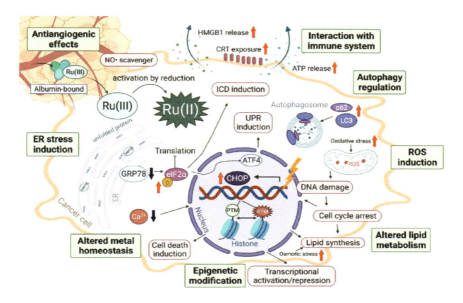

FIGURE 6   Different reported intracellular modes of action of BOLD-100.

The vast majority of Ru-containing anticancer drug development occurs in the area of "piano stool" Ru(II)-arene complexes [91]. Similar to Pt(II) complexes, aquation *via* hydrolysis in the tumor microenvironment applies as the activation mechanism. Nevertheless, also for some Ru(II) complexes, redox-responsive mechanisms have been reported. For example, complex **8** containing a phenylazopyridine ligand increased intracellular ROS levels by reaction with GSH in a redox cycle (Figure 7a) [92]. Detailed analysis showed that **8** was able to oxidize GSH to GSSG, thereby reducing the azo-bond of the phenylazopyridine ligand to a hydrazo group (**8a** and **8b**). The authors proposed that concomitant hydrogenation of O_2 regenerates the azo-functionality in **8** with the subsequent release of H_2O_2. Although in this example the Ru(II) metal center itself did not change its oxidation state, it shows that reaction with GSH can also lead to subsequent redox reactions facilitating DNA binding or ROS generation. A more complex strategy has been reported by Lin et al., which conjugated an *N*-heterocyclic carbene (NHC)-containing Ru(II)-arene complex to 17α-ethynyl testosterone *via* a disulfide linker to design a drug targeting progesterone receptor (PR)-positive breast cancer (Figure 7b) [93]. The cancer-selective redox responsiveness was achieved by cleavage of the disulfide linker by GSH in the tumor microenvironment. Antiproliferative activity *in vitro* was investigated in MCF-7 (PR-expressing) and MDA-MB-231 (PR-negative) cells. In these experiments, it was demonstrated that the Ru-steroid conjugate (Te–S–S–NHC–Ru) was superior to the free Ru(II) complex (NHC-Ru) with significantly improved

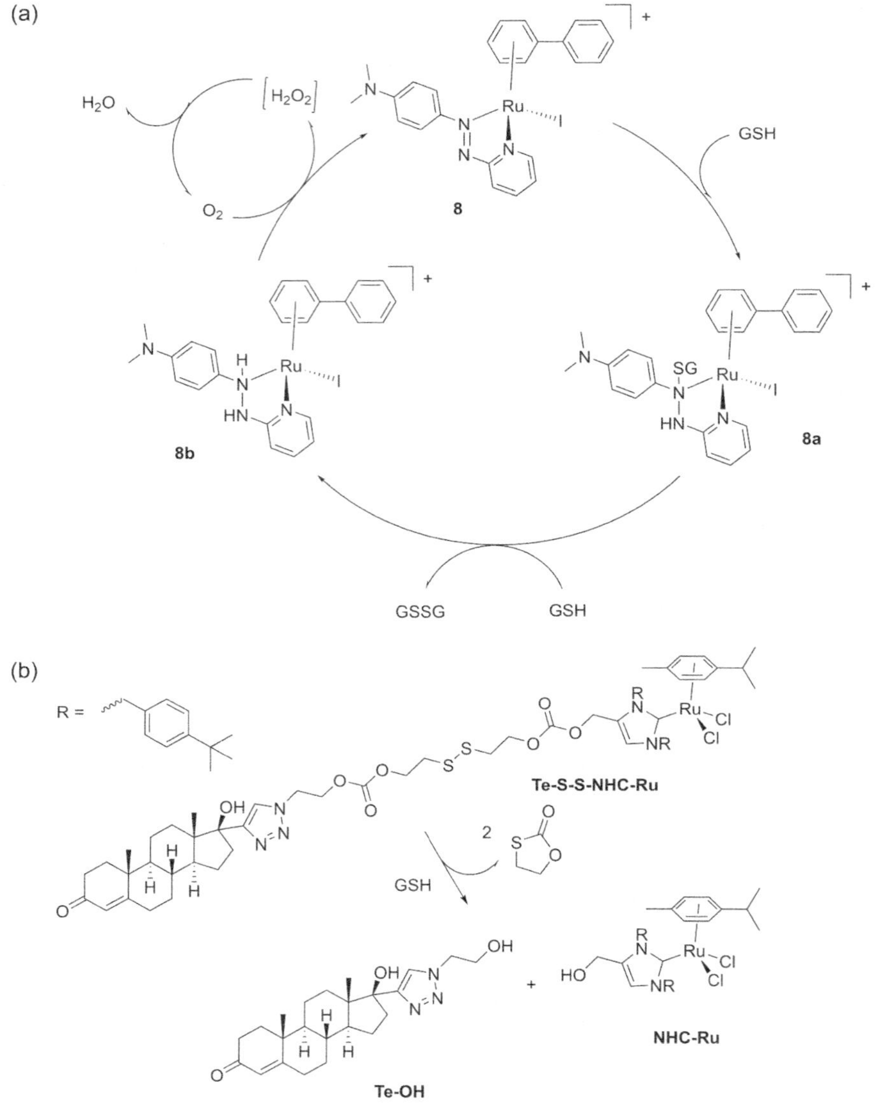

(a)

(b)

FIGURE 7 GSH-mediated redox-responsive Ru(II)-arene complexes. (a) Phenylazopyridine-containing Ru(II)-arene complex; (b) NHC-17α-ethynyl testosterone Ru(II)-arene complex.

cytotoxicity compared to cisplatin. The cellular uptake of Te–S–S–NHC–Ru was vastly improved compared to NHC–Ru in MCF-7 cells. Finally, Te–S–S–NHC–Ru showed slightly enhanced tumor regression, prolonged survival, and improved tolerability in a xenograft mouse model.

2.4 REDOX-RESPONSIVE NANOMATERIALS OF Ru COMPOUNDS

Comparable to Pt(IV) drugs, embedding Ru complexes into nanomaterials was applied as a strategy to improve cancer selectivity and accumulation [73]. Most investigations on Ru nanomaterials focus either on improved passive targeting *via* the EPR effect using a variety of carrier vehicles [94], or on active targeting *via* conjugation of Ru drugs to peptides with cancer-specific properties [95, 96]. Yet, to the best of our knowledge, there is only one example of the preparation of a stimuli-responsive Ru-containing nanomaterial to overcome these problems. Chen et al. reported the promising anticancer activity of Ru(III) prodrugs loaded on mesoporous silica nanoparticles (MSNs) incorporated into fusion protein-loaded liposomes (PLip) specifically targeting H1299 lung cancer cells [97]. Two mer-[Ru(III)Cl$_3$(DMSO)(L$_2$)] (L=1,10-phenanthroline-5-amino-1,8-naphthalimide or 1,10-phenanthroline) prodrug complexes were synthesized (RuDPNI and RuDPH), dispersed in MSNs (Ru-MSNs), and finally encapsulated in fluorescent PLips to yield Ru-MSN-PLip. In addition to the activation by reduction of the Ru(III) complexes, previous investigations showed that PLip-coated MSNs can release their cargo under acidic conditions [98]. Initial, *in vitro* DNA-binding studies revealed that Ru-DPNI exerted a 14 times stronger affinity compared to Ru-DPH. Therefore, only Ru-DPNI and Ru-DPNI-MSN-PLip were evaluated against several cancer cell lines and Ru-DPNI-MSN-PLip was ~400-fold more cytotoxic than Ru-DPNI. Furthermore, as desired, the cytotoxicity of Ru-DPNI-MSN-PLip was significantly more pronounced against H1299 cells compared to the other cell lines due to the presence of the H1299-targeting fusion protein on the liposome surface. The antitumor efficacy was investigated in H1299 tumor-bearing mice, and Ru-DPNI-MSN-PLip showed strong tumor growth inhibition together with good tolerability.

2.5 REDOX-RESPONSIVE Cu COMPLEXES AND THEIR NANOFORMULATIONS

Cu is an essential element for many organisms and is involved in a broad variety of biological pathways [99]. It is well known that the deregulation in Cu homeostasis frequently occurs in cancer [100]. Consequently, several Cu chelators (including trientine and *D*-penicillamine) have been developed to reduce the excessive Cu levels in cancerous tissue [101]. However, despite some rather early reports regarding the activity of Cu complexes *in vivo*, the development of Cu-containing compounds as anticancer agents remained in most cases at a very early stage of preclinical development [81]. An exception is [Cu(4,4′-dimethyl-2,2′-bipyridine)(acetylacetonato)] NO$_3$ (Casiopeina CasIII-ia), which has been tested in a clinical phase I study [102]. Scientific interest in Cu complexes as anticancer agents is still growing and multiple new Cu complexes have been synthesized during the last decades [103, 104].

With regard to this chapter, Cu(II) complexes are worthy of mention, as it is widely accepted that many Cu(II) complexes are reduced by diverse biological reducing agents, including cytochrome P450 and GSH. Frequently, the complexes can be re-oxidized resulting in redox cycling and ROS generation *via* Fenton-like reactions [81]. However, the formed Cu(I) complexes are often unstable and subsequently the attached ligands can also dissociate (Figure 3). In specific cases with appropriate redox potentials, this process only occurs under hypoxic conditions. Consequently, such Cu(II) complexes are also considered as "hypoxia-activated," which will be discussed in more detail in Section 3.

With regard to activation by reduction, the best-studied Cu(II) complexes carry either 1,10-phenanthroline or α-N-heterocyclic thiosemicarbazones as ligands. For 1,10-phenanthroline, the respective Cu complexes have been in most cases investigated in cell-free settings only. The reason for this is the intercalation of 1,10-phenanthroline into the DNA minor groove which enables redox reactions of the Cu core with DNA and RNA. Consequently, the Cu complexes have been used as foot-printing reagents for the evaluation of protein-DNA interactions as well as probe for DNA and RNA secondary structures [81]. In contrast, in case of some thiosemicarbazones, the interaction with Cu was suggested to play a crucial role in the mode of action, e.g., for Dp44mT, DpC, COTI-2, or Me$_2$NNMe$_2$. However, no stimuli-responsive activation steps are involved in their mode of action as, on the contrary, the Cu(II) complexes of these ligands are especially inert and hard to reduce [105, 106]. Interestingly, for other thiosemicarbazones like Triapine, the ligand is readily released from the complex after reduction to Cu(I) [107]. Consequently, there are attempts to exploit this feature also for the preparation of stimuli-responsive nanoformulations [108]. In more detail, Cu-Triapine could be stably encapsulated into liposomes, which resulted in a distinctly prolonged plasma half-life in mice compared to the free complex. In addition, methemoglobinemia formation, a main side effect of Triapine in clinical studies, could be prevented.

3 HYPOXIA-RESPONSIVE METAL-BASED PRODRUGS

Another microenvironmental characteristic in solid tumors are oxygen-lacking hypoxic areas, leading to a more reductive milieu [109]. As hypoxic cancer cells are often resistant to conventional radio- and chemotherapy, hypoxia-activated prodrugs represent a potential targeting strategy [110]. Within this subclass, the most prominent anticancer drugs are organic molecules like nitroimidazoles, quinones, or aromatic N-oxides-containing compounds. Their hypoxic activation is based on oxidoreductase-catalyzed two-step or one-electron reductions generating products that are unstable under hypoxia, whereas in the presence of oxygen, the compounds are immediately re-oxidized. Some of these drugs already entered clinical trials such as the nitroimidazole-based evofosfamide (TH-302) [110]. In a phase I/II study of TH-302 in combination with bortezomib (proteasome inhibitor), promising anticancer activity was observed in heavily pretreated patients with refractory multiple myeloma [111]. However, the phase III study of the combination of TH-302 and doxorubicin against soft-tissue sarcoma did not show prolonged overall survival compared to doxorubicin mono-treatment [112]. Concerning metal-based therapeutics, the development of hypoxia-responsive drugs based on Co(III) complexes is the most frequently followed strategy.

Prodrugs Activated by Cancer-Specific Stimuli

In addition, Cu(II)- and Fe(III)-based substances have the potential for specific reduction under low oxygen levels.

3.1 HYPOXIA-RESPONSIVE Co COMPLEXES

Co is for all animals an essential trace element (usually as vitamin B12; cobalamin), which is involved in numerous biologically important processes [113]. The potential of Co complexes as anticancer agents has been examined for more than 30 years. These studies included simple Co coordination complexes, Schiff base complexes, Co-carbonyl clusters, and hypoxia-responsive Co(III) systems [114]. With regard to this chapter, the latter strategy is the most interesting one, as it gives the possibility to couple (and thereby "deactivate") bioactive agents to the metal to allow tumor-specific, synergistic drug release, especially in the hypoxic areas of the tumor tissue. This often proposed mechanism for Co(III) prodrugs is associated with a reversible redox behavior of these complexes [114]. In more detail, Co(III) complexes are commonly present in octahedral geometries and are highly inert. In contrast, Co(II) complexes exhibit higher lability and are prone to ligand substitution. Under normoxic conditions, the reduced Co(II) complex will immediately be re-oxidized by oxygen to the inert Co(III) analogs, which prevents the release of the bioactive ligand (Figure 3). In contrast, under hypoxic conditions, the Co(II) remains reduced and the (bioactive) ligands are released. Noteworthy, the exact redox properties of the individual Co drugs vary depending on the ligand, which allows fine-tuning of such prodrugs for the specific conditions of the malignant tumor. Interestingly, however, for most reported Co(III) prodrugs, irreversible redox processes in aqueous solutions occurred [115]. This already indicates that the redox chemistry and hypoxia selectivity are more complex than assumed so far and that there are many open questions, when it comes to the clinical development of Co(III) drugs.

Over the last three decades, several Co(III) prodrug candidates have been reported with reduction potentials suitable for hypoxic activation. These compounds harbored various biologically active ligands including nitrogen mustards, tyrosine kinase inhibitors (TKIs), or matrix metalloproteinase (MMP) inhibitors [115–123]. As examples, the mustard agents- and the TKI-releasing complexes will be discussed in more detail.

Nitrogen mustard agents are clinically approved purine DNA base-alkylating anticancer drugs [124]. The first Co(III) complex with the nitrogen mustard bis(2-chloroethyl)amine (BCA) was reported by Teicher et al. (Figure 8; 9) [125]. In the inert Co(III) state, the DNA alkylation by BCA was prevented, as its nitrogen lone pair was engaged in coordination with the Co core. After reduction to Co(II), BCA was released, which enabled cytotoxic effects. Indeed, cell culture experiments revealed promising anticancer activity of 9, which also overcame nitrogen mustard-related resistance in squamous cell carcinoma. However, 9 showed no hypoxia selectivity due to the lack of complex stability [125]. With the aim to develop kinetically more stable hypoxia-activatable Co(III) complexes, Ware et al. used the bidentate mustard ligands N,N'-bis(2-chloroethyl)ethylenediamine (BCE) and

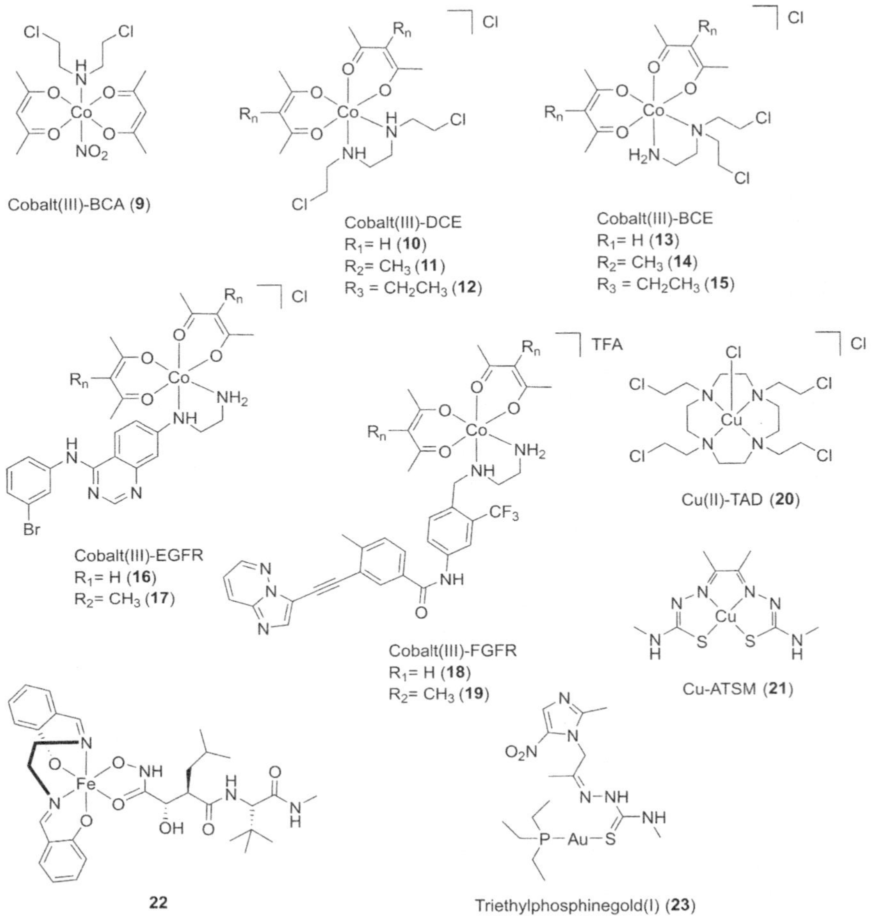

FIGURE 8 Different types of hypoxia-activatable metal drugs.

N,N-bis(2-chloroethyl)ethylenediamine (DCE) to form different types of Co(III) DCE (**10–12**) and Co(III) BCE (**13–15**) complexes (Figure 8) [116–118]. Indeed, low oxygen levels resulted in 6-fold higher cytotoxicity of **11** against Chinese hamster ovary fibroblast cells (AA8 and UV4). In another study, the hypoxic selectivity of **11** was reported to be as high as 20-fold [126]. This complex also showed distinct activity against spheroids of EMT6 mammary carcinoma cells, which were characterized by hypoxic centers. Therefore, the induced toxicity by **11** was believed to result from DCE release within the spheroid core [116]. Structure-activity relationship studies revealed that the exact nature of the ancillary ligand, usually acetylacetonate, was crucial for hypoxic selectivity. While Co(III) DCE complexes with unsubstituted acetylacetonate ligands displayed no hypoxia selectivity, methyl and ethyl analogs showed substantial selectivity up to one order of magnitude [116].

Prodrugs Activated by Cancer-Specific Stimuli 21

Another class of bioactive ligands used for Co(III) complexes are TKIs, that target altered or overexpressed receptor tyrosine kinases, which are well-known growth factor receptors and oncogenes in cancer cells [12, 14]. Similar to conventional chemotherapies, this substance class often lacks tumor selectivity, causing severe side effects. Therefore, strategies for improved tumor targeting are of high interest. For the development of hypoxia-responsive Co(III) complexes, TKIs inhibiting the epidermal growth factor receptor (EGFR; erlotinib analogs; **16–17**) [115, 119] or fibroblast growth factor receptor (FGFR, ponatinib analogs; **18–19**) [108] were employed (Figure 8). The complexation of the TKIs with Co(III) prevents their binding into the ATP-binding pocket of the receptor under normoxic conditions. Only after reduction of the Co(III) complex and release of the active TKI under hypoxia, the drug is able to reach and inhibit its (intracellular) target. All synthesized complexes showed hypoxic selectivity *in vitro* against cancer cell models expressing the corresponding target receptor tyrosine kinase [108, 115, 119]. Likewise, first *in vivo* experiments exhibited promising results [108, 119]. Comparable to the above-discussed nitrogen mustard-releasing substances, methylation of acetylacetonate increased the redox potential and thus the stability of the drugs, which was beneficial for hypoxic activation as well as the stability in serum [108, 115]. However, the FGFR inhibitor-containing Co(III) complex **19** with the highest stability revealed a lower *in vivo* activity, most likely because of insufficient activation by reduction. Consequently, the ideal balance between redox potential, stability, and reduction ability seems to be essential.

3.2 Hypoxia-Responsive Cu, Fe, and Au Complexes

As mentioned already above, analogous to Co(III), some Cu(II) complexes also have the potential to be activated specifically under the low oxygen levels of the malignant tissue *via* reduction to the unstable Cu(I) form, followed by dissociation/release of the ligands [25]. An example is the Cu(II) complex of a mustard derivative of 1,4,7,10-tetraazacyclododecane (Cu-TAD; **20**), which showed 24-fold hypoxic vs. normoxic selectivity against human K562 and A549 cancer cells due to the reduction-induced release of toxic mustard (Figure 8) [127]. The same mode of action is also exploited for Cu(II) bis(thiosemicarbazone) complexes labeled with Cu-60/62/64 which are currently undergoing clinical trials as radiopharmaceuticals for positron emission tomography (PET) imaging of hypoxia (Figure 8). One well-investigated example is Cu-diacetyl-bis(N^4-methylthiosemicarbazone) (Cu-ATSM; **21**), which was suggested to have reduction selectivity in the hypoxic tumor microenvironment based on its lower, biologically accessible reduction potential [128]. Cu-ATSM is currently tested (with subsequent PET/CT imaging) as a screening agent before neo-adjuvant chemo-radiotherapy treatment (capecitabine combined with 50 Gy radiotherapy) in patients with rectal cancer. The aim of this phase II study is to determine the capability of the Cu-ATSM PET/CT scan to predict the response of the neo-adjuvant chemo-radiotherapy treatment by monitoring different parameters (e.g., histological response, progression-free survival) (NCT03951337).

For Fe(III) complexes, only one example which shows hypoxia selectivity has been reported so far. In more detail, Hambley et al. developed Fe(III) complexes containing hydroxamic acids and the MMP inhibitor marimastat (Figure 8; **22**) [129]. Due to their very low reduction potentials, partial reversibility of the re-oxidation, and their good stability in non-reducing biological environments, these complexes were suggested as possible candidates for hypoxia-responsive therapy. However, *in vitro* and *in vivo* proof is still missing [129].

Besides Fe, diverse Au(I, III) complexes have already shown promising pre-clinical results in cell culture as well as *in vivo* [130]. In the case of Au(I, III) complexes containing thiosemicarbazones and bis(thiosemicarbazone) ligands, anticancer activity in different cancer models has been observed. In these cases, inhibition of the seleno-enzyme thioredoxin reductase was suggested as mode of action [131–133]. In order to increase tumor specificity of these potent complexes, Oliveira et al. developed hypoxia-activatable triethylphosphine Au(I) complexes with secnidazole-derived thiosemicarbazone ligands [134]. Due to the 5-nitro-imidazole moiety of the secnidazole, the newly designed drugs were expected to have the ability to switch from a non-toxic into a toxic species *via* a one-electron reduction in the hypoxic tumor environment. Indeed, one investigated triethylphosphine Au(I) complex incorporating a (E)-*N*-methyl-2-(1-(2-methyl-5-nitro-1H-imidazole-1-yl)propan-2-ylidene)hydrazinecarbothioamide ligand (Figure 8; **23**) had promising anticancer activity under hypoxia against HCT-116 colorectal cancer compared to normoxic conditions or to the non-malignant cell model HEK-293 [134]. Of note, in this example, only the nitroimidazole-bearing ligand is activated *via* hypoxia and the Au(I) oxidation state remains unaffected.

3.3 HYPOXIA-RESPONSIVE NANOSYSTEMS RELEASING METAL DRUGS

As already mentioned earlier, nanoformulations are a promising strategy to improve the plasma half-life time, bioavailability, and tumor accumulation of drugs [75]. However, to the best of our knowledge, no nanoformulation has been reported so far which contains hypoxia-responsive metal complexes. In contrast, nanosystems harboring a hypoxia-responding moiety have been designed, which additionally release a metal drug. For example, Yang et al. developed a unique type of hypoxia-responsive human serum albumin-based nanosystem, which is characterized by a cross-link between the hypoxia-sensitive azobenzene group of photosensitizer chlorin e6-conjugated albumin and an oxaliplatin(IV) prodrug. The newly devel-oped nanosystem (100–150 nm) was stable under normal oxygen levels, but when exposed to hypoxic conditions, quickly dissociated into ultra-small albumin and prodrug therapeutic nanoparticles with a <10 nm size, enabling their enhanced intratumoral penetration. After dissociation, the quenched fluorescence of chlorin e6 in the produced albumin nanoparticles was able to recover for bio-imaging and at the same time the photosensitizer generated singlet oxygen species. Thus, com-bined PDT and chemotherapy could be realized with high antitumor efficacy *in vivo* [135]. Another example was developed by Zahang et al., who reported a multi-step drug release nanosystem [136]. On the one hand, it targeted tumor hypoxia

Prodrugs Activated by Cancer-Specific Stimuli 23

via a bifunctional prodrug (including a HIF-1 alpha and a histone deacetylase inhibitor) functionalized by a hypoxia-responsive azobenzene linker. On the other hand, it harbored a photo-responsive Ru complex-derived polymer, which led to the release of a Ru anticancer agent after irradiation with red light (in addition to singlet oxygen). Together, the combinational delivery of the different bioactive reagents resulted in a synergistic cancer therapy approach [136].

4 pH-RESPONSIVE METAL-BASED PRODRUGS

Numerous studies have shown that the extracellular environment of both human and animal tumors is consistently more acidic compared to healthy tissues with pH values reaching as low as 5.5–6.0 [137]. Based on these phenomena, the development of pH-responsive, metal-based anticancer drugs has become an attractive research area in the past decades. Generally, pH-active metal complexes can be designed *via* two main strategies: (1) functionalization of metal complexes with pH-sensitive chemical bonds or moieties, or (2) complexation of anticancer agents with pH-responsive nanocarriers [25]. Ideally, *via* both pathways, a drug is designed that is stable under physiological conditions (pH 7.4), but activated in the acidic tumor microenvironment, which leads to the liberation of the cytotoxic metal core.

4.1 pH-Responsive Pt Complexes

The majority of publications on pH-responsive Pt-based drugs focus on Pt(II) complexes [25]. To the best of our knowledge, pH-activated Pt(IV) prodrugs are not reported in the literature, probably because for such compounds the "activation by reduction" is expected to be sufficient. A popular strategy is the coordination of two bidentate, pH-sensitive moieties to a Pt(II) precursor to yield an inert Pt(II) complex, which turns active *via* hydrolysis in the acidic tumor microenvironment. An early example includes bis-(0-ethyldithiocarbonato)Pt(II) (thioplatin, **24**), which employs ethylxanthate as a pH-sensitive ligand [138]. It was postulated that hydrolysis of the dithiocarbonato ligands under acidic conditions (pH < 7.0) formed the reactive bisaqua complex **24a**, able to bind plasmid DNA (Figure 9). In contrast, at pH 7.4, the intact thioplatin was stable and did not exert cytotoxicity because of the higher affinity of Pt for sulfur over nitrogen in DNA. The activity of **24** was 2–8 fold enhanced at pH 6.8 compared to pH 7.4 in the tested cell lines, in contrast to cisplatin that exhibited higher activity at physiological pH. Thioplatin was more active and better tolerable in H16 and SW707 xenograft experiments compared to cisplatin. In more detail, based on the pH-dependent reactivity of thioplatin, 4–5 fold higher doses could be administered without severe side effects. Another class of pH-responsive metal-based anticancer drugs are 2-aminoalcoholatoplatinum(II) complexes with a particular focus on bis(2-aminoethanol)dichloroplatinum(II) (**25**) and bis[(R)-(-)-2-aminobutanol)] dichloroplatinum(II) (**26**) [139]. For these drugs, a pH-induced equilibrium was suggested in which protonation of the bidentate aminoalcohol at lower pH yields the "open," active dichloridoplatinum(II) species **25a** or **26a** (Figure 9).

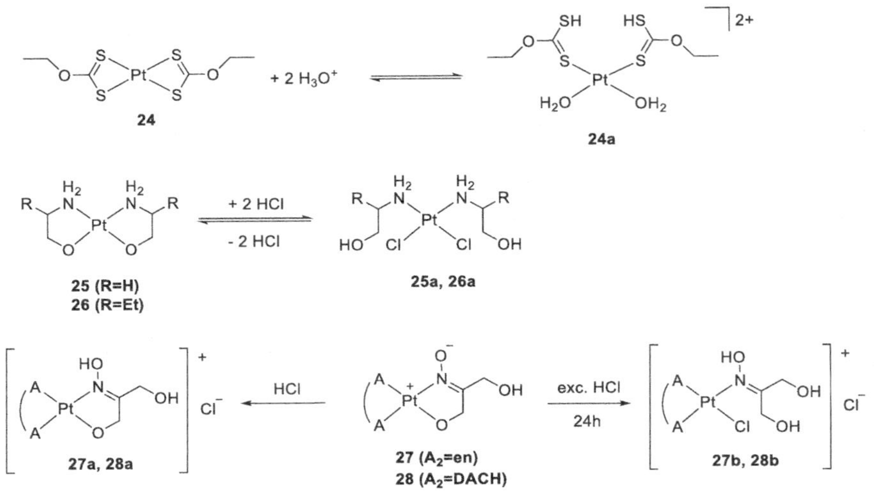

FIGURE 9 Examples of pH-activatable Pt(II) complexes.

No DNA-binding activity at pH 7.4 of both **25** and **26** was apparent. However, they readily formed DNA adducts at pH 6.0. Enhanced DNA binding at lower pH and subsequent crosslinking was suggested as the main cause of their cytotoxicity. The antiproliferative activity in HT-29 and A549 cells revealed a factor of 3–11 higher activity at pH 6.0 compared to pH 7.4 [140]. Although both compounds did not exert higher cytotoxicity than cisplatin or oxaliplatin in cell culture, the authors clearly demonstrated their improved properties due to their pH-responsiveness.

Also, the antitumor activity of various Pt(II)-oxime complexes was reported in the past decades and since then oxime ligands gained significant interest in the development of pH-sensitive Pt(II) complexes [141]. For example, the pH-dependent anticancer activity of a series of 1,3-dihydroxyacetoneoximatoplatinum(II) complexes (**27** and **28**) was investigated (Figure 9) [141]. Acid-mediated protonation of the oximato group and subsequent ring opening was proven by addition of an excess HCl, whereas fast deprotonation and oximato ring-closure occurred at pH 7.4. *In vitro* cytotoxicity was evaluated in the human cancer cell lines CH1, SW480, and A549 compared to cisplatin and oxaliplatin. The IC$_{50}$ values for both open-forms **27b/28b** were slightly higher than oxaliplatin and cisplatin, but were up to 10-fold lower compared to the closed protonated forms **27a/28a** and up to 40-fold lower than the closed zwitterionic species **27/28**. These results strongly support the hypothesis that **27** and **28** are activated in a pH-dependent manner.

4.2 pH-Responsive Pt Nanomaterials

Typically, acid-sensitive release of drugs from carrier vehicles in malignant cells is controlled *via* two strategies. One the one hand, the protonation (ionization) of

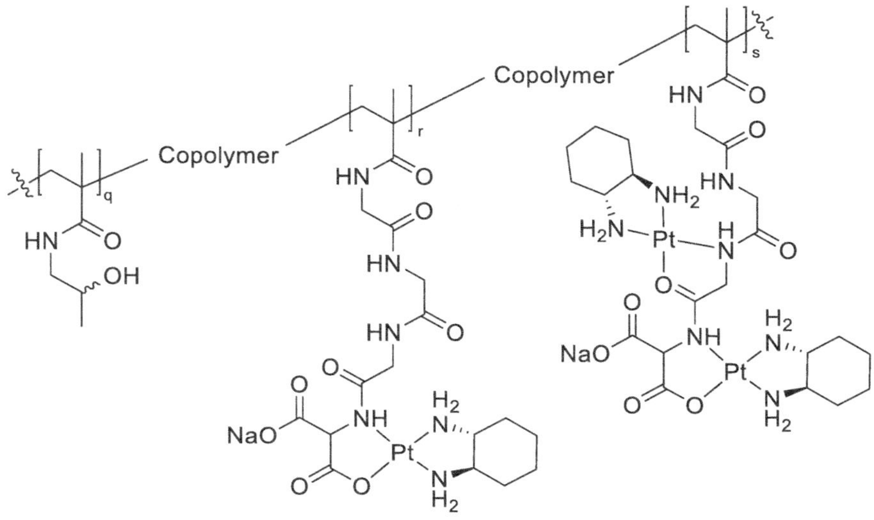

Prodrugs Activated by Cancer-Specific Stimuli

FIGURE 10 Chemical structure of ProLindac.

carrier-incorporated functional groups (like amines or carboxylic acids) in cancerous tissue leads to a change in surface charge and, subsequently, the nanoparticles collapse (due to an alteration in physiochemical properties) and release the active anticancer drugs in the tumor [142]. On the other hand, cleavage of acid-sensitive covalent bonds in the nanomaterial leads to the disintegration of the outer shell and controlled deliverance of the anticancer agent intratumorally [143].

Perhaps the most famous example of a pH-responsive Pt(II)-based nanomaterial is ProLindac™ (AP5346), a diaminocyclohexane (DACH)-Pt prodrug based on a hydroxypropylmethacrylamide copolymer (Figure 10) that advanced to phase II clinical trials for the treatment of ovarian cancer in the past decade [144]. The copolymer backbone contains a linker to an acid-sensitive amidomalonato moiety, which serves as a Pt(II) chelator, in approximately 10:1 ratio. Ultrafiltration experiments showed that Pt release is about seven times higher at pH 5.4 compared to pH 7.4, although the authors suggest that other biological ligands, most likely small sulfur-containing molecules, could also catalyze the detachment of the DACH-Pt(II) species from the polymer [145]. In several tumor xenograft mouse models, the growth inhibition was remarkably better compared to carboplatin or oxaliplatin [146]. Clinical phase I studies demonstrated that high doses of ProLindac could be administered safely. In 2009, the company Access Pharmaceuticals announced positive results in a phase II study against ovarian cancer [147]. However, no further clinical studies or results have been reported since then.

More recently, in contrast to the passive targeting mechanism of ProLindac *via* the EPR effect, pH-sensitive Pt-cored and panitumumab-conjugated apoferritin nanocages were prepared for the treatment of colorectal cancer based on active EGFR targeting [148]. Ferritin is the main iron storage protein of the body, but is also well known for its potential as nanocarrier for medicines owing to its hollow spherical structure. Panitumumab is an antibody specific for the EGFR and is clinically applied for the treatment of metastatic colorectal cancer. The pH-responsive design of the nanoformulation is based on the specific biological characteristics of apoferritin (ferritin without incapsulated iron): the protein complex collapses under acidic conditions and reassembles at physiological pH. This concept was exploited for oxaliplatin and after encapsulation inside the apoferritin, a PEGylated panitumumab unit was conjugated to the carrier protein to yield AFPO. Active targeting and cytotoxicity of AFPO was demonstrated in the colorectal cell models SW-620 (low EGFR expression) versus HCT-116 (EGFR overexpression). Comparable cytotoxicity values were observed for apoferritin and AFPO in SW-620 cells, whereas the cytotoxicity and apoptosis-inducing potential of AFPO in HCT-116 cell lines was significantly increased. The higher cytotoxicity of free oxaliplatin confirmed the prodrug nature of AFPO and the controlled intracellular release of oxaliplatin. Finally, *in vivo* antitumor activity was evaluated in mice bearing SW-620 or HCT-116 tumors and significantly increased tumor growth inhibition was observed for AFPO compared to apoferritin and oxaliplatin in HCT-116-bearing mice only. For more examples of pH-responsive Pt-based nanoparticles with delivery *via* active targeting, the reader is referred to specific reviews [25, 73].

4.3 pH-Responsive Ru Drugs and Nanomaterials

With the exception of several existing publications that report the pH-dependent activation of Ru complexes *via* reduction [149] or *via* light irradiation [150, 151], there is only one example of a pH-responsive Ru drug based on pH-sensitive ligands: an imidazole-containing Ru(II)-bipyridyl complex conjugated to a cRGD peptide (Figure 11a) [152]. As mentioned above, RGD peptides are well known for their high binding affinity to $\alpha_v\beta_3$ integrins [153]. Previous mechanistic investigations by the same authors on similar Ru(II) complexes highlighted that protonation of the imidazole moiety under acidic conditions is crucial for the activation by aquation with release of the cytotoxic Ru(II) bisaqua core (Ru-2) [154]. Anticancer efficacy *in vitro* of Ru-2 and Ru-RGD was screened against various cervical carcinoma and non-malignant cell lines and both Ru-2 and Ru-RGD had cytotoxicity in the low micromolar range similar to cisplatin. In addition, the prodrug nature of the Ru-peptide conjugate was indicated by 2–4 fold higher IC_{50} values. The *in vivo* activity was investigated in CaSki xenografts in mice and higher tumor growth inhibition rates as well as strongly reduced side effects were observed for Ru-RGD compared to Ru-2. In addition, the complex is strongly luminescent. Therefore, Ru-RGD was suggested as fast and economic tool for theranostic tumor diagnosis and therapy.

A very popular strategy in Ru anticancer research is the development of pH-sensitive Ru-based nanomaterials. However, the majority of these investigations focuses on the delivery of PDT-active Ru(II)polypyridyl complexes into the tumor

Prodrugs Activated by Cancer-Specific Stimuli

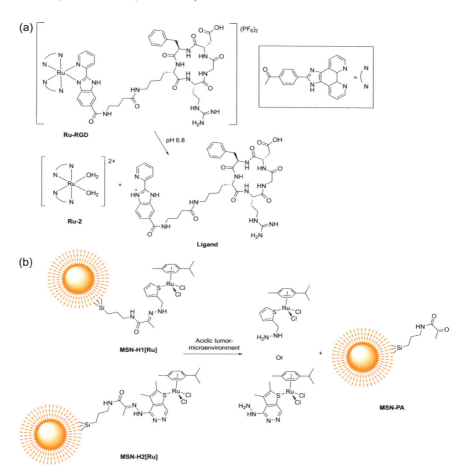

FIGURE 11 pH-responsive Ru-containing nanomaterials. (a) cRGD-containing Ru(II)-bipyridyl complex; (b) MSN-conjugated Ru(II)-arene complex with a pH-sensitive hydrazone linker

microenvironment, which will not be discussed in this chapter [155–157]. Yet, there are a few reports on the pH-triggered intratumoral release of organometallic Ru complexes. For example, recently, Ru(II)-arene complexes were coupled to MSNs *via* pH-sensitive hydrazone linkers (Figure 11b) [158]. The MSN was initially functionalized with 3-aminopropyltriethoxysilane, followed by coupling to pyruvic acid and, subsequently, condensated with two thiophene-functionalized hydazone linkers (H1 and H2) to yield two MSN nanoparticles (MSN-H1 and H2) suitable for coordination to the cytotoxic dichloro(p-cymene)Ru(II) complex ([MSN-H1]Ru and [MSN-H2]Ru). Investigations at different pH values proved the crucial role of the hydrazone linkage and increased Ru(II) release at lower pH. *In vitro* anticancer activity was evaluated against B16F1 melanoma cells.

Both [MSN-H1]Ru and [MSN-H2]Ru were inactive at pH 7.2, but showed MC_{50} values up to the low micromolar range at pH 5.0. However, an *in vivo* proof of anticancer activity is still missing.

5 ENZYME-ACTIVATABLE METAL-BASED DRUGS AND NANOMATERIALS

Besides distinct physicochemical properties, the tumor microenvironment is also characterized by specific protein expression patterns, which can be exploited for cancer targeting and activation of prodrugs. Particularly in the case of organic compounds, several catalytic enzymes such as MMPs or cathepsins need to be mentioned, which are involved in malignant tissue remodeling. As these enzymes have proteolytic functions, prodrug activation often is based on (self-immolative) linkers, which basically offer specific cleavage sites (amino acid sequences) for the proteases [159]. In more detail, several very efficient systems have been already (clinically) developed, such as brentuximab vedotin (INN, Adcetris), a cathepsin B-activated antibody conjugate. This drug selectively targets CD30-overexpressing cancer cells, where it releases the antimitotic agent monomethyl auristatin E [160]. Brentuximab vedotin is approved for several lymphoma types including Hodgkin lymphoma, diverse T-cell lymphoma as well as anaplastic large cell lymphoma.

However, for anticancer metal drugs such prodrug concepts are not easy to translate. Nevertheless, several attempts to employ overexpressed enzymes for metal-based prodrug activation have been reported, which are discussed in the following section.

5.1 ENZYME-ACTIVATABLE PRODRUGS

An established tumor-associated enzyme, which has been frequently exploited for the tumor-specific activation, is β-glucuronidase [161]. Several classes of organic cytotoxic agents have been functionalized with glucuronide moieties that are activated upon cleavage by this enzyme [162]. To the best of our knowledge, with respect to metal-based drugs, only one β-glucuronyl-Pt(II) prodrug has been synthesized [163]. However, this oxaliplatin-releasing prodrug was never investigated biologically. Hence, this field of research might offer a high potential for future drug development.

In addition, different approaches involving combinations of tumor-targeting and enzyme-mediated prodrug activation, such as the antibody-directed enzyme prodrug therapy (ADEPT), should be mentioned briefly [164]. This therapy depends on two separately delivered components: (1) an exogenous enzyme, which is delivered to the cancer cells through conjugation to monoclonal antibodies directed against tumor-specific antigens and (2) a prodrug that is activated by the delivered enzyme. For example, in 1992, Hanessian and Wang synthesized a compound, which releases carboplatin and cephalosporin upon exogenous β-lactamase activation [165]. However, as this method does not rely on endogenous cancer-specific triggers, we will not discuss this approach in more detail.

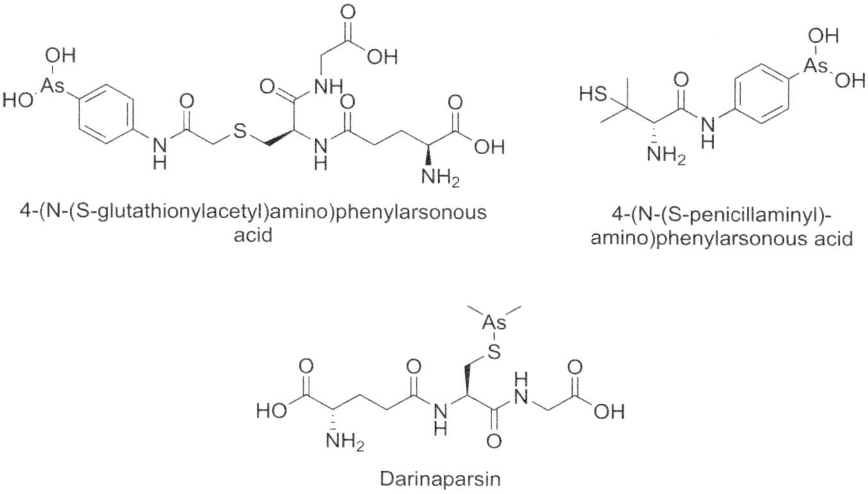

Prodrugs Activated by Cancer-Specific Stimuli

4-(N-(S-glutathionylacetyl)amino)phenylarsonous acid

4-(N-(S-penicillaminyl)-amino)phenylarsonous acid

Darinaparsin

FIGURE 12 Investigational As-containing prodrugs.

Noteworthy, there are some examples of prodrugs derived from the metalloid As, which show promising anticancer activity. These prodrugs are activated by γGSH transferase, a key enzyme involved in GSH metabolism, which is frequently overexpressed in cancer tissue. Three representatives have already been tested in clinical trials (Figure 12): 4-(N-(S-glutathionylacetyl)amino)phenylarsonous acid, 4-(N-(S-penicillaminyl)-amino)phenylarsonous acid, and darinaparsin (S-dimethylarsion-glutathione, ZIO-101) [166, 167]. The first two are As analogs of GSH, which are only activated by proliferating cells, where they follow the same metabolic route as GSH [168]. In more detail, these drugs are applied in a non-permeable form, which is activated by the γGSH transferase at the cell surface by cleavage of the γ-glutamyl group. Subsequently, the dipeptide metabolite is able to enter the cancer cell, where it is further processed by dipeptidases to its single amino acid form. In turn, this crosslinks the cysteine residues of the mitochondrial adenoside nucleotide translocator, resulting in loss of mitochondrial integrity and cell death [36]. In contrast, darinaparsin is an organic arsenical, which has been originally developed to design a better tolerable As-based drug. Subsequent analysis revealed that darinaparsin was not only more active against cancer cells than arsenic trioxide in cell culture but also exerted a different spectrum of activity [169]. Thus, while the PML/RARα fusion gene, a known target of arsenic trioxide, remained unaffected, the activity of darinaparsin was based on ROS generation and oxidative damage in a manner different from arsenic trioxide. Darinaparsin has been tested for its tolerability and anticancer activity in 14 clinical phase I/II trials. The latest multi-center phase II study in relapsed or refractory patients with peripheral T-cell lymphoma has been completed in mid of 2021 (NCT02653976).

5.2 Enzyme-Activatable Nanomaterials Releasing Metal Drugs

Kim et al. reported an elegant method of MMP-2-responsive cisplatin delivery. Cisplatin was conjugated to a self-assembling gel consisting of fatty acids and peptide amphiphiles mimicking the natural extracellular matrix. In addition, a specific peptidase sequence was incorporated into the peptide amphiphiles to facilitate cisplatin release by the enzymatic activity of MMP-2 [170]. Unfortunately, even though this MMP-responsive system has a high potential for further drug development, it has not yet been tested for its anticancer activity.

In addition, telomerase, an enzyme that prolongs telomere length, which is normally deactivated in healthy cells but reactivated in the majority of malignant cells, has been employed as trigger for nanoformulations. Recently, Ma et al. reported on an innovative approach of telomerase-mediated drug release [171]. The authors constructed an icosahedral DNA nanostructure carrying Pt nanoparticles and demonstrated significantly improved anticancer activity in mice in comparison to cisplatin.

Finally, perhaps one of the most successful examples of enzyme-mediated drug release is the secretory phospholipase A2 (sPLA2)-sensitive liposomal cisplatin formulation LiPlaCis, which is currently investigated in a clinical phase II trial (NCT01861496) [172]. sPLA2 is an extracellular enzyme playing a crucial role in tissue inflammation as well as a downstream effector of NF-κB [173]. The anticancer activity of LiPlaCis is based on sPLA2-mediated hydrolysis of the ester linkage of the sn-2-acyls of the phospholipids, which yields free fatty acids and 1-acyl-lysophospholipids. This leads to the destabilization of the liposome membrane, which not only liberates the encapsulated cisplatin, but also results in high local concentrations of lysolipids and free fatty acids at the activation site. These molecules are supposed to function as permeability enhancers across membranes, or at higher amounts, to directly induce toxicity by forming aggregated structures with detergent-like properties [172].

6 GENERAL CONCLUSION

Cancer is a globally growing burden that may affect every second to third person at some point in their lifetime [174]. Consequently, this disease is one of the most investigated in human history and present times. Accordingly, an overwhelming amount of scientific data and reports have accumulated over the years trying to elucidate various mechanisms and common denominating (biological) characteristics [13]. However, based on the diversity and complexity of the disease, the probability of ever finding a single, panacean anticancer drug will probably remain a wishful fantasy. Nevertheless, we may develop highly effective drugs by breaking down the problem and focusing on certain cancer characteristics. Consequently, the search and exploitation of cancer-specific stimuli may represent a promising strategy to successfully develop novel anticancer (metal) drugs. By this approach, not only an enhanced cancer selectivity but also increased tolerability and the potential to circumvent certain resistance mechanisms can be

Prodrugs Activated by Cancer-Specific Stimuli

achieved. With regard to metal complexes, exploitation of the very elegant "activation by reduction" principle is by far the mostly employed strategy, but there are also attempts to use the altered pH and reduced oxygen levels in the malignant microenvironment. However, also in these examples, the underlying mechanisms are often based on "activation by reduction". Consequently, strategies frequently used to develop pure organic drugs such as activation by tumor-specific enzymes are widely neglected. In addition, there are several open questions in the field of metal-based drug development: for example, it is often unclear where and how activation by reduction indeed takes place and if this is sufficient for tumor-specific activity. Therefore, (smart) nanomaterials could serve as powerful partners to finally reach the goal of true tumor specificity in the patient.

ACKNOWLEDGMENTS

We thank the Austrian Science Fund (FWF) project AP32886 and FG3 for financial support.

ABBREVIATIONS

ADEPT	antibody-directed enzyme prodrug therapy
BCA	bis(2-chloroethyl)amine
BCE	N,N'-bis(2-chloroethyl)ethylenediamine
cRGD	cyclic RGD
Cu-ATSM	Cu-diacetyl-bis(N4-methylthiosemicarbazone)
DACH	diaminocyclohexane
DCE	N,N-bis(2-chloroethyl)ethylenediamine
EGFR	epidermal growth factor receptor
en	ethylenediamine
EPR	enhanced permeability and retention
FGFR	fibroblast growth factor receptor
GSH	glutathione
GSSG	glutathione disulfide
IDOi	indolamine-2,3-dioxygenase inhibitor
LDH	layered double hydroxide
MMP	matrix metalloproteinase
MSN	mesoporous silica nanoparticle
NHC	N-heterocyclic carbene
PBMC	peripheral blood mononuclear cells
PDT	photodynamic therapy
PET	positron emission tomography
PLip	protein-loaded liposomes
PR	progesterone receptor
ROS	reactive oxygen species
sPLA2	secretory phospholipase A2
TKI	tyrosine kinase inhibitor

REFERENCES

[1] M. A. Zoroddu, J. Aaseth, G. Crisponi, S. Medici, M. Peana, V. M. Nurchi, *J. Inorg. Biochem.* **2019**, *195*, 120–129.

[2] S. Dasari, P. B. Tchounwou, *Eur. J. Pharmacol.* **2014**, *740*, 364–378.

[3] C. S. Allardyce, P. J. Dyson, *Dalton Trans.* **2016**, *45* (8), 3201–3209.

[4] Y. Xue, S. Gao, J. Gou, T. Yin, H. He, Y. Wang, Y. Zhang, X. Tang, R. Wu, *Expert Opin. Drug Deliv.* **2021**, *18* (2), 187–203.

[5] M. Hoonjan, V. Jadhav, P. Bhatt, *J. Biol. Inorg. Chem.* **2018**, *23* (3), 313–329.

[6] I. Pötsch, D. Baier, B. K. Keppler, W. Berger, in *Metal-Based Anticancer Agents*, Eds A. V. A. Casini, S. M Meier-Menches, RSC Publishing, **2019**, pp. 308–347.

[7] M. Marloye, G. Berger, M. Gelbcke, F. Dufrasne, *Future Med. Chem.* **2016**, *8* (18), 2263–2286.

[8] R. Oun, Y. E. Moussa, N. J. Wheate, *Dalton Trans.* **2018**, *47* (19), 6645–6653.

[9] D. J. Norman, E. González-Fernández, J. Clavadetscher, L. Tucker, M. Staderini, A. R. Mount, A. F. Murray, M. Bradley, *Chem. Commun.* **2018**, *54* (66), 9242–9245.

[10] Y. Wang, D. S. Kohane, *Nat. Rev. Mater.* **2017**, *2* (6), 1–14.

[11] Y. Zhang, J. Yu, H. N. Bomba, Y. Zhu, Z. Gu, *Chem. Rev.* **2016**, *116* (19), 12536–12563.

[12] D. Hanahan, R. A. Weinberg, *Cell* **2000**, *100* (1), 57–70.

[13] D. Hanahan, *Cancer Discov.* **2022**, *12* (1), 31–46.

[14] D. Hanahan, R. A. Weinberg, *Cell* **2011**, *144* (5), 646–674.

[15] T. Wu, Y. Dai, *Cancer Lett.* **2017**, *387*, 61–68.

[16] L. L. Policastro, I. L. Ibañez, C. Notcovich, H. A. Duran, O. L. Podhajcer, *Antioxid. Redox Signal.* **2013**, *19* (8), 854–895.

[17] J. W. Ivey, M. Bonakdar, A. Kanitkar, R. V. Davalos, S. S. Verbridge, *Cancer Lett.* **2016**, *380* (1), 330–339.

[18] M. Forkink, J. A. Smeitink, R. Brock, P. H. Willems, W. J. Koopman, *Biochim. Biophys. Acta* **2010**, *1797* (6–7), 1034–1044.

[19] D. Zhou, L. Shao, D. R. Spitz, *Adv. Cancer. Res.* **2014**, *122*, 1–67.

[20] V. Nogueira, N. Hay, *Clin. Cancer. Res.* **2013**, *19* (16), 4309–4314.

[21] G. Saito, J. A. Swanson, K. D. Lee, *Adv. Drug. Deliv. Rev.* **2003**, *55* (2), 199–215.

[22] J. B. Zhou, Y. Kang, L. Chen, H. Wang, J. Q. Liu, S. Zeng, L. S. Yu, *Front Pharmacol.* **2020**, *11*, 1–17.

[23] M. T. Kuo, *Antioxid. Redox Signal.* **2009**, *11* (1), 99–133.

[24] A. V. Klein, T. W. Hambley, *Chem. Rev.* **2009**, *109* (10), 4911–4920.

[25] X. Wang, X. Wang, S. Jin, N. Muhammad, Z. Guo, *Chem. Rev.* **2019**, *119* (2), 1138–1192.

[26] H. Maeda, J. Wu, T. Sawa, Y. Matsumura, K. Hori, *J. Control. Release* **2000**, *65* (1–2), 271–284.

[27] M. V. Liberti, J. W. Locasale, *Trends Biochem. Sci.* **2016**, *41* (3), 211–218.

[28] L. Xia, L. Oyang, J. Lin, S. Tan, Y. Han, N. Wu, P. Yi, L. Tang, Q. Pan, S. Rao, J. Liang, Y. Tang, M. Su, X. Luo, Y. Yang, Y. Shi, H. Wang, Y. Zhou, Q. Liao, *Mol. Cancer* **2021**, *20* (1), 1–21.

[29] A. Rosenzweig, J. Blenis, A. P. Gomes, *Front. Cell Dev. Biol.* **2018**, *6*, 1–7.

[30] S. K. Parks, J. Mueller-Klieser, J. Pouysségur, *Annu. Rev. Cancer Biol.* **2020**, *4* (1), 141–158.

[31] C. Stefanadis, C. Chrysohoou, D. B. Panagiotakos, E. Passalidou, V. Katsi, V. Polychronopoulos, P. K. Toutouzas, *BMC Cancer* **2003**, *3*, 1–5.

[32] H. T. Nia, L. L. Munn, R. K. Jain, *Clin. Cancer. Res.* **2019**, *25* (7), 2024–2026.

[33] D. Wirtz, K. Konstantopoulos, P. C. Searson, *Nat. Rev. Cancer.* **2011**, *11* (7), 512–522.

[34] T. Risler, *New J. Phys.* **2015**, *17* (5), 1–9.
[35] N. Jessani, Y. Liu, M. Humphrey, B. F. Cravatt, *Proc. Natl. Acad. Sci.* **2002**, *99* (16), 10335–10340.
[36] A. Valente, A. Podolski-Renić, I. Poetsch, N. Filipović, Ó. López, I. Turel, P. Heffeter, *Drug Resist. Updat.* **2021**, *58*, 1–33.
[37] T. C. Johnstone, K. Suntharalingam, S. J. Lippard, *Chem. Rev.* **2016**, *116* (5), 3436–3486.
[38] Z. H. Siddik, *Oncogene* **2003**, *22* (47), 7265–7279.
[39] A. Kastner, I. Poetsch, J. Mayr, J. V. Burda, A. Roller, P. Heffeter, B. K. Keppler, C. R. Kowol, *Angew. Chem. Int. Ed.* **2019**, *58* (22), 7464–7469.
[40] R. G. Kenny, C. J. Marmion, *Chem. Rev.* **2019**, *119* (2), 1058–1137.
[41] J. Mayr, P. Heffeter, D. Groza, L. Galvez, G. Koellensperger, A. Roller, B. Alte, M. Haider, W. Berger, C. R. Kowol, *Chem. Sci.* **2017**, *8* (3), 2241–2250.
[42] J. J. Wilson, S. J. Lippard, *Inorg. Chem.* **2011**, *50* (7), 3103–3115.
[43] J. L. Carr, M. D. Tingle, M. J. McKeage, *Cancer Chemother. Pharmacol.* **2006**, *57* (4), 483–490.
[44] A. Nemirovski, Y. Kasherman, Y. Tzaraf, D. Gibson, *J. Med. Chem.* **2007**, *50* (23), 5554–5556.
[45] S. Choi, C. Filotto, M. Bisanzo, S. Delaney, D. Lagasee, J. L. Whitworth, A. Jusko, C. R. Li, N. A. Wood, J. Willingham, A. Schwenker, K. Spaulding, *Inorg. Chem.* **1998**, *37* (10), 2500–2504.
[46] E. Wexselblatt, D. Gibson, *J. Inorg. Biochem.* **2012**, *117*, 220–229.
[47] J. Z. Zhang, E. Wexselblatt, T. W. Hambley, D. Gibson, *Chem. Commun.* **2012**, *48* (6), 847–849.
[48] S. Dilruba, G. V. Kalayda, *Cancer Chemother. Pharmacol.* **2016**, *77* (6), 1103–1124.
[49] T. J. O'Rourke, G. R. Weiss, P. New, H. A. Burris, 3rd, G. Rodriguez, J. Eckhardt, J. Hardy, J. G. Kuhn, S. Fields, D. D. Von Hoff, *Anticancer Drugs* **1994**, *5* (5), 520–526.
[50] H. Anderson, J. Wagstaff, D. Crowther, R. Swindell, M. J. Lind, J. McGregor, M. S. Timms, D. Brown, P. Palmer, *Eur. J. Cancer Clin. Oncol.* **1988**, *24* (9), 1471–1479.
[51] C. N. Sternberg, P. Whelan, J. Hetherington, B. Paluchowska, P. H. Slee, K. Vekemans, P. Van Erps, C. Theodore, O. Koriakine, T. Oliver, D. Lebwohl, M. Debois, A. Zurlo, L. Collette, Genitourinary Tract Group of the EORTC, *Oncology*, **2005**, *68* (1), 2–9.
[52] M. J. McKeage, P. Mistry, J. Ward, F. E. Boxall, S. Loh, C. O'Neill, P. Ellis, L. R. Kelland, S. E. Morgan, B. Murrer, P. Santabarbara, K. R. Harrap, I. R. Judson, *Cancer Chemother. Pharmacol.* **1995**, *36* (6), 451–458.
[53] A. Bhargava, U. N. Vaishampayan, *Expert Opin. Investig. Drugs* **2009**, *18* (11), 1787–1797.
[54] N. Graf, S. J. Lippard, *Adv. Drug. Deliv. Rev.* **2012**, *64* (11), 993–1004.
[55] D. Gibson, *Dalton Trans.* **2016**, *45* (33), 12983–12991.
[56] D. Gibson, *J. Inorg. Biochem.* **2021**, 1–10.
[57] J. Zajac, H. Kostrhunova, V. Novohradsky, O. Vrana, R. Raveendran, D. Gibson, J. Kasparkova, V. Brabec, *J. Inorg. Biochem.* **2016**, *156*, 89–97.
[58] S. Dhar, S. J. Lippard, *Proc. Natl. Acad. Sci.* **2009**, *106* (52), 22199–22204.
[59] V. Venkataramani, C. Rossner, L. Iffland, S. Schweyer, I. Y. Tamboli, J. Walter, O. Wirths, T. A. Bayer, *Int. J. Biol. Chem.* **2010**, *285* (14), 10678–10689.
[60] J. Yang, X. Sun, W. Mao, M. Sui, J. Tang, Y. Shen, *Mol. Pharm.* **2012**, *9* (10), 2793–2800.
[61] V. Novohradsky, L. Zerzankova, J. Stepankova, O. Vrana, R. Raveendran, D. Gibson, J. Kasparkova, V. Brabec, *J. Inorg. Biochem.* **2014**, *140*, 72–79.
[62] C. S. Kue, A. Kamkaew, K. Burgess, L. V. Kiew, L. Y. Chung, H. B. Lee, *Med. Res. Rev.* **2016**, *36* (3), 494–575.

[63] J. Ma, H. Liu, Z. Xi, J. Hou, Y. Li, J. Niu, T. Liu, S. Bi, X. Wang, C. Wang, J. Wang, S. Xie, P. G. Wang, *Front Chem.* **2018**, *6*, 1–15.

[64] N. Muhammad, N. Sadia, C. Zhu, C. Luo, Z. Guo, X. Wang, *Chem. Commun.* **2017**, *53* (72), 9971–9974.

[65] F. Kratz, *J. Control. Release* **2008**, *132* (3), 171–183.

[66] E. Miele, G. P. Spinelli, E. Miele, F. Tomao, S. Tomao, *Int. J. Nanomed.* **2009**, *4*, 99–105.

[67] L. D. Cranmer, *Onco. Targets Ther.* **2019**, *12*, 2047–2062.

[68] V. Pichler, J. Mayr, P. Heffeter, O. Dömötör, É. A. Enyedy, G. Hermann, D. Groza, G. Köllensperger, M. Galanksi, W. Berger, *Chem. Commun.* **2013**, *49* (22), 2249–2251.

[69] H. Schueffl, S. Theiner, G. Hermann, J. Mayr, P. Fronik, D. Groza, S. van Schonhooven, L. Galvez, N. S. Sommerfeld, A. Schintlmeister, S. Reipert, M. Wagner, R. M. Mader, G. Koellensperger, B. K. Keppler, W. Berger, C. R. Kowol, A. Legin, P. Heffeter, *Chem. Sci.* **2021**, *12* (38), 12587–12599.

[70] T. C. Johnstone, N. Kulak, E. M. Pridgen, O. C. Farokhzad, R. Langer, S. J. Lippard, *ACS Nano.* **2013**, *7* (7), 5675–5683.

[71] J. Lu, X. Liu, Y.-P. Liao, F. Salazar, B. Sun, W. Jiang, C. H. Chang, J. Jiang, X. Wang, A. M. Wu, *Nat. Commun.* **2017**, *8* (1), 1–14.

[72] S. G. Awuah, Y.-R. Zheng, P. M. Bruno, M. T. Hemann, S. J. Lippard, *J. Am. Chem. Soc.* **2015**, *137* (47), 14854–14857.

[73] J. F. Machado, T. S. Morais, *Dalton Trans.* **2022**, *51*, 2593–2609.

[74] Y. Han, P. Wen, J. Li, K. Kataoka, *J. Control. Release.* **2022**, *345*, 709–720.

[75] Q. Peña, A. Wang, O. Zaremba, Y. Shi, H. W. Scheeren, J. M. Metselaar, F. Kiessling, R. M. Pallares, S. Wuttke, T. Lammers, *Chem. Soc. Rev.* **2022**, *51* (7), 2544–2582.

[76] N. Wang, Z. Wang, Z. Xu, X. Chen, G. Zhu, *Angew. Chem. Int. Ed. Engl.* **2018**, *57* (13), 3426–3430.

[77] A. L. Mellor, D. B. Keskin, T. Johnson, P. Chandler, D. H. Munn, *J. Immunol.* **2002**, *168* (8), 3771–3776.

[78] J. Della Rocca, R. C. Huxford, E. Comstock-Duggan, W. Lin, *Angew. Chem. Int. Ed. Engl.* **2011**, *50* (44), 10330–10334.

[79] A. Dasargyri, C. D. Kümin, J. C. Leroux, *Adv. Mater.* **2017**, *29* (7), 1–17.

[80] J. P. Coverdale, T. Laroiya-McCarron, I. Romero-Canelón, *Inorganics* **2019**, *7* (3), 1–15.

[81] U. Jungwirth, C. R. Kowol, B. K. Keppler, C. G. Hartinger, W. Berger, P. Heffeter, *Antioxid. Redox Signal.* **2011**, 1085–1127.

[82] R. Trondl, P. Heffeter, C. R. Kowol, M. A. Jakupec, W. Berger, B. K. Keppler, *Chem. Sci.* **2014**, *5* (8), 2925–2932.

[83] S. Leijen, S. A. Burgers, P. Baas, D. Pluim, M. Tibben, E. van Werkhoven, E. Alessio, G. Sava, J. H. Beijnen, J. H. Schellens, *Investig. New Drugs* **2015**, *33* (1), 201–214.

[84] S. Monro, K. L. Colon, H. Yin, J. Roque, III, P. Konda, S. Gujar, R. P. Thummel, L. Lilge, C. G. Cameron, S. A. McFarland, *Chem. Rev.* **2018**, *119* (2), 797–828.

[85] M. Sulyok, S. Hann, C. Hartinger, B. Keppler, G. Stingeder, G. Koellensperger, *J. Anal. At. Spectrom.* **2005**, *20* (9), 856–863.

[86] A. R. Timerbaev, C. G. Hartinger, S. S. Aleksenko, B. K. Keppler, *Chem. Rev.* **2006**, *106* (6), 2224–2248.

[87] C. G. Hartinger, M. A. Jakupec, S. Zorbas-Seifried, M. Groessl, A. Egger, W. Berger, H. Zorbas, P. J. Dyson, B. K. Keppler, *Chem. Biodivers.* **2008**, *5* (10), 2140–2155.

[88] B. Neuditschko, A. A. Legin, D. Baier, A. Schintlmeister, S. Reipert, M. Wagner, B. K. Keppler, W. Berger, S. M. Meier-Menches, C. Gerner, *Angew. Chem., Int. Ed.* **2021**, *60* (10), 5063–5068.

[89] F. Piccioli, S. Sabatini, L. Messori, P. Orioli, C. G. Hartinger, B. K. Keppler, *J. Inorg. Biochem.* **2004**, *98* (6), 1135–1142.

Prodrugs Activated by Cancer-Specific Stimuli

[90] A. R. Timerbaev, L. S. Foteeva, A. V. Rudnev, J. K. Abramski, K. Połeć-Pawlak, C. G. Hartinger, M. Jarosz, B. K. Keppler, *Electrophoresis* **2007**, *28* (13), 2235–2240.

[91] S. Swaminathan, J. Haribabu, N. Balakrishnan, P. Vasanthakumar, R. Karvembu, *Coord. Chem. Rev.* 2022, *459*, 1–32.

[92] S. J. Dougan, A. Habtemariam, S. E. McHale, S. Parsons, P. J. Sadler, *Proc. Natl. Acad. Sci.* **2008**, *105* (33), 11628–11633.

[93] G. Lv, L. Qiu, K. Li, Q. Liu, X. Li, Y. Peng, S. Wang, J. Lin, *New J. Chem.* 2019, *43* (8), 3419–3427.

[94] L. Zeng, P. Gupta, Y. Chen, E. Wang, L. Ji, H. Chao, Z.-S. Chen, *Chem. Soc. Rev.* **2017**, *46* (19), 5771–5804.

[95] B. M. Blunden, R. Chapman, M. Danial, H. Lu, K. A. Jolliffe, S. Perrier, M. H. Stenzel, *Chem. Eur. J.* **2014**, *20* (40), 12745–12749.

[96] J. F. Machado, M. Machuqueiro, F. Marques, M. P. Robalo, M. F. M. Piedade, M. H. Garcia, J. D. Correia, T. S. Morais, *Dalton Trans.* **2020**, *49* (18), 5974–5987.

[97] F. Chen, F. Zhang, D. Shao, W. Zhang, L. Zheng, W. Wang, W. Yang, Z. Wang, J. Chen, W.-F. Dong, *Appl. Mater. Today* **2020**, *19*, 1–12.

[98] P. N. Durfee, Y.-S. Lin, D. R. Dunphy, A. E. J. Muñiz, K. S. Butler, K. R. Humphrey, A. J. Lokke, J. O. Agola, S. S. Chou, I.-M. Chen, *ACS Nano.* **2016**, *10* (9), 8325–8345.

[99] A. K. Boal, A. C. Rosenzweig, *Chem. Rev.* **2009**, *109* (10), 4760–4779.

[100] Y. Li, *IUBMB Life* **2020**, *72* (9), 1900–1908.

[101] P. Lelièvre, L. Sancey, J.-L. Coll, A. Deniaud, B. Busser, *Cancers,* **2020**, *12* (12), 1–25.

[102] L. Ruiz-Azuara, G. Bastian, M. E. Bravo-Gómez, R. C. Cañas, M. Flores-Alamo, I. Fuentes, C. Mejia, J. C. García-Ramos, A. Serrano. Abstract CT408: Phase I study of one mixed chelates copper (II) compound, Casiopeína CasIIIia with antitumor activity and its mechanism of action, Vol. 74 (in series), AACR, 2014.

[103] C. Santini, M. Pellei, V. Gandin, M. Porchia, F. Tisato, C. Marzano, *Chem. Rev.* **2014**, *114* (1), 815–862.

[104] X. Chen, Q. P. Dou, J. Liu, D. Tang, *Front. Mol. Biosci.* **2021**, *8*, 1–9.

[105] S. Hager, V. F. Pape, V. Pósa, B. Montsch, L. Uhlik, G. Szakács, S. Tóth, N. Jabronka, B. K. Keppler, C. R. Kowol, *Antioxid. Redox Signaling* **2020**, *33* (6), 395–414.

[106] J. H. Bormio Nunes, S. Hager, M. Mathuber, V. Pósa, A. Roller, E. V. A. Enyedy, A. Stefanelli, W. Berger, B. K. Keppler, P. Heffeter, *J. Med. Chem.* **2020**, *63* (22), 13719–13732.

[107] A. Popović-Bijelić, C. R. Kowol, M. E. Lind, J. Luo, F. Himo, E. A. Enyedy, V. B. Arion, A. Gräslund, *J. Inorg. Biochem.* **2011**, *105* (11), 1422–1431.

[108] M. Mathuber, M. Gutmann, M. La Franca, P. Vician, A. Laemmerer, P. Moser, B. K. Keppler, W. Berger, C. R. Kowol, *Inorg. Chem. Front.* **2021**, *8* (10), 2468–2485.

[109] M. C. Brahimi-Horn, J. Chiche, J. Pouysségur, *J. Mol. Med. (Berl)* **2007**, *85* (12), 1301–1307.

[110] Y. Li, L. Zhao, X. F. Li, *Front. Oncol.* **2021**, *11*, 1–13.

[111] J. P. Laubach, C. J. Liu, N. S. Raje, A. J. Yee, P. Armand, R. L. Schlossman, J. Rosenblatt, J. Hedlund, M. Martin, C. Reynolds, K. H. Shain, I. Zackon, L. Stampleman, P. Henrick, B. Rivotto, K. T. V. Hornburg, H. J. Dumke, S. Chuma, A. Savell, D. R. Handisides, S. Kroll, K. C. Anderson, P. G. Richardson, I. M. Ghobrial, *Clin. Cancer. Res.* **2019**, *25* (2), 478–486.

[112] W. D. Tap, Z. Papai, B. A. Van Tine, S. Attia, K. N. Ganjoo, R. L. Jones, S. Schuetze, D. Reed, S. P. Chawla, R. F. Riedel, A. Krarup-Hansen, M. Toulmonde, I. Ray-Coquard, P. Hohenberger, G. Grignani, L. D. Cranmer, S. Okuno, M. Agulnik, W. Read, C. W. Ryan, T. Alcindor, X. F. G. Del Muro, G. T. Budd, H. Tawbi, T. Pearce, S. Kroll, D. K. Reinke, P. Schöffski, *Lancet Oncol.* **2017**, *18* (8), 1089–1103.

[113] L. Leyssens, B. Vinck, C. Van Der Straeten, F. Wuyts, L. Maes, *Toxicology* **2017**, *387*, 43–56.

[114] C. R. Munteanu, K. Suntharalingam, *Dalton Trans.* **2015**, *44* (31), 13796–13808.
[115] M. Mathuber, H. Schueffl, O. Dömötör, C. Karnthaler, É. A. Enyedy, P. Heffeter, B. K. Keppler, C. R. Kowol, *Inorg. Chem.* **2020**, *59* (23), 17794–17810.
[116] D. C. Ware, B. D. Palmer, W. R. Wilson, W. A. Denny, *J. Med. Chem.* **1993**, *36* (13), 1839–1846.
[117] D. C. Ware, W. R. Wilson, W. A. Denny, C. E. F. Rickard, *J. Chem. Soc., Chem. Commun.* **1991**, (17), 1171–1173.
[118] A. J. Clarkson, A. G. Blackman, C. R. Clark, A. M. Sargeson, *Aust. J. Chem.* **2009**, *62* (10), 1221–1225.
[119] C. Karnthaler-Benbakka, D. Groza, K. Kryeziu, V. Pichler, A. Roller, W. Berger, P. Heffeter, C. R. Kowol, *Angew. Chem. Int. Ed. Engl.* **2014**, *53* (47), 12930–12935.
[120] M. V. Palmeira-Mello, A. B. Caballero, J. M. Ribeiro, E. M. de Souza-Fagundes, P. Gamez, M. Lanznaster, *J. Inorg. Biochem.* **2020**, *211*, 1–9.
[121] T. W. Failes, C. Cullinane, C. I. Diakos, N. Yamamoto, J. G. Lyons, T. W. Hambley, *Chemistry* **2007**, *13* (10), 2974–2982.
[122] I. C. de Souza, L. V. Faro, C. B. Pinheiro, D. T. Gonzaga, C. da Silva Fde, V. F. Ferreira, S. Miranda Fda, M. Scarpellini, M. Lanznaster, *Dalton Trans.* **2016**, *45* (35), 13671–13674.
[123] M. Kozsup, X. Zhou, E. Farkas, A. C. Bényei, S. Bonnet, T. Patonay, K. Kónya, P. Buglyó, *J. Inorg. Biochem.* **2021**, *217*, 1–12.
[124] Y. Chen, Y. Jia, W. Song, L. Zhang, *Front. Pharmacol., Review*, **2018**, *9*, 1–12.
[125] B. A. Teicher, M. J. Abrams, K. W. Rosbe, T. S. Herman, *Cancer Res.* **1990**, *50* (21), 6971–6975.
[126] D. C. Ware, P. J. Brothers, G. R. Clark, W. A. Denny, B. D. Palmer, W. R. Wilson, *Dalton Trans.* **2000**, (6), 925–932.
[127] L. L. Parker, S. M. Lacy, L. J. Farrugia, C. Evans, D. J. Robins, C. C. O'Hare, J. A. Hartley, M. Jaffar, I. J. Stratford, *J. Med. Chem.* **2004**, *47* (23), 5683–5689.
[128] R. I. Maurer, P. J. Blower, J. R. Dilworth, C. A. Reynolds, Y. Zheng, G. E. Mullen, *J. Med. Chem.* **2002**, *45* (7), 1420–1431.
[129] T. W. Failes, T. W. Hambley, *J. Inorg. Biochem.* **2007**, *101* (3), 396–403.
[130] C. Nardon, G. Boscutti, D. Fregona, *Anticancer Res.* **2014**, *34* (1), 487–492.
[131] J. A. Lessa, J. C. Guerra, L. F. de Miranda, C. F. Romeiro, J. G. Da Silva, I. C. Mendes, N. L. Speziali, E. M. Souza-Fagundes, H. Beraldo, *J. Inorg. Biochem.* **2011**, *105* (12), 1729–1739.
[132] V. Rodríguez-Fanjul, E. López-Torres, M. A. Mendiola, A. M. Pizarro, *Eur. J. Med. Chem.* **2018**, *148*, 372–383.
[133] J. A. Lessa, K. S. Ferraz, J. C. Guerra, L. F. de Miranda, C. F. Romeiro, E. M. Souza-Fagundes, P. J. Barbeira, H. Beraldo, *Biometals* **2012**, *25* (3), 587–598.
[134] A. P. A. Oliveira, J. T. J. Freitas, R. Diniz, C. Pessoa, S. S. Maranhão, J. M. Ribeiro, E. M. Souza-Fagundes, H. Beraldo, *ACS Omega* **2020**, *5* (6), 2939–2946.
[135] G. Yang, S. Z. F. Phua, W. Q. Lim, R. Zhang, L. Feng, G. Liu, H. Wu, A. K. Bindra, D. Jana, Z. Liu, Y. Zhao, *Adv. Mater.* **2019**, *31* (25), 1–9.
[136] B. Zhang, Z. Xu, W. Zhou, Z. Liu, J. Zhao, S. Gou, *Chem. Sci.* **2021**, *12* (35), 11810–11820.
[137] R. A. Gatenby, R. J. Gillies, *Nat. Rev. Cancer* **2004**, *4* (11), 891–899.
[138] E. Amtmann, M. Zöller, H. Wesch, G. Schilling, *Cancer Chemother. Pharmacol.* **2001**, *47* (6), 461–466.
[139] S. Zorbas-Seifried, C. G. Hartinger, K. Meelich, M. Galanski, B. K. Keppler, H. Zorbas, *Biochemistry* **2006**, *45* (49), 14817–14825.
[140] S. M. Valiahdi, A. E. Egger, W. Miklos, U. Jungwirth, K. Meelich, P. Nock, W. Berger, C. G. Hartinger, M. Galanski, M. A. Jakupec, *J. Biol. Inorg. Chem.* **2013**, *18* (2), 249–260.

Prodrugs Activated by Cancer-Specific Stimuli 37

[141] Y. Y. Scaffidi-Domianello, A. A. Legin, M. A. Jakupec, V. B. Arion, V. Y. Kukushkin, M. S. Galanski, B. K. Keppler, *Inorg. Chem.* **2011**, *50* (21), 10673–10681.
[142] A. K. Varkouhi, M. Scholte, G. Storm, H. J. Haisma, *J. Control. Release* **2011**, *151* (3), 220–228.
[143] J. Du, L. A. Lane, S. Nie, *J. Control. Release* **2015**, *219*, 205–214.
[144] D. P. Nowotnik, E. Cvitkovic, *Adv. Drug. Deliv. Rev.* **2009**, *61* (13), 1214–1219.
[145] S. Van der Schoot, B. Nuijen, P. Sood, K. Thurmond, II, D. Stewart, J. Rice, J. Beijnen, *Pharmazie*, **2006**, *61* (10), 835–844.
[146] J. M. Rademaker-Lakhai, C. Terret, S. B. Howell, C. M. Baud, R. F. De Boer, D. Pluim, J. H. Beijnen, J. H. Schellens, J.-P. Droz, *Clin. Cancer Res.* **2004**, *10* (10), 3386–3395.
[147] D. P. Nowotnik, *Curr. Bioact. Compd.* **2011**, *7* (1), 21–26.
[148] C.-Y. Lin, S.-J. Yang, C.-L. Peng, M.-J. Shieh, *ACS Appl. Mater. Interfaces* **2018**, *10* (7), 6096–6106.
[149] M. Caterino, M. Herrmann, A. Merlino, C. Riccardi, D. Montesarchio, M. A. Mroginski, D. Musumeci, F. Ruffo, L. Paduano, P. Hildebrandt, *Inorg. Chem.* **2019**, *58* (2), 1216–1223.
[150] K. T. Hufziger, F. S. Thowfeik, D. J. Charboneau, I. Nieto, W. G. Dougherty, W. S. Kassel, T. J. Dudley, E. J. Merino, E. T. Papish, J. J. Paul, *J. Inorg. Biochem.* **2014**, *130*, 103–111.
[151] F. Qu, S. Park, K. Martinez, J. L. Gray, F. S. Thowfeik, J. A. Lundeen, A. E. Kuhn, D. J. Charboneau, D. L. Gerlach, M. M. Lockart, *Inorg. Chem.* **2017**, *56* (13), 7519–7532.
[152] Z. Zhao, X. Zhang, C.-E. Li, T. Chen, *Biomaterials* **2019**, *192*, 579–589.
[153] M. A. Dechantsreiter, E. Planker, B. Mathä, E. Lohof, G. Hölzemann, A. Jonczyk, S. L. Goodman, H. Kessler, *J. Med. Chem.* **1999**, *42* (16), 3033–3040.
[154] Z. Zhao, P. Gao, Y. You, T. Chen, *Chem. Eur. J.* **2018**, *24* (13), 3289–3298.
[155] L. He, Y. Huang, H. Zhu, G. Pang, W. Zheng, Y. S. Wong, T. Chen, *Adv. Funct. Mater.* **2014**, *24* (19), 2754–2763.
[156] L. Chen, C. Fu, Y. Deng, W. Wu, A. Fu, *Pharm. Res.* **2016**, *33* (12), 2989–2998.
[157] D. Sun, Z. Wang, P. Zhang, C. Yin, J. Wang, Y. Sun, Y. Chen, W. Wang, B. Sun, C. Fan, *J. Nanobiotechnol.* **2021**, *19* (1), 1–16.
[158] M. Mladenović, I. Morgan, N. Ilić, M. Saoud, M. V. Pergal, G. N. Kaluđerović, N. Ž. Knežević, *Pharmaceutics* **2021**, *13* (4), 1–13.
[159] U. H. Weidle, G. Tiefenthaler, G. Georges, *Cancer Genom. Proteom.* **2014**, *11* (2), 67–79.
[160] H. Franzyk, S. B. Christensen, *Molecules* **2021**, *26* (5), 1–23.
[161] M. de Graaf, E. Boven, H. W. Scheeren, H. J. Haisma, H. M. Pinedo, *Curr. Pharm. Des.* **2002**, *8* (15), 1391–1403.
[162] I. Tranoy-Opalinski, T. Legigan, R. Barat, J. Clarhaut, M. Thomas, B. Renoux, S. Papot, *Eur. J. Med. Chem.* **2014**, *74*, 302–313.
[163] R. A. Tromp, S. S. van Boom, C. Marco Timmers, S. van Zutphen, G. A. van der Marel, H. S. Overkleeft, J. H. van Boom, J. Reedijk, *Bioorg. Med. Chem. Lett.* **2004**, *14* (16), 4273–4276.
[164] K. D. Bagshawe, *Expert Rev. Anticancer Ther.* **2006**, *6* (10), 1421–1431.
[165] S. Hanessian, J. Wang, *Can. J. Chem.* **1993**, *71* (6), 896–906.
[166] L. Horsley, J. Cummings, M. Middleton, T. Ward, A. Backen, A. Clamp, M. Dawson, H. Farmer, N. Fisher, G. Halbert, S. Halford, A. Harris, J. Hasan, P. Hogg, G. Kumaran, R. Little, G. J. Parker, P. Potter, M. Saunders, C. Roberts, D. Shaw, N. Smith, J. Smythe, A. Taylor, H. Turner, Y. Watson, C. Dive, G. C. Jayson, *Cancer Chemother. Pharmacol.* **2013**, *72* (6), 1343–1352.
[167] M. Ogura, W. S. Kim, T. Uchida, N. Uike, Y. Suehiro, K. Ishizawa, H. Nagai, F. Nagahama, Y. Sonehara, K. Tobinai, *Jpn. J. Clin. Oncol.* **2021**, *51* (2), 218–227.

[168] A. S. Don, O. Kisker, P. Dilda, N. Donoghue, X. Zhao, S. Decollogne, B. Creighton, E. Flynn, J. Folkman, P. J. Hogg, *Cancer Cell* **2003**, *3* (5), 497–509.

[169] S. M. Matulis, A. A. Morales, L. Yehiayan, C. Croutch, D. Gutman, Y. Cai, K. P. Lee, L. H. Boise, *Mol. Cancer. Ther.* **2009**, *8* (5), 1197–1206.

[170] J. K. Kim, J. Anderson, H. W. Jun, M. A. Repka, S. Jo, *Mol. Pharm.* **2009**, *6* (3), 978–985.

[171] Y. Ma, Z. Wang, Y. Ma, Z. Han, M. Zhang, H. Chen, Y. Gu, *Angew. Chem. Int. Ed. Engl.* **2018**, *57* (19), 5389–5393.

[172] H. Pourhassan, G. Clergeaud, A. E. Hansen, R. G. Østrem, F. P. Fliedner, F. Melander, O. L. Nielsen, C. K. O'Sullivan, A. Kjær, T. L. Andresen, *J. Control. Release* **2017**, *261*, 163–173.

[173] E. Kupert, M. Anderson, Y. Liu, P. Succop, L. Levin, J. Wang, K. Wikenheiser-brokamp, P. Chen, S. M. Pinney, T. Macdonald, Z. Dong, S. Starnes, S. Lu, *BMC Cancer* **2011**, *11*, 1–10.

[174] R. L. Siegel, K. D. Miller, H. E. Fuchs, A. Jemal, *CA: Cancer J. Clin.* **2022**, *72* (1), 7–33.

2 Light-Activated Drugs for Photodynamic and Photoactivated Therapy

Dmytro Havrylyuk and
Austin Hachey
Department of Chemistry, University of
Kentucky, Lexington, KY 40506, USA

Edith Glazer*
Department of Chemistry
North Carolina State University
Raleigh, NC, USA
eglazer@ncsu.edu

CONTENTS

1 Introduction..40
   1.1 A Short History of Photosensitizers and Photoactivators 40
   1.2 Mechanisms of Photophysical and Photochemical Action 42
   1.3 Recent Progress in Metal-Based Light-Activated
       Drug Discovery 43
   1.4 Highlights of Successful Drugs for Photodynamic Therapy 44
   1.5 Ongoing Challenges and Missed Opportunities 45
2 Traditional Medicinal Chemistry Guidelines...45
3 Proposed Guidelines for Light-Activated Systems.....................................46
4 Example Systems Based on Different Mechanism of Action......................50
   4.1 Organic vs. Metal Containing Photosensitizers 50
       4.1.1 Photocatalysts That Generate $^1O_2$ 50
       4.1.2 Other Types of Photocatalysts 50
   4.2 Organic vs. Metal Containing Photoactivated Agents 51
       4.2.1 Organic Photocages 51
       4.2.2 Inorganic Photocages...53
       4.2.3 Organic Photocages Activated by $^1O_2$.....................................55
       4.2.4 Organic Photoswitches 55
       4.2.5 Inorganic Photoswitches...56

---

*Corresponding author

DOI: 10.1201/9781003272250-2

4.2.6   Cofactor Mimics for Prodrug Activation 57
4.2.7   Exploiting Endogenous Biosynthetic Pathways:
          Protoporphyrin IX Formation 57
4.2.8   Gasotransmitter Release from Inorganic Molecules 58
4.2.9   Nanomedicine 58
4.2.10   Covalent Biomolecule Modification 58
5   General Conclusions 59
Acknowledgments 59
Abbreviations and Definitions 59
References 61

ABSTRACT

Phototherapy occupies a unique position in the health sciences, as it combines features of several different treatment modalities, including traditional chemotherapy, medical physics, and theranostics. Accordingly, new agents for phototherapy require biological properties that are appropriate for their function as drug molecules, photophysical and photochemical properties that enable triggered activity, and even reporting features for the detection of disease and monitoring of treatment efficacy. This poses challenges from early-stage development through clinical application, as all these characteristics are interdependent, but tend to be evaluated and optimized independently. With this chapter we aim to identify and discuss the features that are required for successful photoactive agents, with a particular emphasis on the comparison of inorganic and organic systems. We provide a historical perspective on the field and compare two agents with successful clinical data, use contemporary examples that showcase the versatility of light-activated systems, and revisit some traditional rules used in medicinal chemistry in order to propose characteristics that might be required for the successful development of new photosensitizers and photoactivators that may be translated for use to improve human health.

KEYWORDS

Light; Photosensitizer; Photocage; Photoswitch; Metal-Based Drugs; Cancer; Medicinal Chemistry

1   INTRODUCTION

1.1   A SHORT HISTORY OF PHOTOSENSITIZERS AND PHOTOACTIVATORS

Photoactive molecules have played a role in human health and disease throughout history. Early medical applications date from 1550 BC, and exploited photoreactions facilitated by both endogenous and exogenous natural products, such as psoralens [1]. The beneficial effects of photons were well established by the 20th century, and had reached the level of a cliché, as reflected by Louis Brandeis's 1913 quote, "sunlight is said to be the best of disinfectants" when speaking of the importance of transparency to guard against financial and political corruption [2]. In modern medicine, the story of Sister Jean Ward's serendipitous discovery of phototherapy as a treatment for jaundiced newborns

Light-Activated Drugs for Photodynamic and Photoactivated Therapy

stands as a testament to the transformative impact that one perceptive individual can have on healthcare.

Sister Ward, the director of the premature nursery at Rochford General Hospital in Essex, UK, made a habit of taking jaundiced infants outside for exposure to sunlight, and observed fading of the yellow color in skin that had been irradiated. The distinctive yellow skin and sclera of jaundice is a result of the abnormal buildup of bilirubin, the product of the second step in the porphyrin catabolic pathway. In healthy individuals, this by-product is cleared from the body, but it can cause irreversible neurological damage in infants. Sister Ward's light treatment is now known to result from the photochemical isomerization of the (4Z, 15Z)-bilirubin, a toxic porphyrin metabolite, to the more polar and soluble (4Z, 15E) isomer, along with photooxidation to other products [3] which facilitates their excretion. While this simple light therapy was initially viewed with reservation, it is now widely applied, and an estimate from 2015 indicated that approximately 120 million infants had received phototherapy for jaundice since the treatment was established in 1970 [4]!

However, while photons can be a form of medical treatment, they can also exacerbate specific medical disorders, particularly dermatological diseases such as lupus and rosacea. A severe, inborn error of metabolism in the porphyrin and heme biosynthetic pathway causes cutaneous porphyria, which is believed to be the source of the vampire myth [5]. In this disorder, a deficiency in the uroporphyrinogen III synthase enzyme results in accumulation of photoreactive, and toxic, heme precursors called uroporphyrins. Patients experience damaging effects from this endogenous photocatalyst, resulting in photosensitivity, damage to the skin, and chronic hemolytic anemia associated with vampirism.

The first report of exogenous agents inducing the "photodynamic effect" was in 1900, with the observation by a medical student, Oscar Raab, that the combination of light and acridine orange caused cytotoxicity to a microorganism [6, 7]. This was rapidly followed by the application of the dye eosin to skin cancer lesions for a patient with basal cell carcinoma; moreover, the authors recognized the importance of molecular oxygen for the efficacy of the so-called "photodynamic effect." Soon, however, these organic molecules were replaced by porphyrins, which may or may not bind metals. In addition to appealing photophysical and photobiological properties, different porphyrins had been observed to localize in tumors [8, 9], providing an added component of selectivity for the photodynamic effect.

The first and only photosensitizer approved for cancer therapy by the FDA is Porfimer sodium (Photofrin), a mixture of porphyrin polymers. This agent, when activated with red light, effectively eliminated implanted tumors in mice, and later, in human subjects. Photodynamic therapy (PDT) was extensively developed and championed by Thomas Dougherty from Roswell Park Cancer Center [10], and is now used to treat patients with high-grade dysplasia in Barrett's esophagus, obstructive esophageal cancer, and lung cancer. Photofrin has various drawbacks, but it has exhibited irrefutable success in various applications.

These historical perspectives highlight the fact that organic natural products, both derived from plants or created within the human body, have long been known to act as photosensitizers or photoreactive entities. By comparison, the field of inorganic phototherapy is much younger, as inorganic photosensitizers have no natural source, but it is developing at a rapid pace. In the past few years, there have been several excellent reviews on the topic, addressing diverse systems for biologically active photocatalysts and photoreagents. However, there is still much that is not well understood about these systems, including the photochemical or photophysical mechanisms of action, their resulting biological effects, structure-activity relationships (SAR) that regulate these processes, and how best to harness these features for medical applications.

As a step toward new insights, we have chosen to compare and contrast specific features of organic and inorganic systems used for phototherapeutic applications. Our hope is to identify features shared in common, but also to define non-overlapping assets unique to each of these classes of molecules.

1.2 MECHANISMS OF PHOTOPHYSICAL AND PHOTOCHEMICAL ACTION

Photoactive molecules, particularly photocatalysts, are often termed photosensitizers (PS), and can be rationally designed to manipulate or damage a wide array of biological systems. The operating modality of each system is dictated by its basic photophysical and photochemical properties. In general, the photoexcitation of a molecule leads to relaxation to the ground state *via* radiative decay, vibrational relaxation, energy transfer, or heterolytic/homolytic bond dissociation [11]. Photoactive molecules harness these basic properties to induce a chemical or energetic change in a substrate molecule to impart a biological effect.

Most PS are used for PDT applications, like Photofrin, where the generation of singlet oxygen ($^1O_2$), superoxide ($O_2^{\cdot-}$), or other reactive oxygen species (ROS) leads to direct cell killing. This is an area that has been extensively reviewed [12–14], and the interested reader is particularly encouraged to start with the excellent educational review of McFarland and coworkers [15]. For these applications, desirable properties of the PS include high yields of the triplet excited state, which requires efficient intersystem crossing, as the initially populated excited state is normally a singlet state. The triplet state is required to transfer the energy to $^3O_2$, and it has the added advantage of enjoying a long lifetime (τ) in many cases. The longer the lifetime of the excited state, the greater the odds are of a productive encounter with molecular oxygen, increasing the yield of the toxic species, usually assumed to be $^1O_2$ (quantified as Φ_Δ). Energy transfer to oxygen commonly competes with emission, so these systems can be used for both imaging and treatment, making them theranostic agents.

If the PS contains a metal center, this significantly influences the statistical distribution of relaxation pathways. The heavy metal effect increases spin-orbit coupling, allowing for more intersystem crossing. However, effective photoreagents do not all rely on a long-lived triplet excited state, nor this particular mechanism of $^1O_2$-mediated cell killing. Instead, $^1O_2$ can be used to cleave self-immolating linkers, liberating drugs; other excited states can be accessed that result in electron transfer; and other processes for prodrug activation are available to molecules in their excited states, as shown in Figure 1. While these general mechanisms appear limited in scope, in practice, their application in biological contexts has evolved into a highly diverse spectrum of activities, with several

Light-Activated Drugs for Photodynamic and Photoactivated Therapy 43

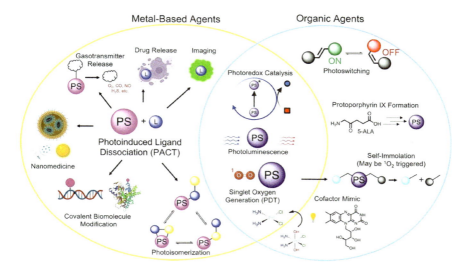

FIGURE 1 Venn diagram illustrating the diverse biological mechanisms that may be utilized with photoactive organic and metal-based molecules. Photoactivated chemotherapy (PACT) falls under the broader mechanistic descriptor of photocaging or photoinduced ligand dissociation.

distinct modes of action not fully defined by simple photochemical or photophysical descriptors alone.

1.3 Recent Progress in Metal-Based Light-Activated Drug Discovery

In order to estimate the research effort and progress associated with the development of new organic vs. inorganic agents and techniques for PDT, we conducted a SciFinder search using the search terms "Phototherapy" vs. the combination of "Photodynamic Therapy" and "Metal Complex." The term "phototherapy" was chosen as it captured the more recent publications on "photodynamic therapy," but also included several early publications from before the time that Photodynamic Therapy entered common usage. While there is a long history of "Phototherapy," literature reports of metal complexes use in PDT emerged only in the 1980s. Organic systems still dominate the field, with 1,693 publications in 2021, compared to 251 for inorganic agents.

We also analyzed the number of clinical trials based on the term "Photodynamic Therapy." The total number of clinical trials was impressive, at 667, although 187 did not define the phase. The majority were Phase II trials, at 40%, but there were >27% in early Phase I or Phase I. In preclinical studies, various metals have been investigated, with contributions from molecules containing ruthenium, copper, platinum, iridium, and osmium in decreasing order. Overall, the analysis of the literature and clinical trials revealed a robust field with significant molecular diversity for inorganic systems, and extensive efforts for translation to the clinic.

1.4 HIGHLIGHTS OF SUCCESSFUL DRUGS FOR PHOTODYNAMIC THERAPY

Porfimer sodium (Photofrin) is a photosensitizer approved worldwide to treat patients with high-grade dysplasia in Barrett's esophagus, obstructive esophageal cancer, and lung cancer. Two porphyrin precursors, 5-aminolevulinic acid (5-ALA; Lexulan) and the ester methyl 5-aminolevulinate (MAL, Metvix), are also approved for topical PDT for actinic keratosis. These serve as prodrugs, where uptake into cells and metabolism leads to their conversion into PpIX, and thus, they induce the photophysical properties associated with this endogenous cofactor. All of these porphyrin-based compounds can be activated with blue light for emission, and red light for photosensitization. Notably, they exhibit enhanced uptake in cancerous tumors, and can be used for visualization during resection, intraoperative PDT, or regular PDT.

Verteporfin (Visudyne), a benzoporphyrin derivative, is approved for use to ablate abnormal vasculature in the eye for wet macular degeneration. Two photosensitizers, temoporfin and LUZ111, have been approved in the European Union (EU), and talaporfin in Japan. All the clinically approved photosensitizers for cancer therapy contain the tetrapyrrolic structural scaffold; thus all these drugs have similar photophysical and photobiological properties, but also share similar issues, including low water solubility, poor photostability, slow body clearance, and relatively low selectivity for cancerous tissues. The coordination of the tetrapyrrolic scaffold to a metal center produced systems that overcome some of these limitations, and has been shown to improve the metabolic stability and photostability of clinical candidates [16]. In addition, macrocyclic extension and coordination to a metal for compounds such as texaphyrins result in bathochromic shifts in absorption, facilitating the use of longer wavelength, deeper penetrating light. One member of this class, Motexafin Lutetium, contains the lanthanide lutetium, and was activated at 732 nm when studied in phase I clinical trials for the treatment of prostate cancer. Another successful example of metal coordination is TOOKAD® soluble (Padeliporfin), a palladium complex of a bacteriochlorophyll derivative, which is now approved for use in 31 European countries, Israel, and Mexico for treatment of prostate cancer. Padeliporfin is activated by laser light at 753 nm with a fixed power of 150 mW cm^{-2} [17].

Recently, polypyridine complexes of transition metals have received increasing attention as preclinical candidates for PDT. The success of TLD1433, a polypyridyl Ru(II) complex for the treatment of bladder cancer [15], inspired inorganic medicinal chemists to develop new PDT and PACT agents based on ruthenium(II) [18, 19], osmium(II) [20, 21], iridium(III) [22], and platinum(IV) [23] complexes. Currently, TLD1433 is in Phase II clinical trials conducted in Canada, the United States, and internationally for "Intravesical Photodynamic Therapy (PDT) in BCG Refractory/Intolerant Non-Muscle Invasive Bladder Cancer (NMIBC) Patients." The molecule was synthesized in May 2011 by

Light-Activated Drugs for Photodynamic and Photoactivated Therapy **45**

McFarland and entered clinical trials within ~6 years. As mentioned in the exceptional story of the TLD1433 development [15], the fast progress from "the bench to a clinical trial" was possible thanks to a variety of factors, including (a) multidisciplinary team efforts, (b) the early identification of the NMIBC as a target, and most significantly, (c) the parallel development of compound, medical device, and PDT package via a "tumor-centered approach." This required rational design criteria to be established prior to compound development and optimization. Notably, however, these design criteria were based on characteristics of both the tumor type and the planned therapeutic strategy, rather than focusing on specific features for a generalized "optimal" photosensitizer.

1.5 Ongoing Challenges and Missed Opportunities

While some clinical trials fail due to poor trial design, a particular challenge for PDT is that it is only used as a last resort in heavily pretreated patients. This reduces the chances that the trial will achieve standard measures of success for new cancer therapies, as the patients in the study suffer disease that is highly refractory, and have already been subjected to many taxing treatments. A clinical trial design that addresses patients who do not have advanced disease would be anticipated to have a greater likelihood of demonstrating positive results. Additional issues in PDT trials include misdiagnosis of the stage of the patients, and challenges in achieving accurate dosimetry. An unusual onus placed on PDT is the significant time delay between treatments, or only one treatment is planned, as for intraoperative PDT, in contrast to the repeated treatments used in chemotherapy or radiation therapy. Given the fractional kill theory commonly used in standard chemotherapy, there is a low likelihood that a single treatment can induce prolonged suppression of malignancies that have high proliferative capacities and continuously evolve.

The best plan, as proposed by McFarland, is that the photosensitizer and phototherapy package be developed with the plan of treatment to provide the best chance of success so that clinical trials can progress to more challenging experiments. There are also missed opportunities if the treatment focus fails to address unmet needs, such as palliative care and interstitial PDT, or targets cancer types for which there are established and successful standard-of-care treatments. Finally, for photocaging approaches, systems should be designed based on rational features where phototherapy confers significant advantages to the particular drug that is delivered, either by reducing issues of systemic toxicity or low selectivity, or by providing a multimodal effect.

2 TRADITIONAL MEDICINAL CHEMISTRY GUIDELINES

Almost 25 years ago, Christopher Lipinski and coworkers at Pfizer provided an analysis of the physicochemical properties of clinical candidates in Phase II clinical trials. Based on their review, they introduced the Lipinski (Pfizer) rule of 5 (Ro5) for the development of orally bioavailable drug candidates. The Ro5 became one of the most used guidelines for the evaluation of drug-likeness in medicinal chemistry. In the original paper, the authors predicted "that poor absorption or permeation is more likely when there are more than 5 H-bond donors, 10 H-bond acceptors, the molecular weight (MWT) is greater than 500 and the calculated Log P (CLogP) is greater than 5" [24]. Later these rules were enhanced and other parameters were identified as important for oral bioavailability, such as a number of rotatable bonds $\leq$ 10 and a polar surface area for passively absorbed molecules equal to or less than $140\,\text{Å}^2$ [25].

While the Ro5 is for orally bioavailable compounds, this evaluation system is applied to define and select hit compounds, and is useful in part due to the consideration that the next stages of drug discovery—hit-to-lead, and lead optimization—involve synthetic efforts that result in an increase in molecular weight of the drug candidate and can lead to safety and tolerability issues. Hughes and co-authors later summarized key *in vitro* assays in early drug discovery, providing target values for physicochemical and *in vitro* ADME properties [26]. Some of these features include (a) aqueous solubility (values >$100\,\mu M$), (b) Log $D_{7.4}$ (values of 0–3; the value is ca. 2 for blood-brain barrier (BBB) penetration), (c) microsomal stability, with intrinsic clearance (CL_{int}) values <30 μL $min^{-1} mg^{-1}$ protein), (d) lack of hepatic CYP450 inhibition (IC_{50} > $10\,\mu M$), and (e) absence of Hep G2 hepatotoxicity (i.e., no effect at $50 \times IC_{50}$). The next step, the authors stated, is that lead compounds with a high potency and selectivity, as well as satisfactory physicochemical and *in vitro* ADME properties, should be subject to pharmacokinetic evaluation in rats, with a target half-life value of >60min for agents applied via intravenous administration [26]. These "rules" and experimental parameters provide a useful workflow and system for optimization in traditional medicinal chemistry.

Lipinski's rules focused on features that impact pharmacokinetics and ADME, assuming passive transport. As a result, the rules do not apply to a variety of effective drugs, including biologics, substrates of biological transporters, and natural products. They also don't apply to most photoactive systems, which generally require higher molecular weights and are lipophilic, due to being highly conjugated. While it is one thing to recognize that some rules may be ignored, it is challenging to perform research in a drug discovery area in the complete absence of guidelines or standardized systems for evaluation. Accordingly, we have considered a variety of features that could be loosely formulated as "rules" for inorganic systems, which we have modified to encompass the required features of light-activated systems.

3 PROPOSED GUIDELINES FOR LIGHT-ACTIVATED SYSTEMS

The development of new candidates for phototherapy applications is usually focused on improved photophysical properties for new compounds, while neglecting the general principles and rules of traditional drug discovery. Moreover, the properties of an "ideal photosensitizer" are often referenced, but the proposed values are inconsistent, or numerical values for various key features are absent. For example, different values for the "PDT window" have been reported, ranging from 600 to 1200nm; nonetheless, TLD1433 is highly successful and is irradiated

Light-Activated Drugs for Photodynamic and Photoactivated Therapy 47

with green light (525 nm) for treatment of NMIBC in clinical trials, where the limited tissue penetration is a significant advantage.

Based on the analysis of clinical drugs and candidates, various promising compounds from the recent literature, and our own experience, we wish to provide our best ideas for the key properties and features for future light-active agents. We hope this will be useful for the inorganic medicinal chemistry community, serving not only as a filter for the hit and lead discovery process, but also as a motivator for the development of new PDT and PACT agents with improved properties that are enabled to reach clinical evaluation and, finally, the market.

We compare six key properties of Photofrin and TLD1433 in Figure 2, including photophysical (1–3), physicochemical (4), and biological parameters (5–6). Photofrin is activated with red (630 nm) light, and the value of its molar extinction coefficient at this wavelength, ε, varies in the literature from 1,170 [27] to 3,000 [15] $M^{-1}cm^{-1}$. A molar extinction coefficient of 2,000 $M^{-1}cm^{-1}$ is reported for TLD1433 at its excitation wavelength of 525 nm [15]. Both drugs exhibit high quantum yields for the generation of $^1O_2$, with $\Phi_\Delta > 0.85$. The comparison of molar weight is only approximate, as Photofrin is a mixture of oligomers formed by ether and ester linkages of up to eight porphyrin units (in contrast to TLD1433, which is a single molecular entity, albeit currently generated as a racemic mixture

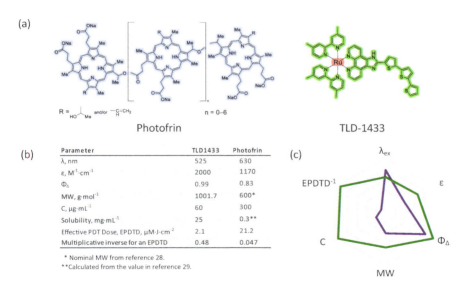

FIGURE 2 (a) Structures of Photofrin (purple) and TLD1433 (green). (b) Table of values for Photofrin and TLD1433. (c) Radar charts for comparison of the key features for Photofrin (solid purple) and TLD1433 (solid green). The axes scale from center to perimeter as follows: λ_{ex}, 0–800 nm; ε, 0–3,000 $M^{-1}cm^{-1}$; Φ_Δ, 0–1; MW, 0–1,500 g mol^{-1}; C, the highest concentration used for evaluation of cytotoxicity *in vitro*, reflecting the solubility of compounds in the assay conditions, 0–300 µg mL^{-1}; and EPDTD^{-1}, a multiplicative inverse for an effective PDT dose, 0–0.5. Note: low values of MW are preferred.

of enantiomers). Therefore, we adopted the nominal MW of 600 g mol^{-1} that is commonly used in the literature for Photofrin [28].

Solubility is a crucial parameter for potential drug candidates. Photofrin is administered as a slow intravenous injection, with a final concentration of 2.5 mg mL^{-1} in either 5% dextrose or 0.9% sodium chloride injection, while TLD1433 is under evaluation at 0.7 mg TLD1433 per cm^2 bladder surface area. As we could not ascertain the solubility limit for either compound, we compared the top concentration (C) for both drugs that were used for *in vitro* evaluations. We used this as an estimate of the solubility of the compounds under biological conditions, as well as the highest concentration where there is no cytotoxic effect without irradiation. While TLD1433 was tested starting from 300 μM (~300 μg mL^{-1}) [29], the highest value for Photofrin we found in the literature was 60 μg mL^{-1} [30]. Finally, we analyzed the data for *in vitro* cytotoxicity. We were not able to find any publication where these two drugs were tested under the same conditions, likely due to the difficulty for scientists to obtaining Photofrin. The conditions, including cell lines, incubation time, and light source and dose, were highly variable (Table 1), so a direct comparison of a biological efficacy based on IC$_{50}$ values would be inappropriate. Inspired by Hasan's work [31], we considered an "effective PDT dose" (EPDTD), a product of the IC$_{50}$ value and light dose, for a more accurate estimation of the potency of the two PDT agents.

As is apparent from the radar plot of Figure 2c, TLD1433 exhibits some superior properties to Photofrin. This multicomponent analysis allows for a more holistic evaluation of molecular features and highlights the fact that focusing on specific photophysical properties is insufficient. For example, both compounds have the same high value for Φ_Δ, but the EPDTD for each compound is radically different. This does not even begin to take into account potential variations in immunological effects, as TLD1433 can confer antitumor immunity [32–34]. Thus, while we recognize that it is not possible to predict *in vivo* biological efficacy, we propose a few features that should be considered in early-stage compound design and optimization.

This first feature we propose is a requirement for absorption over 400 nm, as irradiation at shorter wavelengths is known to be mutagenic. While some molecules may have the ability to be activated via two photon absorption, this is currently not an accessible approach in the clinic. Second, we advise a decreased focus on attaining specific values of ε, Φ_Δ, and Φ_{PS}, the quantum yield of photosubstitution. While reasonable absorption at the excitation wavelength is required, it also should be recognized that this value, and Φ_Δ and Φ_{PS}, can change as a function of environment and upon association with biomolecules. Moreover, the requirements for Φ_Δ and Φ_{PS} are dependent on the type of phototherapy, i.e., a catalytic system vs. an irreversible, stoichiometric system like a photocage, the nature of the light applied, the biological environment, and many other features. For example, a photocage that releases a highly potent reagent, with IC$_{50}$ values in the pM or nM range, requires a lower effective dose than a system that liberates a less active ligand. The combined impact of these factors can be evaluated if the EPDTD is provided.

Light-Activated Drugs for Photodynamic and Photoactivated Therapy 49

TABLE 1
PDT Parameters for *in vitro* Cytotoxicity of Photofrin and TLD-1433

Cancer	Cell Line	IC_{50}, μM	Light Dose, J cm^{-2}	Effective PDT Dose, μM J cm^{-2}	Reference
		Photofrin			
Human leukemia	HL-60	10	5	50	[133]
Human colorectal adenocarcinoma	HT29	12.5	5	62.5	[134]
Mouse colon adenocarcinoma	Colo-26	9	0.9	8.1	[135]
Human glioblastoma	A172	16.7	0.5	8.3	[30]
Human glioblastoma	U118MG	16.7	0.5	8.3	[30]
Human glioblastoma	U87MG	16.7	0.5	8.3	[30]
Human epidermoid carcinoma	A431	1.94	1.5	2.91	[28]
			Average	**21.2**	
		TLD-1433			
Human lung adenocarcinoma	A549	0.099	20	1.98	[136]
Human leukemia	HL-60	0.2	100	20	[29]
Mouse colon fibroblast	CT26.WT	0.021	45	0.94	[137]
Mouse colon fibroblast	CT26.CL25	0.011	45	0.49	[137]
Human brain glioblastoma	U87	0.051	45	2.29	[137]
Human conjunctival malignant melanoma	CRMM1	0.0059	19	0.11	[138]
Human conjunctival malignant melanoma	CRMM2	0.0048	19	0.091	[138]
Human conjunctival malignant melanoma	CM2005.1	0.0058	19	0.11	[138]
Human uveal melanoma	OMM1	0.014	19	0.26	[138]
Human uveal melanoma	OMM2.5	0.013	19	0.24	[138]
Human uveal melanoma	MEL270	0.01	19	0.19	[138]
Epidermoid carcinoma	A431	0.049	19	0.93	[138]
Cutaneous melanoma	A375	0.05	19	0.95	[138]
Human bladder carcinoma	T24	0.077	22.5	1.73	[139]
Rat urothelial-derived tumor	AY-27	0.039	22.5	0.87	[139]
			Average	**2.1**	

Third, we recommend evaluating physiochemical and *in vitro* ADME properties [26] at an early stage of research for agents that are expected to be applied systemically. Compounds that are not sufficiently stable in biological media and serum to conduct experiments that require hours to days are unlikely to progress, and the best photocage in the world will not be effective if it is rapidly and extensively metabolized. In addition, the potential toxicity of the metabolic products should be considered, as illustrated by the examples of damaging effects of endogenous heme metabolism.

4 EXAMPLE SYSTEMS BASED ON DIFFERENT MECHANISM OF ACTION

This section aims to classify and provide contemporary examples for each of numerous biological mechanisms described for inorganic and organic photoactive molecules, with special attention dedicated to the increasing importance of metal-based photocages for photoactivated chemotherapy (PACT, also termed photochemotherapy, PCT) and related applications.

4.1 Organic vs. Metal Containing Photosensitizers

4.1.1 Photocatalysts That Generate $^1O_2$

Both organic and inorganic compounds share basic photochemical and photophysical mechanisms that have long been utilized for interrogating biological systems, including photoluminescence and $^1O_2$ generation. These are very mature fields, with agents that efficiently generate $^1O_2$ in clinical use for PDT. Rather than review these topics, we discuss the prototypical porphyrin-based PDT agent, Photofrin, and the most promising inorganic PDT agent, TLD1433, in the "Success highlights" section.

4.1.2 Other Types of Photocatalysts

In contrast to photogeneration of $^1O_2$, photoredox catalysis in living systems is an emerging and fast-growing field. Historically, this has been the domain of precious metal complexes, but recently, competitive organophotoredox catalysts have emerged [35]. There are limited examples of successful application in cells, but one demonstrated the production of NAD$^{\bullet}$ radicals from redox cycling of **1** (Figure 3a) in hypoxic A549 human lung adenocarcinoma cells upon irradiation with 450 nm light (10 J cm^{-2}) [36], achieving a phototoxicity index (PI) value of 27.2 in normoxia, and a PI value of 18.5 in hypoxia. The photocatalytic redox mechanism offers the prospect of alternative strategies to circumventing the barrier of sensitizing $^1O_2$ within the hypoxic tumor microenvironment.

Li *et al.* expanded the strategy of NAD radical production in cancer cells to incorporate organophotoredox catalysis. They utilized a prodrug strategy, which required the enzymatic unmasking of photoredox catalyst **2** by the enzyme nitroreductase, a protein that is overexpressed in cancer tissues [37]. The active agent then enabled the generation of NAD$^{\bullet}$ radicals in cells using low-energy red or NIR light. Their strategy was expanded into mice, and demonstrated light-dependent reduction of xenograft tumor growth to 95% vs. control; to our knowledge this is the first application of a targeted photoredox process in a living organism.

Photoredox catalysis in cells is expanding beyond anticancer strategies to other areas of chemical biology, with applications as a fundamental research tool.

Light-Activated Drugs for Photodynamic and Photoactivated Therapy 51

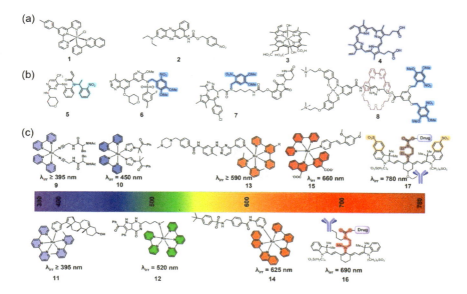

FIGURE 3 Diversity of organic and inorganic photoactive agents. (a) Examples of photoredox catalysts employed in living systems, including the naturally occurring photosensitizer PpIX (4). (b) Recent examples of organic photocaging groups used for anticancer applications. The photocaging groups are shown in blue. (c) Structures of PACT agents discussed, with reference to their activation wavelengths. The Ru(II) complexes act via dissociation of a metal-ligand bond, while the red light-sensitive cyanine photocages function by C-C cleavage by photosensitized $^1O_2$.

Buksh et al. debuted μMap-Red, a photoredox proximity labeling system centered around the red-light-activated tin porphyrinoid catalyst **3** (Figure 3) [38]. This system enables unbiased labeling and speciation of the local chemical environment in biological systems through short-lived biotin-linked nitrogen radical species generated at the antibody-conjugated photocatalyst. These exciting applications of targeted, light-controlled catalysis in living systems demonstrate a promising future for this emerging field. While it was previously believed that rationally designed, small-molecule catalysts would not function in the complex reaction medium of the cell, these and other examples are reversing such assumptions.

4.2 Organic vs. Metal Containing Photoactivated Agents

4.2.1 Organic Photocages

Photocaging has proven to be a highly successful approach to mask the activity of a reagent by forming a prodrug. This approach is assumed to be oxygen-independent, which addresses the limitation of O_2 that is commonly a concern for treatment of solid tumors that contain hypoxic regions. While photocages are generally stoichiometric reagents, in contrast to photocatalysts, an advantage is that photocaging can be used for nontoxic biological effectors, such as neuro-modulator agents like dopamine, serotonin, and saxitoxin [39–41]. Organic and inorganic photocaged agents have been reviewed [42–44], and the subject was recently celebrated in a diverse collection of articles in a journal special issue [45]. Photocaging can also be used to regulate the structure, location, and activity of proteins [46, 47] and nucleic acids [48], but we will not address these areas. Related to this concept is the field of photopharmacology [49, 50] which more broadly involves the activation (not just release) of molecules, including non-chemotherapeutic payloads, and other regulators of fundamental biology [51, 52]. This topic is discussed in a separate section below on photoswitches.

Commonly used organic photocages include nitro-benzyl and coumarin-4-yl-methyl groups. Recently, nitro-benzyl groups were used for photocontrol of the proteosome [53], and for KDAC [54], B-Raf^{V600E} [55], ERK1/2 [56], and PI3K [57] inhibition. The organic photocaging group resulted in reduced inhibitor activity; for example, the protected ERK1/2 inhibitor **5**, shown in Figure 3b, exhibited half-maximal inhibitory concentration (IC_{50}) values at the micromolar level without irradiation. Upon irradiation with 365 nm UV light, the active inhibitor was released, which exhibited IC_{50} values of 45–270 nM, providing a photoactivity index (PI, the ratio between activity in the dark and light conditions) of up to 250 [56]. Similarly, photocaging of PI3K inhibitor **6** with PI3Kα IC_{50}=0.6 nM yielded a prodrug with significantly reduced activity without irradiation, with IC_{50}=343 nM. The IC_{50} value was 0.58 nM after UV light irradiation at 365 nm, providing a PI value of >590 [57].

Photocaging is not limited to enzyme inhibitors, and can be applied to molecules that regulate protein:protein interactions (PPIs). Both nitro-benzyl and coumarin-4-ylmethyl groups were utilized for photocaging of PROteolysis TArgeting Chimeras (PROTACs) to gain spatiotemporal control of protein degradation [58–62]. However, it should be noted that the caging groups are less effective in reducing protein degradation than they are for blocking enzyme inhibition, and thus provide lower PI values. For example, photocaging of the dBET1 PROTAC, which is an active Brd4 degrader at 0.1 μM in Ramos cells, resulted in pc-PROTAC1 **7** that did not show Brd4 degradation at 3 μM. Irradiation with 365 nm UV light reduced Brd4 levels at 0.3 μM concentrations, similar to the effects of 0.1 μM dBET1, yielding a PI of only <10.

Organic photocages have also been used for protecting inorganic anticancer agents. Lewis and Vilar proposed an elegant approach for photocontrol of cyto-toxicity for a Pt(II)-salphen complex, a known G-quadruplex DNA binder, by the combination of organic photocaging groups and incorporation of a rotaxane as a stoppering unit [63]. The prodrug **8** showed enhanced cell permeability and no cytotoxicity against osteosarcoma cells in the absence of irradiation. Activation with 365 nm light resulted in release of Pt(II)-salphen complex and increased cytotoxicity, with IC_{50}=3.8 μM.

While organic photocages have demonstrated success for photocontrol of protein inhibition, protein degradation, and cytotoxic small molecules, there are several challenges for these systems, including (a) many organic photocages require

Light-Activated Drugs for Photodynamic and Photoactivated Therapy 53

irradiation with the high energy UV light that has very limited tissue penetration, can lead to sample overheating, and causes phototoxic or photoallergic reactions [64], (b) photoactivation can be nonselective and produce off-target photoproducts, and (c) the introduction of organic caging groups decreases the solubility and metabolic stability of compounds. The development of metal-based photocages may overcome these issues.

4.2.2 Inorganic Photocages

A property of some transition metal complexes is that irradiation with light can induce excitation of electrons to antibonding molecular orbitals, followed by photochemical ligand loss. This characteristic is the basic mechanism behind PACT/PCT, in which the light-triggered dissociation of a molecule produces an active chemotherapeutic agent. These terms both fall under the umbrella descriptor of photoinduced ligand dissociation, and include additional mechanisms such as photoisomerization, gasotransmitter release, covalent biomolecule modification, and diverse applications in nanomedicine. This section will briefly describe notable metal-based examples within this mechanistic class, and speculate on future directions of the field.

Ru(II) complexes are frequently used for photocaging, where a biologically active monodentate ligand is masked by coordination to a metal center. Photorelease of this ligand allows for temporal and spatial control over its activity. The seminal work in this area was performed by Etchenique, who developed phototriggered Ru(II) complexes that released nitrogen-containing neurotransmitters [65–69]. In 2012, our group described the use of intrinsically strained Ru(II) complexes as potent light-triggered cytotoxins, where the metal released bidentate ligands and induced DNA damage analogous to cisplatin [70]. In the same year, we demonstrated the tunable photophysics of such Ru(II) systems, as switching the ligand from 2,2′-bipyridine (bpy) to 2,2′-biquinoline (biq) created complexes that could be activated with red and near-IR light [71]. In the following decade, the field of metal-based PACT has experienced explosive growth [72–81], and is now a well-developed branch of medicinal inorganic chemistry. Different "caged" groups have been coordinated to ruthenium scaffolds, including imidazole, pyridine, diazines, amines, nitriles, and thioethers [82]. Each of these functionalities can be incorporated in more sophisticated organic molecules for light-triggered release. For example, the Bonnet group demonstrated that thioethers can be caged and released [83], and Renfrew has used imidazole-containing drugs for photodelivery [84–86].

Ru(II) scaffolds have been exploited for photocontrol of enzyme inhibition, as exemplified by compounds **9–15** in Figure 3c. Kodanko and Turro have shown a variety of nitriles can be caged, such as peptide-based protease inhibitors [82, 87]. Inhibition of the cysteine protease papain was studied for [Ru(bpy)$_2$] complex **9** in the dark and the light ($\lambda_{irr} \geq 395$ nm). Notably, the Ru(II) complex exhibited enzyme inhibition without irradiation, with IC$_{50}$=9.5 µM, but there was a 32-fold enhancement in potency with visible light (IC$_{50}$=0.295 µM) [87]. We used the same Ru(II) scaffold for caging of metyrapone, etomidate, and a new P450 inhibitor [88], and all demonstrated triggerable enzyme inhibition. The Ru(II) complex with the novel P450 inhibitor, **10**, exhibited IC_{50} values for enzyme inhibition of 6.8 in the dark and 0.05 µM with indigo light ($\lambda_{irr} = 450$ nm), providing a PI value of 136.

One challenge for chemists using [Ru(bpy)$_2$] and other *bis*-bidentate complexes is the fact that either one or two monodentate ligands could be "caged", and the values of Φ_{PS} for the first and second ligand are highly variable. Alternatively, the combination of tridentate ligands and strain-inducing bidentate ligands creates stoichiometric photocages that have more predictable photochemistry [89]. The [Ru(tpy)(NN)] scaffold, where tpy is the tridentate 2,2';6',2"-terpyridine ligand, and NN are bidentate ligands, has been used for caging of abiraterone (**11**, a CYP17A1 inhibitor) [90], a microtubule targeting agent (**12**) [91], imatinib (**13**, a tyrosine kinase inhibitor) [92], inhibitors of cathepsin B [93], nicotinamide phosphoribosyltransferase (NAMPT, **14**) [94], CYP3A4 [95], and CYP1B1 (**15**) [96]. In contrast to [Ru(tpy)(dmbpy)(abiraterone)] (dmbpy, 6,6'-dimethylbipyridine, compound **11**) that was activated with blue light ($\lambda_{irr} \geq 395$ nm) in a cell cytotoxicity assay against the DU145 cell line [90], the Ru(II) complex with the microtubule targeting agent **12** was tested with green light ($\lambda_{irr} = 520$ nm) under normoxia and hypoxia. The largest PI values of 21 and 29 were observed against the A375 and A431 skin cancer cell lines under normoxia, and they were slightly reduced under hypoxia (PI > 12) [91], highlighting the fact that even photocages exhibit reduced efficacy under hypoxic conditions.

As anticipated, the inclusion of the biq ligand in Ru(II) photocages in compounds **13–15** shifted the absorption profile to longer wavelengths compared to analogous bpy systems [71, 97]. This is due to the lower energy of the metal-to-ligand charge transfer (MLCT) transitions, which depend on the lowest unoccupied molecular orbital (LUMO) of the conjugated biq ligand. Thus, [Ru(tpy)(biq)] photocages can be activated with longer wavelengths of light, which is appealing for the ability to achieve greater depths of penetration into tissues. The [Ru(tpy)(biq)] scaffold was used for the development of photoactive inhibitor of NAMPT [94], with compound **14** exhibiting a dark IC_{50} of 4.8 µM, and an 18-fold increase in potency upon irradiation with 625 nm light, resulting in $IC_{50} = 0.26$ µM. In an effort to preserve the favorable photophysics but eliminate some of the issues with [Ru(tpy)(biq)], we undertook optimization of Ru(tpy) scaffold. The addition of carboxylic acids, using the [2,2'-biquinoline]-4,4'-dicarboxylic acid ligand (bca), reduced cellular toxicity caused by the metal complex, such that no adverse effects were observed up to 100 µM concentrations [97]. This scaffold was used in compound **15** for photocaging of a potent CYP1B1 inhibitor ($IC_{50} = 310$ pM), which resulted in precise control over enzyme activity with red light ($\lambda_{irr} = 660$ nm). The key features that enable a PI value of >6,300 were the sub-nanomolar potency of the caged molecule, the high purity and thermal stability of the intact Ru(II) complex, and a high degree of photosubstitution upon activation with red light [96].

Rather than changing the chromophore features of the metal complex, an alternative approach to use lower energies of light with photocages is the "reverse" FRET effect, exploiting Förster energy transfer from an appended chromophore. This approach was pioneered by Etchenique to uncage nitrile and chloride ligands

Light-Activated Drugs for Photodynamic and Photoactivated Therapy

[98, 99], and has been used to liberate thioethers [100]. Triplet-triplet annihilation has also been successfully and creatively demonstrated for photorelease from Ru(II), with 620 nm light activation through 7 mm of a pork fillet, used as a model of patient tissue [101].

4.2.3 Organic Photocages Activated by $^1O_2$

Singlet oxygen may be used as the active agent to cleave self-immolating linkers, thus providing an alternative approach to "photo-uncaging" a previously inactive compound. By tethering a pharmacological payload to a photosensitizer through a $^1O_2$-sensitive aminoacrylate linker, Hossion et al. achieved the release of 99% of anticancer agents 7-ethyl-10-hydroxycamptothecin (SN-38) and combretastatin A-4 (CA-4) after irradiation with 540 nm light [102]. Their strategy resulted in PI values of 4.8 for photouncaged SN-38 and 14.5 for photouncaged CA-4 in MCF-7 breast cancer cells.

Another elegant example of linker cleavage induced by $^1O_2$ is the development of drug delivery systems based on the highly tunable cyanine caging groups by Schnermann and colleagues [103–105]. The mechanism of activation includes photoinduced cleavage of C–C bond, following by thermal hydrolysis and intramolecular cyclization with the release of the caged drug. The caging of an estrogen receptor antagonist, 4-hydroxycyclofen, produced a prodrug with low cytotoxicity against MCF-7 cells, with an IC_{50} value of 150 μM without irradiation and 16-fold improved activity upon irradiation with 690 nm light [103]. Next, this cleavage strategy was combined with antibody drug conjugates (ADCs) using panitumumab, a monoclonal anti-EGFR antibody. This yielded compound **16**, a cyanine-panitumumab conjugate with combretastatin A4, a potent inhibitor of microtubule polymerization [104]. The cytotoxicity of the prodrug was tested against MDA-MB-468 cells (EGFR+), both in the dark and with 690 nm light; the activity was enhanced by 69-fold upon irradiation. Subsequent optimization of the cyanine caging group and linker resulted in caged ADC **17** with improved photophysical and biological properties. In addition, systems with caged duocarmycin were effectively activated with both 690 and 780 nm light. The compounds were tested for cytotoxicity against MDA-MB-468 and EGFR- (MCF-7) cells, and a PI value of >300 was observed for MDA-MB-468 cell line [105]. The high thermal stability of the prodrugs, the pM potency of the uncaged duocarmycin, and the high yield of released drug upon irradiation made these compounds some of the most efficient systems among organic photocages.

4.2.4 Organic Photoswitches

Unlike photocaging groups, which are permanently in an "on" state once they are activated, photoswitchable groups allow biological activity to be reversed with different wavelengths of light. The most common organic mechanism to achieve this switching is *cis-trans* isomerization, typically of azobenzene moieties. Photoswitches have been successfully generated for a variety of medically relevant compounds [49, 50, 106], and recently, several examples of photoswitching PROTACs have been reported.

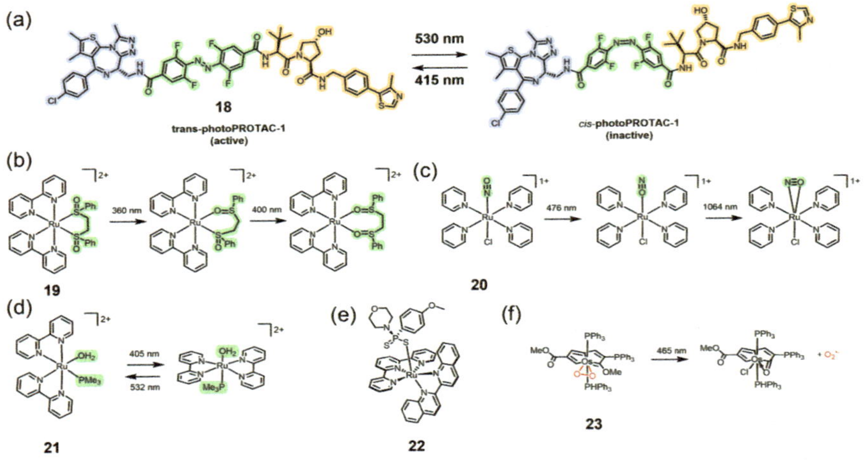

FIGURE 4 Photoswitching and gas-releasing molecules. (a) The photochemical behavior *cis-trans* isomerization of an azobenzene-containing photoswitchable PROTAC. The photoswitching group is shown in green, the E3 ligase ligand is orange, and the bait for the protein of interest, Brd4, is purple. (b–d) Examples of photoisomerization in Ru(II) complexes. (b) Linkage isomerism in a sulfoxide ligand. (c) Photoisomerization of the nitrosyl ligand in $[Ru(py)_4NOCl]^{2+}$. Isomerization to the η-1 Ru-O isomer occurs with 476 nm light. Isomerization to the η-2 isomer occurs from the η-1 Ru-O isomer with 1,064 nm light. (d) *Cis-trans* isomerization, in which irradiation induces exchange of axial and equatorial ligands. (e) Photoactivated gas-releasing metal complex. Upon irradiation with red light, the sulfur ligand is ejected and hydrolyzed to form H_2S. (f) An osmium complex that liberates superoxide even under hypoxic conditions.

Crews and coworkers presented the first example in 2019 with compound **18**, Figure 4 [107], and achieved selective degradation of Brd2 upon irradiation with 415 nm light at concentrations as low as 0.25 μM. Trauner and coworkers reported a series of Brd2–4 degraders activated by 390 nm light at concentrations as low as 10 nM [108]. You and Jiang observed anticancer activity by targeting the Brc-Abl fusion protein with a photoswitchable PROTAC, with degradation activity at levels as low as 100 nM, and an EC_{50} value of 28 nM in a BRC-ABL + K562 cell viability assay [109]. Overall, the major disadvantages of these systems are their requirement for UV light for activation, which is a barrier to application in most living systems. Potentially, metal-based systems based on photoswitchable linkage isomerism accessible at longer wavelengths could provide a solution to these challenges.

4.2.5 Inorganic Photoswitches

Transition metal complexes can undergo an interesting subclass of photoisomerization, in which the linkage of a ligand rearranges upon irradiation (Figure 4b and c). In the case of Ru(II), linkage photoisomerism is frequently encountered for sulfoxide ligands as in compound **19**; this behavior has been recently reviewed by Rack, who pioneered this chemistry [110]. As the Ru(II) MLCT excited state can be thought of as a Ru(III) center ligated by a radical ligand anion, the "harder"

Light-Activated Drugs for Photodynamic and Photoactivated Therapy   57

oxygen atom can be induced to bind the oxidized metal, while in the ground state the "softer" sulfur atom binds preferentially. Other ambient ligands, such as NO, can also rearrange upon irradiation, as for compound **20** [111]. In addition, certain metal complexes such as **21** can undergo *cis-trans* isomerization [112], in which axial ligands become equatorial, and vice versa. While there is yet to be an example of photoisomerization in a metal complex used to induce a biological effect, linkage isomerization in transition metal complexes may be a promising route to generate inorganic analogs of classical photoswitches.

4.2.6 Cofactor Mimics for Prodrug Activation

Proteins that naturally bind to cofactors may be targeted by photoactive synthetic cofactor mimics [46]. Recent work from Salassa and colleagues took advantage of the natural photoredox catalytic activity of flavoproteins that can bind and activate flavin-conjugated prodrugs. It was demonstrated that Pt(IV) and Ru(II) prodrugs that were appended to flavin adenine dinucleotide (FAD) and flavin adenine mononucleotide (FMN) could be converted into their cytotoxic Pt(II) and Ru(II)-OH_2 forms using a variety of endogenous electron donors, including nicotinamide adenine dinucleotide (NADH) [113]. By employing various combinations of one of four flavoproteins, five metallo-prodrugs, and two electron donors, up to 100% conversion of both Pt(IV) and Ru(II) prodrugs was achieved with good catalytic efficiency upon irradiation with 460 nm light, including in cell culture media [114]. The promising *in vitro* results encourage translation to biological systems.

Inorganic cofactor mimics can also be exploited when protein binding can be achieved. For example, Zn(II) porphyrins were incorporated into iron heme-binding proteins such as myoglobin [115] and bacterioferritin [116]. However, it is not clear how versatile this approach may be, given that heme is cytotoxic, so there are tightly regulated mechanisms for its cellular trafficking and protein insertion [117]. As a result, significant structural perturbations of a synthetic cofactor analog may not be possible.

4.2.7 Exploiting Endogenous Biosynthetic Pathways: Protoporphyrin IX Formation

An alternative pseudo "prodrug" approach is to take advantage of the natural biosynthetic machinery of the host to synthesize photoactive molecules *in vivo*. This is the basis of the mechanism of action for the amino acid 5-aminolevulinic acid (5-ALA; Lexulan) and the ester methyl 5-aminolevulinate (MAL, Metvix), which are both approved for PDT. These molecules are processed through the endogenous intracellular biochemical pathway into protoporphyrin IX, compound **4**, a photosensitizer. The prodrugs MAL and 5-ALA are used as topical PDT agents for several conditions [118], including acne [119], gynecological cancers [120], and keratosis [121].

Protoporphyrin IX possesses fluorescent properties and thus 5-ALA is currently in regular clinical use as a visual guide for tumor resection procedures [122–124]. This opens the possibility of intraoperative PDT, as exemplified by the INDYGO clinical trial of 5-ALA for patients with glioblastoma. An early analysis of outcomes demonstrated an average time for progression-free survival of 17 months [125], which is twice that for the standard therapy, and is continuing to increase, as participants in the trial continue to survive. Given the notoriously poor prognosis for these patients, these results are particularly compelling [126]. Notably, this clinical trial has similarities to that for TLD1433 in bladder cancer, as it also relied on the parallel development of compound, medical device, and PDT package, including real-time assessment of dosimetry.

The approach of using synthetic precursors as prodrug is limited by the selectivity of the endogenous biosynthetic enzymes, restricting the chemical structures that can be successfully incorporated. This makes organic systems more straightforward than inorganic substrates, particularly as metal ions are under tight regulation in biological systems due to their potential toxicity.

4.2.8 Gasotransmitter Release from Inorganic Molecules

Some transition metal complexes possess the property of being able to ligate molecular gases, effectively trapping them in condensed phases under conditions at which they would otherwise diffuse. These gases can be released upon irradiation to effect biological processes. In general, the largest classes of photocaged gasotransmitters are carbon monoxide releasing molecules (CORMs) and nitric oxide releasing molecules (NORMs). While both organic and inorganic examples of these two classes have been reviewed [42], we wish to highlight two recent and exotic metal-based gasotransmitter releasing agents.

Serving as a "prodrug" for a gas, Ru(II) complex **22** releases a ligand upon irradiation with red light that is readily hydrolyzed in cells to form H_2S [127]. This strategy is laudable, as other difficult-to-handle gases such as PH_3 may be suitably formulated as prodrugs in this fashion for release by metal complexes. Recently, Lu *et al.* developed an osmium-peroxo complex **23** which readily ejects superoxide upon irradiation with 465 nm light and demonstrated antitumor activity in mice [128]. The ROS-generating ability of traditional PDT agents is built into the complex, thus enabling activity in hypoxic conditions.

4.2.9 Nanomedicine

Nanomedicine is one of the fastest growing fields in modern science. As with molecular medicines, spatiotemporal control and deployment of nanotechnology are paramount to successful translation to the clinic. The use of inorganic photoactive materials in nanomedicine is addressed in reviews [129, 130] and a book chapter by Parracino *et al.* [131].

4.2.10 Covalent Biomolecule Modification

Development of photoactivatable molecules for the covalent modification of biomolecules is an attractive method to install imaging agents, to develop artificial catalytic metalloenzymes, and to modify nucleic acids in living systems. While many metals have the ability to form covalent adducts with biomolecules, the largest group of inorganic covalent binders in this class are the platinum agents

Light-Activated Drugs for Photodynamic and Photoactivated Therapy   59

[132]. It is our hope that future work in this area will enable the site-selective formation of metal-biomolecule bonds under optical control for such diverse applications as mentioned above.

5 GENERAL CONCLUSIONS

Despite the fact that phototherapy has exhibited great promise for decades, and over several clinical trials, it remains a marginalized therapeutic approach. The challenge of simultaneously delivering the appropriate therapeutic dose of compound and light creates complications for medical practitioners, and phototherapy trial designs in cancer are further endangered by serving as a last resort for patients with highly resistant tumors. However, these drawbacks are mitigated by the multiple effective mechanisms of action that can be harnessed in photoactive systems, and the creativity of the scientists and doctors involved in their development. We anticipate that the utilization of some general guidelines, heavily inspired by practices in traditional medicinal chemistry, will accelerate progress in this field and improve the rate of successful translation of light-responsive systems.

ACKNOWLEDGMENTS

We gratefully acknowledge the support of the National Institute of General Medical Sciences of the National Institutes of Health under Award Numbers R01GM138882 and 5R01GM107586.

ABBREVIATIONS AND DEFINITIONS

ADC	antibody drug conjugate
ADME	absorption, distribution, metabolism, and excretion
5-ALA	5-aminolevulinic acid
BBB	blood-brain barrier
bca	[2,2'-biquinoline]-4,4'-dicarboxylic acid
BCG	bacillus calmette-guerin
Bcr-Able	fusion of break point cluster (Bcr) and Abelson (Abl) tyrosine kinase protein
biq	2,2'-biquinoline
bpy	2,2'-bipyridine
B-RafV600E	B-rapidly accelerated fibrosarcoma mutant
Brd2, 4	bromodomain-containing protein 2, 4
CA-4	combretastatin A-4
CLint	intrinsic clearance
CLogP	calculated log P
CORM	carbon monoxide releasing molecule
CYP	cytochrome P450
dmbpy	6,6'-dimethyl-2,2'-bipyridine
EGFR+	epidermal growth factor receptor

EPDTD	effective PDT dose
ERK1/2	extracellular signal-regulated kinase
FAD	flavin adenine dinucleotide
FDA	U.S. Food and Drug Administration
FMN	flavin adenine mononucleotide
FRET	Förster (Fluorescence) Resonance Energy Transfer
IC$_{50}$	half-maximal inhibitory concentration
KDAC	lysine deacetylase
Log D7.4	n-octanol/buffer solution distribution coefficient at pH = 7.4
LUMO	lowest unoccupied molecular orbital
MAL	methyl 5-aminolevulinate
MLCT	metal-to-ligand charge transfer
MW	molecular weight
NADH	nicotinamide adenine dinucleotide
NAD	nicotinamide adenine dinucleotide radical
NAMPT	nicotinamide phosphoribosyltransferase
NIR	near-infrared
nM	nanomolar
nm	nanometer
NMIBC	non-muscle invasive bladder cancer
NN	bidentate ligands
NORM	nitric oxide releasing molecules
PACT	photoactivated chemotherapy
PDT	photodynamic therapy
PI	phototoxicity index, photoactivity index
PI3K	phosphatidylinositol 3-kinase
pM	picomolar
PPIs	protein:protein interactions
PpIX	protoporphyrin IX
PROTAC	PROteolysis TArgeting Chimera
PS	photosensitizer
ROS	reactive oxygen species
Ro5	rule of 5
SAR	structure-activity relationship
SN-38	7-ethyl-10-hydroxycamptothecin
tpy	2,2′;6′,2″-terpyridine
UV	ultraviolet
VIN	vulvar intraepithelial neoplasia
$^1O_2$	singlet oxygen
$O_2{}^{\cdot-}$	superoxide
Φ_Δ	singlet oxygen quantum yield
Φ_{PS}	photosubstitution quantum yield
τ	lifetime
ε	molar extinction coefficient
λ_{irr}	wavelength of light used for irradiation

REFERENCES

[1] P. Wyss, *Photomedicine in Gynecology and Reproduction*, 1st edn., Karger, Basel, New York, 2000, pp. 4–11.

[2] L. Brandeis, *Harper's Weekly* **1913,** December 20, 10–13.

[3] L. C. Cardoso, R. M. L. Savedra, M. M. Silva, G. R. Ferreira, R. F. Bianchi, M. F. Siqueira, *J. Phys. Chem. A* **2015**, *119*, 9037–9042.

[4] M. J. Maisels, *J. Perinatol.* **2015**, *35*, 671–675.

[5] R. P. P. W. M. Maas, P. J. G. M. Voets, *QJM* **2014**, *107*, 945–946.

[6] S. K. Sharma, P. Mroz, T. H. Dai, Y. Y. Huang, T. G. St Denis, M. R. Hamblin, *Israel J. Chem.* **2012**, *52*, 691–705.

[7] O. Raab, *Z. Biol.* **1900**, *39*, 524–526.

[8] L. O. Manganiello, F. H. Figge, *Bull. Sch. Med. Univ. Md.* **1951**, *36*, 3–7.

[9] D. S. Rassmussen-Taxdal, G. E. Ward, F. H. Figge, *Cancer* **1955**, *8*, 78–81.

[10] M. R. Hamblin, *Photochem. Photobiol.* **2020**, *96*, 506–516.

[11] J. R. Lakowicz, *Principles of Fluorescence Spectroscopy*, 3rd edn., Springer, New York, 2006, pp. 1–25.

[12] T. C. Pham, V. N. Nguyen, Y. Choi, S. Lee, J. Yoon, *Chem. Rev.* **2021**, *121*, 13454–13619.

[13] X. Zhao, J. Liu, J. Fan, H. Chao, X. Peng, *Chem. Soc. Rev.* **2021**, *50*, 4185–4219.

[14] J. F. Algorri, M. Ochoa, P. Roldan-Varona, L. Rodriguez-Cobo, J. M. Lopez-Higuera, *Cancers (Basel)* **2021**, *13*, 4447. https://doi.org/10.3390/cancers13174447

[15] S. Monro, K. L. Colon, H. Yin, J. Roque, III, P. Konda, S. Gujar, R. P. Thummel, L. Lilge, C. G. Cameron, S. A. McFarland, *Chem. Rev.* **2019**, *119*, 797–828.

[16] J. Karges, *Angew. Chem. Int. Ed. Engl.* **2022**, *61*, e202112236.

[17] A. R. Azzouzi, S. Vincendeau, E. Barret, A. Cicco, F. Kleinclauss, H. G. van der Poel, C. G. Stief, J. Rassweiler, G. Salomon, E. Solsona, A. Alcaraz, T. T. Tammela, D. J. Rosario, F. Gomez-Veiga, G. Ahlgren, F. Benzaghou, B. Gaillac, B. Amzal, F. M. Debruyne, G. Fromont, C. Gratzke, M. Emberton, *Lancet Oncol.* **2017**, *18*, 181–191.

[18] Y. Chen, L. Bai, P. Zhang, H. Zhao, Q. Zhou, *Molecules* **2021**, *26*, 5679–5699.

[19] S. Banerjee, *Chembiochem* **2021**, *22*, 2407–2409.

[20] E. C. Glazer, *Photochem. Photobiol.* **2017**, *93*, 1326–1328.

[21] P. Zhang, H. Huang, *Dalton Trans.* **2018**, *47*, 14841–14854.

[22] R. Guan, L. Xie, L. Ji, H. Chao, *Eu. J. Inorg. Chem.* **2020**, *2020*, 3978–3986.

[23] C. Imberti, P. Zhang, H. Huang, P. J. Sadler, *Angew. Chem. Int. Ed. Engl.* **2020**, *59*, 61–73.

[24] C. A. Lipinski, F. Lombardo, B. W. Dominy, P. J. Feeney, *Adv. Drug. Deliv. Rev.* **1997**, *23*, 3–25.

[25] D. F. Veber, S. R. Johnson, H. Y. Cheng, B. R. Smith, K. W. Ward, K. D. Kopple, *J. Med. Chem.* **2002**, *45*, 2615–2623.

[26] J. P. Hughes, S. Rees, S. B. Kalindjian, K. L. Philpott, *Br. J. Pharmacol.* **2011**, *162*, 1239–1249.

[27] A. E. O'Connor, W. M. Gallagher, A. T. Byrne, *Photochem. Photobiol.* **2009**, *85*, 1053–1074.

[28] J. Berlanda, T. Kiesslich, V. Engelhardt, B. Krammer, K. Plaetzer, *J. Photochem. Photobiol. B* **2010**, *100*, 173–180.

[29] G. Shi, S. Monro, R. Hennigar, J. Colpitts, J. Fong, K. Kasimova, H. Yin, R. DeCoste, C. Spencer, L. Chamberlain, A. Mandel, L. Lilge, S. A. McFarland, *Coord. Chem. Rev.* **2015**, *282–283*, 127–138.

[30] M. Chakrabarti, N. L. Banik, S. K. Ray, *PLoS One* **2013**, *8*, e55652.

[31] I. Rizvi, S. Anbil, N. Alagic, J. Celli, L. Z. Zheng, A. Palanisami, M. D. Glidden, B. W. Pogue, T. Hasan, *Photochem. Photobiol.* **2013**, *89*, 942–952.

[32] P. Konda, L. M. Lifshits, J. A. Roque, 3rd, H. D. Cole, C. G. Cameron, S. A. McFarland, S. Gujar, *Oncoimmunology* **2020**, *10*, 1863626.

[33] L. M. Lifshits, J. A. Roque, III, P. Konda, S. Monro, H. D. Cole, D. von Dohlen, S. Kim, G. Deep, R. P. Thummel, C. G. Cameron, S. Gujar, S. A. McFarland, *Chem. Sci.* **2020**, *11*, 11740–11762.

[34] P. Konda, J. A. Roque, III, L. M. Lifshits, A. Alcos, E. Azzam, G. Shi, C. G. Cameron, S. A. McFarland, S. Gujar, *Am. J. Cancer. Res.* **2022**, *12*, 210–228.

[35] T. Bortolato, S. Cuadros, G. Simionato, L. Dell'Amico, *Chem. Commun.* **2022**, *58*, 1263–1283.

[36] H. Y. Huang, S. Banerjee, K. Q. Qiu, P. Y. Zhang, O. Blacque, T. Malcomson, M. J. Paterson, G. J. Clarkson, M. Staniforth, V. G. Stavros, G. Gasser, H. Chao, P. J. Sadler, *Nat. Chem.* **2019**, *11*, 1041–1048.

[37] M. L. Li, K. H. Gebremedhin, D. D. Ma, Z. J. Pu, T. Xiong, Y. J. Xu, J. S. Kim, X. J. Peng, *J. Am. Chem. Soc.* **2022**, *144*, 163–173.

[38] B. F. Buksh, S. D. Knutson, J. V. Oakley, N. B. Bissonnette, D. G. Oblinsky, M. P. Schwoerer, C. P. Seath, J. B. Geri, F. P. Rodriguez-Rivera, D. L. Parker, G. D. Scholes, A. Ploss, D. W. C. MacMillan, *J. Am. Chem. Soc.* **2022**, *144*, 6154–6162.

[39] A. V. Elleman, G. Devienne, C. D. Makinson, A. L. Haynes, J. R. Huguenard, J. Du Bois, *Nat. Commun.* **2021**, *12*, 1–9.

[40] R. Araya, V. Andino-Pavlovsky, R. Yuste, R. Etchenique, *ACS Chem. Neurosci.* **2013**, *4*, 1163–1167.

[41] R. Cabrera, O. Filevich, B. Garcia-Acosta, J. Athilingam, K. J. Bender, K. E. Poskanzer, R. Etchenique, *ACS Chem. Neurosci.* **2017**, *8*, 1036–1042.

[42] R. Weinstain, T. Slanina, D. Kand, P. Klan, *Chem. Rev.* **2020**, *120*, 13135–13272.

[43] L. Josa-Culleré, A. Llebaria, *ChemPhotoChem* **2021**, *5*, 296–314.

[44] P. Klán, T. Šolomek, C. G. Bochet, A. Blanc, R. Givens, M. Rubina, V. Popik, A. Kostikov, J. Wirz, *Chem. Rev.* **2013**, *113*, 119–191.

[45] M. J. Schnermann, Y. You, *Photochem. Photobiol.* **2022**, *98*, 287.

[46] A. E. Mangubat-Medina, Z. T. Ball, *Chem. Soc. Rev.* **2021**, *50*, 10403–10421.

[47] D. C. F. Monteiro, E. Amoah, C. Rogers, A. R. Pearson, *Acta Crystallogr. D Struct. Biol.* **2021**, *77*, 1218–1232.

[48] N. Klöcker, F. P. Weissenboeck, M. van Dülmen, P. Špaček, S. Hüwel, A. Rentmeister, *Nat. Chem.* **2022**, *14*, 905–913.

[49] W. A. Velema, W. Szymanski, B. L. Feringa, *J. Am. Chem. Soc.* **2014**, *136*, 2178–2191.

[50] K. Hull, J. Morstein, D. Trauner, *Chem. Rev.* **2018**, *118*, 10710–10747.

[51] D. Kolarski, C. Miró-Vinyals, A. Sugiyama, A. Srivastava, D. Ono, Y. Nagai, M. Iida, K. Itami, F. Tama, W. Szymanski, T. Hirota, B. L. Feringa, *Nat. Commun.* **2021**, *12*, 1–12.

[52] M. Ricart-Ortega, J. Font, A. Llebaria, *Mol. Cell Endocrinol.* **2019**, *488*, 36–51.

[53] E. Uhl, F. Wolff, S. Mangal, H. Dube, E. Zanin, *Angew. Chem. Int. Ed. Engl.* **2021**, *60*, 1187–1196.

[54] K. S. Troelsen, E. D. D. Calder, A. Skwarska, D. Sneddon, E. M. Hammond, S. J. Conway, *ChemMedChem* **2021**, *16*, 3691–3700.

[55] Z. Chen, R. Ke, Z. Song, Y. Zhou, X. Ren, W. Huang, Z. Wang, K. Ding, *Bioorg. Med. Chem. Lett.* **2022**, *64*, 128683.

[56] R. Chen, Z. Wang, L. Liu, Z. Pan, *Chem. Commun.* **2022**, *58*, 4901–4904.

[57] K. Zhang, M. Ji, S. Lin, S. Peng, Z. Zhang, M. Zhang, J. Zhang, Y. Zhang, D. Wu, H. Tian, X. Chen, H. Xu, *J. Med. Chem.* **2021**, *64*, 7331–7340.

[58] G. Xue, K. Wang, D. Zhou, H. Zhong, Z. Pan, *J. Am. Chem. Soc.* **2019**, *141*, 18370–18374.

[59] Y. Naro, K. Darrah, A. Deiters, *J. Am. Chem. Soc.* **2020**, *142*, 2193–2197.

Light-Activated Drugs for Photodynamic and Photoactivated Therapy 63

[60] C. S. Kounde, M. M. Shchepinova, C. N. Saunders, M. Muelbaier, M. D. Rackham, J. D. Harling, E. W. Tate, *Chem. Commun.* **2020**, *56*, 5532–5535.

[61] J. Liu, H. Chen, L. Ma, Z. He, D. Wang, Y. Liu, Q. Lin, T. Zhang, N. Gray, H. Kaniskan, J. Jin, W. Wei, *Sci. Adv.* **2020**, *6*, eaay5154. doi: 10.1126/sciadv.aay5154.

[62] Z. Li, S. Ma, X. Yang, L. Zhang, D. Liang, G. Dong, L. Du, Z. Lv, M. Li, *Eur. J. Med. Chem.* **2021**, *222*, 113608.

[63] T. Kench, P. A. Summers, M. K. Kuimova, J. E. M. Lewis, R. Vilar, *Angew. Chem. Int. Ed.* **2021**, *60*, 10928–10934.

[64] R. Weinstain, T. Slanina, D. Kand, P. Klán, *Chem. Rev.* **2020**, *120*, 13135–13272.

[65] L. Zayat, C. Calero, P. Albores, L. Baraldo, R. Etchenique, *J. Am. Chem. Soc.* **2003**, *125*, 882–3.

[66] V. Nikolenko, R. Yuste, L. Zayat, L. M. Baraldo, R. Etchenique, *Chem. Commun.* **2005**, *13*, 1752–1754.

[67] L. Zayat, M. Salierno, R. Etchenique, *Inorg. Chem.* **2006**, *45*, 1728–1731.

[68] L. Zayat, O. Filevich, L. M. Baraldo, R. Etchenique, *Philos. Trans. A Math Phys. Eng. Sci.* **2013**, *371*, 20120330.

[69] V. San Miguel, M. Alvarez, O. Filevich, R. Etchenique, A. del Campo, *Langmuir* 2012, *28*, 1217–1221.

[70] B. S. Howerton, D. K. Heidary, E. C. Glazer, *J. Am. Chem. Soc.* **2012**, *134*, 8324–8327.

[71] E. Wachter, D. K. Heidary, B. S. Howerton, S. Parkin, E. C. Glazer, *Chem. Commun.* **2012**, *48*, 9649–9651.

[72] Y. J. Chen, W. H. Lei, G. Y. Jiang, Y. J. Hou, C. Li, B. W. Zhang, Q. X. Zhou, X. S. Wang, *Dalton Trans.* **2014**, *43*, 15375–15384.

[73] J. A. Cuello-Garibo, M. S. Meijer, S. Bonnet, *Chem. Commun.* **2017**, *53*, 6768–6771.

[74] Q. X. Zhou, X. S. Wang, *Acta Chim. Sinica* **2017**, *75*, 49–59.

[75] S. Bonnet, *Dalton Trans.* **2018**, *47*, 10330–10343.

[76] C. Zhang, R. L. Guan, X. X. Liao, C. Ouyang, T. W. Rees, J. P. Liu, Y. Chen, L. N. Ji, H. Chao, *Chem. Commun.* **2019**, *55*, 12547–12550.

[77] R. Boerhan, W. Z. Sun, N. Tian, Y. C. Wang, J. Lu, C. Li, X. X. Cheng, X. S. Wang, Q. X. Zhou, *Dalton Trans.* **2019**, *48*, 12177–12185.

[78] A. Busemann, I. Flaspohler, X. Q. Zhou, C. Schmidt, S. K. Goetzfried, V. H. S. van Rixel, I. Ott, M. A. Siegler, S. Bonnet, *J. Biol. Inorg. Chem.* **2021**, *26*, 667–674.

[79] S. Kuang, F. M. Wei, J. Karges, L. B. Ke, K. Xiong, X. X. Liao, G. Gasser, L. N. Ji, H. Chao, *J. Am. Chem. Soc.* **2022**, *144*, 4091–4101.

[80] L. Gourdon, K. Cariou, G. Gasser, *Chem. Soc. Rev.* **2022**, *51*, 1167–1195.

[81] Q. C. Chen, J. A. Cuello-Garibo, L. Bretin, L. Y. Zhang, V. Ramu, Y. Aydar, Y. Batsiun, S. Bronkhorst, Y. Husiev, N. Beztsinna, L. P. Chen, X. Q. Zhou, C. Schmidt, I. Ott, M. J. Jager, A. M. Brouwer, B. E. Snaar-Jagalska, S. Bonnet, *Chem. Sci.* **2022**, *13*, 6899–6919.

[82] A. Li, C. Turro, J. J. Kodanko, *Chem. Commun.* **2018**, *54*, 1280–1290.

[83] R. E. Goldbach, I. Rodriguez-Garcia, J. H. van Lenthe, M. A. Siegler, S. Bonnet, *Chem. Eur. J.* **2011**, *17*, 9924–9929, S9924/1-S9924/21.

[84] J. Wei, A. K. Renfrew, *J. Inorg. Biochem.* **2018**, *179*, 146–153.

[85] H. Chan, J. B. Ghrayche, J. Wei, A. K. Renfrew, *Eur. J. Inorg. Chem.* **2017**, *2017*, 1679–1686.

[86] N. Karaoun, A. K. Renfrew, *Chem. Commun.* **2015**, *51*, 14038–14041.

[87] T. Respondek, R. N. Garner, M. K. Herroon, I. Podgorski, C. Turro, J. J. Kodanko, *J. Am. Chem. Soc.* **2011**, *133*, 17164–17167.

[88] A. Zamora, C. A. Denning, D. K. Heidary, E. Wachter, L. A. Nease, J. Ruiz, E. C. Glazer, *Dalton Trans.* **2017**, *46*, 2165–2173.

[89] S. Bonnet, J.-P. Collin, J.-P. Sauvage, E. Schofield, *Inorg. Chem.* **2004**, *43*, 8346–8354.

[90] A. Li, R. Yadav, J. K. White, M. K. Herroon, B. P. Callahan, I. Podgorski, C. Turro, E. E. Scott, J. J. Kodanko, *Chem. Commun.* **2017**, *53*, 3673–3676.

[91] V. H. S. van Rixel, V. Ramu, A. B. Auyeung, N. Beztsinna, D. Y. Leger, L. N. Lameijer, S. T. Hilt, S. E. Le Dévédec, T. Yildiz, T. Betancourt, M. B. Gildner, T. W. Hudnall, V. Sol, B. Liagre, A. Kornienko, S. Bonnet, *J. Am. Chem. Soc.* **2019**, *141*, 18444–18454.

[92] T. N. Rohrabaugh, A. M. Rohrabaugh, J. J. Kodanko, J. K. White, C. Turro, *Chem. Commun.* **2018**, *54*, 5193–5196.

[93] K. Arora, M. Herroon, M. H. Al-Afyouni, N. P. Toupin, T. N. Rohrabaugh, Jr., L. M. Loftus, I. Podgorski, C. Turro, J. J. Kodanko, *J. Am. Chem. Soc.* **2018**, *140*, 14367–14380.

[94] L. N. Lameijer, D. Ernst, S. L. Hopkins, M. S. Meijer, S. H. C. Askes, S. E. Le Devedec, S. Bonnet, *Angew. Chem. Int. Ed. Engl.* **2017**, *56*, 11549–11553.

[95] N. Toupin, S. J. Steinke, S. Nadella, A. Li, T. N. Rohrabaugh, Jr., E. R. Samuels, C. Turro, I. F. Sevrioukova, J. J. Kodanko, *J. Am. Chem. Soc.* **2021**, *143*, 9191–9205.

[96] D. Havrylyuk, A. C. Hachey, A. Fenton, D. K. Heidary, E. C. Glazer, *Nat. Commun.* **2022**, *13*, 3636.

[97] D. Havrylyuk, K. Stevens, S. Parkin, E. C. Glazer, *Inorg. Chem.* **2020**, *59*, 1006–1013.

[98] O. Filevich, B. García-Acosta, R. Etchenique, *Photochem. Photobiol. Sci.* **2012**, *11*, 843–847.

[99] G. Carrone, F. Gantov, L. D. Slep, R. Etchenique, *J. Phy. Chem. A* **2014**, *118*, 10416–10424.

[100] A. Bahreman, J.-A. Cuello-Garibo, S. Bonnet, *Dalton Trans.* **2014**, *43*, 4494–4505.

[101] S. H. C. Askes, M. S. Meijer, T. Bouwens, I. Landman, S. Bonnet, *Molecules* **2016**, *21*, 1460.

[102] A. M. Hossion, M. Bio, G. Nkepang, S. G. Awuah, Y. You, *ACS Med. Chem. Lett.* **2013**, *4*, 124–127.

[103] A. P. Gorka, R. R. Nani, J. Zhu, S. Mackem, M. J. Schnermann, *J. Am. Chem. Soc.* **2014**, *136*, 14153–14159.

[104] R. R. Nani, A. P. Gorka, T. Nagaya, H. Kobayashi, M. J. Schnermann, *Angew. Chem. Int. Ed. Engl.* **2015**, *54*, 13635–13638.

[105] R. R. Nani, A. P. Gorka, T. Nagaya, T. Yamamoto, J. Ivanic, H. Kobayashi, M. J. Schnermann, *ACS Cent. Sci.* **2017**, *3*, 329–337.

[106] M. J. Fuchter, *J. Med. Chem.* **2020**, *63*, 11436–11447.

[107] P. Pfaff, K. T. G. Samarasinghe, C. M. Crews, E. M. Carreira, *ACS Cent. Sci.* **2019**, *5*, 1682–1690.

[108] M. Reynders, B. S. Matsuura, M. Berouti, D. Simoneschi, A. Marzio, M. Pagano, D. Trauner, *Sci. Adv.* **2020**, *6*, eaay5064. DOI: 10.1126/sciadv.aay5064

[109] Y.-H. Jin, M.-C. Lu, Y. Wang, W.-X. Shan, X.-Y. Wang, Q.-D. You, Z.-Y. Jiang, *J. Med. Chem.* **2020**, *63*, 4644–4654.

[110] S. B. Vittardi, R. Thapa Magar, D. J. Breen, J. J. Rack, *J. Am. Chem. Soc.* **2021**, *143*, 526–537.

[111] I. Stepanenko, M. Zalibera, D. Schaniel, J. Telser, V. B. Arion, *Dalton Trans.* **2022**, *51*, 5367–5393.

[112] Y. Rojas Pérez, L. D. Slep, R. Etchenique, *Inorg. Chem.* **2019**, *58*, 11606–11613.

[113] S. Alonso-de Castro, A. L. Cortajarena, F. Lopez-Gallego, L. Salassa, *Angew. Chem. Int. Ed.* **2018**, *57*, 3143–3147.

[114] J. Gurruchaga-Pereda, V. Martínez-Martínez, E. Rezabal, X. Lopez, C. Garino, F. Mancin, A. L. Cortajarena, L. Salassa, *ACS Catalysis* **2020**, *10*, 187–196.

Light-Activated Drugs for Photodynamic and Photoactivated Therapy   65

[115] P. Delcanale, C. Montali, B. Rodríguez-Amigo, S. Abbruzzetti, S. Bruno, P. Bianchini, A. Diaspro, M. Agut, S. Nonell, C. Viappiani, *J. Agric. Food. Chem.* **2016**, *64*, 8633–8639.

[116] B. S. Benavides, S. Valandro, D. Cioloboc, A. B. Taylor, K. S. Schanze, D. M. Kurtz, Jr., *Biochemistry* **2020**, *59*, 1618–1629.

[117] R. K. Donegan, C. M. Moore, D. A. Hanna, A. R. Reddi, *Free Radic. Biol. Med.* **2019**, *133*, 88–100.

[118] P. Foley, *J. Dermatolog. Treat.* **2003**, *14 (Suppl 3)*, 15–22.

[119] Y. Yao, J. Zuo, L. Chen, *Am. J. Transl. Res.* **2021**, *13*, 10816–10822.

[120] Y. Su, Y. Zhang, Y. Tong, L. Zhang, P. Li, H. Zhang, X. Zhang, Y. Tang, L. Qin, Y. Shen, B. Wang, Y. Zhou, L. Cao, M. Zhang, T. Zhang, *Photodiagn. Photodyn. Ther.* **2022**, *37*, 102634.

[121] J. C. Bai-Habelski, A. Ko, C. Ortland, M. Stocker, A. Ebeling, U. Reinhold, *Exp. Dermatol.* **2022**, 31, 1385–1391.

[122] B. Kiesel, J. Freund, D. Reichert, L. Wadiura, M. T. Erkkilae, A. Woehrer, S. Hervey-Jumper, M. S. Berger, G. Widham, *Front. Oncol.* **2021**, *11*, 699301.

[123] B. Kiesel, L. I. Wadiura, M. Mischkulnig, J. Makolli, V. Sperl, M. Borkovec, J. Freund, A. Lang, M. Millesi, A. S. Berghoff, J. Furtner, A. Woehrer, G. Widhalm, *Cancers (Basel)* **2021**, *13*, 6119.

[124] T. A. Eatz, D. G. Eichberg, V. M. Lu, L. Di, R. J. Komotar, M. E. Ivan, *J. Neurooncol.* **2022**, *156*, 233–256.

[125] M. Vermandel, C. Dupont, F. Lecomte, H. A. Leroy, C. Tuleasca, S. Mordon, C. G. Hadjipanayis, N. Reyns, *J. Neurooncol.* **2021**, *152*, 501–514.

[126] ClinicalTrials.gov website of National Library of Medicine (NLM). Study identifier: NCT03048240.

[127] J. J. Woods, J. Cao, A. R. Lippert, J. J. Wilson, *J. Am. Chem. Soc.* **2018**, *140*, 12383–12387.

[128] N. Lu, Z. Deng, J. Gao, C. Liang, H. Xia, P. Zhang, *Nat. Commun.* **2022**, *13*, 2245.

[129] H. P. Lee, A. K. Gaharwar, *Adv. Sci.* **2020**, *7*, 2000863.

[130] M. J. Mitchell, M. M. Billingsley, R. M. Haley, M. E. Wechsler, N. A. Peppas, R. Langer, *Nat. Rev. Drug. Discov.* **2021**, *20*, 101–124.

[131] J. Pérez Prieto, M. A. González Béjar, *Photoactive Inorganic Nanoparticles: Surface Composition and Nanosystem Functionality*, Elsevier, Amsterdam; Oxford, Cambridge, MA, 2019.

[132] Z. W. Dai, Z. G. Wang, *Molecules* **2020**, *25*, 5167; https://doi.org/10.3390/molecules25215167.

[133] M. Nonaka, H. Ikeda, T. Inokuchi, *Photochem. Photobiol.* **2004**, *79*, 94–98.

[134] A. Hajri, S. Wack, C. Meyer, M. K. Smith, C. Leberquier, M. Kedinger, M. Aprahamian, *Photochem. Photobiol.* **2002**, *75*, 140–148.

[135] D. G. Hilmey, M. Abe, M. I. Nelen, C. E. Stilts, G. A. Baker, S. N. Baker, F. V. Bright, S. R. Davies, S. O. Gollnick, A. R. Oseroff, S. L. Gibson, R. Hilf, M. R. Detty, *J. Med. Chem.* **2002**, *45*, 449–461.

[136] S. Chamberlain, H. D. Cole, J. Roque, III, D. Bellnier, S. A. McFarland, G. Shafirstein, *Pharmaceuticals (Basel)* **2020**, *13,* 137. https://doi.org/10.3390/ph13070137

[137] J. Fong, K. Kasimova, Y. Arenas, P. Kaspler, S. Lazic, A. Mandel, L. Lilge, *Photochem. Photobiol. Sci.* **2015**, *14*, 2014–2023.

[138] Q. Chen, V. Ramu, Y. Aydar, A. Groenewoud, X. Q. Zhou, M. J. Jager, H. Cole, C. G. Cameron, S. A. McFarland, S. Bonnet, B. E. Snaar-Jagalska, *Cancers (Basel)* **2020**, *12*(3), 587. https://doi.org/10.3390/cancers12030587.

[139] L. Lilge, S. Roufaiel, S. Lazic, P. Kaspler, M. A. Munegowda, M. Nitz, J. Bassan, A. Mandel, *Transl. Biophotonics* **2020**, *2*, e201900032.

3 Mitochondria as a Metallo-Drug Target for Therapeutic Purposes

Andrea Erxleben
School of Biological and Chemical Sciences, University of Galway, University Road, Galway, H91TK33, Ireland
andrea.erxleben@nuigalway.ie

CONTENTS

1 Introduction 68
   1.1 Mitochondria as Unusual Cell Organelles 68
   1.2 Role of the Mitochondria in Cell Death Pathways 69
      1.2.1 Apoptosis 69
      1.2.2 Non-Apoptotic Cell Death 70
   1.3 Mitochondrial Diseases 71
   1.4 Mitochondria and Cancer 72
2 Mitochondria as Drug Targets 72
3 Mechanistic Studies of Mitochondria-Targeting Metallo-Drugs 74
4 Accumulation of Metallo-Drugs in the Mitochondria 75
5 Mitochondria-Targeting Metal-Based Cancer Drugs 76
   5.1 Platinum Complexes 76
   5.2 Gold Complexes 82
   5.3 Ruthenium, Iridium, and Rhenium Complexes 86
   5.4 Copper Complexes 90
   5.5 Photoactivated Metallo-Drugs and Metal-Based Photosensitizers 92
6 Concluding Remarks and Perspectives 97
Acknowledgments 98
Abbreviations 98
References 99

ABSTRACT

As the cell's power plants, the mitochondria provide the cell with ATP through oxidative phosphorylation. However, they are also key players in biosynthesis and regulated cell death. It is therefore not surprising that they have emerged as promising drug targets in cancer chemotherapy. Mitochondria-targeting drugs can bypass resistance mechanisms and (re-)activate cell death programs in tumor cells. The mitochondria

DOI: 10.1201/9781003272250-3

are ideal targets of metallo-drugs, as many metal complexes tend to accumulate in the mitochondria because of their lipophilicity and positive charge or can be conveniently functionalized with mitochondria-directing entities. This chapter starts with an overview on the role of the mitochondria in cell death, disease, and cancer. We then discuss recent developments of mitochondria-targeting platinum, gold, ruthenium, iridium, rhenium, and copper complexes as well as metal-based photosensitizers.

KEYWORDS

Mitochondria; Cancer; Metal Complexes; Photosensitizers; Chemotherapy

1 INTRODUCTION

The mitochondria are the cell's powerhouses. They synthesize ATP via respiration and are therefore essential for the cellular energy metabolism. Besides their role in bioenergetics, they also control redox homeostasis, participate in the biosynthesis of heme, nucleotides, cholesterol, and cardiolipin and have important functions in calcium homeostasis and apoptosis. The citric acid cycle, the β-oxidation of fatty acids, the metabolism of certain amino acids, and the formation of Fe/S clusters take place in the mitochondria. The proper functioning of these cell organelles is thus critical for normal cell function and human health. The mitochondria not only play a fundamental role in oncogenesis, tumor progression, and the immortality of cancer cells but are also involved in the response to treatment.

In the following sections, key features of the mitochondria will be described with an emphasis on their role in cancer and cell death signaling as well as strategies to kill cancer cells by interfering with their bioenergetics or mitochondrial metabolism using metallo-drugs including platinum, gold, ruthenium, iridium, rhenium, and copper complexes. Experimental methods to study mitochondria-targeting metallo-drugs will also be briefly summarized.

1.1 MITOCHONDRIA AS UNUSUAL CELL ORGANELLES

In electron microscopy images, the mitochondria appear as ovoid or rod-shaped structures, 1–10 μm in length and about 0.7 μm in diameter. Cells can contain hundreds to thousands of mitochondria depending on the tissue and cell type. Mitochondria are dynamic organelles that undergo continuous fusion and fission and their morphology and size vary between different cell types and within the cellular population. They are composed of the outer mitochondrial membrane (OMM), the inner mitochondrial membrane (IMM), the intermembrane space (IMS) and the mitochondrial matrix (MM). In the MM the citric acid cycle produces NADH and $FADH_2$ that deliver the electrons to the electron transport chain (ETC). The IMM is subdivided into the inner boundary membrane and the cristae which accommodate the protein complexes of the ETC and ATPase for oxidative phosphorylation (OXPHOS). The electron transfer along the ETC releases energy which is used to pump protons from the MM to the IMS. The resulting H^+ gradient provides the energy to drive the synthesis of ATP [1].

The mitochondria are unusual organelles in that they have their own genome that is different from the nuclear genome of the cell. The mitochondria contain multiple copies of circular DNA (mtDNA), about 16.6 kb long in humans, that is maternally inherited. Human mtDNA encodes 13 proteins of the ETC as well as 22 transfer RNAs and 2 ribosomal RNAs [2]. The mitochondria divide independently of the cell cycle by simple fission.

The mitochondria play a fundamental role in apoptosis. While they are not directly involved in the cell death signaling cascades of non-apoptotic regulated cell death pathways such as paraptosis, ferroptosis, necroptosis, and autophagic cell death, these cell death modalities can be triggered by cellular stressors resulting from the disruption of mitochondrial function.

1.2 ROLE OF THE MITOCHONDRIA IN CELL DEATH PATHWAYS

1.2.1 Apoptosis

Apoptosis as a form of programmed cell death occurs via two distinct pathways, the death-receptor-mediated or extrinsic pathway and the mitochondria-mediated or intrinsic pathway (Figure 1) [3]. In the mitochondria-mediated pathway, the so-called mitochondrial permeability transition (MPT) pore, a high conductance channel, is opened upon a pro-apoptotic signal or a pathological trigger (e.g., ROS, radiation, DNA damage). The sudden increase in the permeability of the IMM induces the loss of the mitochondrial transmembrane potential ($\Delta\Psi_m$), swelling of the MM due to the osmotic influx of water, rupture of the OMM,

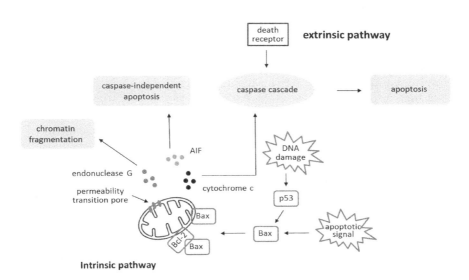

FIGURE 1 Mitochondrial and death-receptor-mediated pathways of apoptosis.

and the release of apoptogenic proteins such as cytochrome c, apoptosis-inducing factor (AIF), and endonuclease G that initiate the death-signaling cascade, DNA fragmentation, and chromatin condensation. The loss of $\Delta\Psi_m$ represents a point of no return in the death cascade. Mitochondrial membrane permeabilization can also result from a process called mitochondrial outer membrane permeabilization (MOMP) that is regulated by members of the Bcl-2 protein family such as Bax. On a pro-apoptotic signal, Bax translocates from the cytosol to the mitochondria and inserts into the OMM where it homo- or heterodimerizes with other pro-apoptotic proteins of the Bcl-2 family which leads to the formation of mitochondrial pores. Bax can also be activated by the tumor-suppressor p53 in response to DNA damage. Apoptotic cell death is accompanied by mitochondrial fragmentation, and in fact, mitochondrial fission seems to be important for the execution of apoptosis [3].

1.2.2 Non-Apoptotic Cell Death

Ferroptosis. Agents that induce ferroptosis are of interest as they are able to eradicate cancer cells that have developed mechanisms to escape apoptosis. The mechanism of ferroptosis is iron-dependent and involves the accumulation of lipid peroxides. It can be induced by dysfunction of system x_c^- and cysteine deprivation. Cysteine is a building block of glutathione (GSH), a key reductant in mammalian cells and a cofactor for glutathione peroxidase 4 (GPX4). Cysteine can be taken up into cells in its reduced form via a neutral amino acid transporter or in its oxidized cystine form by the system x_c^- cystine/glutamate antiporter. GPX4 protects the cell from the peroxidation of membrane lipids. The formation of lipid peroxides is catalyzed by free intracellular Fe via the Fenton reaction. A key feature of ferroptosis is thus the loss of the integrity of the cell membrane and organelle membranes due to impaired GSH-dependent antioxidant defense mechanisms [4].

Autophagy-dependent cell death. Autophagy is a catabolic homeostatic process that is associated with the degradation of cytoplasmic material by the lysosomes. Proposed mechanisms of autophagy-dependent cell death include excessive autophagy, excessive mitophagy, and autosis. Excessive autophagy involves the extreme formation of autophagosomes, the double membrane vesicles that transport damaged organelles or cellular components to the lysosomes for degradation. Excessive mitophagy refers to the excessive autophagic destruction of mitochondria [4].

Paraptosis. The key feature of paraptosis is dilation of the endoplasmic reticulum (ER) and/or mitochondria. Typical apoptotic characteristics such as DNA condensation and fragmentation, membrane blebbing, and the formation of apoptotic bodies are absent. Paraptosis is not well understood at the molecular level. Perturbations of ion homeostasis and cellular proteostasis as a consequence of proteasome inhibition or disruption of thiol homeostasis seem to be important. It has been proposed that Ca^{2+}-mediated communication between the ER and the mitochondria, mitochondrial Ca^{2+} overload, Ca^{2+} depletion in the ER, and the accumulation of misfolded proteins in the ER contribute to mitochondrial dilation and ER stress during paraptosis [5].

Mitochondria as a Metallo-Drug Target for Therapeutic Purposes   71

Necroptosis. Necroptosis is the regulated, caspase-independent form of necrosis (uncontrolled or accidental cell death). One of the signaling molecules involved is the receptor-interacting protein kinase RIPK3 that upregulates PYGL, PDC-E1, and mitochondrial NOX4 which enhances the mitochondrial energy metabolism, ROS generation, and mitochondrial damage. Furthermore, phosphate glycerin mutase 5 located in the OMM disrupts the mitochondrial metabolism, inhibits GSH, and activates dynamin-protein 1. However, there is also evidence that the mitochondria are not necessary for necroptosis [4, 6].

1.3 MITOCHONDRIAL DISEASES

A number of chronic and serious diseases are linked to mutations in mtDNA or nuclear genes that impair mitochondrial function. These include mitochondrial myopathy, Leber's hereditary optic neuropathy, mitochondrial diabetes, and cardiovascular disease. Abnormal mitochondria are involved in the pathogenesis of neurodegenerative disorders such as Alzheimer's disease, Huntington's disease, Parkinson's disease, and amyotrophic lateral sclerosis. The mitochondria play a role in the activation of immune cells and the production of immune mediators in autoimmune inflammatory diseases. Mitochondrial dysfunction mediates the death of cardiac muscle cells during ischemia-reperfusion injury [7].

Cells and individual mitochondria can contain a mixture of wild-type and mutant mtDNA genomes (heteroplasmy) [8]. When the mitochondria are divided between the daughter cells during cell division, a daughter cell can inherit a population of mitochondria with a higher ratio of mutant to wild-type mtDNA. As mutant mtDNA levels increase, eventually a threshold is reached beyond which mitochondrial dysfunction manifests itself. The progressive accumulation of mutations in mtDNA is likely to contribute to the process of ageing [9]. Furthermore, reduced mitochondrial biogenesis and mitophagy seem to play a role in ageing [10]. The earlier hypothesis that ageing is linked to the effects of ROS production has been challenged recently [11, 12]. Increased ROS levels in mitochondria are a consequence of electron leakage from the respiratory chain. While low levels of ROS have important signaling roles, excess ROS leads to oxidative stress and damage. It has been argued that mtDNA is particularly vulnerable to ROS-induced mutations due to its close proximity to the source and lack of histone protection [13]. Furthermore, one important DNA repair mechanism, nucleotide excision repair, is missing in the mitochondria. MtDNA mutations not only impair respiration but also affect the accuracy of electron transfer. This, in turn, further enhances ROS production and mutation creating a vicious cycle of oxidative stress and impaired bioenergetics ultimately resulting in the progressive decline of mitochondrial respiration [14]. However, more recent studies showed that mtDNA is protein coated and packaged into protein-DNA complexes, so-called mitochondrial nucleoids, and thus is not overly accessible to ROS [11, 12].

The cellular mitochondrial population is maintained through mitochondrial turnover, cycles of fission and fusion during which dysfunctional parts are fragmented and degraded by mitophagy [15]. Imbalanced mitochondrial dynamics, i.e., excessive or deficient fragmentation and impaired mitophagy, lead to cell damage and apoptosis and are linked to the development of various pathologies [16]. The hallmarks of cancer, resistance to apoptosis, insensitivity to anti-growth signals, and unlimited proliferation have been attributed to mitochondrial dysfunction [17].

1.4 MITOCHONDRIA AND CANCER

The mitochondria are involved in the recognition of cancer cells by the immune system and in the activation of the anticancer immune response. On the other hand, they can have a direct role in tumorigenesis [18]. The three main mechanisms by which mitochondria contribute to malignant transformation are as follows:

1. Accumulation of potentially oncogenic DNA mutations via excessive ROS production. ROS can also act as signaling agents and activate oncogenic pathways.
2. Abnormal accumulation of mitochondrial metabolites such as fumarate, succinate, and 2-hydroxyglutarate that inhibit enzymes controlling gene expression leading to the expression of a potentially oncogenic transcriptional program.
3. Impaired MOMP or MPT enabling malignant precursors to escape apoptosis (e.g., via the overexpression of anti-apoptotic proteins or mutations of pro-apoptotic proteins).

Cancer cells are able to alter their metabolism to support their high energy demand and biosynthesis. A common feature of this metabolic reprogramming is the switch from OXPHOS to glycolysis under normoxic conditions, known as the Warburg effect ("aerobic glycolysis") [19]. Aerobic glycolysis is less efficient for ATP generation than OXPHOS, but is advantageous for the formation of nucleotides, amino acids, and lipids required by rapidly proliferating cells. The shift to glycolysis to produce ATP has been linked to resistance to apoptosis [20]. In some tumors $\Delta\Psi_m$ is increased which enhances resistance to regulated cell death. Old or damaged mitochondria are normally removed by mitophagy. Impaired mitophagy promotes malignant transformation. Various mitochondrial metabolites facilitate the epithelial-to-mesenchymal transition, the process by which malignant cells gain increased invasive and migratory potential [21]. It has been emphasized that the genetic and epigenetic alterations that lead to aberrant growth and proliferation do not affect mitochondrial function [22]. In fact, properly functional mitochondrial respiration is essential for tumorigenesis and impaired mitochondrial respiration is not the cause of the Warburg effect.

2 MITOCHONDRIA AS DRUG TARGETS

From the above it is clear that the mitochondria present therapeutic opportunities for a range of pathological conditions including degenerative disorders and hyperproliferative diseases. In fact, the mitochondria are now considered a major

Mitochondria as a Metallo-Drug Target for Therapeutic Purposes 73

drug target in cancer therapy. About 10 years ago the term "mitocan" was introduced as the acronym for "mitochondria and cancer" [23]. The eight classes of mitocans are: (1) hexokinase inhibitors (Hexokinase II is overexpressed in cancer cells and is involved in the first step of glycolysis), (2) agents that interact with proteins of the Bcl-2 family, (3) thiol redox modulators, (4) voltage-dependent anion channel/adenine nucleotide translocase targeting compounds, (5) agents inhibiting the ETC (either directly by interacting with a protein subunit of the enzyme complexes or by accepting electrons flowing across the ETC), (6) lipophilic cations targeting the IMM, (7) agents targeting the tricarboxylic acid cycle, and (8) drugs interacting with mtDNA.

In contrast to cancer drugs that induce mitochondrial apoptosis indirectly via nuclear DNA damage, mitocans that act on the mitochondria directly have the advantage of a typically low genotoxicity. Antimitochondrial agents that disrupt the $\Delta\Psi_m$ and facilitate mitochondrial membrane permeabilization (MMP) directly can bypass resistance mechanisms and (re)activate cell death programs.

Reduced antitumor immunity and resistance to (drug-induced) apoptosis is linked to cancer cell hypoxia [24]. OXPHOS inhibition decreases oxygen consumption and thus hypoxia so that agents that inhibit the ETC can alleviate antitumor resistance. OXPHOS inhibitors are particularly interesting for chemosensitization and for combination with other therapies [24].

The mitochondrial proteins thioredoxin reductase (TrxR), pyruvate dehydrogenase kinase (PDK), and the translocator protein 18 kDa (TSPO) are established drug targets.

TrxR as drug target. The ubiquitous NADPH-dependent flavoprotein TrxR plays a critical role in the cellular redox homeostasis. It exists in three isoforms: cytosolic TrxR1, mitochondrial TrxR2, and testis-specific TrxR3. TrxR maintains the cellular redox state by reducing the disulfide protein thioredoxin (Trx) to its dithiol form:

$$NADPH + H^+ + Trx\text{-}S_2 \rightarrow NADP^+ + Trx\text{-}(SH)_2 \qquad (1)$$

In addition to its role as an intracellular antioxidant, reduced Trx is involved in various essential redox processes including the reduction of ribonucleotides to deoxyribonucleotides by ribonucleotide reductase, a critical step in DNA synthesis and hence in cell proliferation. Furthermore, the Trx system is important in the regulation of transcription factors and protein biosynthesis. The overexpression of TrxR in many cancers is associated with accelerated tumor growth and evasion of apoptosis leading to chemoresistance. Tumor cells upregulate TrxR expression to meet their demand of deoxyribonucleotides for DNA synthesis and to protect themselves from NK-lysin, tumor necrosis factor-α, and ROS [25]. A redox-active selenocysteine in the C-terminal sequence has a pivotal role in the catalytic mechanism and also provides a binding site for soft metal centers of metallo-drugs. Specifically, the inhibition of TrxR2 decreases the level of mitochondrial thiols which in turn alters the mitochondrial membrane permeability and thus initiates apoptosis. Given the multifactorial role of the TrxR/Trx system,

TrxR inhibitors can simultaneously target DNA synthesis, the antioxidant defense system of the tumor cell, and autocrine growth stimulation.

PDK as drug target. The pyruvate dehydrogenase complex in the mitochondrial membrane converts the glycolysis product pyruvate to acetyl-CoA. Acetyl-CoA delivers the acetyl group to the citric acid cycle. PDK inactivates pyruvate dehydrogenase by phosphorylation. Inhibition of PDK increases the flux of pyruvate into the mitochondria, thereby shifting the metabolism from glycolysis to complete glucose oxidation.

TSPO as drug target. TSPO is abundant in peripheral organs such as liver, kidney, and lung and in the glial cells of the central nervous system. It is located at the OMM and plays a regulatory role in mitochondria-mediated cell death pathways. It is also involved in the regulation of mitochondrial energy metabolism, mitochondrial quality control, steroidogenesis, immunomodulation, and cell proliferation [26]. TSPO-specific ligands have been shown to chemosensitize solid tumors and to induce apoptosis and cell cycle arrest in cancer cells [27]. TSPO is overexpressed in many tumor types including breast, prostate, ovarian, colorectal, and brain cancers and the level of overexpression is linked to malignancy and cancer progression [28].

A few non-metal mitochondria-targeting drugs are currently used in the clinic (e.g., venetoclax) or are undergoing clinical trial (e.g., MitoTam). Antimitochondrial metallo-drugs have not yet reached this stage of development, but are an active research field in medicinal inorganic chemistry [29]. For almost all of the different classes of mitocans there are examples of metal-based agents with promising *in vitro* and sometimes *in vivo* activity. The most studied are metal complexes that target mtDNA, TrxR, dissipate $\Delta\Psi_m$, interact with Bcl-2 proteins or cause the accumulation of ROS either directly through a redox-active metal center or indirectly through the inhibition of a redox-modulating enzyme.

3 MECHANISTIC STUDIES OF MITOCHONDRIA-TARGETING METALLO-DRUGS

The mitochondrial accumulation of a metallo-drug containing a non-endogenous metal ion can be quantitatively determined by inductively coupled plasma mass spectrometry (ICP-MS) after isolation of the mitochondrial fraction using commercially available extraction kits [30]. Besides ICP-MS analysis as a sensitive and the most widely used technique, less common methods are high-resolution atomic absorption spectroscopy and energy-dispersive X-ray spectroscopy of the mitochondrial lysates. Many mitochondria-targeting metallo-drugs are emissive and their subcellular localization can be tracked *in situ* in live cells using confocal fluorescence microscopy [31]. Costaining with mitochondria-specific dyes such as Mitotracker Green gives merged images of the fluorescence emissions from the metal complex and from the dye. The degree of colocalization can be quantified by correlation analysis. Synchrotron X-ray fluorescence nanoprobe is an emerging technique to study the distribution of metallo-drugs in cellular

Mitochondria as a Metallo-Drug Target for Therapeutic Purposes 75

organelles. It has been recently used to confirm the localization of an organo-metallic half-sandwich Os(II) complex in the mitochondria [32]. For a detailed discussion of methods for tracking metal complexes in cells, see also Chapter 10.

Morphological damage of the mitochondria and changes of their membrane ultrastructure can be visualized by transmission electron microscopy (TEM).

Mitochondrial dysfunction is linked to altered mitochondrial parameters including $\Delta\Psi_m$, O_2 consumption rate (OCR), ATP production, basal respiration, maximum respiration, and ROS levels. $\Delta\Psi_m$, in particular, is a measure of mitochondrial integrity. $\Delta\Psi_m$ is generally determined using a lipophilic cationic fluorescent dye, e.g., rhodamine 123 or JC-1, that equilibrates across the mitochondrial membrane in a Nernstian fashion [33]. The accumulation of the dye in the mitochondria can be monitored by confocal microscopy, flow cytometry, or using a plate reader. JC-1, for example, normally emits a green fluorescence. When it accumulates to high concentrations in the mitochondria, it aggregates to give so-called J aggregates that emit a red fluorescence. A decrease in $\Delta\Psi_m$ results in the release of JC-1 into the cytosol leading to a shift from red to the original green fluorescence.

Cell-based assays to detect ROS use a non-fluorescent dye that is oxidized by ROS and then becomes fluorescent. The extracellular acidification rate (ECAR) is an indicator of metabolic status and metabolic alterations. The Seahorse assay measures the flux of H^+ production (i.e., the ECAR) along with the OCR. The total cellular ATP production rate, ATP production rate via OXPHOS, and ATP production rate via the glycolytic pathway are calculated from the ECAR and OCR under basal conditions and after the serial addition of mitochondrial inhibitors.

Damage to mtDNA manifests itself in a reduction of copy number and transcription levels of genes encoded by mtDNA. The copy number and transcription level are determined by quantitative polymerase chain reaction (qPCR) and reverse transcription-qPCR. Pico Green staining is an assay to visualize mtDNA and to estimate the degree of mtDNA depletion [34]. The intercalating dye has been used to study mtDNA binding in live cells.

For mitochondria-mediated apoptosis, Western blots can detect caspase activity, Bax and Bcl-2 expression, and the release of cytochrome c from the mitochondria into the cytosol.

4 ACCUMULATION OF METALLO-DRUGS IN THE MITOCHONDRIA

One of the challenges in the development of antimitochondrial drugs is the delivery to the affected mitochondria. To accumulate in the mitochondria, drug molecules have to pass both the cell membrane and the double-layer mitochondrial membrane. While the OMM is relatively permeable due to the presence of large protein-based pores, the IMM is highly impermeable and presents a rigid barrier to molecular diffusion. The high negative potential of -120 to $-180\,$mV of the IMM, which is 3- to 5-fold higher than that of the cell membrane [35], provides a driving force for the accumulation of cationic molecules in the negatively charged MM. Because of the downregulation of ATP synthase in cancer cells, H^+ ions accumulate in the IMS resulting in a higher mitochondrial membrane potential (ca. $-220\,mV$) compared to healthy cells [36]. This offers an opportunity for the preferential uptake of antimitochondrial drugs into the mitochondria of cancer cells. Many metal complexes accumulate in the mitochondria due to their lipophilicity and positive charge. It has been proposed that a $\log P_{o/w}$ value between 0 and +5 and a charge >0 results in a high probability of mitochondrial localization [37]. There are two main strategies to direct cancer drugs to the MM: direct conjugation to a targeting ligand via a covalent bond and use of a nanocarrier with an attached targeting ligand. The oldest and most widely used mitochondria-directing ligands are delocalized lipophilic cations such as triphenylphosphonium (TPP), rhodamine 123, guanidinium, and dequalinium. TPP is particularly popular because of its stability in biological systems, low reactivity toward cellular components, and facile synthesis and purification [38]. Other targeting ligands are peptides, specifically mitochondria-penetrating peptides such as (L-cyclohexyl alanine-D-arginine)$_3$, mitochondria-targeting sequence, and Szeto-Schiller peptides [39]. The latter are water-soluble tetrapeptides that accumulate in the IMM, scavenge ROS, and inhibit the opening of the MPT pores. In the case of metallo-drugs, lipophilic metal entities have also been utilized as mitochondria-targeting ligands.

5 MITOCHONDRIA-TARGETING METAL-BASED CANCER DRUGS

5.1 PLATINUM COMPLEXES

Platinum complexes are traditionally associated with DNA interaction. The binding of cis-Pt(NH$_3$)$_2^{2+}$ to guanine, following the loss of the leaving group ligands, is generally considered the key event in the anticancer action of the three worldwide approved Pt drugs, cisplatin (cis-[PtCl$_2$(NH$_3$)$_2$]), carboplatin (cis-[Pt(cbdca)(NH$_3$)$_2$]; cbdca = 1,1-cyclobutanedicarboxylic acid) and oxaliplatin ([Pt(dach)(ox)]; dach = (1R, 2R)-1,2-cyclohexanediamine, ox = oxalate). The formation of 1,2-intrastrand crosslinks of type cis-[Pt(NH$_3$)$_2$(dGpG)] and cis-[Pt(NH$_3$)$_2$(dApG)] inhibits replication and transcription and triggers the DNA damage response leading to apoptosis if repair fails [40]. However, there is increasing evidence that the mitochondria are also a direct target of cisplatin. Cellular studies found higher platination levels of mtDNA compared to nuclear DNA (nDNA) under certain conditions [41] and experimental data that corroborate a direct role of the mitochondria in the mode of action of cisplatin in the specific case of head and neck cancer have been published [42]. The recent development of a mitochondria-targeting, cisplatin-selective fluorescent sensor led to compelling evidence for the direct interaction of cisplatin with the mitochondria [43]. Cisplatin is transported and delivered to the mitochondria by the Cu chaperone COX17 [43, 44]. Knockdown of COX17 results in the decreased mitochondrial accumulation of

Mitochondria as a Metallo-Drug Target for Therapeutic Purposes

cisplatin and a significantly reduced cytotoxicity confirming the mitochondria as a target.

A number of Pt complexes have been reported to accumulate in the mitochondria (Figure 2). The cationic complex **Pt-1** is an example. This monofunctional complex with a pendant DNA-intercalating naphthalimide moiety was designed as an anticancer agent capable of damaging both nuclear and mitochondrial DNA. It showed a high *in vitro* and *in vivo* cytotoxicity with a better selectivity for cancer cells than cisplatin and a low systemic toxicity. Mechanistic studies confirmed the induction of mtDNA damage, the hypopolarization of the mitochondria, generation of ROS, and the induction of apoptosis following the upregulation of pro-apoptotic proteins and downregulation of anti-apoptotic proteins as well as the reduced transcription of mtDNA-encoded genes [45].

Cells treated with the glucose-modified terpyridine complex **Pt-2** internalize Pt-containing self-assembled superstructures into the mitochondria. The mitochondria swell and have disordered cristae and a decreased $\Delta\Psi_m$ [46].

Several Pt(II) and Pt(IV) complexes have been specifically designed to accumulate in the mitochondria. Targeting entities used to direct Pt agents to the mitochondria comprise lipophilic ligands, such as TPP and rhodamine,

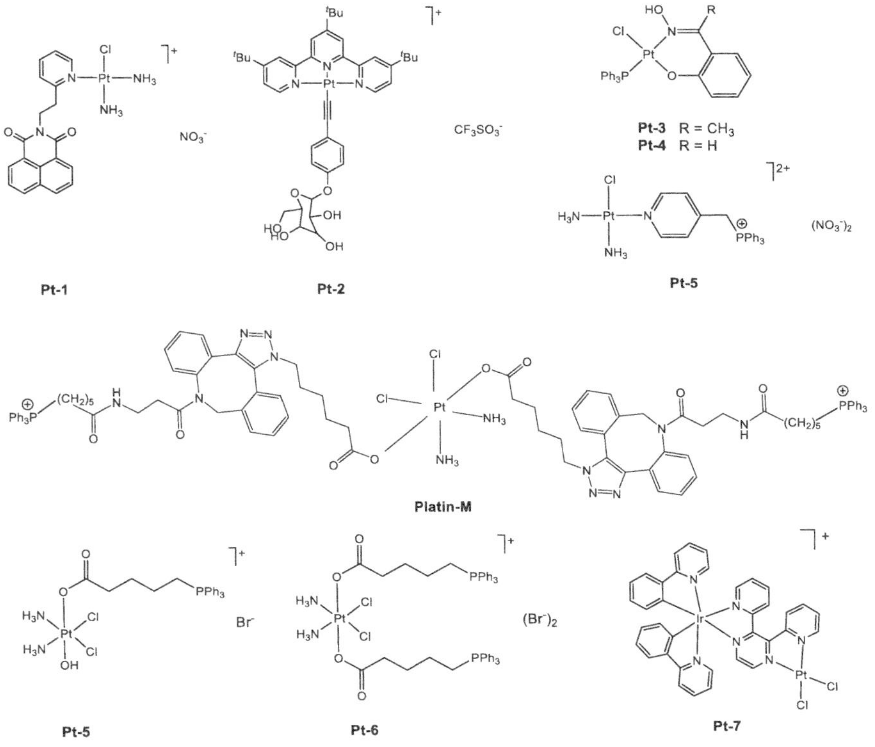

FIGURE 2 Mitochondria-targeting Pt complexes.

mitochondria-penetrating peptides, nucleotides, and metal-based units. In complexes **Pt-3a** and **Pt-3b**, lipophilic TPP is attached to the Pt(II) center. Both compounds accumulate in the mitochondria, decrease $\Delta\Psi_m$, and increase intracellular ROS levels. The complexes are potent cytotoxins, with **Pt-3a** being remarkably active in the cisplatin-resistant A2780cis ovarian carcinoma cell line [47]. In complex **Pt-4**, the pyridine ligand of monofunctional pyriplatin is functionalized with a TPP group. **Pt-4** is more active against A549 cells and less toxic to non-cancerous cells than cisplatin. It also effectively slows down tumor growth in a mouse model. The mode of action is multifactorial and includes damage to mtDNA, reduction of basal and maximal respiration levels, inhibition of ATP synthesis and OXPHOS, increase of the citrate level, and depolarization of $\Delta\Psi_m$. A decrease in the number of mitochondria and changes in the ultrastructure and membrane of the mitochondria further indicate that the mitochondria are the main target of **Pt-4** [48].

Dhar and coworkers designed the Pt(IV) complex **Platin-M** with two axial TPP-functionalized ligands in order to redirect cisplatin to mtDNA [49]. Pt(IV) complexes are prodrugs that are converted to the active Pt(II) species by biological reducing agents such as ascorbate, cysteine, GSH, or biomacromolecules (Figure 3). Pt(IV) prodrugs were originally developed to tackle the high systemic toxicity of cisplatin and to enable oral administration. Due to their d^6 electronic configuration and octahedral coordination geometry, Pt(IV) complexes are inert and do not react with DNA or off-target biomolecules. They require "activation by reduction" upon which the additional "axial" ligands and cisplatin are released.

To further enhance the affinity for the mitochondria, **Platin-M** was encapsulated into triblock copolymer-based nanoparticles functionalized with another TPP group. This dual-targeting approach led to a 30 times higher Pt concentration in the mitochondria compared to the nucleus and to the formation of cis-Pt(NH$_3$)$_2^{2+}$-mtDNA crosslinks. Cytotoxicity studies were performed in cisplatin-resistant A2780/CP70 cells that have hyperpolarized mitochondria and an efficient cisplatin-DNA repair machinery, in SH-SY5Y neuroblastoma cells that have an increased number of mitochondria and in androgen-independent PCa cells. Up to 85 times higher cytotoxicities compared to cisplatin were observed [49].

The cytotoxicities and antimitochondrial activities of the mono- and bisfunctionalized Pt(IV) prodrugs **Pt-5** and **Pt-6** were compared with those of cisplatin and a physical mixture of cisplatin and the TPP ligand [50]. **Pt-6** is more efficiently internalized by cancer cells and is therefore more active than **Pt-5**. In

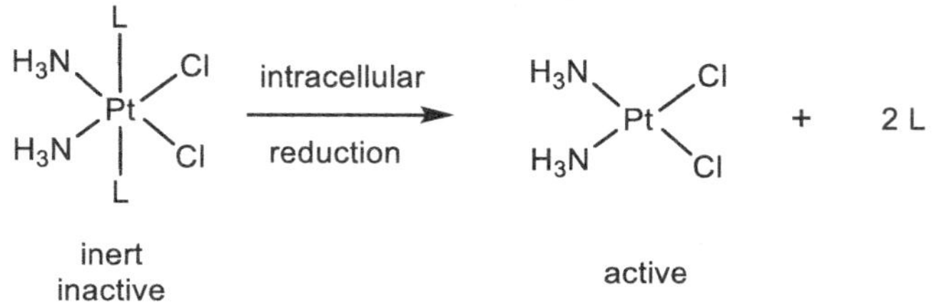

FIGURE 3 Pt(IV) complexes as prodrugs for cisplatin.

Mitochondria as a Metallo-Drug Target for Therapeutic Purposes 79

contrast to cisplatin, **Pt-6** affects the morphology of the mitochondria, inhibits OXPHOS and aerobic glycolysis, and reduces ATP synthesis. The complex also has an effect on the cell cycle that is different from that of cisplatin confirming a distinct mechanism of action. **Pt-6** is less active than cisplatin and this can be attributed to its decreased reactivity to DNA. The platination levels of nDNA in cells treated with **Pt-5**, **Pt-6**, and cisplatin correlate with the cytotoxicity which indicates that DNA interaction is still a key event in the anticancer action of these mitochondria-targeted prodrugs.

Wisnovsky *et al.* coordinated the *cis*-Pt(NH$_3$)$_2$$^{2+}$ entity to a mitochondria-penetrating peptide. The conjugate accumulates in the mitochondria of HeLA and ovarian cancer cells and overcomes resistance in cisplatin-insensitive cancer cells. It damages mtDNA, but not nDNA, leads to an increase in mitochondrial superoxide levels, and triggers apoptosis [51].

MtDNA synthesis requires the import of deoxynucleotides. The uptake of the platinated deoxynucleotide [Pt(dien)(5′-dGTP-*N7*)] into isolated mitochondria was shown to be mediated by the mitochondrial deoxynucleotide carrier, a transporter at the IMM. The model platinated nucleotide can be incorporated to some extent into mtDNA by polymerase γ [52].

Heterodinuclear Ir(III)-Pt(II) complexes of type [PtCl$_2$(diimine-diimine)Ir(L-*N,C*)$_2$]$^+$ or [PtCl(terpyridine-diimine)Ir(L-*N,C*)$_2$]$^{2+}$, where L is a cyclometalating ligand, can accumulate in the mitochondria due to the positive charge of the Ir(III)(diimine)(L-*N,C*)$_2$ entity. For example, 80% of complex **Pt-7** taken up by cancer cells is found in the mitochondria. Cells lose the $\Delta\Psi_m$, have damaged DNA, increased superoxide levels, reduced ATP production and basal respiration, and switch from OXPHOS to glycolysis on incubation with **Pt-7**. The complex triggers cell death via necrosis in cisplatin-resistant cancer cells [53].

Rhodaplatin 2 is a prodrug for oxaliplatin with a lipophilic, positively charged rhodamine ligand in axial position. Besides facilitating the accumulation of the complex in the mitochondria, rhodamine acts as an internal photocatalyst that promotes the activation of the prodrug on irradiation [54]. MtDNA damage is observed, while nDNA is not a target as evidenced by the lacking triggering of the DNA damage response.

The axial positions of Pt(IV) complexes have not only been used to functionalize the prodrug with a targeting entity but also to attach an organic anti-mitochondrial agent to the metallo-drug enabling simultaneous nDNA damage and disruption of mitochondrial function. The first example of such dual-action agents was **mitaplatin**, which contains two axial dichloroacetate (DCA) ligands [55]. DCA is a chemosensitizer. It reverses the Warburg effect by inhibiting PDK and acts as a pro-apoptotic agent by decreasing $\Delta\Psi_m$ and promoting the opening of the mitochondrial transition pore [56]. **Mitaplatin** overcomes cisplatin resistance and shows selectivity for cancer cells. Pt levels in both the nucleus and the mitochondria are higher in cells incubated with **mitaplatin** than in cells treated with cisplatin, and mitochondrial damage and dysfunction have been confirmed [57]. Likewise, analogous Pt(IV) derivatives of oxaliplatin with one or two axial DCA ligands are active in oxaliplatin-resistant cancer cell lines [58].

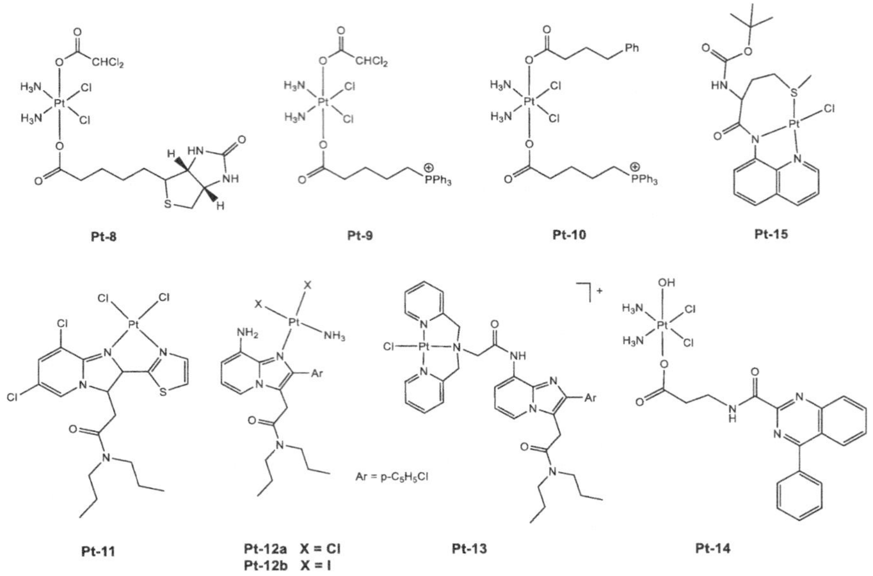

FIGURE 4 Pt(II) and Pt(IV) complexes with antimitochondrial axial ligands.

Recently Pt(IV) prodrugs have been developed with both targeting and bioactive ligand functionalization (Figure 4). In complex **Pt-8** biotin was attached to the cisplatin scaffold in addition to DCA to accumulate the prodrug in tumor cells that overexpress the biotin receptor [59]. A comparison with the corresponding biotin-hydroxido complex demonstrated that DCA significantly enhances the cytotoxicity in a number of cancer cell lines. Loss of $\Delta\Psi_m$, increase in cellular ROS, inhibition of both glycolysis and OXPHOS, and changes to the mitochondrial morphology were observed. Differences in the effect of **Pt-8** and cisplatin on the cell cycle support distinct modes of action. Complexes **Pt-9** and **Pt-10** containing a TPP ligand and DCA or 4-phenylbutyrate as antimitochondrial agents were designed to ensure that prodrug activation takes place in the mitochondria instead of the cytoplasm [60]. Additionally, **Pt-9** was encapsulated into a liposomic carrier for general tumor-targeting. The synergistic action of DCA and cisplatin led to an improved *in vitro* anticancer activity and complete tumor remission in animal studies. The fact that a higher Pt content was found in mtDNA than in nDNA confirmed the design concept.

α-Tocopherol succinate (α-toc) is a vitamin E analog that promotes mitochondria-mediated apoptosis by activating pro-apoptotic Bax and inhibiting Bcl-xL-Bax interactions. An α-toc Pt(IV) complex was shown to be 220 times more cytotoxic against A2780 ovarian cancer cells than a mixture of cisplatin and α-toc. At the same time the complex was 265 times less toxic to non-tumorigenic MRC-5 cells compared to A2780 cells [61]. α-Toc has also been used as a ligand for Pt(II) and synergistic effects due to the simultaneous damage to DNA and the mitochondria were reported [62].

Mitochondria as a Metallo-Drug Target for Therapeutic Purposes

Lonidamine inhibits hexokinase and complex II of the ETC. It also suppresses the functions of the mitochondrial pyruvate carrier and monocarboxylate transporter. The latter mediates the efflux of lactic acid so that its inhibition leads to the acidification of the cancer cell. A Pt(IV) derivative of cisplatin with an axial lonidamine ligand showed good cytotoxicity in various cell lines. However, it was also very active in non-cancerous cells [63].

Another class of bioactive ligands that target the mitochondria are ligands that interact with TSPO. Alpidem and PK11195 are two examples of TSPO-targeting ligands. Derivatives of these compounds have been coordinated to Pt(II) and Pt(IV). The Pt(II) complexes **Pt-11–Pt-13** have a high affinity for TSPO [64]. While **Pt-13** is only modestly cytotoxic, **Pt-12a** and **Pt-12b** have IC_{50} values in the micromolar range, comparable to cisplatin. These two Pt complexes accumulate in glioma cells and are active in cisplatin-resistant cells. In **Pt-14** a derivative of PK11195 is attached to the axial position of the cisplatin scaffold. The Pt(IV) prodrug is 13 times more active against MCF-7 breast cancer cells than cisplatin. Mechanistic studies including cell death kinetic assessment, immunodetection of γ-H2AX foci, comet assay, ROS production, mitochondrial membrane potential and respiration, morphological analysis by TEM, and TSPO binding docking studies indicated a multimodal mechanism combining the effects of DNA damage and antimitochondrial effects [65].

Terpyridine (terpy) Pt(II) complexes have been identified as potent cytotoxins. The mode of action of complexes of type $[Pt(terpy)L](NO_3)_2$ and $[\{Pt(terpy)\}_2(\mu\text{-}L)]$ $(NO_3)_3$ involves the inhibition of TrxR, probably by binding to the selenocysteine residue. This is not surprising given the high affinity of Pt(II) for soft sulfur and selenium ligands. The complexes inactivate TrxR irreversibly in almost stoichiometric quantity and are active against glioblastoma and head and neck squamous carcinoma cell lines [66]. Recently, a terpy complex tagged with TPP has been synthesized to direct the terpy-Pt entity to mitochondrial TrxR2 [67]. The TPP-modified complex causes morphological damage to the mitochondria and mitochondrial dysfunction and induces mitophagy. Detailed mechanistic studies revealed that the mode of action includes the dissipation of $\Delta\Psi_m$, a decrease of mitochondrial and cellular ROS, basal respiration, and ATP production, as well as the reduction of mitochondrial and cellular TrxR activity by 70 and 50%, respectively. The inhibition of both the mitochondrial and glycolytic metabolism means that also the cancer cell's metabolic adaption is blocked. No damage to nDNA was observed. The complex showed enhanced cytotoxicity against cisplatin-insensitive ovarian cancer cells.

There are a growing number of reports on Pt complexes that induce oxidative stress which in turn triggers mitochondrial depolarization and mitochondria-mediated apoptosis [68–70].

Pt-15 has been shown to induce ER stress [71]. ER stress activates the unfolded protein response which impacts the mitochondrial function and triggers mitophagy. **Pt-15** does not damage nDNA but accumulates in the mitochondria. Cells treated with **Pt-15** have a dissipated $\Delta\Psi_m$, increased mitochondrial ROS levels, and decreased ATP levels and ATPase activity. Inhibition of mtDNA is observed and TEM shows the formation of mitophagic vacuoles and mitophago-somes. Unfortunately, **Pt-15** is not selective to cancer cells but is also quite toxic to normal cells.

5.2 GOLD COMPLEXES

Au(I) and Au(III) complexes are widely studied as potential anticancer metallo-drugs and over the years many interesting examples with promising *in vitro* and *in vivo* activity have been published [72]. Biological studies often indicate a com-plex mechanism that includes mitochondrial dysfunction. While all mechanistic studies suggest that the mechanism of Au-based cancer drugs is multifactorial, TrxR has been identified as the common primary target. As typical soft Lewis acids, Au(I) and Au(III) have a high affinity for selenium donor sites and bind strongly to the selenocysteine side chain in the C-terminal active site of TrxR. For a number of Au(I) complexes a higher binding affinity to cytosolic TrxR than to mitochondrial TrxR was reported which was attributed to sequence variations that lead to a greater acidity of the active site of the cytosolic isoform [72]. A com-bination of MALDI-TOF mass spectrometry and biochemical studies indicated that TrxR inhibition by Au(I) and Au(III) complexes requires the conversion of cysteine/selenocysteine residues to their thiol/selenol "gold-reactive" form, i.e., the pre-reduction of TrxR [73]. Binding of Au(I) to RSe^- in the active site results in the irreversible inhibition of TrxR. In the case of Au(III), oxidative damage to active site cysteine and selenocysteine seems to be more important than the formation of a coordinative bond. Inhibition of cytosolic and mitochondrial TrxR unbalances the cellular redox homeostasis and affects the oxidation state of mito-chondrial thiols, ultimately resulting in mitochondrial dysfunction. Often, but not always the cytotoxicities of a series of related Au complexes correlate with the TrxR inhibitory activities, in line with the multifactorial mode of action of Au metallo-drugs [74, 75].

Linear Au(I) complexes were originally used in the treatment of rheu-matoid arthritis. The first routinely applied anti arthritic drug, auranofin, S-triethylphosphinegold(I)-2,3,4,6-tetra-O-acetyl-1-thio-β-D-glucopyranoside (Figure 5), has recently raised significant attention as an antitumor agent. Auranofin is active against B16 cells and overcomes resistance in cisplatin-resis-tant ovarian cancer cells. It was also shown to have *in vivo* activity against P388 murine leukemia. Auranofin has entered phase I/II clinical trial for the treatment of chronic lymphocytic leukemia, small lymphocytic lymphoma, and prolympho-cytic lymphoma [76]. A problem of auranofin and related complexes that needs to be tackled for further clinical development is the low *in vivo* stability.

Auranofin inhibits isolated mitochondrial TrxR at 20 nM concentration. Rat liver mitochondria were shown to swell and to lose their mitochondrial mem-brane potential on treatment with auranofin [77]. Cox *et al.* demonstrated that auranofin-induced mitochondrial oxidative stress due to TrxR inhibition results in the oxidation of mitochondrial peroxiredoxin Prx3 [78]. A recent study strongly suggests that the mitochondrial protein NADH kinase Pos5 is a primary target

Mitochondria as a Metallo-Drug Target for Therapeutic Purposes

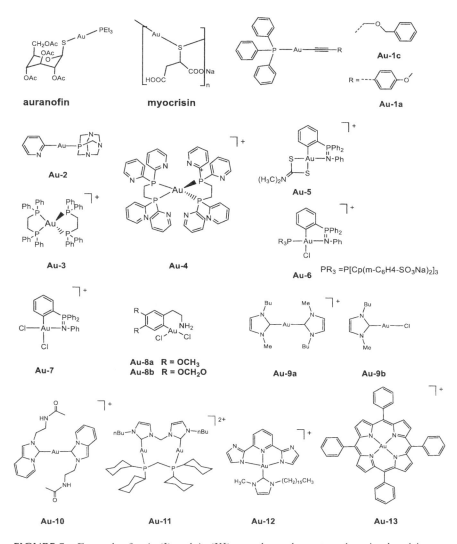

FIGURE 5 Examples for Au(I) and Au(III) complexes that act on the mitochondria.

of auranofin [79]. Two other examples of anti arthritic Au(I) complexes that can act on the mitochondria are aurothiomalate and Et$_3$PAuCl [72]. Both complexes inhibit mitochondrial TrxR and stimulate the MMP transition.

Au complexes that are investigated as (antimitochondrial) cancer drugs can be classified as (1) linear, neutral, auranofin-type complexes, (2) tetrahedral cationic Au(I) complexes with chelating bis(phosphine) ligands, (3) linear, neutral or cationic Au(I) complexes with one or two *N*-heterocyclic carbene ligands, and (4) square-planar Au(III) complexes [72, 80]. Au(I) is highly labile and auranofin-type complexes with phosphine ligands undergo rapid ligand exchange with biological sulfur ligands resulting in a low *in vivo* stability and fast metabolization. In particular, the facile reaction with cysteine and methionine residues in off-target proteins leads to side effects such as nephrotoxicity. These complexes often also have a poor selectivity for cancer cells.

More recently, there is growing interest in organometallic Au(I) compounds with alkynyl ligands and several [Au(I)(alkynyl)(phosphine)] complexes were found to have promising *in vitro* and *in vivo* activities. Figure 5 shows representative examples that act on the mitochondria. Alkynylgold(I)phosphine complexes can achieve high cellular uptake, high selectivity for TrxR, and strong antiproliferative activity with IC_{50} values in the low micromolar or even submicromolar range [74, 81]. Complexes with a triphenylphosphine ligand are generally taken up more efficiently by cells than alkylphosphine complexes. Mass spectrometry analysis of the reaction of complexes **Au-1a** and **Au-1b** with a selenocysteine-containing model peptide showed binding of a "naked" Au atom as well as binding of the gold(alkynyl) and gold(triphenylphosphine) fragments, suggesting that both ligands are replaced and that there is no strong preference for the replacement of either the alkynyl or phosphine ligand [74]. Complex **Au-2** contains the water-soluble 1,3,5-triaza-7-phosphaadamantane (PTA) ligand instead of triphenylphosphine. PTA enhances the water solubility and therefore facilitates the administration and pharmacokinetics of the gold drug. **Au-2** was shown to enter the mitochondria, disrupt mitochondrial function, increase ROS production, and trigger necroptosis. The complex is active against tumor spheroids [82].

Au(I) complexes with bis(phosphine) chelate ligands have long been investigated with the aim of increasing the stability of the Au-P coordination [80]. These complexes have a tetrahedral geometry. **Au-3** and **Au-4** were studied by Berners-Price and coworkers and are two of the first representatives of this type of anticancer gold compound [72, 80].

Square-planar Au(III) complexes with anticancer properties comprise complexes with dithiocarbamate, polyamine, cyclometalating, and porphyrin ligands. Chelating dithiocarbamato ligands form stable complexes with Au(III) and several examples have been reported that overcome cisplatin resistance and cause TrxR inhibition, mitochondrial swelling, depolarization of the mitochondria, and ROS generation [80]. The cyclometalated complexes **Au-5–Au-7** have been shown to induce oxidative stress leading to the loss of $\Delta\Psi_m$, apoptosis, and necrosis [80, 83]. However, differences in the involvement of pro-apoptotic proteins have been observed that were ascribed to the different redox properties of the three complexes. **Au-6** is slowly reduced to [AuCl(PR$_3$)] which might be the active species [83]. Two other examples of Au(III) complexes with cyclometalating ligands are **Au-8a** and **Au-8b**. Accumulation in the mitochondria was confirmed and mitochondrial dysfunction was shown to result in high ROS levels in the ER and in the induction of the ER stress response, ultimately leading to autophagy and apoptosis. Cytotoxicity studies demonstrated a lower resistance factor compared to cisplatin. **Au-8b** proved to be less toxic and more active in a mouse model than cisplatin [84]. **Au-8a** and **8b** inhibit TrxR, but are less efficient inhibitors than auranofin. This is often the case for Au(III) complexes and may

Mitochondria as a Metallo-Drug Target for Therapeutic Purposes   85

be related to the observation that Au(III) probably inactivates TrxR via oxidative damage rather than by forming a coordinative bond.

The best-studied groups of mitochondria-targeting (cationic) lipophilic complexes are Au(I) complexes with *N*-heterocyclic carbene (NHC) ligands and Au(III) porphyrin complexes [80]. NHCs are electron-rich, neutral ligands that are strong σ donors. They have similar donor properties as phosphines and form strong bonds with Au(I), thus conferring a high stability toward blood thiols such as serum albumin and GSH. NHCs are relatively easy to synthesize and their lipophilicity can be readily tuned by introducing different substituents on the ring nitrogens. Since the pioneering work by Berners-Price and coworkers in 2004 [85] a large number of Au(I) NHC-halide, NHC-pseudohalide, NHC-thiolate, NHC-phosphine, and bis-NHC complexes have been investigated. In particular, cationic bis-NHC Au(I) complexes are taken up efficiently by the mitochondria. Bis-NHC complexes are more stable toward thiols than NHC-halide complexes, but the presence of two strong coordinative bonds also decreases the TrxR inhibition activity [86]. Nevertheless, bis-NHC complexes can be more cytotoxic than the corresponding mono-NHC complexes, possibly due to the enhanced mitochondrial accumulation. **Au-9a** is an example. Its IC_{50} value is 20 times lower than that of the mono-NHC complex **Au-9b**. A detailed proteomic study was performed confirming that **Au-9a** impairs the mitochondrial respiration and increases mitochondrial ROS levels as a consequence of mitochondrial dysfunction. Cells treated with **Au-9a** undergo a metabolic shift toward glycolysis. **Au-9a** and **9b** both inhibit TrxR, upregulate Bax, and downregulate Bcl2. Interestingly, the bis-NHC complex is the more potent TrxR inhibitor [87]. A reduction in tumor size in mice bearing highly aggressive B16F10 melanoma was observed on treatment with the bis-NHC complex **Au-10** [88].

A number of bidentate ligands have been developed to generate highly stable, metallacycle-type dinuclear Au complexes [85, 89]. Complex **Au-11**, for example, was shown to inhibit tumor growth in two independent mouse models [89].

Au(III) complexes with NHC ligands are less abundant than their well-explored Au(I) counterparts. One example is **Au-12** that was evaluated in a mouse model [90]. Au(III) NHC complexes can be reduced under physiological conditions.

Cationic, lipophilic Au(III) porphyrin complexes are another promising class of antimitochondrial cancer drugs [91–94]. IC_{50} values as low as 0.03 μM were obtained for Au(III) complexes of tetraarylporphyrins and a correlation with the lipophilicity and cellular uptake was observed. Porphyrin ligands stabilize the +III oxidation state of gold and tetraarylporphyrinato complexes were found to be stable toward reduction by GSH. Complex **Au-13**, usually known as **gold-1a**, is a TrxR inhibitor and is highly active in cisplatin-resistant and multidrug-resistant cancer cell lines. IC_{50} values up to 100-fold lower than those of cisplatin and significant *in vivo* activity were reported [94]. Accumulation of the complex in the mitochondria was confirmed by costaining with MitoTracker Orange. In addition to TrxR inhibition, **gold-1a** decreases the expression of the anti-apoptotic bcl-2 protein [91]. A possible interaction of the Au(III) porphyrin complex with bcl-2 is supported by molecular docking. A proteomic study revealed ROS generation, depletion of $\Delta\Psi_m$ within 3 h after cellular uptake, and caspase-dependent and caspase-independent mitochondrial apoptosis [95]. There is also evidence that the mitochondrial chaperone Hsp60 is a target of **gold-1a**. Hsp60, heat-shock protein 60, plays a role in the regulation of apoptosis and tumor maintenance and is overexpressed in primary malignant tumors [93]. Furthermore, **gold-1a** was shown to transcriptionally upregulate pro-apoptotic PMS2 gene expression [96]. Remarkably, the Au(III) porphyrin complex is able to inhibit the self-renewal ability of cancer stem cells and may therefore have potential for the treatment of relapsed cancers [97]. To enhance the cellular uptake, selectivity, and efficacy, **gold-1a** was encapsulated in mesoporous silica nanoparticles decorated with an integrin-recognizing tripeptide [92]. The nanoparticle formulation caused an overproduction of ROS and eventually triggered ROS-mediated cell death signaling.

Up to date, the conjugation of mitochondria-directing entities to Au complexes is not well explored. Three different Au(I)(phosphine) fragments were attached to mitochondria-targeting di- and tetrapeptides. Cells treated with the conjugates had elevated ROS levels, lost their mitochondrial membrane potential, and underwent apoptosis as a result of TrxR inhibition. Importantly, an effect on the respiration rate of highly aggressive and cisplatin-resistant p53-mutant MDA-MB231 breast cancer cells was observed [98].

5.3 RUTHENIUM, IRIDIUM, AND RHENIUM COMPLEXES

Octahedral Ru(II) complexes with three bidendate or two tridentate pyridyl ligands were initially studied as DNA or RNA probes [99]. However, Ru(II) polypyridyl complexes are lipophilic cations and as such can accumulate in the mitochondria and exert cytotoxicity via the mitochondrial dysfunction pathway. Often a lower cytotoxicity in healthy cells is observed compared to cisplatin. Ru(II) polypyridyl complexes are also luminescent and their application in photoactivated chemotherapy and photodynamic tumor therapy will be discussed in Section 5.5.

It was proposed that the hydrophobic dipyridophenazine ligands of complex **Ru-1** (Figure 6) intercalate into the mitochondrial membrane leading to the perturbance of $\Delta\Psi_m$ [100]. Surprisingly, attaching a mitochondria-targeting peptide to **Ru-1** did not enhance the mitochondrial uptake but on the contrary, resulted in a nonspecific intracellular distribution and loss of the cytotoxic activity [101]. The cyclometalated complex **Ru-2** kills cisplatin-resistant A549 cancer cells at submicromolar concentration. Fifty-five percent of the total cellular uptake is localized in the mitochondria. The complex is able to inhibit TrxR [102]. Some Ru complexes with polypyridyl ligands were also shown to downregulate pro-survival proteins and to upregulate pro-apoptotic Bcl-2 proteins [103, 104].

Like their Ru(II) counterparts, Ir(III) complexes with di- or tridentate polypyridyl or cyclometalating ligands are effectively internalized by the mitochondria [105–109]. One of the heterocyclic ligands in **Ir-1** and **Ir-2** has a pendant indenoisoquinoline moiety. Indenoisoquinoline derivatives are inhibitors of nuclear

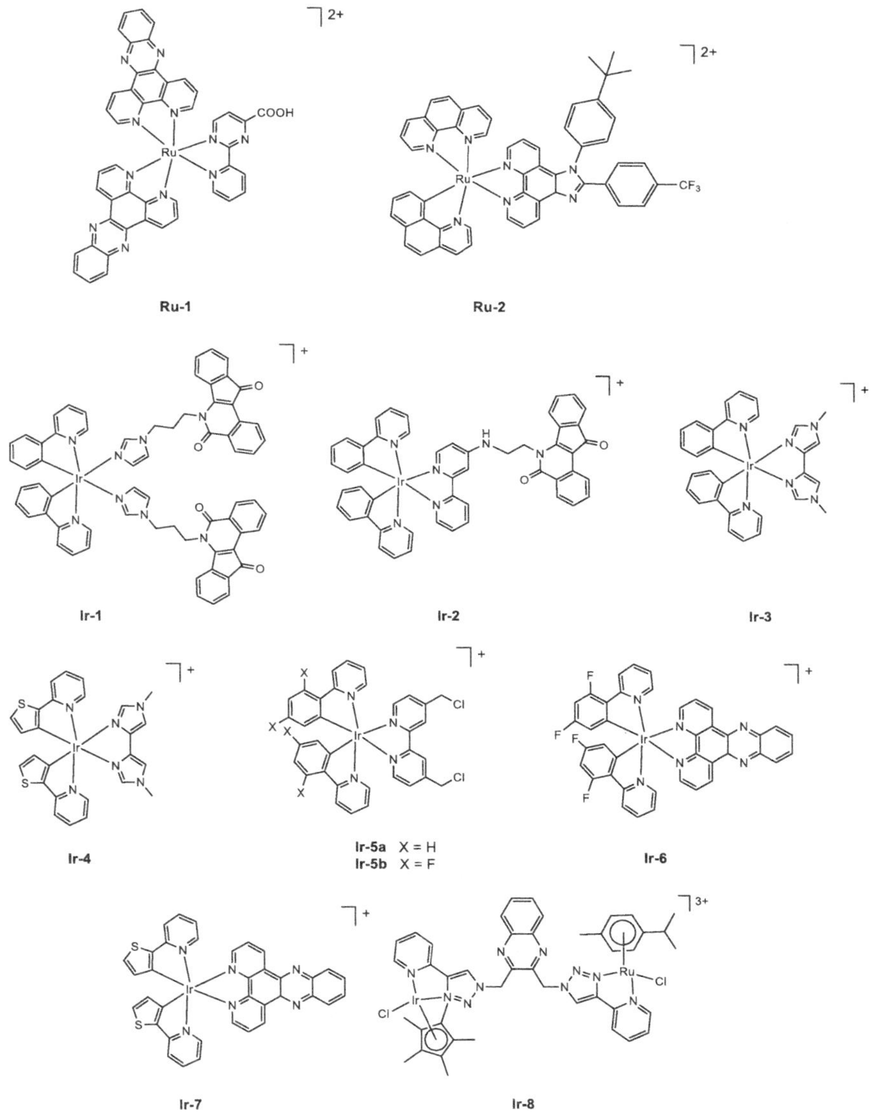

Mitochondria as a Metallo-Drug Target for Therapeutic Purposes

FIGURE 6 Mitochondria-targeting Ru(II) and Ir(III) polypyridyl complexes.

topoisomerase I (TOP1). Topoisomerases have a critical role in DNA replication and transcription by controlling DNA supercoiling. They are therefore over-expressed in tumor cells. Topoisomerase I poisons such as indenoisoquinoline trap the transient covalent topoisomerase-DNA complex. The Ir entities of **Ir-1** and **Ir-2** divert indenoisoquinoline from nuclear to mitochondrial topoisomerase I (TOP1MT) that acts on mtDNA. The complexes poison TOP1MT, thereby inhibiting mtDNA replication. They also cause ROS overload, mitochondrial dysfunction, and caspase 3/7-dependent cell death. **Ir-1** and **Ir-2** are twofold more cytotoxic than free indenoisoquinoline. This was attributed to the different repair capacities for the trapped TOP1-nDNA and TOP1MT-mtDNA complexes [105].

Ir complexes have also been shown to induce cancer cell death by mitophagy. **Ir-3** and **Ir-4** trigger mitophagy by oxidative stress, mitochondrial depolarization, ATP depletion, and alteration of the mitochondrial metabolism [108].

Complexes **Ir-5a** and **Ir-5b** contain reactive chloromethyl substituents that react with thiol groups in mitochondrial proteins and thus have a prolonged retention in the mitochondria. Potent cytotoxicity was observed in various cell lines with IC_{50} values in the 0.2–1.8 µM range. As expected, **Ir-5a** and **Ir-5b** provoke mitochondrial damage and raised ROS levels, inhibit mitochondrial respiration, diminish ATP production, and induce apoptosis [107].

Due to the extended aromatic systems, **Ir-6** and **Ir-7** intercalate into mtDNA and cause mtDNA damage. Evidence that mtDNA is the primary target of the complexes is the reduction in mtDNA copy number, the suppression of mtDNA transcription, and the increase in IC_{50} value in mtDNA free cells compared to wild-type cells. As a result of mtDNA damage, **Ir-6** and **Ir-7** lead to a loss of $\Delta\Psi_m$, ATP depletion, decreased basal OCR, and reduced maximum and non-mitochondrial respiration, eventually leading to mitophagy [109].

Accumulation in the mitochondria and the induction of mitochondrial dysfunction was also reported for heterodinuclear Ru and Ir complexes. **Ir-8** is a potent and selective cytotoxin for colorectal adenocarcinoma (Caco-2) and cervical carcinoma HeLa cells [110].

The promising anticancer properties of Re(I) complexes have only recently been discovered. Re(I) compounds can trigger various cell death mechanisms including apoptosis, paraptosis, ferroptosis, and necroptosis, often in combination. Anticancer Re(I) complexes are usually based on the stable $Re(CO)_3$ core. They are easily accessible by well-established and chemically robust synthetic routes. Positively charged $Re(CO)_3$ complexes with diimine and monofunctional heterocyclic ligands of type fac-$[Re(CO)_3(N^\wedge N)L]^+$ are lipophilic and preferentially accumulate in the mitochondria where they provoke mitochondrial dysfunction-mediated cell death through oxidative stress, loss of $\Delta\Psi_m$, and ATP depletion [111–116]. They are luminescent with good photostability, long-lived emission states, high quantum yields, and large Stokes shifts and thus enable simultaneous therapeutic activity and monitoring of the mitochondrial morphology. The dinuclear complexes **Re-1a** and **Re-1b** (Figure 7) were shown to disturb the GSH metabolism, to damage mtDNA, and to reduce the copy number of mtDNA. The complexes inhibit tumor growth in a mouse model [111].

The monodentate ligands in fac-$[Re(CO)_3(N^\wedge N)L]^+$ complexes have been functionalized with bioactive moieties. In **Re-2**, DCA is conjugated to the axial pyridine ligand. The complex inhibits PDK and treated cells undergo a metabolic shift from glycolysis to glucose oxidation. Coculture experiments with normal cells confirmed that malignant cells are selectively killed. Furthermore, **Re-2** exhibits anti-metastatic, anti-invasion, and anti-angiogenic activity and inhibits tumor growth

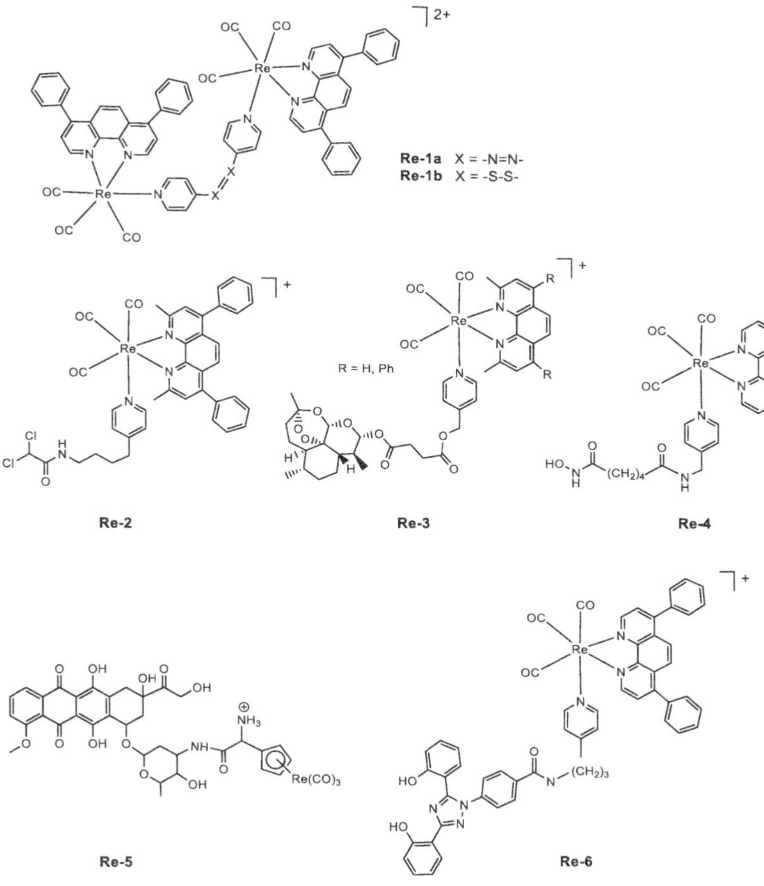

Mitochondria as a Metallo-Drug Target for Therapeutic Purposes

FIGURE 7 Mitochondria-targeting Re(I) complexes.

in MCF-7 tumor-bearing mice. As the phosphorescence lifetime of the complex is O_2-sensitive, the intracellular O_2 consumption, i.e., changes of the mitochondrial metabolic status can be tracked in cells [112]. The artesunate entity in **Re-3** has antiproliferative and pro-apoptotic properties. In addition to the depletion of GSH the complex was shown to inactivate GPX4 leading to lipid peroxidation accumulation. **Re-3**-mediated cell death occurs via a combination of apoptosis and ferroptosis [113]. **Re-4** contains a derivative of the histone deacetylase (HDAC) inhibitor SAHA (where SAHA is suberoylanilide hydroxamic acid). The complex inhibits the HDAC7 isoform that is located in the mitochondrial inner membrane space. HDAC7 is involved in the proliferation of cancer cells and in the regulation of apoptosis. **Re-4** is active in the cisplatin-resistant A549R cell line [113]. The CpRe(CO)$_3$$^+$-doxorubicin conjugate **Re-5** was synthesized to redirect doxorubicin from the nucleus to the mitochondria [115]. The complex led to a depletion of $\Delta\Psi_m$ and activated caspase 3/7 three-fold more efficiently than doxorubicin. While large amounts of **Re-5** are found in the mitochondria, the complex is also taken up by the nucleus and inhibits topoisomerase. In **Re-6**, a Fe chelator is appended to the tricarbonyl diimine Re(I) core to simultaneously target the mitochondrial metabolism and Fe homeostasis. The complex causes immunogenic apoptotic cell death in breast cancer cells and inhibits tumor growth in a murine breast cancer model. The mode of action includes the relocation of cellular Fe to the mitochondria and the downregulation of the expression of $Fe^{II}/2$-oxoglutarate-dependent demethylases. This results in an increase in the methylation levels of DNA, RNA, and histone which leads to epigenetic changes, in particular alterations in RNA polymerase activity. Furthermore, cells incubated with **Re-6** have a hypopolarized $\Delta\Psi_m$ and diminished ATP levels, maximum respiration, non-mitochondrial respiration, glycolytic capacity, and glycolytic reserve as well as elevated mitochondrial ROS levels due to the accumulation of Fe in the mitochondria [116].

5.4 COPPER COMPLEXES

Cancer cells typically have a higher Cu uptake than normal cells and elevated Cu concentrations are observed in cancerous tissue. Cu is involved in angiogenesis which in turn is implicated in tumor growth, invasion, and metastasis [117]. The anticancer properties of Cu complexes are generally attributed to the redox properties of Cu and thus the ability to generate ROS. The ligand in anticancer Cu complexes can modulate the redox potential, lipophilicity, cellular uptake, and cellular distribution. The largest and most prominent class of cytotoxic Cu compounds are complexes of type [Cu(N^O)(diimine)] and [Cu(O^O)(diimine)], the so-called Casiopeinas® [117]. Many Casiopeinas have high *in vitro* and *in vivo* activities, [Cu(glycinate)(4,7-dimethyl-1,10-phenanthroline)]NO$_3$ (CasIIgly, Figure 8) is investigated in phase I clinical trials [118]. Casiopeinas were developed as DNA cleavage agents; however, they have also been shown to impair the function of isolated mitochondria by inhibiting respiration and ATP synthesis [119].

Cu thiosemicarbazones are another class of Cu compounds that act on the mitochondria. Thiosemicarbazones alone are often potent cytotoxins, and 3-aminopyridine-2-carboxaldehyde thiosemicarbazone (Triapine®) has entered clinical trials for advanced-stage malignancies. Cu coordination usually enhances the cytotoxicity of thiosemicarbazones. **Cu-1** inhibits the mitochondrial respiration in isolated mitochondria by targeting the ubiquinone binding site of complex I of the ETC [120]. Cu(II) bis(thiosemicarbazone) complexes have a physiologically accessible redox potential and are susceptible to the intracellular reduction of the Cu center followed by dissociation into free Cu(I) and ligand. The released Cu(I) can react with cellular thiols. However, this does not seem to be the case for **Cu-1**, as evidence has been obtained that the intact Cu complex interacts with complex I of the respiratory chain [120].

The trinuclear complex **Cu-2** contains a dithiocarbazate Schiff base ligand that is structurally related to heterocyclic thiosemicarbazones. The complex induces ferroptotic cell death in pancreatic cancer cells, bypassing the notorious resistance of pancreatic cancer cell lines to apoptosis, one of the reasons for the

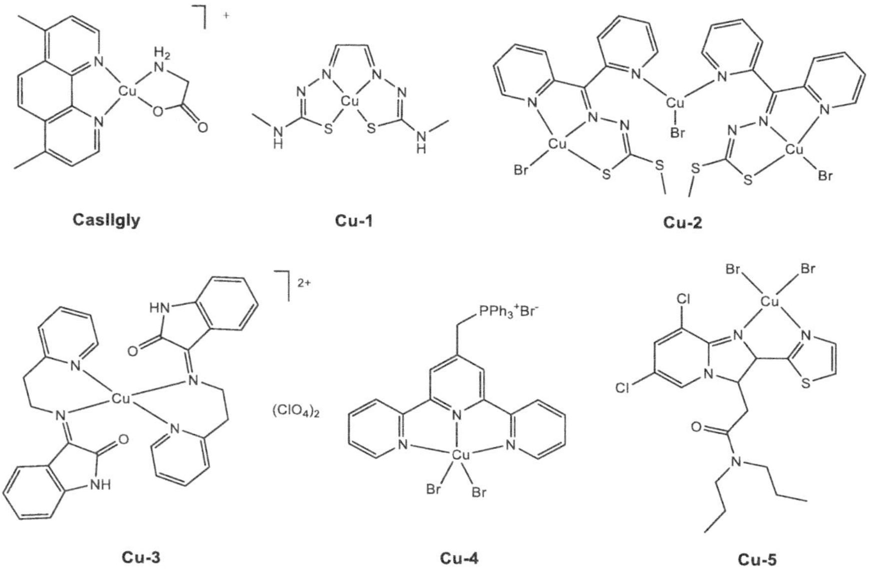

Mitochondria as a Metallo-Drug Target for Therapeutic Purposes

FIGURE 8 Mitochondria-targeting Cu complexes.

frequent treatment failure of this type of cancer. **Cu-2** exerts cytotoxic activity in three pancreatic cancer cell lines at submicromolar concentrations and reduces the tumor volume in ASPC-1 tumor-bearing mice. As the complex is fluorescent, its accumulation in the mitochondria could be confirmed by colocalization studies with MitoTracker. Cells treated with **Cu-2** show morphological changes of the mitochondria typical for ferroptotic cells such as decreased size, reduced cristae, increased mitochondrial membrane density, and ruptured OMM [121]. The Schiff base complex **Cu-3** increases mitochondrial ROS levels and affects the activity of complex I of the respiratory chain. The mitochondrial damage due to ETC impairment triggers apoptosis via the mitochondrial route [122]. The TPP-appended terpy complex **Cu-4** achieves an approximately twofold higher mitochondrial uptake than [Cu(terpy)Br$_2$]. The complex proved highly effective against cisplatin-resistant cancer cell lines and suppresses the growth of liver cancer xenografts *in vivo* [123]. **Cu-4** intercalates into DNA and causes oxidative DNA cleavage and dissipation of $\Delta\Psi_m$. A later detailed mechanistic study demonstrated that mitochondria-mediated apoptosis is triggered via the loss of $\Delta\Psi_m$, ROS production, increase in Bax levels, decrease in Bcl-2 levels and cytochrome c release. The complex promotes the translocation of p53 to the mitochondria. Furthermore, ROS-mediated activation of Drp1 was observed. Drp1 plays a role in the regulation of mitochondrial fission so that **Cu-4** unbalances the mitochondrial dynamics [124]. Liu, Wang, and coworkers developed a Cu complex of a peptide consisting of the Cu-binding gly-gly-his domain and a mitochondria-penetrating peptide domain [125]. The peptide complex is selectively taken up by the mitochondria and produces ROS via the Fenton reaction with endogenous H$_2$O$_2$

leading to mitochondrial dysfunction and opening of the MPT pore. As cancer cells have higher H_2O_2 levels than normal cells, a metallo-drug acting as a Fenton catalyst has inherent selectivity. **Cu-5** was designed to target the TSPO protein on the OMM. The complex proved to be a potent cytotoxin against various cancer cell lines including multidrug-resistant colon cancer cells and led to a 98% reduction in a murine LLC solid tumor. **Cu-5** binds with nanomolar affinity to TSPO and the cytotoxicity correlates with the TSPO expression levels. Impairment of the respiratory chain was observed leading to a reduction in OCR and elevated ROS levels. Cells treated with **Cu-5** had depolarized and swollen mitochondria with disrupted cristae [126].

5.5 PHOTOACTIVATED METALLO-DRUGS AND METAL-BASED PHOTOSENSITIZERS

Metallo-drugs that are inactive in the dark and are activated by illumination with visible or near-infrared light enable highly selective tumor therapy, as healthy tissue not exposed to irradiation is protected. In photodynamic therapy (PDT) a photosensitizer (PS) mediates the formation of highly reactive and cytotoxic $^1O_2$ that then causes irreversible damage to the cancer cell. On absorption of light, the PS is excited to the $^1S^*$ state which undergoes an intersystem crossing (ISC) to the $^3S^*$ state. The collision of the excited $^3S^*$ PS with $^3O_2$ and energy transfer generate $^1O_2$ (type II photoprocess):

$$PS(^1S) + h\nu \rightarrow PS(^1S^*) \rightarrow PS(^3S^*) \tag{2}$$

$$PS(^3S^*) + {}^3O_2 \rightarrow PS(^1S) + {}^1O_2 \tag{3}$$

The short lifetime (<40 ns) and diffusion range (<20 nm) of $^1O_2$ limits its radius of action and allows a spatially and temporally controlled therapy. While $^1O_2$ is the main ROS involved in PDT, PSs can also produce superoxide and hydroxyl radicals in a type I photoprocess. The advantage of the formation of $^1O_2$ compared to other ROS such as peroxides or superoxide is the lack of any cellular defense mechanism. Cancer cell mitochondria are particularly vulnerable to PDT-induced oxidative stress because of their unstable redox balance. The main challenge in PDT is the development of PSs that work within the phototherapeutic absorption window of 700–850 nm for deep tissue penetration.

The most prominent and best-studied class of mitochondria-targeting PDT agents are Ru(II) and Ir(III) complexes with polypyridyl and cyclometalating ligands. The Ru complex TLD-1433, developed by McFarland and coworkers, has entered clinical trials for PDT treatment of bladder cancer [127]. A few illustrative examples of Ru- and Ir-based PDT agents that show recent developments in the field are shown in Figure 9.

Complex **PDT-Ru1** is functionalized with a TPP group to enhance the mitochondria-targeting properties. The compound is inactive in the dark, but becomes a potent cytotoxin in multicellular tumor HeLa spheroids on irradiation with NIR light [128]. Complexes **PDT-Ru2**-**PDT-Ru5** are dual-mode-of-action agents that

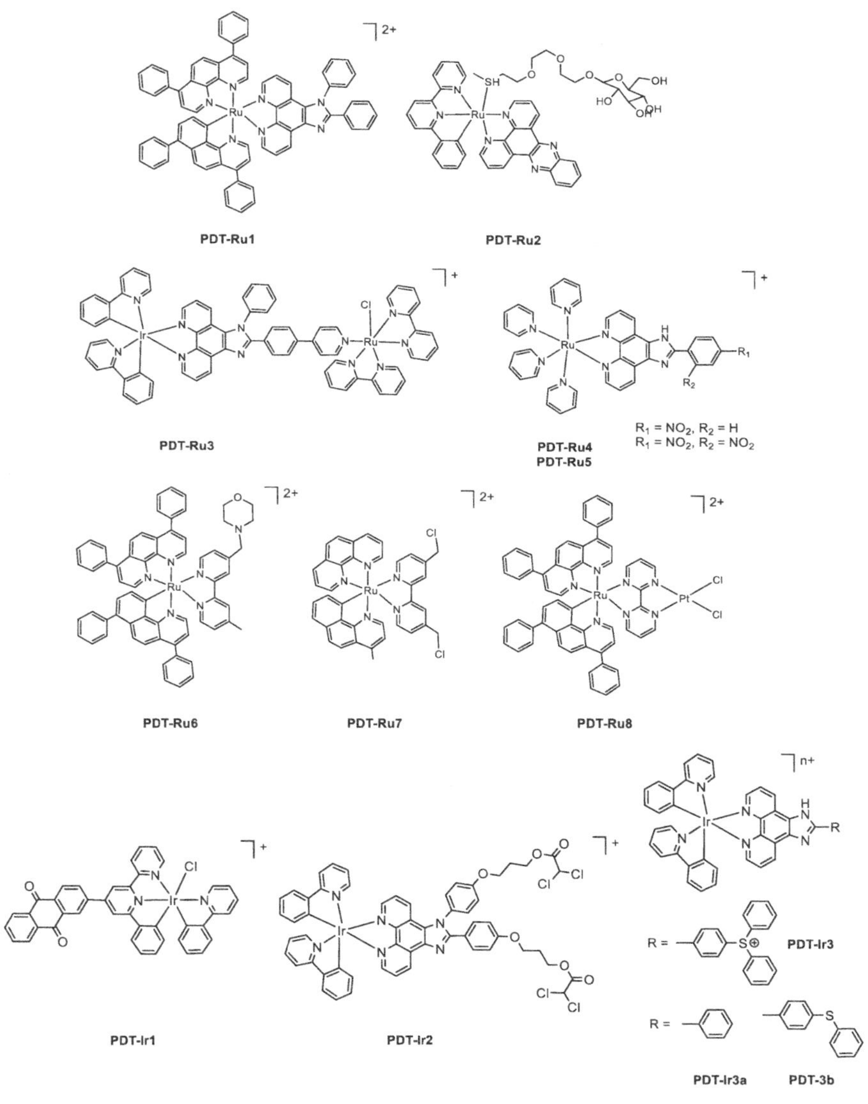

Mitochondria as a Metallo-Drug Target for Therapeutic Purposes

FIGURE 9   Ru(II)- and Ir(III)-based PDT agents.

combine PDT activity and photoactivated chemotherapeutic activity. Besides photostable polypyridyl ligands, they contain photolabile monodentate ligands that are released on illumination enabling covalent binding of Ru(II)polypyridyl to mtDNA. Both **PDT-Ru2** and its photoproduct generate $^1O_2$ that mediates photocleavage of mtDNA [129]. In **PDT-Ru3** an Ir(III)polypyridyl moiety is linked to the Ru(II) center as a mitochondria-directing group and PS. On photoirradiation the Ru-N bond to the pyridyl linker is cleaved. MtDNA damage was confirmed by qPCR and PicoGreen staining, while no damage to nDNA was observed. MtDNA cleavage along with mitochondrial dysfunction trigger apoptosis in cisplatin-resistant A549R cells treated with the complex. **PDT-Ru3** has a phototherapeutic index (ratio of IC_{50} values in the dark and under irradiation) of 25.2 in A549R cells [130]. The dual-mode mechanism of **PDT-Ru4** and **PDT-Ru5** includes coordination to mtDNA following photo-induced dissociation of the monodentate pyridyl ligands and photocatalysis of the oxidation of NADH to NAD^+. NADH depletion combined with mtDNA damage provokes mitochondrial dysfunction [131]. **PDT-Ru6** is an interesting example of a PS owing to its ability to cause stepwise photodamage to the acidic lysosomes and to the more alkaline mitochondria. Because of the ionizable morpholine substituent, the photophysical properties of the complex are pH-dependent. **PDT-Ru6** localizes in the lysosomes first. When the lysosomes are damaged by photo-induced $^1O_2$, the PS is released from the damaged organelles and translocates to the mitochondria where it leads to the loss of mitochondrial integrity and $\Delta\Psi_m$ [132].

Due to the dependence on sufficient O_2 concentrations, PDT is less efficient in hypoxic tumors. The chloromethyl-substituted bipyridine ligand in **PDT-Ru7** undergoes a dehalogenation reduction on irradiation with visible light in the presence of NADH leading to the generation of highly reactive carbon radicals and NADH depletion in the mitochondria. The complex triggers apoptosis in ovarian carcinoma cells under hypoxic conditions [133].

The heterodinuclear Pt, Ru-PS **PDT-Ru8** was shown to bind to mtDNA, to suppress the transcription of mtDNA-encoded genes, and to affect the nucleoid remodeling, amplification, and copy number of mtDNA. Knockdown of mtDNA in HeLa cells reduced the cytotoxicity confirming mtDNA as a primary target. **PDT-Ru8**-mediated PDT led to a reduction in the basal OCR, ATP production, maximum respiration, and non-mitochondrial respiration, to an increase in mitochondrial ROS, G_0/G_1 cell cycle arrest, and caspase-dependent apoptosis. The complex has a low dark toxicity and shows potent *in vivo* activity in a mouse model [134].

Representative examples of Ir-based mitochondria-targeting PSs are displayed in Figure 9. The majority of Ir(III) PSs generate $^1O_2$. **PDT-Ir1** is of special interest, as the reduced form of the anthraquinone pendant presents a photoactivatable carbon radical generator. The reduction of the anthraquinone moiety at low O_2 concentration switches on the two-photon emissive properties of the complex. The complex is thus an efficacious PDT agent under hypoxia. The requirement for hypoxic conditions for the activation makes **PDT-Ir1** highly selective. A phototherapeutic index of 19.4 was determined in A549 cells [135]. In the cyclometalated complex **PDT-Ir2** DCA is conjugated to the diimine ligand via an esterase-labile ester bond. A 33-fold higher photocytotoxicity in cancer cells compared to normal cells was observed. More than 87% of the complex is taken up into the mitochondria. Cells treated with **PDT-Ir2** undergo a metabolic shift from glycolysis to glucose oxidation [136]. The idea of **PDT-Ir3** is to disturb the pH balance of the mitochondria through the use of a photoacid generator. The pendant triphenylsulfonium group is a common functional group in photoacid

Mitochondria as a Metallo-Drug Target for Therapeutic Purposes	95

generators. The complex is highly photocytotoxic in cisplatin-sensitive A549 and cisplatin-resistant A549R cells with phototherapeutic indices of 588 and 583 under hypoxic conditions. Irradiation of **PDT-Ir3** produces photoacid and complexes **PDT-Ir3a** and **3b**. The latter act as $^1O_2$ PSs and reinforce the photodamage to the mitochondria manifested through a decrease in $\Delta\Psi_m$, suppression of ATP synthesis and elevated ROS production [137]. A different type of mitochondria-targeting Ir(III) complex was prepared by the reaction of an aldehyde-functionalized diimine complex with α, ω-diamines followed by reduction of the imine to the amine. The resulting luminescent triple-stranded chiral metallohelicates and achiral mesocates were shown to target mtDNA [138]. In particular, the mesocate derived from 1,5-diaminopentane has a strong affinity for the minor groove of DNA and exerts a strong photocytotoxicity in MCF-7 cells. It was proposed that apoptosis is triggered by $^1O_2$-mediated cleavage of mtDNA. Lee *et al.* used a multifunctional Ir(III) diimine complex containing a hydrophobic energy donor to study oxidative-stress-induced mitochondrial dysfunction and cell death. The complex localizes in the outer surface of the OMM and IMM. Oxidative stress produced by the complex not only affects mitochondrial proteins but also proteins of the ER and peroxisomes that are in contact with the mitochondria. Oxidative stress leads to the crosslinking of proteins and formation of protein aggregates which increases the viscosity of the microenvironment, thus affecting metabolite diffusion which then hinders mitochondrial respiration and metabolism. Furthermore, the oxidation of channel and translocase proteins disturbs the movement of ions and the transport of metabolites. The accumulation of Ca^{2+} ions in the MM opens the MPT pores. The oxidation of mitochondrial and ER proteases and chaperones leads to an accumulation of misfolded or damaged proteins causing mitochondrial fission/fusion and swelling [139].

There are a growing number of cytotoxic Os complexes, some of which were shown to target the mitochondria [32, 140]. A half-sandwich Os(II) complex was reported that represents a photoactivatable anticancer agent that undergoes photodissociation accompanied by oxidation of the Os(II) center to Os(III) under blue UVA light. The complex localizes mainly in the mitochondria in the dark but translocates to the nucleus on irradiation provoking damage of both the mitochondria and nuclear DNA [141].

Difluoro-boraindacene dyes, commonly known as BODIPY dyes, are extensively used in cellular imaging due to their favorable photophysical and photochemical properties and stability in the tumor microenvironment. Furthermore, BODIPY conjugates are well known to accumulate in the mitochondria. The BODIPY entity has been attached to pyridine or imidazole ligands of cationic monofunctional Pt(II) complexes to combine the effects of DNA platination and PDT. Some examples are shown in Figure 10. In addition to acting as dual-action agents, the presence of Pt also enhances the PDT effect of BODIPY. For all compounds preferential uptake into the mitochondria was confirmed. Complexes **PDT-Pt1a-c** are analogs of pyriplatin with a pendant BODIPY group. The complexes have excellent photocytotoxicity in lung cancer (A549), breast cancer (MCF-7), and skin keratinocyte (HaCaT) cells with IC_{50} values in

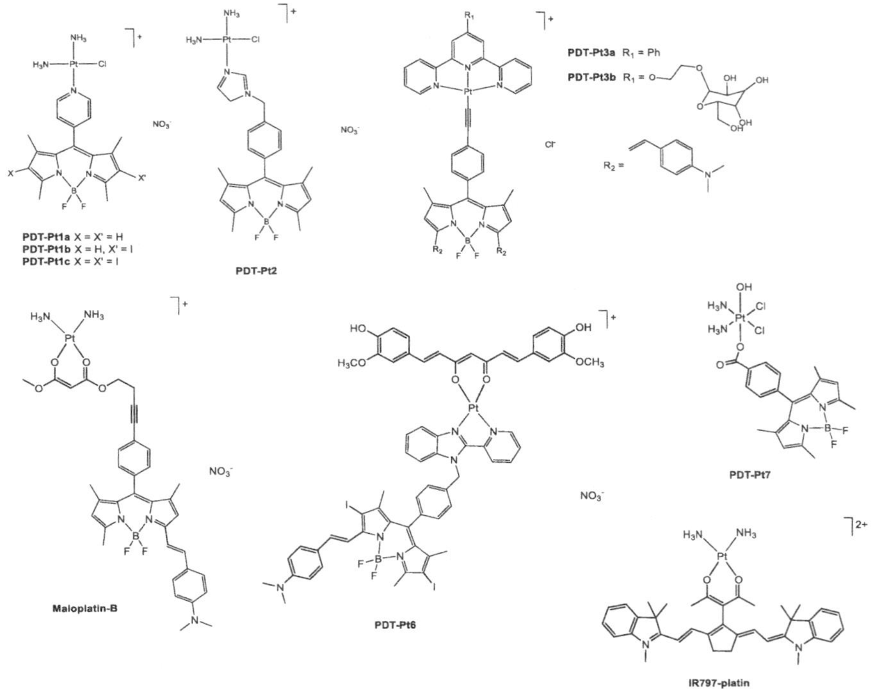

96 Erxleben

FIGURE 10 Pt complexes with pendant photosensitizers.

the 0.05–1.7 µM range, while they are essentially non-toxic in the dark [142]. The heavy atom effect of the iodine substituents in **PDT-Pt1b** and **PDT-Pt1c** increases the $^1O_2$-generating ability of these two complexes. The $^1O_2$-generating ability correlates with the photocytotoxicity. **PDT-Pt1b** is emissive and cellular imaging confirmed its accumulation in the mitochondria. Treated cells lose their $\Delta\Psi_m$ and undergo apoptosis. In the imidazoplatin-BODIPY conjugate **PDT-Pt2** the BODIPY core and Pt-coordinating heterocycle are separated by a CH_2 space which reduces the efficiency of the ISC and thus the quantum yield and ROS formation [143].

The mitochondria-targeting complex **PDT-Pt3b** has been additionally modified with a glucose moiety to enhance the solubility and the general uptake into cancer cells [144]. This resulted in a higher activity in cervical, breast, and lung cancer cells compared to **PDT-Pt3a**. On red light exposure the Pt-C≡CR bond is cleaved and the BODIPY ligand is released. In **Maloplatin-B** a BODIPY-functionalized ligand is attached to a bifunctional Pt(II) complex. The BODIPY group is appended to an *O,O*-donor leaving group ligand allowing the combination of DNA crosslinking and photo-mediated ROS formation. $\Delta\Psi_m$ is affected on irradiation with red light, but not in the dark. Excellent photocytotoxicity in the 650–850 nm window was confirmed in HeLA and A549 cancer cells [145].

Complex **PDT-Pt4** contains curcumin as a second PS. DNA photocleavage studies revealed that the two PSs generate two different types of ROS, $^1O_2$ (BODIPY), and OH (curcumin). **PDT-Pt4** affects $\Delta\Psi_m$ and induces apoptosis via the mitochondrial pathway. The complex accumulates mainly in the ER and causes mitochondrial dysfunction via ER stress [146]. Chakravarty and coworkers combined PDT with the Pt(IV) prodrug approach [147]. **PDT-Pt5** having an axial BODIPY ligand is preferentially taken up by the mitochondria and exerts photocytotoxicity in MCF-7 breast, cervical HeLa, and A549 lung cancer cells with IC_{50} values in the low micromolar range. A different type of PS is used in **IR797-platin**. The cis-Pt(NH$_3$)$_2$$^{2+}$ entity is coordinated to the β-keto-enol group of heptamethine cyanine. Like BODIPY, heptamethine cyanine dyes localize preferentially in the mitochondria. **IR797-platin** generates $^1O_2$ and releases cis-[Pt(NH$_3$)$_2$(H$_2$O)$_2$]$^{2+}$ on illumination with near-IR light giving rise to submicromolar IC_{50} values. Confocal microscopy showed the accumulation of **IR797-platin** in the mitochondria and lysosomes [148].

6 CONCLUDING REMARKS AND PERSPECTIVES

Owing to the central role of nDNA in the mode of action of the blockbuster metallo-drug cisplatin, the design of new metallo-drugs has long been guided by metal complex DNA interactions. However, in recent years the role of signaling pathways and cellular stressors other than DNA damage in the mechanisms of anticancer metallo-drugs has come more and more into focus. The examples discussed in this chapter are clear evidence that mitochondria-targeting metallo-drugs are an effective strategy for chemotherapy. Agents that disrupt the mitochondrial bioenergetics and redox homeostasis offer the unique opportunity to bypass resistance mechanisms and many of the described antimitochondrial metal complexes are highly potent in cisplatin-resistant cancer cell lines. Due to the altered mitochondrial metabolism in cancer cells, antimitochondrial metallo-drugs possess an inherent selectivity. Their mechanisms are complex and varied but all converge on the induction of mitochondrial dysfunction-mediated cell death pathways. While mitochondria-targeting metallo-drugs are a promising class of chemotherapeutic drugs, there are a number of challenges to be met before their clinical translation: Many antimitochondrial metal complexes are cationic. The positive charge that facilitates accumulation in the mitochondria also promotes the interaction with negatively charged proteins, thus reducing the targeting efficiency. Moreover, mitochondria-targeting metallo-drugs can still accumulate in healthy cells where off-target binding can cause side effects. Dissociation of the ligands or exchange of the ligands with blood serum thiols can lead to premature drug loss and excretion *in vivo*. Future work should therefore focus on effective strategies for the delivery of antimitochondrial agents to cancer tissue. Other important future directions are multi-targeting antimitochondrial metal complexes, e.g., metal complexes that simultaneously act on the mitochondria and the nucleus. A small number of such dual-target agents have been discussed in this chapter, but this is certainly an avenue that should be pursued further.

In particular, paraptosis-inducing metallo-drugs that target both the mitochondria and the ER are of interest as an approach to tackle resistance to apoptosis. There is significant elevated protein folding activity in the ER of rapidly proliferating cells and the ER of cancer cells is already under stress.

In conclusion, there is no doubt that mitochondria-targeting metallo-drugs for therapeutic purposes will remain an active field of research in the foreseeable future.

ACKNOWLEDGMENTS

This review was supported in part by grants from Science Foundation Ireland (12/RC/2275) and the European Commission (REP-749621-1, PIEF-GA-2011–298099).

ABBREVIATIONS

AIF	apoptosis-inducing factor
ATP	adenosine triphosphate
BODIPY	difluoro-boraindacene
DCA	dichloroacetate
$\Delta\Psi_m$	mitochondrial transmembrane potential
dGTP	deoxyguanosine triphosphate
dien	diethylenetriamine
ECAR	extracellular acidification rate
ER	endoplasmic reticulum
ETC	electron transport chain
FADH$_2$	dihydroflavine-adenine dinucleotide
dApG	2′-deoxyadenyl(3′→5′)-2′-deoxyguanosine
dGpG	2′-deoxyguanylyl(3′→5′)-2′-deoxyguanosine
GSH	glutathione
GPX4	glutathione peroxidase 4
HDAC	histone deacetylase
ICP-MS	inductively coupled plasma mass spectrometry
IMM	inner mitochondrial membrane
IMS	intermembrane space
ISC	intersystem crossing
$\log P_{o/w}$	octanol-water partition coefficient
MALDI-TOF	matrix-assisted laser desorption/ionization-time of flight
MM	mitochondrial matrix
MMP	mitochondrial membrane permeabilization
MOMP	mitochondrial outer membrane permeabilization
MPT	mitochondrial permeability transition
mtDNA	mitochondrial DNA
NADH	reduced nicotinamide adenine dinucleotide
NADPH	reduced nicotinamide adenine dinucleotide phosphate
nDNA	nuclear DNA

Mitochondria as a Metallo-Drug Target for Therapeutic Purposes

NHC	*N*-heterocyclic carbene
OCR	O_2 consumption rate
OMM	outer mitochondrial membrane
OXPHOS	oxidative phosphorylation
PDK	pyruvate dehydrogenase kinase
PDT	photodynamic therapy
PS	photosensitizer
PTA	1,3,5-triaza-7-phosphaadamantane
qPCR	quantitative polymerase chain reaction
ROS	reactive oxygen species
SAHA	suberoylanilide hydroxamic acid
TEM	transmission electron microscopy
terpy	terpyridine
α-toc	α-tocopherol succinate
TPP	triphenylphosphonium
Trx	thioredoxin
TrxR	thioredoxin reductase
TSPO	translocator protein 18 kDa

REFERENCES

[1] T. G. Frey, C. A. Mannella, *Trends Biochem. Sci.* **2000**, *25*, 319–324.

[2] J.-W. Taanman, *Biochim. Biophys. Acta* **1999**, *1410*, 103–123.

[3] S. Y. Jeong, D. W. Seol, *BMB Rep.* **2008**, *41*, 11–22.

[4] C. Tian, Y. Liu, Z. Li, P. Zhu, M. Zhao, *Front. Cell Dev. Biol.* **2022**, *10*, 832356.

[5] E. Kim, D. M. Lee, M. J. Seo, H. J. Lee, K. S. Choi, *Front. Cell. Dev. Biol.* **2021**, *8*, 607844.

[6] Q. Han, Y. Ma, H. Wang, Y. Dai, C. Chen, Y. Liu, L. Jing, X. Sun, *J. Trans. Med.* **2018**, *16*, 201.

[7] S. R. Pieczenik, J. Neustadt, *Exp. Mol. Pathol.* **2007**, *83*, 84–92.

[8] D. C. Wallace, D. Chalkia, *Cold Spring Harb. Perspect. Biol.* **2013**, *5*, a021220.

[9] K. Szczepanowska, A. Trifunovic, *Essays Biochem.* **2017**, *61*, 325–337.

[10] R. Shi, M. Guberman, L. A. Kirshenbaum, *Trends Cardiovasc. Med.* **2018**, *28*, 246–260.

[11] X. J. Chen, R. A. Butow, *Nat. Rev. Genet.* **2005**, *6*, 815–825.

[12] C. Kukat, C. A. Wurm, H. Spahr, M. Falkenberg, N. G. Larsson, S. Jakobs, *Proc. Natl. Acad. Sci. U.S.A.* **2011**, *108*, 13534–13539.

[13] B. Bandy, A. J. Davison, *Free Radic. Biol. Med.* **1990**, *8*, 523–539.

[14] W. Linnane, S. Marzuki, T. Ozawa, M. Tanaka, *Lancet* **1989**, *1*, 642–645.

[15] L. Tilokani, S. Nagashima, V. Paupe, J. Prudent, *Essays Biochem.* **2018**, *62*, 341–360.

[16] A. M. Bertholet, A. Delerue, A. M. Millet, M. F. Moulis, C. David, M. Daloyau, L. Arnauné-Pelloquin, N. Davezac, V. Mils, M. C. Miquel, M. Rojo, P. Belenguer, *Neurobiol. Dis.* **2016**, *90*, 3–19.

[17] L. Galluzzi, E. Morselli, O. Kepp, I. Vitale, A. Rigoni, E. Vacchelli, M. Michaud, H. Zischka, M. Castedo, G. Kroemer, *Mol. Aspects Med.* **2010**, *31*, 1–20.

[18] P. E. Porporato, N. Filigheddu, J. M. Bravo-San Pedro, G. Kroemer, L. Galluzzi, *Cell Res.* **2018**, *28*, 265–280.

[19] O. Warburg, *Science* **1956**, *123*, 309–314.

[20] F. Marcucci, C. Rumio, *Neoplasia* **2021**, *23*, 234–245.

[21] M. A. Nieto, R. Y. Huang, R. A. Jackson, J. P. Thiery, *Cell* **2016**, *166*, 21–45.

[22] W.-X. Zong, J. D. Rabinowitz, E. White, *Mol. Cell* **2016**, *61*, 667–676.

[23] J. Neuzil, L. F. Dong, J. Rohlena, J. Truksa, S. J. Ralph, *Mitochondrion* **2013**, *13*, 199–208.

[24] K. Klein, K. He, A. I. Younes, H. B. Barsoumian, D. Chen, T. Ozgen, S. Mosaffa, R. R. Patel, M. Gu, J. Novaes, A. Narayanan, M. A. Cortez, J. W. Welsh, *Front. Immunol.* **2020**, *11*, 573326.

[25] D. T. Lincoln, E. M. Ali Emadi, K. F. Tonissen, F. M. Clarke, *Anticancer Res.* **2003**, *23(3B)*, 2425–2433.

[26] S. Galiegue, N. Tinel, P. Casellas, *Curr. Med. Chem.* **2003**, *10*, 1563–1572.

[27] D. Decaudin, M. Castedo, F. Nemati, A. Beurdeley-Thomas, G. De Pinieux, A. Caron, P. Pouillart, J. Wijdenes, D. Rouillard, G. Kroemer, M. F. Poupon, *Cancer Res.* **2002**, *62*, 1388–1393.

[28] Z. Han, R. S. Slack, W. Li, V. Papadopoulos, *J. Recept. Signal Transduct. Res.* **2003**, *23*, 225–238.

[29] A. Erxleben, *Curr. Med. Chem.* **2019**, *26*, 694–728.

[30] D. Proefrock, A. Prange, *Appl. Spectrosc.* **2012**, *66*, 843–868.

[31] B. Chazotte, *Cold Spring Harb. Protoc.* **2011**, *8*, 990–992.

[32] C. Sanchez-Cano, I. Romero-Canelon, Y. Yang, I. J. Hands-Portman, S. Bohic, P. Cloetens, P. J. Sadler, *Chem. Eur. J.* **2017**, *23*, 2512–2516.

[33] F. Sivandzade, A. Bhalerao, L. Cucullo, *Bio Protoc.* **2019**, *9*, e3128.

[34] N. Ashley, D. Harris, J. Poulton, *Exp. Cell Res.* **2005**, *303*, 432–446.

[35] J. Zielonka, J. Joseph, A. Sikora, M. Hardy, O. Ouari, J. Vasquez-Vivar, G. Cheng, M. Lopez, B. Kalyanaraman, *Chem. Rev.* **2017**, *117*, 10043–10120.

[36] H. Cho, Y.-Y. Cho, M. S. Shim, J. Y. Lee, H. S. Lee, H. C. Kang, *Biochim. Biophys. Acta Mol. Basis Dis.* **2020**, *1866*, 165808.

[37] N. Jiang, J. Fan, T. Liu, J. Cao, B. Qiao, J. Wang, P. Gao, X. Peng, *Chem. Commun.* **2013**, *49*, 10620–10622.

[38] M. T. Jeena, S. Kim, S. Jin, J.-H. Ryu, *Cancers* **2020**, *12*, 4.

[39] G. Battogtokh, Y.-Y. Cho, J. Y. Lee, H. S. Lee, H. C. Kang, *Front. Pharmacol.* **2018**, *9*, 922.

[40] K. Kohno, T. Uchiumi, I. Niina, T. Wakasugi, T. Igarashi, Y. Momii, T. Yoshida, K. Matsuo, N. Miyamoto, H. Izumi, *Eur. J. Cancer* **2005**, *41*, 2577–2586.

[41] O. A. Olivero, C. Semino, A. Kassim, D. M. Lopez-Larraza, M. C. Poirier, *Mutat. Res.* **1995**, *346*, 221–230.

[42] K. J. Cullen, Z. Yang, L. Schumaker, Z. Guo, *J. Bioenerg. Biomembr.* **2007**, *39*, 43–50.

[43] J. X. Ong, H. V. Le, V. E. Y. Lee, W. H. Ang, *Angew. Chem. Int. Ed.* **2021**, *60*, 9264–9269.

[44] L. Zhao, Q. Cheng, Z. Wang, Z. Xi, D. Xu, Y. Liu, *Chem. Comm.* **2014**, *50*, 2667–2669.

[45] Y. Guo, Y. He, S. Wu, S. Zhang, D. Song, Z. Zhu, Z. Guo, X. Wang, *Inorg. Chem.* **2019**, *58*, 13150–13160.

[46] K.-C. Tong, P.-K. Wan, C.-N. Lok, C.-M. Che, *Chem. Sci.* **2021**, *12*, 15229–15238.

[47] M. Hyeraci, M. Colalillo, L. Labella, F. Marchetti, S. Samaritani, V. Scalcon, M. P. Rigobello, L. Dalla Via, *ChemMedChem* **2020**, *15*, 1464–1472.

[48] Z. Zhu, C. Wang, C. Zhang, Y. Wang, H. Zhang, Z. Gan, Z. Guo, X. Wang, *Chem. Sci.* **2019**, *10*, 3089–3095.

[49] S. Marrache, P. K. Pathak, S. Dhar, *Proc. Natl. Acad. Sci. USA* **2014**, *111*, 10444–10449.

Mitochondria as a Metallo-Drug Target for Therapeutic Purposes   101

[50] S. Jin, Y. Hao, Z. Zhu, N. Muhammad, Z. Zhang, K. Wang, Y. Guo, Z. Guo, X. Wang, *Inorg. Chem.* **2018**, *57*, 11135–11145.

[51] S. P. Wisnovsky, J. J. Wilson, R. J. Radford, M. P. Pereira, M. R. Chan, R. R. Laposa, S. J. Lippard, S. O. Kelley, *Chem. Biol.* **2013**, *20*, 1323–1328.

[52] P. Lunetti, A. Romano, C. Carrisi, D. Antonucci, T. Verri, G. E. De Benedetto, V. Dolce, F. P. Fanizzi, M. Benedetti, L. Capabianco, *ChemistrySelect* **2016**, *1*, 4633–4637.

[53] C. Ouyang, L. Chen, T. W. Rees, Y. Chen, J. Liu, L. Ji, J. Long, H. Chao, *Chem. Commun.* **2018**, *54*, 6268–6271.

[54] Z. Deng, C. Li, S. Chen, Q. Zhou, Z. Xu, Z. Wang, H. Yao, H. Hirao, G. Zhu, *Chem. Sci.* **2021**, *12*, 6536–6542.

[55] S. Dhar, S. J. Lippard, *Proc. Natl. Acad. Sci. USA* **2009**, *106*, 22199–22204.

[56] P. W. Stacpole, *Metab. Clin. Exp.* **1989**, *38*, 1124–1144.

[57] X. Xue, S. You, Q. Zhang, Y. Wu, G.-z. Zou, P. C. Wang, Y.-l. Zhao, Y. Xu, L. Jia, X. Zhang, X.-J. Liang, *Mol. Pharmaceutics* **2012**, *9*, 634–644.

[58] J. Zajak, H. Kostrhunova, V. Novohradsky, O. Vrana, R. Raveendran, D. Gibson, J. Kasparkova, V. Brabec, *J. Inorg. Biochem.* **2016**, *156*, 89–97.

[59] S. Jin, Y. Guo, D. Song, Z. Zhu, Z. Zhang, Y. Sun, T. Yang, Z. Guo, X. Wang, *Inorg. Chem.* **2019**, *58*, 6507–6516.

[60] M. V. Babak, Y. Zhi, B. Czarny, T. B. Toh, L. Hooi, E. K.-H. Chow, W. H. Ang, D. Gibson, G. Pastorin, *Angew. Chem. Int. Ed.* **2019**, *58*, 8109–8114.

[61] K. Suntharalingam, Y. Song, S. J. Lippard, *Chem. Commun.* **2014**, *50*, 2465–2468.

[62] A. Mallick, P. More, S. Ghosh, R. Chippalkatti, B. A. Chopade, M. Lahiri, S. Basu, *ACS Appl. Mater. Interfaces* **2015**, *7*, 7584–7598.

[63] H. Chen, F. Chen, W. Hu, S. Gou, *J. Inorg. Biochem.* **2018**, *180*, 119–129.

[64] N. Denora, R. M. Iacobazzi, G. Natile, N. Margiotta, *Coord. Chem. Rev.* **2017**, *341*, 1–18.

[65] L. Tabrizi, K. Thompson, K. Mnich, C. Chintha, A. Gorman, L. Morrison, J. Luessing, N. Lowndes, P. Dockery, A. Samali, A. Erxleben, *Mol. Pharmaceutics* **2020**, *7*, 3009–3023.

[66] K. Becker, C. Herold-Mende, J. J. Park, G. Lowe, R. H. Schirmer, *J. Med. Chem.* **2001**, *44*, 2784–2792.

[67] K. Wang, C. Zhu, Y. He, Z. Zhang, W. Zhou, N. Muhammad, Y. Guo, X. Wang, Z. Guo, *Angew. Chem. Int. Ed.* **2019**, *58*, 4638–4643.

[68] D. Tolan, V. Gandin, L. Morrison, A. El-Nahas, C. Marzano, D. Montagner, A. Erxleben, *Sci. Rep.* **2016**, *6*, 29367.

[69] L. Dalla Via, S. Santi, V. Di Noto, A. Venzo, E. Agostinelli, A. Calcabrini, M. Condello, A. Toninello, *J. Biol. Inorg. Chem.* **2011**, *16*, 695–713.

[70] C. Icsel, V. T. Yilmaz, B. Cevatemre, M. Aygun, E. Ulukaya, *J. Biol. Inorg. Chem.* **2020**, *25*, 75–87.

[71] Y. Guo, S. Jin, H. Yuan, T. Yang, K. Wang, Z. Guo, X. Wang, *J. Med. Chem.* **2022**, *65*, 520–530.

[72] A. Bindoli, M. P. Rigobello, G. Scutari, C. Gabbiani, A. Casini, L. Messori, *Coord. Chem. Rev.* **2009**, *253*, 1692–1707.

[73] C. Gabbiani, G. Mastrobuoni, F. Sorrentino, B. Dani, M. P. Rigobello, A. Bindoli, M. A. Cinellu, G. Pieraccini, L. Messori, A. Casini, *Med. Chem. Commun.* **2011**, *2*, 50–54.

[74] A. Meyer, C. P. Bagowski, M. Kokoschka, M. Stefanopoulou, H. Alborzinia, S. Can, D. H. Vlecken, W. S. Sheldrick, S. Wölfl, I. Ott, *Angew. Chem. Int. Ed.* **2012**, *51*, 8895–8899.

[75] P. Hikisz, L. Szczupak, A. Koceva-Chyla, A. Guspiel, L. Oehninger, I. Ott, B. Therrien, J. Solecka, K. Kowalski, *Molecules* **2015**, *20*, 19699–19718.

[76] F. H. Abdalbari, C. M. Telleria, *Discov. Onc.* **2021**, *12*, : 42.

[77] M. P. Rigobello, G. Scutari, R. Boscolo, A. Bindoli, *Br. J. Pharmacol.* **2002**, *136*, 1162–1168.

[78] G. Cox, K. K. Brown, E. S. J. Arner, M. B. Hampton, *Biochem. Pharmacology* **2008**, *76*, 1097–1109.

[79] T. Gamberi, T. Fiaschi, A. Modesti, L. Massai, L. Messori, M. Balzi, F. Magherini, *Int. J. Biochem. Cell. Biol.* **2015**, *65*, 61–71.

[80] P. J. Barnard, S. J. Berners-Price, *Coord. Chem. Rev.* **2007**, *251*, 1889–1902.

[81] J.-J. Zhang, M. A. Abu el Maaty, H. Hofmeister, C. Schmidt, J. K. Muenzner, R. Schobert, S. Wölfl, I. Ott, *Angew. Chem. Int. Ed.* **2020**, *59*, 16795–16800.

[82] I. Marmol, M. Virumbrales-Munoz, J. Quero, C. Sanchez-de-Diego, L. Fernandez, I. Ochoa, E. Cerrada, M. J. R. Yoldi, *J. Inorg. Biochem.* **2017**, *176*, 123–133.

[83] L. Vela, M. Contel, L. Palomera, G. Azaceta, I. Marzo, *J. Inorg. Biochem.* **2011**, *105*, 1306–1313.

[84] K.-B. Huang, F.-Y. Wang, X.-M. Tang, H.-W. Feng, Z.-F. Chen, Y.-C. Liu, Y.-N. Liu, H. Liang, *J. Med. Chem.* **2018**, *61*, 3478–3490.

[85] P. J. Barnard, M. V. Baker, S. J. Berners-Price, D. A. Day, *J. Inorg. Biochem.* **2004**, *98*, 1642–1647.

[86] R. Rubbiani, I. Kitanovic, H. Alborzinia, S. Can, A. Kitanovic, L. A. Onambele, M. Stefanopoulou, Y. Geldmacher, W. S. Sheldrick, G. Wolber, A. Prokop, S. Wölfl, I. Ott, *J. Med. Chem.* **2010**, *53*, 8608–8616.

[87] F. Magherini, T. Fiaschi, E. Valocchia, M. Becatti, A. Pratesi, T. Marzo, L. Massai, C. Gabbiani, I. Landini, S. Nobili, E. Mini, L. Messori, A. Modesti, T. Gamberi, *Oncotarget* **2018**, *9*, 28042–28068.

[88] A. Nandy, S. K. Dey, S. Das, R. N. Munda, J. Dinda, K. D. Saha, *Mol. Cancer* **2014**, *13*, 57.

[89] T. Zou, C. T. Lum, C.-N. Lok, W.-P. To, K.-H. Low, C.-M. Che, *Angew. Chem. Int. Ed.* **2014**, *53*, 5810–5814.

[90] T. Zou, C. T. Lum, S. S.-Y. Chui, C.-M. Che, *Angew. Chem. Int. Ed.* **2013**, *52*, 2930–2933.

[91] R.W.-Y. Sun, C. K.-L. Li, D.-L. Ma, J. J. Yan, C.-N. Lok, C.-H. Leung, N. Zhu, C. M. Che, *Chem. Eur. J.* **2010**, *16*, 3097–3113.

[92] L. He, T. Chen, Y. You, H. Hu, W. Zheng, W.-L. Kwong, T. Zou, C.-M. Che, *Angew. Chem. Int. Ed.* **2014**, *53*, 12532–12536.

[93] D. Hu, Y. Liu, Y-T. Lai, K.-C. Tong, Y.-M. Fung, C.-N. Lok, C.-M. Che, *Angew. Chem. Int. Ed.* **2016**, *55*, 1387–1391.

[94] C.-M. Che, R.W.-Y. Sun, W.-Y. Yu, C.-B. Ko, N. Zhu, H. Sun, *Chem. Commun.* **2003**, 1718–1719.

[95] Y. Wang, Q. Y. He, R. W.-Y. Sun, C.-M. Che, J.-F. Chiu, *Cancer Res.* **2005**, *65*, 11553–11564.

[96] C. T. Lum, R. W.-Y. Sun, T. Zou, C.-M. Che, *Chem. Sci.* **2014**, *5*, 1579–1584.

[97] C. T. Lum, A. S.-T. Wong, M. C. M. Lin, C.-M. Che, R. W.-Y. Sun, *Chem. Commun.* **2013**, *49*, 4364–4366.

[98] S. D. Köster, H. Alborzinia, S. Can, I. Kitanovic, S. Wölfl, R. Rubbiani, I. Ott, P. Riesterer, A. Prokop, K. Merz, N. Metzler-Nolte, *Chem. Sci.* **2012**, *3*, 2062–2072.

[99] K. E. Erkkila, D. T. Odom, J. K. Barton, *Chem. Rev.* **1999**, *99*, 2777–2796.

[100] V. Pierroz, T. Joshi, A. Leonidova, C. Mari, J. Schur, I. Ott, L. Spiccia, S. Ferrari, G. Gasser, *J. Am. Chem. Soc.* **2012**, *134*, 20376–20387.

[101] T. Joshi, V. Pierroz, S. Ferrari, G. Gasser, *ChemMedChem* **2014**, *9*, 1419–1427.

[102] L. Zeng, Y. Chen, J. Liu, H. Huang, R. Guan, L. Ji, H. Chao, *Sci. Rep.* **2016**, *6*, 19449.

Mitochondria as a Metallo-Drug Target for Therapeutic Purposes 103

[103] T. Chen, Y. Liu, W.-J. Zheng, J. Liu, Y.-S. Wong, *Inorg. Chem.* **2010**, *49*, 6366–6368.

[104] X. Yang, L. Chen, Y. Liu, Y. Yang, T. Chen, W. Zheng, J. Liu, Q.-Y. He, *Biochimie* **2012**, *94*, 345–353.

[105] L. He, K. Xiong, L. Wang, R. Guan, Y. Chen, L. Ji, H. Chao, *Chem. Commun.* **2021**, *57*, 8308–8311.

[106] N. Roy, U. Sen, S. R. Chaudhuri, V. Muthukumar, P. Moharana, P. Paira, B. Bose, A. Gauthaman, A. Moorthy, *Dalton Trans.* **2021**, *50*, 2268–2283.

[107] J.-J. Cao, C.-P. Tan, M.-H. Chen, N. Wu, D.-Y. Yao, X.-G. Liu, L.-N. Ji, Z.-W. Mao, *Chem. Sci.* **2017**, *8*, 631–640.

[108] M.-H. Chen, F.-X. Wang, J.-J. Cao, C.-P. Tan, L.-N. Ji, Z.-W. Mao, *ACS Appl. Mater. Interfaces* **2017**, *9*, 13304–13314.

[109] J.-J. Cao, Y. Zheng, X.-W. Wu, C.-P. Tan, M.-H. Chen, N. Wu, L.-N. Ji, Z.-W. Mao, *J. Med. Chem.* **2019**, *62*, 3311–3322.

[110] N. Roy, U. Sen, Y. Madaan, V. Methukumar, S. Varddhan, S. K. Sahoo, D. Panda, B. Bose, P. Paira, *Inorg. Chem.* **2020**, *59*, 17689–17711.

[111] F.-X. Wang, J.-H. Liang, H. Zhang, Z.-H. Wang, Q. Wan, C.-P. Tan, L.-N. Ji, Z.-W. Mao, *ACS Appl. Mater. Interfaces* **2019**, *11*, 13123–13133.

[112] J. Yang, Q. Cao, H. Zhang, L. Hao, D. Zhou, Z. Gan, Z. Li, Y.-X. Tong, L.-N. Ji, Z.-W. Mao, *Biomaterials* **2018**, *176*, 94–105.

[113] R.-R. Ye, B.-C. Chen, J.-J. Lu, X.-R. Ma, R.-T. Li, *J. Inorg. Biochem.* **2021**, *223*, 111537.

[114] R.-R. Ye, C.-P. Tan, Y.-N. Lin, L.-N. Ji, Z.-W. Mao, *Chem. Commun.* **2015**, *51*, 8353–8356.

[115] S. Imstepf, V. Pierroz, R. Rubbiani, M. Felber, T. Fox, G. Gasser, R. Alberto, *Angew. Chem. Int. Ed.* **2016**, *55*, 2792–2795.

[116] Z.-Y. Pan, C.-P. Tan, L.-S. Rao, H. Zhang, Y. Zheng, L. Hao, L.-N. Ji, Z.-W. Mao, *Angew. Chem. Int. Ed.* **2020**, *59*, 18755–18762.

[117] C. Santini, M. Pellei, V. Gandin, M. Porchia, F. Tisato, C. Marzano, *Chem. Rev.* **2014**, *114*, 815–862.

[118] New Cancer Drug Called Casiopeínas Tested at Phase I Clinical Trials, Source: Information Agency CONACYT – http://www.salud.carlosslim.org/english2/new-cancer-drug-called-casiopeinas-tested-at-phase-i-clinical-trials/ 2nd March 2017.

[119] A. Marin-Hernandez, I. Gracia-Mora, L. Ruiz-Ramirez, R. Moreno-Sanchez, *Biochem. Pharmacol.* **2003**, *65*, 1979–1989.

[120] K. Y. Djoko, P. S. Donnelly, A. G. McEwan, *Metallomics* **2014**, *6*, 2250–2259.

[121] Y. Guo, M. Chen, S. Li, J. Deng, J. Li, G. Fang, F. Yang, G. Huang, *J. Med. Chem.* **2021**, *64*, 5485–5499.

[122] G. Filomeni, S. Piccirillo, I. Graziani, S. Cardaci, A. M. Da Costa Ferreira, G. Rotilio, M. R. Ciriolo, *Carcinogenesis* **2009**, *30*, 1115–1124.

[123] W. Zhou, X. Wang, M. Hu, C. Zhu, Z. Guo, *Chem. Sci.* **2014**, *5*, 2761–2770.

[124] J. Shao, M. Li, Z. Guo, C. Jin, F. Zhang, C. Ou, Y. Xie, S. Tan, Z. Wang, S. Zheng, X. Wang, *Cell Commun. Signal.* **2019**, *17*, 19.

[125] X. Li, S. Hao, A. Han, Y. Yang, G. Fang, J. Liu, S. Wang, *J. Mater. Chem. B* **2019**, *7*, 4008–4016.

[126] D. Montagner, B. Fresch, K. Browne, V. Gandin, A. Erxleben, *Chem. Commun.* **2017**, *53*, 134–137.

[127] S. Monro, K. L. Colon, H. Yin, J. Roque, III, P. Konda, S. Gujar, R. P. Thummel, L. Lilge, C. G. Cameron, S. A. McFarland, *Chem. Rev.* **2019**, *119*, 797–828.

[128] J. Liu, Y. Chen, G. Li, P. Zhang, C. Jin, L. Zeng, L. Ji, H. Chao, *Biomaterials* **2015**, *56*, 140–153.

[129] L. N. Lameijer, S. L. Hopkins, T. G. Breve, S. H. C. Askes, S. Bonnet, *Chem. Eur. J.* **2016**, *22*, 18484–18491.

[130] C. Zhang, R. Guan, X. Liao, C. Ouyang, T. W. Rees, J. Liu, Y. Chen, L. Ji, H. Chao, *Chem. Commun.* **2019**, *55*, 12547–12550.

[131] S. Qi, Z. Jin, Y. Jian, Y. Hou, C. Li, Y. Zhao, X. Wang, Q. Zhou, *Chem. Commun.* **2021**, *57*, 4162–4166.

[132] K. Qiu, Y. Wen, C. Ouyang, X. Liao, C. Liu, T. W. Rees, Q. Zhang, L. Ji, H. Chao, *Chem. Commun.* **2019**, *55*, 11235–11238.

[133] N. Tian, W. Sun, X. Guo, J. Lu, C. Li, Y. Hou, X. Wang, Q. Zhou, *Chem. Commun.* **2019**, *55*, 2676–2679.

[134] Y. Zheng, D.-Y. Zhang, H. Zhang, J.-J. Cao, C.-P. Tan, L.-N. Ji, Z.-W. Mao, *Chem. Eur. J.* **2018**, *24*, 18971–18980.

[135] S. Kuang, L. Sun, X. Zhang, X. Liao, T. W. Rees, L. Zeng, Y. Chen, X. Zhang, L. Ji, H. Chao, *Angew. Chem. Int. Ed.* **2020**, *59*, 20697–20703.

[136] J. Liu, C. Jin, B. Yuan, Y. Chen, X. Liu, L. Ji, H. Chao, *Chem. Commun.* **2017**, *53*, 9878–9881.

[137] L. He, M.-F. Zhang, Z.-Y. Pan, K.-N. Wang, Z.-J. Zhao, Y. Li, Z.-W. Mao, *Chem. Commun.* **2019**, *55*, 10472–10475.

[138] X. Li, J. Wu, L. Wang, C. He, L. Chen, Y. Jiao, C. Duan, *Angew. Chem. Int. Ed.* **2020**, *59*, 6420–6427.

[139] C. Lee, J. S. Nam, C. G. Lee, M. Park, C.-M. Yoo, H.-W. Rhee, J. K. Seo, T.-H. Kwon, *Nat. Commun.* **2021**, *12*, 26.

[140] M. Ye, W.-Q. Huang, Z.-X. Li, C.-X. Wang, T. Liu, Y. Z. Chen, C. H.-H. Hor, W.-L. Man, W.-X. Ni, *Chem. Commun.* **2022**, *58*, 2468–2471.

[141] X. Xue, Y. Fu, L. He, L. Salassa, L.-F. He, Y.-Y. Hao, M. J. Koh, C. Soulie, R. J. Needham, A. Habtemariam, C. Garino, K. A. Lomachenko, Z. Su, Y. Qian, M. J. Paterson, Z.-W. Mao, H.-K. Liu, P. J. Sadler, *Inorg. Chem.* **2021**, *60*, 17450–17461.

[142] M. K. Raza, S. Gautam, P. Howlader, A. Bhattacharyya, P. Kondaia, *Inorg. Chem.* **2018**, *57*, 14374–14385.

[143] M. K. Raza, S. Gautam, A. Garai, K. Mitra, P. Kondaia, *Inorg. Chem.* **2017**, *56*, 11019–11029.

[144] V. Ramu, S. Gautam, A. Garai, P. Kondaiah, A. R. Chakravarty, *Inorg. Chem.* **2018**, *57*, 1717–1726.

[145] V. Ramu, P. Kundu, P. Kondaiah, A. R. Chakravarty, *Inorg. Chem.* **2021**, *60*, 6410–6420.

[146] Upadhyay, P. Kundu, V. Ramu, P. Kondaiah, A. R. Chakravarty, *Inorg. Chem.* **2022**, *61*, 1335–1348.

[147] A. Bera, S. Gautam, M. K. Raza, P. Kondaiah, A. R. Chakravarty, *J. Inorg. Biochem.* **2021**, *223*, 11526.

[148] K. Mitra, C. E. Lyons, M. C. T. Hartman, *Angew. Chem. Int. Ed.* **2018**, *57*, 10263–10267.

4 Transition Metal-Based Antiviral Agents Against SARS-CoV-2 and Other Pathogenic Viruses

Maria Gil-Moles

Institute of Medicinal and Pharmaceutical Chemistry
Technische Universität Braunschweig, Beethovenstr. 55
D-38106 Braunschweig, Germany
Departamento de Química, Universidad de La Rioja
Centro de Investigación de Síntesis Química (CISQ),
Complejo Científico Tecnológico, ES- 26004 Logroño, Spain

Ingo Ott*

Institute of Medicinal and Pharmaceutical Chemistry
Technische Universität Braunschweig, Beethovenstr. 55
D-38106 Braunschweig, Germany
ingo.ott@tu-braunschweig.de

CONTENTS

1 Introduction 106
2 Background on Metal-Based Antiviral Agents 107
    2.1 Pathogenic Viruses with Relevance for Metal-Based Antiviral Agents 107
    2.2 Antiviral Drug Targets of Relevance for Metal-Based Compounds 108
3 Period 4 Metal-Based Antiviral Agents 109
    3.1 Scandium to Iron in Antiviral Metal Complexes 109
    3.2 Cobalt Complexes as Antiviral Agents 112
    3.3 Nickel Complexes as Antiviral Agents 113
    3.4 Copper Complexes as Antiviral Agents 114
    3.5 Zinc Complexes as Antiviral Agents 115
        3.5.1 Zinc Complexes Against Different Viruses 116
        3.5.2 Antiviral Properties of Zinc Against Respiratory Viruses 117

---

*Corresponding author

DOI: 10.1201/9781003272250-4

| 4 | Period 5 Metal-Based Antiviral Agents | 119 |

4 Period 5 Metal-Based Antiviral Agents 119
   4.1   Yttrium to Technetium in Antiviral Metal Complexes 119
   4.2   Ruthenium, Rhodium and Palladium Complexes as Antiviral Agents.... 119
   4.3   Silver and Cadmium Complexes as Antiviral Agents 121
5 Period 6 and 7 Metal-Based Antiviral Agents 122
   5.1   Lanthanum to Platinum in Antiviral Metal Complexes 122
   5.2   Gold Complexes as Antiviral Agents 124
       5.2.1   Gold Complexes Against HIV and Other Viruses 124
       5.2.2   Gold Complexes as SARS-CoV-2 Antivirals........................ 126
   5.3   Mercury Complexes as Antiviral Agents 129
6 Summary and Outlook 129
Acknowledgements 131
Abbreviations 131
References 131

ABSTRACT

While metal complexes have been playing an important role in medicinal inorganic chemistry for the development of novel anticancer agents, their application as antiviral agents has been little explored. However, a few very successful developments confirm that there is considerable potential for the development of metal-based antiviral drugs. In this chapter, the recent literature on transition-metal-based antiviral agents is summarized with a special focus on highly pathogenic viruses including SARS-CoV-2, the causative agent of the current COVID-19 pandemic. In particular, cobalt, copper, zinc and gold in antiviral metal complexes have shown very promising preclinical, and partwise clinical, results that suggest more intensive research is warranted on metal-based antiviral agents.

KEYWORDS

Antiviral; HIV; metallo-drug; SARS-CoV-2; Transition Metal Complexes

1 INTRODUCTION

Metals and metal complexes have been used in medicine since ancient times. With the serendipitous discovery of the anticancer effects of the square planar platinum complex cisplatin in the 1960s, the research field of inorganic medicinal chemistry has evolved and nowadays presents an active and prospering area combining and integrating inorganic chemistry with medicinal chemistry. Based on the tremendous success of the platinum-based cancer chemotherapeutics, the focus of inorganic medicinal chemistry research has been largely devoted to the development and study of novel antitumor therapeutics and the elucidation of their mechanism of action. Over time, however, it has been increasingly recognized that metal complexes can also be considered as highly promising drug candidates for other therapeutic indications, such as infectious diseases, and the scientific literature in this area has been steadily increasing with antibiotic metallo-drug development as a leading topic [1]. However, the application of metal complexes as antiviral agents has been relatively little explored and the scientific literature is less rich in comparison with the mentioned other areas.

As a consequence of the outbreak of the current pandemic caused by the severe acute respiratory syndrome coronavirus 2 (SARS-CoV-2) at the end of 2019, antiviral drug development has in general become one of the most urgent tasks of modern medicinal chemistry and some metal complexes have already demonstrated considerable potential, contributing to this global effort. In this chapter, we wish to give an overview on the most important developments of transition metal complexes as antiviral agents with a focus on drug candidates against highly pathogenic viruses including SARS-CoV-2. The medicinal chemistry of antiviral transition metal complexes will be reviewed; however, nanoparticles and polynuclear complexes will generally not be considered with a few exceptions. Complexes of non-transition metals or metalloids are also not within the scope of this chapter. Thus, for example, the excellent works of Hongzhe Sun and colleagues [2, 3] on bismuth antiviral complexes are therefore not included in this chapter but are referred to in Chapter 5 of this book.

2 BACKGROUND ON METAL-BASED ANTIVIRAL AGENTS

There appears to be no systematic evaluation of metal-based compounds as antiviral agents, neither regarding the type of virus nor the type of antiviral drug target. Certainly, this is in part related to aspects of biological laboratory safety as is also the case for other potential classes of drugs. However, for some viruses and the related molecular drug targets, interesting results have been obtained with multiple types of transition metal complexes. With the outbreak of the SARS-CoV-2 pandemic, the interest in metal-based antiviral drugs, in general, has been rediscovered and some very informative review papers have recently been published [4–7].

2.1 Pathogenic Viruses with Relevance for Metal-Based Antiviral Agents

Over time, metal complexes have been evaluated as antiviral drugs against many different types of viruses. Regarding the most frequently studied types of viruses, metal-based antiviral agents have increasingly demonstrated promising activity against herpes simplex virus (HSV), human immunodeficiency virus (HIV) and SARS-CoV-2.

Herpes simplex virus 1 and 2 (HSV-1 and HSV-2) lead to life-long infections in the majority of humans. Most of the infections remain asymptomatic. Blisters are the most common symptom and can occur on mouth, lips or genitals. However, there are also rare severe infections, such as herpes simplex encephalitis, and HSV infections are of concern during pregnancy.

The human immunodeficiency virus (HIV) causes acquired immunodeficiency syndrome (AIDS), which is transmitted mostly by sexual contact, but also during pregnancy, breastfeeding or via contaminated blood transfusions or needles. The virus primarily infects components of the human immune system, such as CD4+ T cells, macrophages and dendritic cells. HIV is a retrovirus and, as such, it is an RNA virus that translates its genetic information from RNA to DNA, integrates the DNA into the genome of the host cell and ultimately transcribes new viral RNA from the integrated DNA. HIV and the resulting disease AIDS have an enormous impact on society and healthcare. Highly active antiretroviral therapy (HAART) offers a treatment to slow down the progression of the infection, however, there is no cure nor an effective vaccine available.

The SARS-CoV-2 is the causative agent of the current COVID-19 (coronavirus disease 2019) pandemic. The outbreak and global spread of this virus has caused an unprecedented and still ongoing global health crisis. SARS-CoV-2 is a positive-sense single-stranded RNA virus, which is contagious in humans and spreads through close contact and via aerosols and respiratory droplets. While vaccines have been available since approximately 1 year after the start of the pandemic, effective therapeutic drugs are still rare and drug development research for curative agents is still ongoing without a significant breakthrough.

2.2 Antiviral Drug Targets of Relevance for Metal-Based Compounds

The number of registered drugs to treat viral infections has been increasing over the last years; however, the overall number of successful drug discovery and development projects remains low in comparison to that of antibacterial drugs. One major reason for this could be due to the fact that viruses, unlike bacteria, do not have their own metabolism and rely on the functional components and organelles of the host cell for their replication. As a consequence, the number of virus-specific molecular drug targets remains comparably low. The key steps of the basic viral life cycle include the entry of the virus particles into the host cell, the uncoating and release of the virus inside the infected cells, viral replication and assembly of new virus particles, and release/exit of the new viruses from the infected cell. In principle, most of the registered antiviral drugs interfere with one of the following mechanisms, enzymes, or events in this viral life cycle:

- virus entry into the host cell (inhibition of adsorption, fusion or uptake into the host cell)
- uncoating of the virus particle inside the host cell
- DNA polymerase, reverse transcriptase (only for retroviruses), DNA or RNA metabolism
- activity of viral proteases
- excretion of new virus particles from the infected cell

Figure 1 shows simplified viral life cycles for SARS-CoV-2 and HIV.

Antiviral Agents Against SARS-CoV-2 and Other Pathogenic Viruses 109

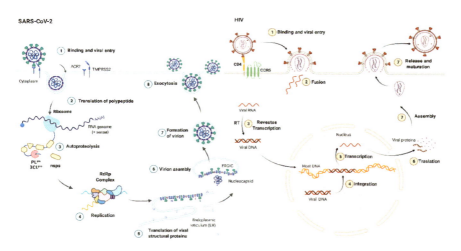

FIGURE 1 Viral life cycles of SARS-CoV-2 (left) and HIV (right). (Adapted from "SARS-CoV-2_life_cycle+HIV Sites for Therapeutic Intervention" by BioRender.com (2022). Retrieved from https://app.biorender.com/biorender-templates.)

Mechanistic studies on antiviral metal complexes have been rare. However, as outlined in this chapter, metal species in principle can act as entry inhibitors or target several steps in the replication process of the virus inside the infected cell. Regarding the mechanisms directed against the intracellular viral replication, the inhibition of some key enzymes in the process could be confirmed. For example, our recent paper demonstrated that the SARS-CoV-2 papain-like protease PL^{pro}, which is essential for processing viral polyproteins, can be inhibited by gold and some other metal-based agents [8]. For several metal complexes that are active against HIV, the enzyme reverse transcriptase, which is essential in retroviruses to translate RNA into DNA, was confirmed as a possible target. In addition to such "direct" antiviral effects, it should be noted that many metal compounds can trigger immunomodulatory effects in the infected cells that "indirectly" help to defend against the viral infection.

3 PERIOD 4 METAL-BASED ANTIVIRAL AGENTS

3.1 Scandium to Iron in Antiviral Metal Complexes

Regarding scandium, there appear to be no studies on antiviral properties available. Titanium complexes have also been extensively studied as anticancer agents with titanocene dichloride as a lead compound. Regarding their antiviral activity, ionic biscyclopentadienyl titanium complexes showed moderate activity against different viruses, such as HSV-1 and HSV-2, vaccinia virus (VV), vesicular stomatitis virus (VSV), Coxsackie virus type B4, sindbis virus (SINV), semliki forest virus (SFV) and parainfluenza virus type 3 [9]. Very recently, Gil-Moles *et al.* studied the activity of titanocene dichloride (**Ti-1**, see Figure 2) against

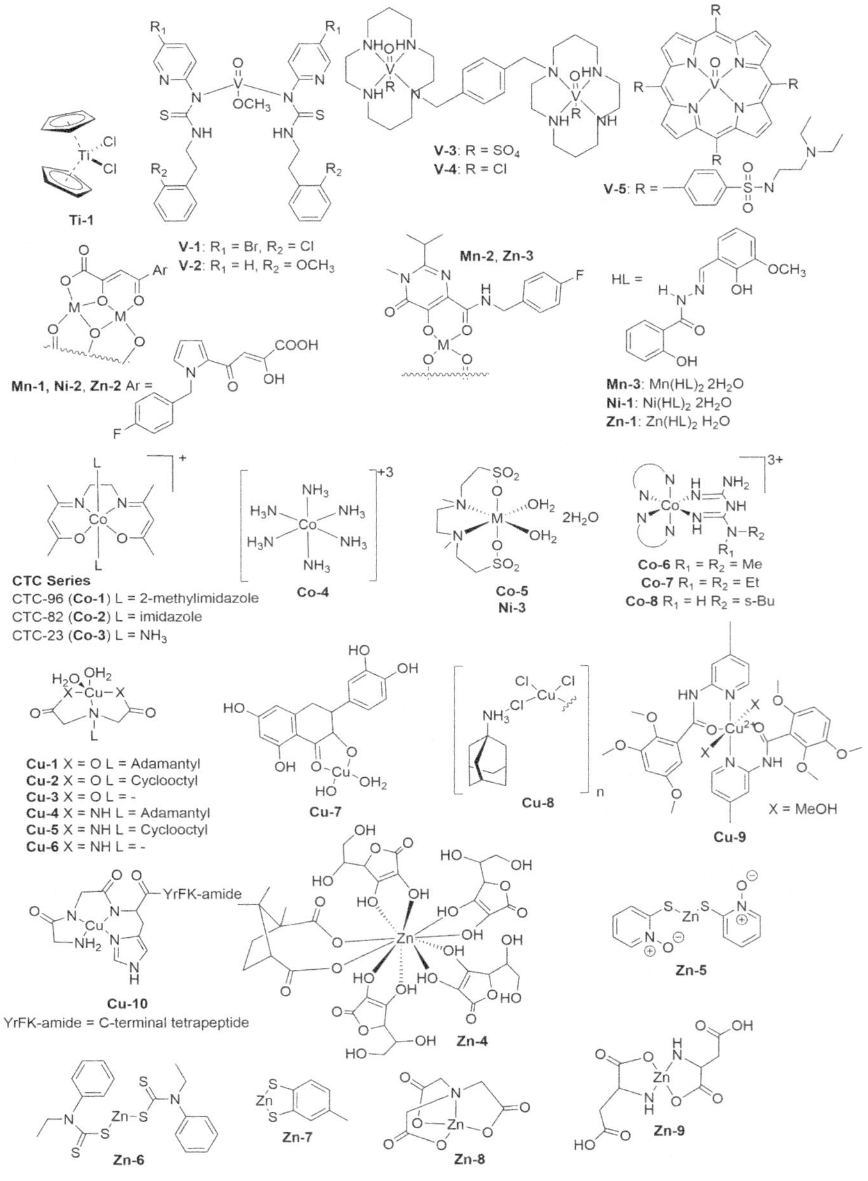

FIGURE 2 Selected period 4 metal complexes with antiviral activity.

SARS-CoV-2 protein targets. Titanocene dichloride showed a strong inhibition of the interaction between the spike protein and the ACE2 receptor at low micromolar dosage, while it proved inactive against the protease PL[pro]. Thus, **Ti-1** might act as an entry inhibitor. In addition, **Ti-1** also showed antiviral activity against

SARS-CoV-2 infected cells at concentrations above 100 µM (non-toxic range) [8]. Another study by Cirri *et al.* showed that **Ti-1** was inactive when tested by a direct yield reduction assay (DYRA); however, it became active when tested by a secondary yield reduction assay (SYRA), which evaluates possible activity at late stages of viral replication undetectable by DYRA. Thus, this may be indicative of **Ti-1** targeting late stages of viral replication [10].

Vanadium complexes have been investigated for different indications, such as cancer or diabetes [11, 12]. The antiviral activity of vanadium is largely unexplored and almost all studies focus on the potential of vanadium against HIV [13]. Oxovanadium complexes **V-1–V-4** (see Figure 2) presented a potent antiviral activity against HIV-1 (drug-resistant strain $HTLV_{IIIB}$) and HIV-2. In addition, it was demonstrated that **V-1** and **V-2** inhibit reverse transcriptase with IC_{50} values in the submicromolar range [14, 15]. A series of physiologically stable vanadium compounds was developed using porphyrins as ligands. All compounds were active when the drug was added to the medium before and after HIV-1 infection. Complex **V-5** (see Figure 2) showed the best results and also proved to be an inhibitor of reverse transcriptase [16].

There are also studies on the potential activity of vanadium complexes against SARS-CoV-2. However, these studies are only theoretical, and no experimental studies have yet been carried out. From these studies it can be suggested that vanadium compounds are potential inhibitors of two important biological targets for SARS-CoV-2, namely, 3CL^{pro} (3C-like protease) and RdRp (RNA-dependent RNA polymerase) [17, 18].

The biological role of chromium is associated with insulin [19], and some studies showed that chromium supplementation can improve insulin resistance and metabolic abnormalities in patients with HIV [20, 21]. Regarding the antiviral activity of chromium complexes, a recent study with $CrCl_3$ against HSV-1 and BVDV (bovine viral diarrhoea virus) confirmed activity against both viruses [22].

Manganese is an essential trace element and plays a vital role in regulation of immune functions, defence against ROS, etc. Its antiviral activity has not been extensively studied. Manganese saturated lactoferrin was active against different types of viruses such as HIV-1 [23], rotavirus [24] and influenza [25]. Manganese compounds with chelating ligands exhibited antiviral activity against HIV-1 and HIV-2 [26]. For example, **Mn-1** (see Figure 2) is active in the low micromolar range and **Mn-2** in the nanomolar range. In addition, **Mn-2** was confirmed to be a potent inhibitor of both HIV-1 integrase and HIV-1 reverse transcriptase. **Mn-3** was evaluated against a panel of diverse DNA- and RNA viruses. It was highly active against HSV-1, HSV-2 and vaccinia virus (VV). On the contrary, **Mn-3** was inactive against adenovirus type 2 (Ad2) and vesicular stomatitis virus (VSV) [27].

Iron plays a very important role in living organisms including viruses. The direct antiviral activity of iron complexes has not been extensively studied and few examples exist. Similar as with manganese, iron saturated lactoferrin was active against HIV-1 [23], rotavirus [24] and influenza [25]. A recent study with $FeCl_3$ showed that this compound presented antiviral activity against HSV-1 and BVDV (bovine viral diarrhoea virus) [22]. In another study, out of 13 iron complexes, which were studied as inhibitors of SARS-CoV-2 protein targets, only two nucleoside derivatives were moderately active as inhibitors of the spike/ACE2 interaction [8].

3.2 Cobalt Complexes as Antiviral Agents

Cobalt is an essential trace element and plays a crucial role in many biological processes. One of the first studies on the biological activity of cobalt complexes dates back to 1952 when Dwyer *et al.* evaluated the toxicity of different cobalt(III) complexes in a mouse model [28]. Numerous biological studies have been carried out using cobalt complexes as agents against cancer or infectious diseases.

The most promising and most extensively studied type of cobalt(III) complexes are complexes based on a chelating Schiff base with the general formula $[Co(acacen)(L)_2]^+$ (acacen=bis(acetylacetone)ethylenediamine) developed by Costa and co-workers [29] and labelled as CTC complexes. Complexes **Co-1–Co-3** are the most intensively studied complexes of this type. In 1998, the possible treatment of epithelial herpetic keratitis caused HSV-1 was evaluated. The study was performed *in vitro* using infected Vero cells and *in vivo* using a rabbit eye model infected with HSV-1 [30]. All compounds inhibited HSV-1 in Vero cells with CTC-96 (**Co-1**) as the most active and selective complex regarding toxicity. Furthermore, in *in vivo* studies, **Co-1** was found to inhibit replication of HSV-1 at concentrations 1,000-fold lower than a clinically approved standard (Viroptic®).

CTC complexes can be strongly coordinated to histidine via ligand exchange and the stability of cobalt(III) complexes with histidine in the axial position is particularly high [31]. For this reason, the authors suggested that CTC-96 might inhibit the herpes virus maturational protease.

The ability of the CTC series of complexes (see Figure 2) to interact with zinc fingers was evaluated and the high affinity for histidine residues was confirmed. It was observed *in vitro* that the CTC compounds reacted irreversibly with zinc finger proteins, including a synthetic peptide representing the first zinc finger region from HIV-1 nucleocapsid protein (NCp7) and Sp1, a DNA-binding zinc finger protein. Both biological targets are important for the transcription of the HIV-1 virus [32].

Further studies on the mechanism of action showed that CTC-96 targets the initial fusion events between the virus and the cell [33]. It appears that the compound targets an event downstream of adhesion. The data reveal that CTC-96 inhibits membrane fusion events but does not provide information on the exact mechanism of inhibition. Furthermore, it was found that CTC-96 also inhibited plaque formation by VSV (vesicular stomatitis virus) and VZV (varicella-zoster virus) as efficiently as that by HSV-1. Taking these results into account, CTC-96 can be regarded as a broad-spectrum inhibitor of enveloped virus infection targeting the infection at the membrane fusion point, regardless of the type of virus and cellular receptors present. In addition, it was noted that CTC-96 does not enter the cells efficiently and, therefore, an intracellular mechanism of action

Antiviral Agents Against SARS-CoV-2 and Other Pathogenic Viruses 113

appears unlikely. The interaction with zinc fingers, such as NCp7 and Sp1, as well as with the maturational protease appears therefore less relevant. Continuing the studies on CTC-96, the activity against keratoconjunctivitis caused by human adenovirus type 5 (HAD type 5) was evaluated *in vitro* in cells and *in vivo* using a rabbit model [34]. The treatment reduced disease severity and viral titres on the corneal surface. For CTC-96, it was shown that the dose needed to treat HAD type 5 was higher than the dose needed to treat HSV-1. This might be the consequence of the fact that HAD type 5 does not have a membrane and it is possible that the inhibitory action of the drug involves one or more capsid or intra-capsid proteins, which are less accessible to the drug than the membrane surface proteins of enveloped viruses. It is important to note that CTC-96 is a promising candidate and reached phase II trials in 2011 for treatment of herpes simplex labialis under the trademark Doxovir™ by REDOX Pharmaceutical Corp, Greenavle, NY.

In addition to CTC type complexes, other types of cobalt derivatives have been studied against different types of viruses. Cobalt(III) complexes were studied against sindbis virus (SINV, genus alphavirus) [31, 35]. While the cobalt(III) complexes with chelate ligand cyclen were not active, **Co-4** (hexammine) exhibited a potent dose-dependent inhibition of sindbis virus replication. Studies have also been carried out on the antiviral activity of cobalt compounds against HIV. Compound **Co-5** showed antiviral activity in pre- and post-infected cells with HIV-1 NL4.3 [36]. This feature may indicate a dual mechanism of action that combines preventive and therapeutic HIV treatment.

Recently, a family of complexes with biguanidine ligands was evaluated against influenza virus (H1N1 pdm09) and herpes simplex virus 2 (HSV-2) (see structures of **Co-6**, **Co-7** and **Co-8** in Figure 2) [37, 38]. The complexes did not show noticeable activity against H1N1 pdm09, but they turned out to be active against HSV-2. The authors proposed that these data, together with the literature, show that the main influence on antiviral activity is exerted by the number of free (uncoordinated) functional groups in the ligands, although the structures of the metal complexes are also important. To reach more reliable conclusions on the anti-influenza and anti-herpetic activity of metal complexes, more extensive studies are necessary.

3.3 Nickel Complexes as Antiviral Agents

Nickel is an essential element for microorganisms and plants; however, the physiological role for mammalians is unclear [39]. Nickel compounds as antiviral agents have not been extensively studied, although there are a few studies on this subject. The nickel compound **Ni-1**, an analogue to **Mn-3**, also showed antiviral activity against HSV-1, HSV-2 and VV (see Figure 2) [27]. **Ni-2** (an analogue of **Mn-1**) was active against HIV-1 and HIV-2. Overall, the behavior was very similar to that of the manganese complexes [26]. The complex **Ni-3** (an analogue **Co-5**) also showed activity against HIV-1 pre- and post-infected cells similar to the cobalt compound [36].

3.4 Copper Complexes as Antiviral Agents

Copper has a long history in medicine and its antimicrobial properties have been known since antiquity. In addition, copper is an essential element for organisms and is involved in many physiological functions. Several studies have demonstrated the potential of copper complexes to act as anticancer antimicrobial, anti-inflammatory and antiviral agents as well as, enzyme inhibitors [40]. Regarding the antiviral properties of copper, there are numerous studies on materials and surfaces that have shown that copper and its alloys have excellent potential to control the spread of infectious diseases [41]. However, here we will focus on the antiviral properties and mechanisms of action of copper(II) and copper(I) complexes.

There are several studies on the antiviral activity of different copper(II) derivatives against various strains of influenza. Busath and co-workers evaluated *in vitro* a series of copper(II) complexes (see Figure 2) with tripodal ligands coordinating bis(carboxymethyl)amino (**Cu-1**, **Cu-2** and **Cu-3**) or bis(carbamoylmethyl)amino groups (**Cu-4**, **Cu-5** and **Cu-6**) as potential antivirals against different strains of influenza [42]. All derivatives exhibited promising antiviral activity and selectivity indices. Further studies focused on the M2 ion channel, which is a proton-selective viral protein integrated in the viral envelope of the influenza and often undergoes multiple mutations. The authors studied the interaction of **Cu-1**–**Cu-6** with different M2 mutations, confirming that copper compounds have the ability to inhibit the native M2 channel and also the M2 S31N mutation, but not the H37A mutation where the histidines are mutated to alanines. These results indicate that the copper complexes bind to the histidines of the M2 channels. Studies in zebrafish showed that the complexes, with the exception of **Cu-3**, were strongly toxic [43].

The complex **Cu-7** showed potent *in vivo* antiviral activity by both oral and intraperitoneal administration. A standard model of lethal influenza virus infection in white mice caused by the influenza virus strain A/Aichi/2/68 (H3N2) was used [44]. Oral administration of compound **Cu-7** resulted in an increase in the protection index for the animals by 20%, while the intraperitoneal injection increased the protection index by 40% compared to the animals that were not treated.

Amantadine is an antiviral drug that is used in the treatment of influenza. However, several strains of influenza virus show resistance to this treatment. In this respect, a copper derivative with amantadine (**Cu-8**) was studied against an amantadine-resistant virus, A/WSN/33 wild virus and several mutations [45]. The mechanism of action involved an increase in membrane permeability greater than that observed for $CuCl_2$ with significantly lower toxicity. *In silico* studies indicated that the complex could effectively block the replication-mediated proton current of the M2 S31N virus.

One important biological target for HIV treatment is the enzyme HIV protease. This enzyme is essential for processing the viral polyproteins and its inhibition will lead to the disruption of viral replication. Leviene *et al.* evaluated the ability of $CuCl_2$ to inhibit HIV protease wild type and one synthetic variant where Cys[67] and Cys[95] were replaced by α-aminobutyric acid. The synthetic protease has a similar three-dimensional structure and very similar activity, so it is possible to assess

Antiviral Agents Against SARS-CoV-2 and Other Pathogenic Viruses

whether cysteine residues are essential in the copper mechanism. The viral protease was inhibited at stoichiometric copper concentrations and the inhibition was very fast and was not reversed by subsequent exposure to ethylenediamine tetraacetic acid EDTA or dithiothreitol. Direct inhibition by copper requires the presence of cysteine residues in the protease. The synthetic protease, lacking cysteine residues, was not inhibited by $CuCl_2$ exposure. However, the addition of a mixture of dithiothreitol as an exogenous thiol together with $CuCl_2$ caused even the synthetic protease to be inactivated [46]. In view of these results, the authors also evaluated if copper(I) complexes could exhibit similar activities. For this purpose, they carried out the same experiment with copper complexes with bathocuproine disulfonic acid and neocuproine. They observed that bathocuproine disulfonic acid copper(I) inhibited the wild-type HIV-1 protease, while neocuproine copper(I) chloride only partially inhibited it. In addition, bathocuproine disulfonic acid copper(I) was also able to inhibit mutant synthetic HIV protease, while neither the free ligand nor copper(I) alone was able to inhibit the mutant HIV protease [47].

Another study evaluated the ability of different copper complexes to inhibit HIV-1 protease [48]. All compounds were active against the wild-type protease; however, against the mutant protease, only compound **Cu-9** showed activity. It was observed that only **Cu-9** was stable under the test conditions and that the inhibition produced by the rest of the compounds against the wild-type protease could be exclusively due to free copper(II) ions. This behavior would agree with the observations by Leviene *et al.*, who found that only copper chelates are able to inhibit the mutant protease.

A study on the virostatic properties of $CuCl_2$ alone or in the presence of reducing agents against HSV was carried out. Copper(II) chloride alone exhibited antiviral activity in the toxic range; however, when reducing agents were added, it was possible to reduce the copper concentration to the non-toxic range with high inhibition of HSV [49, 50].

Another paper describes a possible treatment of hepatitis C virus (HCV) based on the concept of catalytic metallo-drugs that promote irreversible destruction of a therapeutic target, such as the stem-loop IIb (SL IIb) of the internal ribosomal entry site (IRES) RNA of hepatitis C virus (HCV). The approach involves a C-terminal tetrapeptide, which includes a D-configured arginine coupled to metal-binding domain **Cu-10** (see Figure 2). **Cu-10** was very active against SL IIb, while $CuCl_2$ showed virtually no activity. **Cu-10** also exhibited high antiviral activity and very low toxicity [51].

Regarding the possible antiviral activity of copper complexes against SARS-CoV-2, there are still no experimental studies. However, some recent theoretical studies and reviews suggest that copper compounds could be excellent candidates for the development of antivirals against SARS-CoV-2 [52–55].

3.5 Zinc Complexes as Antiviral Agents

Zinc is an essential micronutrient for many organisms. It is an integral part of many proteins and is decisive for their structure and function. Hence, zinc is biologically essential for cellular processes and for the development and function of the immune system. Furthermore, although zinc is essential for a proper immune response to a multitude of microorganisms including viruses, zinc has direct antiviral properties. This section will focus on the direct antiviral activity of zinc compounds rather than their antiviral properties via immunomodulatory effects [56–59].

3.5.1 Zinc Complexes Against Different Viruses

In the 1970s, several studies were carried out with zinc salts against HSV-1 and HSV-2. For example, $ZnSO_4$ can inhibit HSV-1 replication when added at the end of the virus adsorption period with the zinc ions irreversibly inhibiting the replication of HSV-1 in BSC-1 cells [60]. Regarding HSV-2, $ZnSO_4$ prevents the synthesis of virus-induced polypeptides, and the formation of new viruses. However, in these studies the replication of the virus is not inhibited in an irreversible way [61]. Another study demonstrated that zinc acetate ($Zn(OAc)_2$) has the ability to strongly inhibit the DNA polymerase of HSV-1 *in vitro* [62]. Further investigations showed that the mechanism of action was probably not due to intracellular inhibition of virus replication, but rather the consequence of the drastic inactivation of free virus in skin tissues, intercellular vesicles and blisters. Moreover, electron microscopic studies showed massive deposition of zinc on the surfaces of HSV virions, and these zinc deposits apparently interfered with the proper functioning of viral glycoproteins, resulting in blockage of the normal mechanism of penetration by membrane fusion [63].

Zn-1 (see Figure 2) was evaluated against a panel of diverse DNA- and RNA viruses. It was highly active against HSV-1, HSV-2 and VV with EC_{50} values in the low micromolar range. In contrast, it did not show any activity against Ad2 and VSV [27]. Some *in vivo* studies against HSV-2 were carried out and zinc salts (acetate, sulphate, chloride and gluconate) provide significant protection against HSV-2. However, at the concentrations required to obtain protection, the zinc salts produced vaginal epithelial disruption in the mouse models [64]. A series of zinc acetate and carrageenan gels was studied. The gels were effective and showed low toxicity *in vitro* and caused little damage to cervicovaginal and rectal mucosa *in vivo*, and did not induce increased susceptibility to HSV-2 infection in a mouse model [65]. Microbicide gels can also be used for the prevention of human-to-human HIV transmission. In this regard, the authors used a macaque model to test the efficacy of microbicide gel containing zinc acetate and the non-nucleoside reverse transcriptase inhibitor MIV-150. Daily vaginal application of this gel for 2 weeks fully protected the macaques from subsequent SHIV (simian-human immunodeficiency virus) infection induced after 24 h from the last gel application [66].

Previously, some *in vitro* studies on the antiviral activity of zinc complexes against HIV have been carried out. In the early 1990s it was observed that zinc(II) ions can inhibit the correct functioning of HIV-1 protease and renin, two enzymes essential for HIV replication [67]. Zinc salts (acetate, chloride and nitrate) exhibited anti-HIV-1 activities and inhibited HIV-1 RNA transcription and HIV-1 production in the cell culture medium [68]. In a more recent study, the authors studied the

Antiviral Agents Against SARS-CoV-2 and Other Pathogenic Viruses   117

mechanism by which zinc(II) ions derived from $ZnCl_2$ can inhibit reverse transcriptase (RT) activity. Magnesium(II) acts as a cofactor of RT, however, in the presence of zinc(II) it can be substituted. Remarkably, the $RT-Zn^{2+}$-(primer-template) complex was much more stable than the same complex formed with magnesium(II), while the rate of nucleotide incorporation was much slower. This results in an inhibition of RT, as a "dead-end complex" is formed with very slow incorporation kinetics [69]. Zinc compounds with chelating ligands have been shown to exhibit antiviral activity against HIV-1 and HIV-2 with significant differences in antiviral activity being observed depending on the ligand used [26]. The complexes **Zn-2** and **Zn-3** (see Figure 2) were the most potent candidates with EC_{50} in the low micromolar and nanomolar range respectively against both HIV-1 and HIV-2.

Other sexually transmitted viral diseases are caused by the papillomaviridae family, and the HPV is a primary cause of cervical cancers. The requirement for HPV infection to lead to cervical carcinoma is the continuous expression of E6/E7 proteins. Exogenous zinc treatment can effectively inhibit the production of viral oncogenic proteins E6 and E7. The mechanism by which zinc regulates E6 and E7 expression is unknown; however, it is possible that zinc regulates this expression by inhibiting some part of the viral cycle [70, 71]. A clinical trial showed that a 12-week treatment with zinc citrate (CIZAR®) may result in elimination of HR-HPV (high-risk human papilloma virus) infection of the cervix [72].

Other studies showed that oral supplementation with $ZnSO_4$ could be effective in the treatment of viral warts caused by HPV [73]. Arising from this, a recent study evaluated the ability of zinc tetra-ascorbo-camphorate (**Zn-4**, see Figure 2) *in vitro* against HPV-16. When the compound was added to the cells at the same time as the infection, it was able to inhibit the adsorption of HPV-16. Also, when the cells were pre-treated with **Zn-4**, greater anti-HPV activity was observed. These results suggest that **Zn-4** is more effective in preventing HPV attachment to target cells than at other points of the viral replication cycle [74].

The antiviral properties of zinc salts have also been evaluated against other viruses but with a lower intensity. For example, zinc salts such as sulphate and chloride exhibited antiviral activity against HCV (hepatitis C virus). They significantly suppressed the viral replication in the genome-length HCV RNA replication system [75]. Zinc can induce metallothionein (MT) expression and inhibit HCV replication *in vitro*. It is likely that MTs mediate their antiviral effect through modulation of intracellular zinc [76]. Other studies evaluated the potential of zinc(II) ions derived from $ZnCl_2$ against SFV. Zinc(II) ions can inhibit the SFV liposome fusion via interference with the formation of fusion-active E1 homotrimers [77]. Biochemical studies showed that zinc ions strongly inhibit E1 trimer formation in wild-type SFV, while a mutation in H333 in E1 DIII conferred resistance to zinc. These results suggest that zinc ions act by blocking foldback of DIII through its interaction with H333 [78].

3.5.2 Antiviral Properties of Zinc Against Respiratory Viruses

$ZnCl_2$ showed activity against eight types of human rhinoviruses that are common cold triggers [79]. The zinc ions could interact with capsid polypeptides of HRV-1A, and it was observed that normal proteolytic processing of HRV-1A polypeptides was inhibited by the binding of zinc ions to the rhinoviral protein precursors, particularly in regions containing the capsid sequences [80]. However, in another study, zinc salts (including $ZnCl_2$) showed different results against HRV-A1 and HRV-39. The authors concluded that no clear antiviral effects were evident [81]. Different clinical studies suggest than zinc supplementation reduces the common cold duration, although a high dosage was needed [82]. However, the possible beneficial effects reported for zinc supplementation in treating colds may not be related directly to selective antirhinovirus activity.

The effect of different zinc salts (acetate, lactate, sulphate) on replication of respiratory syncytial virus (RSV) was studied. Zinc salts were active *in vitro* during preincubation, adsorption, penetration or egress. In addition, zinc salts prevented efficient RSV infection by preventing cell-to-cell spreading in culture when the HEp-2 cells were pre-treated with zinc salts only prior to infection with RSV, or when zinc salts were added to semisolid overlay media only after infection [83].

Zinc is considered as a potential treatment in the therapy of SARS-CoV-2 infection due to its immunomodulatory effects as well as its direct antiviral effect. To date, there have not been many studies on the antiviral activity of Zn compounds against SARS-CoV-2; however, the few studies that exist, together with the multitude of studies carried out against other types of respiratory viruses, make zinc a potential candidate for the treatment of this infection. The combination of zinc acetate ($Zn(OAc)_2$) and pyrithione can inhibit the replication of SARS-CoV-1 and equine arteritis virus (EAV) in cell culture at low micromolar range. Also, the mixture of pyrithione and zinc(II) was able to inhibit the RNA-dependent RNA polymerase (RdRp) of both viruses. This study revealed that zinc(II) could block the initiation step of EAV RNA synthesis, whereas in the case of the SARS-CoV-1, RdRp elongation was inhibited and template binding reduced [84].

Another important biological target for SARS-CoV-1 replication is the main protease or 3C-like protease (3CL^{pro}) and several studies have been carried out to determine the ability of Zn-conjugates (see Figure 2, **Zn-5–Zn-9**) to inhibit this enzyme [85, 86]. **Zn-5** was a competitive inhibitor with an inhibitory constant of $0.17\,\mu M$. In contrast, **Zn-6** and **Zn-7** were non-competitively active against SARS-CoV-1 protease with similar k_i values [85]. Regarding crystal structures of the zinc-conjugated complexes (**Zn-8**, **Zn-9**) with 3CL^{pro}, the zinc ion plays a key role in targeting the catalytic residues, via binding to the H41–C145 catalytic dyad to give rise to a zinc-central tetrahedral geometry [86].

Taking these results and the structural similarities between SARS-CoV-1 and SARS-CoV-2 into account, several studies on zinc compounds against 3CL^{pro} of SARS-CoV-2 have been carried out [87, 88]. Different zinc salts such as chloride, acetate, glycinate and gluconate strongly inhibited 3CL^{pro} and the mode of inhibition was found to be non-competitive and reversible by adding EDTA. The crystal structures showed that the zinc ion binds to C145 and H41 with a tetrahedral environment as observed in the previous studies with SARS-CoV-1 [86]. Only zinc acetate showed antiviral activity at a non-toxic range. This may be due to varying stability constants and therefore the varying bioavailability of free zinc

Antiviral Agents Against SARS-CoV-2 and Other Pathogenic Viruses **119**

ions at physiological pH of the different salts. Therefore, the authors mixed zinc acetate with quercetin (natural zinc ionophore) at a 1:2 molar ratio and a >2-fold increase in antiviral activity was observed [88].

A recent study has shown that zinc gluconate strongly inhibited both 3CL[pro] and PL[pro] (papain-like protease), two essential proteases for SARS-CoV-2 replication [89]. The biochemical (for PL[pro]) and crystallographic data (only for 3CL[pro]) reveal that zinc gluconate interacted with catalytic site residues. Also, the authors concluded that the treatment with zinc gluconate plus hinokitiol (a zinc ionophore) could lead to elevated intracellular zinc(II) levels and hence significantly impaired the two protease activities *in cellulo*.

4 PERIOD 5 METAL-BASED ANTIVIRAL AGENTS

4.1 YTTRIUM TO TECHNETIUM IN ANTIVIRAL METAL COMPLEXES

None of these metals have demonstrated antiviral properties to date and the most studied biological application for them is as radioisotopes in nuclear medicine [90]. In the case of Mo it is often part of polyoxometalates (POMs) [8, 91], which have been shown to possess antiviral activity. Examples are provided in Chapter 5 of this volume.

4.2 RUTHENIUM, RHODIUM AND PALLADIUM COMPLEXES AS ANTIVIRAL AGENTS

Ruthenium complexes have been extensively studied as anticancer and antibacterial agents. Rhodium complexes have also been increasingly considered for metallo-drug design [92, 93]. However, their potential applications as antiviral agents have not been extensively studied. There are several, albeit limited, studies on the activity of ruthenium complexes against HIV. A family of 18 polypyridyl ruthenium(II) and ruthenium(III) complexes were analysed against HIV-1. However, only one compound (**Ru-1**, see Figure 3) was found to be active and with a good selectivity index [94]. One polyanionic ruthenium oxo oxalato cluster $Na_7[Ru_4(\mu_3\text{-}O)_4(C_2O_4)_6]$ shows anti-HIV activity and inhibits reverse transcriptase (RT) in the nanomolar range [95]. In another study it was observed that ruthenium arenes, such as **Ru-2** and **Ru-3**, strongly inhibit HIV integrase [96]. The complex **Ru-4** showed potent anti-HIV activity and it was also found to inhibit the formation of TAR-TAT complexes. The trans-activation response (TAR) region is a region of high secondary structure within HIV-1 RNA that complexes with the virus-encoded transactivator protein (TAT) and regulates viral transcription [97]. Studies on other types of viruses are even scarcer. There are some examples of ruthenium arenes which have been tested against HSV-1 and polio virus type 1, and only **Ru-5** (see Figure 3) was found to be active against poliovirus [98].

Regarding rhodium complexes, a study on the photo-inactivation of sindbis virus showed that **Rh-1** produces a reduction in viral titre upon irradiation at 355 nm. It was also found that the virus is not affected by irradiation in the absence of the metal complex or by the metal complex in the dark [99]. Several

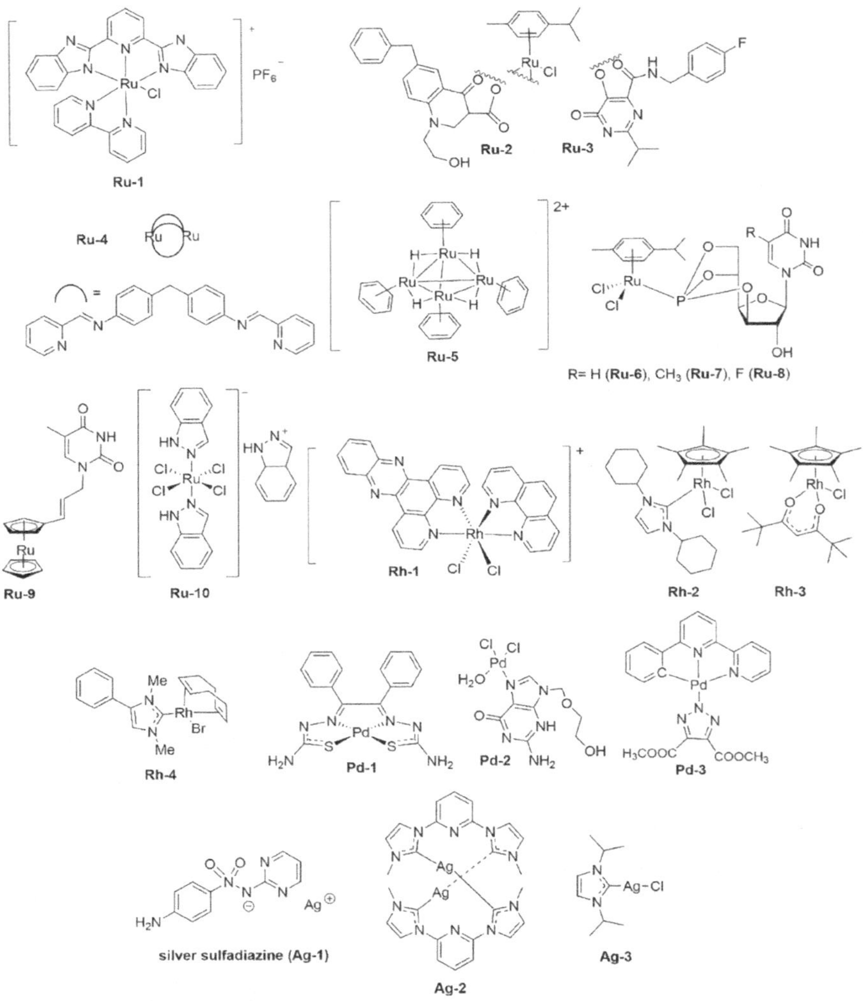

FIGURE 3 Selected period 5 metal complexes with antiviral properties.

recent studies have evaluated different ruthenium and rhodium compounds against SARS-CoV-2. In fact, **Rh-2** and **Rh-3** complexes were found to be very active against this virus. The compounds showed low toxicity in Vero E-6 and CaLu-3 cells, and altogether these results highlight the great potential of rhodium cyclopentadienyl derivatives as agents against SARS-CoV-2 [100]. Gil-Moles *et al.* evaluated 17 ruthenium and 11 rhodium complexes against PL^pro (SARS-CoV-1 and SARS-CoV-2) and the spike/ACE2 interaction. Rhodium complexes showed moderate inhibition of the spike/ACE2 interaction, while all complexes were good inhibitors of both PL^pro enzymes with **Rh-4** as the most active. Ruthenium derivatives with partial nucleoside structure (**Ru-6–Ru-9**) showed moderate inhibition

Antiviral Agents Against SARS-CoV-2 and Other Pathogenic Viruses **121**

of the spike/ACE2 interaction. Messori and colleagues confirmed the antiviral activity of the ruthenium(III) anticancer agent KP1019 (**Ru-10**) against SARS-CoV-2 with an acceptable toxicity profile [10]. In contrast, NAMI-A, another well-established ruthenium metallo-drug candidate, was inactive.

Palladium complexes have been extensively studied as anticancer agents due to their similarity to platinum [101]. On the other hand, studies on the antiviral activity of such compounds are very rare. Palladium compound (**Pd-1**) with thiosemicarbazone as ligand showed great activity against HSV-1 and HSV-2 (acyclovir-resistant strains) with a selectivity index of 8 [102].

In another study, the anti-HSV-1 activity of a palladium complex coordinated with acyclovir (**Pd-2**) was evaluated and a synergistic effect between acyclovir and palladium was observed (100-fold increase in activity compared to acyclovir) [103]. There is also a study against the interaction of spike/ACE2 and PL^{pro} of SARS-CoV-2, where it was observed that **Pd-3** moderately inhibited the PL^{pro} enzyme [8].

4.3 Silver and Cadmium Complexes as Antiviral Agents

Metallic silver, silver ions and also silver nanoparticles have been included in many consumer products (e.g. cosmetics) and medical devices based on their well-known antibacterial properties [104, 105]. The drug silver sulfadiazine is a combination of a silver ion with the antibiotic sulfadiazine and has been applied for topical treatments (see Figure 3). The antibacterial effects of silver compounds are likely due to released Ag$^+$ ions, and several deleterious effects (e.g. disruption of bacterial cell walls, interaction with DNA, enzyme inhibition) have been reported. However, the specific mechanisms of action of silver complexes are still largely unknown.

Notably, there has been an increasing number of literature reports on the emerging importance of silver nanoparticles targeting the viral life cycle and viral replication, including studies against SARS-CoV-2 [106]. Whereas this chapter focuses on ionic silver complexes, the interested reader can find an up-to-date overview on antiviral applications of silver nanoparticles in the review paper by Ghosh *et al.* [107].

The activity of silver nitrate against HSV was described in several reports in the 1970s, including a study using a rabbit eye infection model [108–110]. Silver nitrate was not active against other viruses (e.g. vaccinia virus, adenovirus, poliovirus). Mechanistic studies indicated that it did not affect the rate of attachment to the host cells but rather the multiplication of the virus at steps soon after the attachment.

Early reports on antiviral properties of silver sulfadiazine date back to 1974, when Tokumaru *et al.* described antiviral actions in tissue culture and an ocular infection model, in which herpes simplex (HSV) and vesicular stomatitis viruses (VSV) were shown to be susceptible to the treatment [111]. Other silver(I) complexes with sulfonamide antibiotics (mafenide and ethylmafenide) triggered antibacterial properties and antiviral activity against the Chikungunya virus (CHIKV) in the non-toxic concentration range [112].

Several studies report antiviral activity with multinuclear and polymeric silver compounds. Polymeric silver complexes were reported to inhibit the enzymatic activity of HIV reverse transcriptase and were suggested as a potential antiviral agent [113]. Further studies on polymeric silver complexes against a broad variety of different viruses showed that they were not active at non-toxic concentrations [114]. A polymeric complex of silver with mercaptoethanesulfonate was inactive against a broad panel of viruses; however, it showed good results against respiratory syncytial virus (RSV) [115]. A macrocyclic silver complex with an N-heterocyclic carbene (NHC) ligand (**Ag-2**) was reported to have strong antiviral activity against HIV-1 [116]. The heteronuclear coordination polymer silver bis(citrato)germanate, containing silver and germanium, was more effective against several influenza strains than oseltamivir [117].

Regarding SARS-CoV-2, silver complexes have been rarely studied (see also Chapter 5 of this book). Interaction of silver compounds with the spike protein or the protease M^{pro} was suggested by computational chemistry studies [118, 119]. For example, silver nitrate, silver sulfadiazine and a silver N-heterocyclic carbene complex (**Ag-3**) were evaluated as inhibitors of the interaction of the SARS-CoV-2 spike protein with the ACE2 host cell receptor and the SARS-CoV-2 protease PL^{pro}. While only **Ag-3** showed low activity against the protein-protein interaction, all three complexes were strong inhibitors of SARS-CoV-2 PL^{pro} activity. Notably, they were much less active against the PL^{pro} from the SARS-CoV, indicating that the inhibition could be selective. After toxicity evaluation, complex **Ag-3** was selected for SARS-CoV-2 antiviral studies and was shown to inhibit viral replication at non-toxic concentrations [8].

Cadmium is a non-essential transition metal that is well known for its health risk for both animals and humans and reports on biomedical applications are rare. Cadmium acetate decreased HIV-1 replication at dosages below the strong host cell toxicity and this effect could be attributed to the inhibition of HIV-1 RNA transcription [120, 121]. Amongst several metals, cadmium complexes with 1,10-phenanthroline ligands showed the strongest activity against influenza [122]. Their antiviral activity depended on the kinetic reactivity of the complexes and the lipophilicity of the ligands.

5 PERIOD 6 AND 7 METAL-BASED ANTIVIRAL AGENTS

5.1 Lanthanum to Platinum in Antiviral Metal Complexes

Only few studies report on the antiviral activity of transition metal complexes from lanthanum to platinum.

Interestingly, rare earth ions were reported to block the ion pores generated by class II fusion proteins of alphaviruses [123]. Treatment with several lanthanide ions (La^{3+}, Ce^{3+}, Pr^{3+}, Nd^{3+}) reverted the ability of host cells to replicate flavivirus RNA in experiments with the West Nile virus and Uganda S virus [124].

Radioimmunotherapy is a therapeutic approach that makes use of the specific antigen-antibody interaction to deliver lethal radiation to cells by means of radiolabelled antibodies. This concept has been evaluated for HIV-1 using

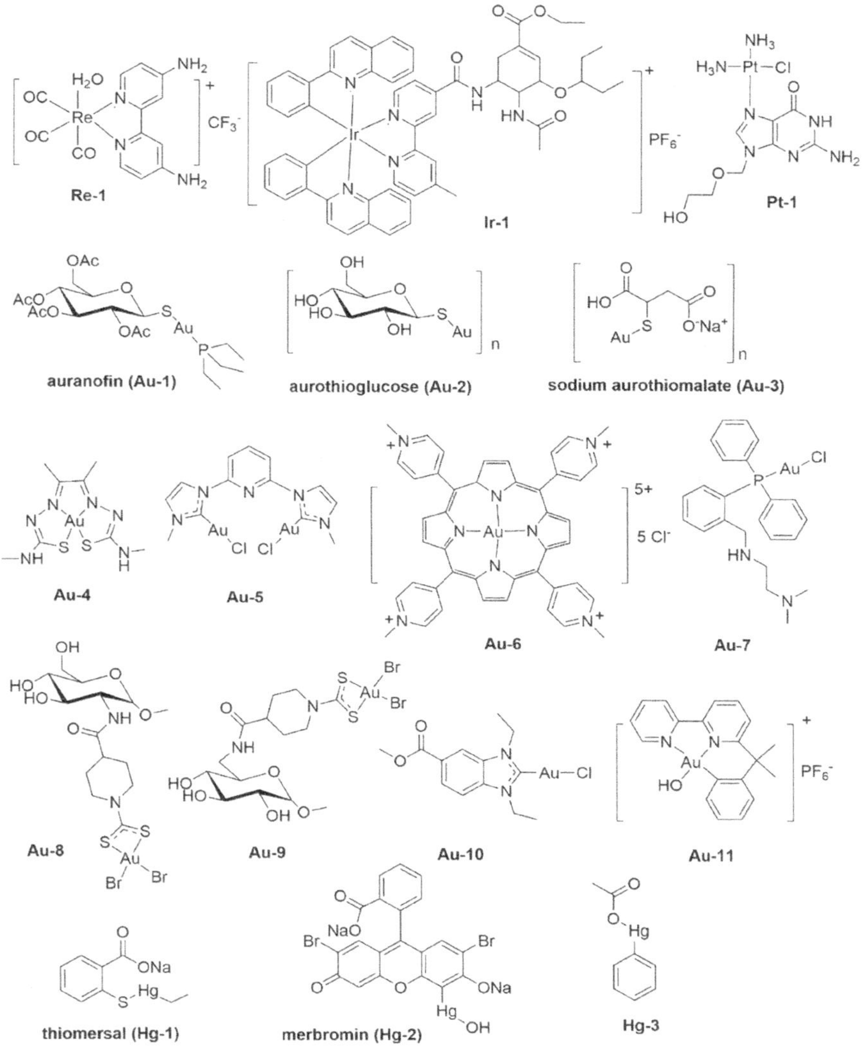

Antiviral Agents Against SARS-CoV-2 and Other Pathogenic Viruses 123

FIGURE 4 Selected period 6 and period 7 metal complexes with antiviral properties.

[188]Re-labelled polyclonal antibodies for the HIV envelope glycoproteins gp-120 and gp-41 [125]. The conjugates selectively killed infected cells *in vitro*. Further *in vivo* studies in mice using the [188]Re-labelled antibody for gp-41 resulted in a substantial reduction of HIV-infected cells in a dose-dependent manner without causing acute haematologic toxicity.

Rhenium(I) tricarbonyl complexes were evaluated as covalent inhibitors of SARS-CoV-2 protease 3CL[pro] targeting the cysteine residue in the active site of the enzyme [126]. Complex **Re-1** (Figure 4) was the most active inhibitor and showed selective inhibition of 3CL[pro] in comparison with other proteases, such as cathepsin. Antiviral studies with infected cells have not yet been reported for this compound.

Dual-functional luminescent iridium(III) complexes conjugated to the anti-influenza drug oseltamivir were reported to inhibit neuraminidase stronger than oseltamivir [127]. While the oseltamivir moiety of these complexes enables binding to the enzyme on the cell surface, the iridium centre has the function of a signalling unit. The most promising compound **Ir-1** (Figure 4) showed also appreciable photophysical properties with long emission lifetime, large Stokes shift, high quantum yield and strong red emission. Other cyclometallated iridium(III) complexes were shown to inhibit the replication of HSV-1 and HSV-2 [128].

Platinum complexes, such as cisplatin or carboplatin, are well known for their impressive anticancer activity and have been extensively used in cancer chemotherapy for many decades. The potential of platinum complexes as antiviral agents has been very recently comprehensively reviewed by de Castro *et al.* [129]. A notable example is the cisplatin-nucleotide conjugate **Pt-1** (Figure 4), which showed good activity against HSV-1. Regarding SARS-CoV-2 antiviral agents, there appear to be no studies with platinum complexes against infected cells available so far. Cisplatin and some cyclometallated platinum(II) species were only weak inhibitors of the SARS-CoV-2 protease PL^{pro} [8].

5.2 Gold Complexes as Antiviral Agents

Gold and gold complexes have been playing an important role in human mankind, not only because of their economic and cultural values, but also to a smaller extent because of their applications in chemistry and in medicine. Although their importance has been declining over the last years, auranofin (**Au-1**), aurothioglucose (**Au-2**) and aurothiomalate (**Au-3**) (Figure 4) have been used for decades for the treatment of symptoms of rheumatoid arthritis. Currently gold complexes belong to the most intensively studied transition metal complexes in inorganic medicinal chemistry for application in cancer chemotherapy and in the treatment of infectious diseases, however, with less focus on viral infections.

5.2.1 Gold Complexes Against HIV and Other Viruses

As early as 1985 the inhibition of herpes simplex and Epstein-Barr virus DNA polymerases by auranofin (**Au-1**) and other gold complexes was reported [130]. However, the concentration required to inhibit HSV-1 replication in cells was also toxic to the non-infected cells. In 1993, Okada *et al.* reported on the *in vitro* anti-HIV-1 activity of reactive intermediates of aurothioglucose (**Au-2**) and aurothiomalate (**Au-3**) [131]. Whereas **Au-2** and **Au-3** showed only little to moderate antiviral effects, their derivatives with a molar equivalent of a thiol ligand, e.g. bis(thioglucose)gold(I), showed significantly higher efficacy. The antiviral activity was attributed to ligand exchange processes at the virus surface with a cysteine residue of the glycoprotein 41 (gp41). This interaction resulted in the release of another glycoprotein, gp120, from gp41, with the consequence of a lowered infectivity. In a cell-free assay, the HIV-1 reverse transcriptase activity was inhibited by bis(thioglucose)gold(I).

Antiviral Agents Against SARS-CoV-2 and Other Pathogenic Viruses **125**

For auranofin the inhibition of gp120 reduction was suggested as a mechanism of HIV entry blockage [132]. Both thioredoxin and the enzyme protein disulphide isomerase catalyse gp120 reduction and hence their inhibitors could affect virus entry. Auranofin was shown to inhibit HIV replication; however, the required dosage was close to the toxicity range of the complex.

Aurothioglucose was also found to inhibit the tumour-necrosis factor α (TNF-α) induced HIV replication in cells [133]. The complex inhibited the TNF-α induced activation of NF-κB, which is a transcription factor and also a potent activator of HIV-1 gene expression.

The immunomodulating effects of aurothiomalate were examined in a mouse AIDS (MAIDS) infection model suggesting the interleukin-2 (IL-2) induction by the drug as an important factor for decreasing the disease progression [134].

Shapiro and Masci in 1996 reported on an exciting case study of a patient with HIV infection and disabling psoriatic arthritis, who was treated with auranofin. The patient showed a significant sustained increase in CD4 cells [135]. This effect strongly indicated a possible impact of auranofin on HIV treatment.

Despite the potency of antiretroviral therapies for AIDS, the treatments do not eradicate the virus from the organism, as memory $CD4^+$ T cells can host a transcriptionally silent but replication competent provirus. Importantly, auranofin restricted the viral reservoir in rhesus macaques in a monkey AIDS model and induced containment of the viral load when the therapy was interrupted [136]. Further studies in rhesus macaques under highly intensified antiretroviral therapy confirmed that auranofin, in combination with the glutathione synthesis inhibitor buthionine sulfoximine (BSO), resulted in long-lasting drug-free control of viremia following therapy suspension [137]. Such "anti-memory" effect of auranofin, caused by affecting redox-sensitive cell death pathways, was further reported in leucocytes [138]. The "indirect" antiviral effects of auranofin, meaning effects related to oxidative stress and the immune response of the host cells, have been nicely reviewed by Benhar *et al.* [139].

The above described findings resulted in a HIV clinical phase II trial of auranofin in combination with antiretroviral therapy. Interim analyses confirmed that auranofin was well tolerated and supported the idea that auranofin might impact the viral reservoir [140, 141].

The gold metabolite dicyanogold(I) was found to inhibit the replication of HIV in a cell culture model [142]. As dicyanogold(I) is a common metabolite of the three, clinically used antirheumatic gold complexes (aurothioglucose, aurothiomalate and auranofin), it can be speculated that it might be the source of the antiviral activity of these three individual gold drugs (see the review of Fonteh *et al.* for a broader discussion of this aspect) [143].

Regarding gold(III) compounds, bis(thiosemicarbazonate) gold(III) complexes (e.g. **Au-4**) were demonstrated to decrease HIV replication at cytostatic concentrations [144]. The authors of the study discussed that cytostatic agents can lower $CD4^+$ expression and T-cell proliferation, and with such cytostatic properties and suppressive effects on the immune activation, they could be part of a combination with antiviral agents. Further studies on two bis(thiosemicarbazonate) gold(III) complexes showed that they were able to reactivate latent HIV via activation of protein kinase c (PKC) with some contribution of exogenous TNF-α induction [145].

Interestingly, gold complexes have also emerged as hit compounds in several screening campaigns for antiviral drugs. In a screening of 774 FDA-registered drugs, auranofin was identified as 1 of 30 promising drug candidates against the Zika virus (ZIKV) [146]. In another high-throughput screening of a compound library of 767 FDA-approved drugs against vaccinia virus (VACV), auranofin was among the 26 top candidates that showed a selectivity index>3 after a toxicity counter screen in non-infected cells [147]. However, it was not among the compounds with a top selectivity index that were investigated further. In this screening, VACV was used as a surrogate for the smallpox virus, which is a virus of concern as potential bioterrorism agent.

Interestingly, with the gold analogue of the silver complex **Ag-2** described earlier, an organometallic gold species, **Au-5**, was generated and showed anti-HIV-1 activity in infected MT-4 leukaemia cells [116].

Regarding "direct" antiviral targets of gold complexes as anti-HIV compounds, the enzyme reverse transcriptase has been considered as a potential target in several studies. The likely first report on the effect of gold complexes on this enzyme is a conference report by Blough *et al.* at the 5th International Conference on AIDS in 1989 as discussed later in a review by Fonteh *et al.* [143]. The gold(III) porphyrin complex **Au-6** reported by Sun *et al.* is another interesting example of a gold-based reverse transcriptase inhibitor [148].

In 2009, Fonteh and Meyer reported 11 gold(I) phosphine complexes as inhibitors of HIV reverse transcriptase and protease [149]. Seven of those complexes inhibited reverse transcriptase activity, while four inhibited protease activity. Of the four complexes with activity against protease only, the one with low activity was active against reverse transcriptase (see **Au-7**). The gold-free ligands were inactive in the assays confirming the importance of the gold ions.

5.2.2 Gold Complexes as SARS-CoV-2 Antivirals

Based on the above outlined promising results as antiviral drug candidates, gold complexes were suggested for SARS-CoV-2 drug discovery and drug repurposing studies soon after the outbreak of the COVID-19 pandemic in 2019 [150]. The first experimental results were reported in 2020 by Rothan *et al.* [151] and Gil-Moles *et al.* [152]. Rothan *et al.* confirmed the antiviral effects of auranofin against SARS-CoV-2 infected cells in several types of assays [151]. Notably, auranofin reduced SARS-CoV-2 infectivity in low micromolar concentration below the level of toxicity. The infection with SARS-CoV-2 triggers acute inflammation and neutrophilia with an overexpression of several cytokines and reactive oxygen species. The so-called cytokine storm causes the devastating inflammatory lung disorder that is characteristic for COVID-19 and is associated with multiple organ dysfunction leading to high mortality of the infectious disease. Thus, inhibition of redox enzymes, such as TrxR, and anti-inflammatory effects with a reduction of cytokine formation triggered by auranofin, could affect SARS-CoV-2 infectivity and replication. In fact, auranofin efficiently decreased the SARS-COV-2-induced

Antiviral Agents Against SARS-CoV-2 and Other Pathogenic Viruses 127

strong up-regulation of key cytokines (IL-6, IL-1β, TNFα and NF-κB), suggesting that it could be a useful drug not only to block virus replication but also to limit the SARS-CoV-2 associated lung injury.

The inhibitory effects of auranofin and a series of five selected organometallic gold compounds against several target proteins of SARS-CoV-2 were studied by Gil-Moles *et al.* [152]. All complexes were moderate inhibitors of the interaction of the spike protein with the angiotensin-converting enzyme 2 (ACE2) of the host cell, indicating that the complexes could act as viral entry inhibitors. Studies on the inhibitory activity of the papain-like proteases (PL^{pro}) of SARS-CoV-2 as well as the PL^{pro} of the SARS outbreak in 2003 (SARS-CoV-1) revealed promising activity and interesting structure-activity relationships. As a cysteine protease, PL^{pro} hosts a cysteine residue in the catalytic site that can be considered as a likely binding partner for the Lewis-soft gold ions of the complexes. In addition, PL^{pro} contains a zinc-binding domain, where zinc is coordinated by several cysteines that are also likely to interact with gold complexes. In fact, the studied gold complexes showed a different pattern of activity between the two PL^{pro} enzymes from SARS-CoV-2 and SARS-CoV-1 with a broad range of activity from highly active (e.g. submicromolar IC$_{50}$ values) to inactive (e.g. >50μM). Mechanistic studies confirmed that the pattern of activity against the two types of PL^{pro} correlated excellently with efficacy of the complexes as zinc ejectors. Overall, regarding the protein targets of SARS-CoV-2, auranofin and some organometallic complexes could be considered as the most promising lead compounds for further inhibitor development.

Based on these promising results, a screening of more than 100 metal complexes, including 36 structurally diverse gold compounds, as inhibitors of the spike/ACE2 interaction and PL^{pro} activity was performed. These studies generally confirmed that gold complexes have a low to moderate efficacy as spike/ACE2 inhibitors; however, there are many examples of strong PL^{pro} inhibitors. With the exception of complexes with bulky side chains, complexes of the type (NHC)Au(I)Cl were among the most effective PL^{pro} inhibitors in a primary single-dosage screening together with some glycoconjugates and several gold(III) complexes. In good agreement with the above described study, biscarbene complexes with firmly coordinated ligands of the type Au(NHC)$_2^+$ or (alkynyl)Au(I)(NHC) were less potent inhibitors. For the ten most promising inhibitors, including the reference drug aurothiomalate, IC$_{50}$ values in the low micromolar nanomolar range were determined, confirming the considerable potential of gold complexes as SARS-CoV-2 PL^{pro} inhibitors. Notably, the strongest SARS-CoV-2 PL^{pro} inhibitor **Au-8** reached an IC$_{50}$ value as low as 90nM. After cell toxicity screening, the complexes aurothiomalate and **Au-8–Au-10** with absent or low cell toxicity were selected for antiviral studies in SARS-CoV-2 infected cells. While aurothiomalate was inactive in this antiviral assay, the (NHC)Au(I)Cl complex **Au-10** at low micromolar (6.25 and 25μM) and the gold(III) dithiocarbamates **Au-8** and **Au-9** at a high non-toxic dosage (500μM) strongly blocked SARS-CoV-2 replication.

Cirri *et al.* studied a panel of selected metallo-drugs, including five gold complexes, for their potential as SARS-CoV-2 antivirals at non-toxic concentration [10]. Of those, the gold(III) complex Aubipyc (**Au-11**) showed promising antiviral activity with a selectivity index over toxicity of 10.6. However, the other studied gold compounds, including auranofin, were not active in the assay. As for auranofin, the authors concluded that this contrast to other reports (see [151]) could be due to different experimental conditions and the almost overlapping dose-response curves for cytotoxicity and antiviral activity. For **Au-11**, computational chemistry supported the involvement of the interaction with reactive cysteine residues in the mechanism of action.

In a report on the relevance of the disulphide bonds of the receptor binding domain of the SARS-CoV-2 spike protein, auranofin was confirmed to prevent syncytia formation, viral entry into cells and infection in a pseudovirus mouse model, while aurothiomalate and aurothioglucose had no effects [153]. However, in addition to the above report about moderate activity in the spike/ACE2 assay [152], auranofin did not prevent binding of the spike protein to the ACE2 receptor and no covalent binding of auranofin to cysteines of the spike protein could be confirmed.

In a screening of a total of 7,039 compounds as inhibitors of the SARS-CoV-2 guanine-N7-methyltransferase auranofin was identified as 1 of the 33 best hit compounds [154]. Auranofin was not active against the human no human guanine-N7-methyltransferase; however, it was not active against viral replication in cells.

In another antiviral screening 1,043 FDA-approved drugs were investigated in a pseudovirus assay and the best candidates were evaluated in an authentic SARS-CoV-2 antiviral assay [155]. Auranofin was identified in the first round of screening among the 44 best candidates; however, it was among the 32 examples that were excluded from further screening because of toxicity.

In a library of 1,600 small molecule active pharmaceutical ingredients that was investigated for inhibition of SARS-CoV-2 main protease (M^{pro}), auranofin and aurothioglucose were identified as efficient inhibitors of the enzyme [156]. Similar to PL^{pro}, M^{pro} is a cysteine protease with an accessible cysteine in the catalytic site.

Aurothioglucose was also identified as 1 of 43 hit compounds in a high-throughput X-ray crystallographic screening of 5,953 compounds as M^{pro} inhibitors [157]. However, it was not active in an antiviral screening assay. In the aurothioglucose/M^{pro} crystal structure the cysteine residue Cys145 became oxidized to a sulfinic acid and a disulphide linkage to thioglucose was only observed at Cys156 on the surface of the enzyme, where thioglucose was located between two lysine residues, indicating that the compound did not lead to the expected formation of a stable gold-cysteine-adduct in the active site.

Importantly, auranofin has also been studied in an animal model. After oral administration in Syrian hamsters in therapeutic as well as prophylactic regimens, it reduced the viral replication, IL-6 production and lung inflammation [158].

Antiviral Agents Against SARS-CoV-2 and Other Pathogenic Viruses 129

5.3 Mercury Complexes as Antiviral Agents

Mercury and its complexes are known for their toxic effects and, as such, have been rarely investigated in metallo-drug design. Notable exceptions are some organomercury derivatives, such as thiomersal (also: thimerosal, **Hg-1**) or merbromin (**Hg-2**), that can be used as preservatives or antiseptics in cosmetic and pharmaceutical products.

Studies in mice indicated that exposure to methylmercury had negative effects on myocarditis caused by coxsackie virus [159]. Regarding antiviral studies against HIV-1, differing results were reported. Whereas neither mercury chloride nor its complex with N-acetylcysteine was active against HIV-1 in one report, mercury chloride was found to be active against HIV-1 in another study, although it triggered toxic effects [120, 121]. After a gene expression analysis in response to influenza A infection and screening of a database of drug-associated gene expression profiles, the topical antiseptic merbromin (**Hg-2**) was identified as a drug candidate and antiviral effects against influenza were confirmed [160].

Interestingly, merbromin was also identified as a nanomolar inhibitor of the pUL50-pUL53 interaction, which is relevant for the egress of the human cytomegalovirus (HCMV) [161]. The inhibitory effect was compound specific, as other mercury compounds, such as thiomersal, were not active. Merbromin also dose-dependently inhibited HCMV infection in human foreskin fibroblast (HFF) cells in the non-toxic range.

Thiomersal and phenylmercuric acetate (**Hg-3**) were identified as very potent inhibitors of the M^{pro} protease of the SARS outbreak from late 2002 in a screening of 960 drugs [85]. Moreover, both complexes also inhibited the replication of SARS-CoV-1 in cells.

The potential of these two complexes as well as merbromin as M^{pro} protease inhibitors was also confirmed for the enzyme of SARS-CoV-2 in several drug screening studies [162–165]. Regarding the enzymatic inhibition mechanism, for merbromin it was concluded that it is a mixed-type M^{pro} inhibitor that binds to the cysteine in the active site as well the interaction interface of the monomers of the enzyme [165].

In contrast to the promising results obtained with M^{pro}, thiomersal was among the inactive complexes in a screening for inhibitors of the spike/ACE2 interaction and the SARS-CoV-2 protease PL^{pro} [8]. Analogously to the results with auranofin (see above), thiomersal was among the most active hit compounds in a screening for inhibitors of the SARS-CoV-2 guanine-N7-methyltransferase; however, it was also not active in the cell-based antiviral assay [154].

6 SUMMARY AND OUTLOOK

The application of metal complexes as antiviral agents is less explored compared to other areas, such as the development of anticancer and antimicrobial agents. However, as a consequence of the current SARS-CoV-2 pandemic outbreak, the development of innovative antiviral drugs has emerged as a very urgent task. In this chapter, we have reviewed the most important developments of transition metal complexes with antiviral properties and given particular attention to SARS-CoV-2.

The most widely studied period 4 transition metals, from which the best conclusions can be extracted are those related to cobalt, copper and zinc complexes. In this respect, cobalt compounds have shown very good results against HSV reaching phase II clinical trials in the case of **Co-1** (CTC-96). Copper complexes have also shown very promising results in the treatment of influenza, their most important biological target being the M2 ion channel. In addition, copper complexes have also been shown to be very good HIV protease inhibitors. Regarding SARS-CoV-2, the studies carried out to date are only theoretical, although they suggest, together with the data against other viruses, that copper complexes may be very good candidates against SARS-CoV-2. Zinc compounds have been very successful against sexually transmitted viruses such as HSV, HIV and HPV. For example, zinc-based microbicidal gels have shown good *in vivo* results against HSV and can even prevent HIV transmission. In terms of activity of zinc salts against respiratory viruses, promising results have been observed against rhinoviruses and SARS-CoV-1/SARS-CoV-2 with RdRp, 3CL^{pro} and PL^{pro} being promising biological targets. In the case of 3CL^{pro}, the Zn-conjugates **Zn-5–Zn-9** were also shown to be potent inhibitors.

The period 5 metal complexes that appear to be most promising in this area contain ruthenium, rhodium and silver. Some ruthenium derivatives have already demonstrated strong HIV reverse transcriptase and HIV integrase inhibition. There are very few studies on rhodium complexes; however, they seem to be very good candidates for PL^{pro} inhibition of SARS-CoV-2. As for silver complexes, studies are also scarce although some studies have shown that silver compounds can be effective against HSV and HIV, among others. Regarding their activity against SARS-CoV-2, some silver complexes were shown to be able to selectively inhibit PL^{pro} of SARS-CoV-2 as the same derivatives hardly inhibited this enzyme of SARS-CoV-1.

In period 6, gold complexes have been the most extensively studied, most likely inspired by the success of auranofin. Gold compounds have demonstrated very promising results in the possible treatment of HIV with gp120/gp41, reverse transcriptase and TNF-α among the possible molecular targets. In addition, auranofin, in combination with antiretroviral therapeutic agents, has reached phase II clinical trials. As for SARS-CoV-2, the scientific community has made great efforts and in a very short period of time it has been possible to identify different gold compounds with potential to treat SARS-CoV-2 infections. Thus, for example, auranofin has shown very good results even in animal models and reduced the viral replication, IL-6 production and inflammation in the lungs. Also, auranofin and aurothioglucose were identified as efficient inhibitors of 3CL^{pro}. Furthermore, different gold(I) and gold(III) compounds have been demonstrated to be efficient inhibitors of PL^{pro} and moderate inhibitors of the spike/ACE2 interaction.

Following this review, we consider that metallo-drugs as antiviral agents have great potential. In addition, given the high number of new viruses that may appear in the future generating new pandemic outbreaks, research in this area is of great importance.

ACKNOWLEDGEMENTS

Financial support of our research by the Ministry of Science and Culture of Lower Saxony (graduate programme iCA "Drug Discovery and Cheminformatics for New Anti-infectives"), the DFG (Deutsche Forschungsgemeinschaft) and NextGenerationEU (Margarita Salas) is gratefully acknowledged.

ABBREVIATIONS

ACE2	angiotensin-converting enzyme 2
Ad2	adenovirus type 2
CHIKV	chikungunya virus
EAV	equine arteritis virus
EDTA	ethylenediamine tetraacetic acid
gp	glycoprotein
HAD type 5	human adenovirus type 5
HAdV-36	human adenovirus 36
HCMV	human cytomegalovirus
HCV	hepatitis C virus
HIV-1	human immunodeficiency virus 1
HIV-2	human immunodeficiency virus 2
HPV	human papilloma virus
HRV	human rhinovirus
HSV-1	herpes simplex virus 1
HSV-2	herpes simplex virus 2
Mpro	main protease/3CLpro (3 C-like protease)
PKC	protein kinase C
PLpro	papain-like protease
RdRp	RNA-dependent RNA polymerase
RSV	respiratory syncytial virus
RT	reverse transcriptase
SARS-CoV-1	severe acute respiratory syndrome coronavirus 1
SARS-CoV-2	severe acute respiratory syndrome coronavirus 2
SFV	Semliki forest virus
SHIV	simian-human immunodeficiency virus
SINV	sindbis virus
VACV	vaccinia virus: smallpox virus surrogate
VSV	vesicular stomatitis virus

REFERENCES

[1] A. Frei, J. Zuegg, A. G. Elliott, M. Baker, S. Braese, C. Brown, F. Chen, C. G Dowson, G. Dujardin, N. Jung, A. P. King, A. M. Mansour, M. Massi, J. Moat, H. A. Mohamed, A. K. Renfrew, P. J. Rutledge, P. J. Sadler, M. H. Todd, C. E. Willans, J. J. Wilson, M. A. Cooper, M. A. T. Blaskovich, *Chem. Sci.* **2020**, *11*, 2627–2639.

[2] S. Yuan, R. Wang, J. F.-W. Chan, A. J. Zhang, T. Cheng, K. K.-H. Chik, Z.-W. Ye, S. Wang, A. C.-Y. Lee, L. Jin, H. Li, D.-Y. Jin, K.-Y. Yuen, H. Sun, *Nature Microbiol.* **2020**, *5*, 1439–1448.

[3] R. Wang, J. F.-W. Chan, S. Wang, H. Li, J. Zhao, T. K.-Y. Ip, Z. Zuo, K.-Y. Yuen, S. Yuan, H. Sun, *Chem. Sci.* **2022**, *13*, 2238–2248.

[4] R. E. F. de Paiva, A. Marçal Neto, I. A. Santos, A. C. G. Jardim, P. P. Corbi, F. R. G. Bergamini, *Dalton Trans.* **2020**, *49*, 16004–16033.

[5] D. Cirri, A. Pratesi, T. Marzo, L. Messori, *Expert Opin. Drug Disc.* **2021**, *16*, 39–46.

[6] K. Ioannou, M. C. Vlasiou, *Biometals* **2022**, *35*, 639–652.

[7] J. Karges, S. M. Cohen, *Chembiochem* **2021**, *22*, 2600–2607.

[8] M. Gil-Moles, S. Türck, U. Basu, A. Pettenuzzo, S. Bhattacharya, A. Rajan, X. Ma, R. Büssing, J. Wölker, H. Burmeister, H. Hoffmeister, P. Schneeberg, A. Prause, P. Lippmann, J. Kusi-Nimarko, S. Hassell-Hart, A. McGown, D. Guest, Y. Lin, A. Notaro, R. Vinck, J. Karges, K. Cariou, K. Peng, X. Qin, X. Wang, J. Skiba, Ł. Szczupak, K. Kowalski, U. Schatzschneider, C. Hemmert, H. Gornitzka, E. R. Milaeva, A. A. Nazarov, G. Gasser, J. Spencer, L. Ronconi, U. Kortz, J. Cinatl, D. Bojkova, I. Ott, *Chem. Eur. J.* **2021**, *27*, 17928–17940.

[9] S. G. Ward, R. C. Taylor, P. Köpf-Maier, H. Köpf, J. Balzarini, E. de Clercq, *Appl. Organometal. Chem.* **1989**, *3*, 491–497.

[10] D. Cirri, T. Marzo, I. Tolbatov, A. Marrone, F. Saladini, I. Vicenti, F. Dragoni, A. Boccuto, L. Messori, *Biomolecules* **2021**, *11*, 1858.

[11] J. C. Pessoa, S. Etcheverry, D. Gambino, Coord. *Chem. Rev.* **2015**, *301*, 24–48.

[12] A. Sigel, H. Sigel, R. K. O. Sigel, Eds., *Interrelations between Essential Metal Ions and Human Diseases*, Springer, Dordrecht, New York, **2013**.

[13] R. W.-Y. Sun, D.-L. Ma, E. L.-M. Wong, C.-M. Che, *Dalton Trans.* **2007**, 43 4884–4892.

[14] O. J. D'Cruz, Y. Dong, F. M. Uckun, *Biochem. Biophys. Res. Commun.* **2003**, *302*, 253–264.

[15] A. Ross, D. C. Soares, D. Covelli, C. Pannecouque, L. Budd, A. Collins, N. Robertson, S. Parsons, E. de Clercq, P. Kennepohl, P. J. Sadler, *Inorg. Chem.* **2010**, *49*, 1122–1132.

[16] S.-Y. Wong, R. Wai-Yin Sun, N. P.-Y. Chung, C.-L. Lin, C.-M. Che, *Chem. Commun.* **2005**, 28 3544–3546.

[17] T. Scior, H. H. Abdallah, S. F. Z. Mustafa, J. A. Guevara-García, D. Rehder, *Inorg. Chim. Acta.* **2021**, *519*, 120287.

[18] M. C. Vlasiou, K. S. Pafti, *Comput. Toxicol.* **2021**, *18*, 100157.

[19] L. Coffee, *Diet and Health; Implications for Reducing Chronic Disease Risk*, National Acad. Press, Washington, DC, **1991**.

[20] E. Aghdassi, I. E. Salit, L. Fung, S. Sreetharan, S. Walmsley, J. P. Allard, *J. Am. Coll. Nutr.* **2006**, *25*, 56–63.

[21] E. Aghdassi, B. M. Arendt, I. E. Salit, S. S. Mohammed, P. Jalali, H. Bondar, J. P. Allard, *Curr. HIV Res.* **2010**, *8*, 113–120.

[22] S. Terpiłowska, A. K. Siwicki, *Biometals* **2017**, *30*, 565–574.

[23] P. Puddu, P. Borghi, S. Gessani, P. Valenti, F. Belardelli, L. Seganti, *Int. J. Biochem. Cell Biol.* **1998**, *30*, 1055–1063.

[24] F. Superti, R. Siciliano, B. Rega, F. Giansanti, P. Valenti, G. Antonini, *Biochim. Biophys. Acta Gen. Subj.* **2001**, *1528*, 107–115.

[25] A. Pietrantoni, M. G. Ammendolia, F. Superti, *Biochem. Cell Biol.* **2012**, *90*, 442–448.

[26] M. Carcelli, D. Rogolino, M. Sechi, G. Rispoli, E. Fisicaro, C. Compari, N. Grandi, A. Corona, E. Tramontano, C. Pannecouque, L. Naesens, *Eur. J. Med. Chem.* **2014**, *83*, 594–600.

Antiviral Agents Against SARS-CoV-2 and Other Pathogenic Viruses   133

[27] D. Rogolino, M. Carcelli, A. Bacchi, C. Compari, L. Contardi, E. Fisicaro, A. Gatti, M. Sechi, A. Stevaert, L. Naesens, *J. Inorg. Biochem.* **2015**, *150*, 9–17.

[28] F. P. Dwyer, E. C. Gyarfas, W. P. Rogers, J. H. Koch, *Nature* **1952**, *170*, 190–191.

[29] G. Costa, G. Mestroni, G. Tauzher, L. Stefani, *J. Organomet. Chem.* **1966**, *6*, 181–187.

[30] S. P. Epstein, J. A. Wallace, D. Epstein, C. C. Stewart, R. M. Burger, *Cornea* **1998**, *17*, 550–557.

[31] E. L. Chang, C. Simmers, D. A. Knight, *Pharmaceuticals (Basel)* **2010**, *3*, 1711–1728.

[32] A. Y. Louie, T. J. Meade, *PNAS* **1998**, *95*, 6663–6668.

[33] J. A. Schwartz, E. K. Lium, S. J. Silverstein, *J. Virol.* **2001**, *75*, 4117–4128.

[34] S. P. Epstein, Y. Y. Pashinsky, D. Gershon, I. Winicov, C. Srivilasa, K. J. Kristic, P. A. Asbell, *BMC Ophthalmol.* **2006**, *6*, 22.

[35] J. B. Delehanty, J. E. Bongard, D. C. Thach, D. A. Knight, T. E. Hickey, E. L. Chang, *Bioorg. Med. Chem.* **2008**, *16*, 830–837.

[36] S. García-Gallego, M. J. Serramía, E. Arnaiz, L. Díaz, M. A. Muñoz-Fernández, P. Gómez-Sal, M. F. Ottaviani, R. Gómez, F. J. de La Mata, *Eur. J. Inorg. Chem.* **2011**, 1657–1665.

[37] V. P. Kirin, A. G. Demkin, A. I. Smolentsev, T. N. Il'icheva, V. A. Maksakov, *Russ. J. Coord. Chem.* **2016**, *42*, 260–266.

[38] V. P. Kirin, A. G. Demkin, T. S. Sukhikh, T. N. Ilyicheva, V. A. Maksakov, *J. Mol. Struct.* **2022**, *1250*, 131486.

[39] S. Kumar, A. V. Trivedi, *Int. J. Curr. Microbiol. App. Sci.* **2016**, *5*, 719–727.

[40] I. Iakovidis, I. Delimaris, S. M. Piperakis, *Mol. Biol. Int.* **2011**, *2011*, 594529.

[41] V. Govind, S. Bharadwaj, M. R. Sai Ganesh, J. Vishnu, K. V. Shankar, B. Shankar, R. Rajesh, *Biometals* **2021**, *34*, 1217–1235.

[42] N. A. Gordon, K. L. McGuire, S. K. Wallentine, G. A. Mohl, J. D. Lynch, R. G. Harrison, D. D. Busath, *Antivir. Res.* **2017**, *147*, 100–106.

[43] K. L. McGuire, J. Hogge, A. Hintze, N. Liddle, N. Nelson, J. Pollock, A. Brown, S. Facer, S. Walker, J. Lynch, R. G. Harrison, D. D. Busath, in *Engineered Nanomaterials – Health and Safety*, Eds S. Marius Avramescu, K. Akhtar, I. Fierascu, S. Bahadar Khan, F. Ali, A. M. Asiri, IntechOpen, London **2020**. DOI: 10.5772/intechopen.88786

[44] N. N. Trofimova, V. A. Babkin, O. I. Kiselev, *Russ. Chem. Bull.* **2015**, *64*, 1430–1436.

[45] C. N. Banti, N. Kourkoumelis, A. G. Hatzidimitriou, I. Antoniadou, A. Dimou, M. Rallis, A. Hoffmann, M. Schmidtke, K. McGuire, D. Busath, A. Kolocouris, S. K. Hadjikakou, *Polyhedron* **2020**, *185*, 114590.

[46] A. R. Karlström, R. L. Levine, *PNAS* **1991**, *88*, 5552–5556.

[47] D. A. Davis, A. A. Branca, A. J. Pallenberg, T. M. Marschner, L. M. Patt, L. G. Chatlynne, R. W. Humphrey, R. Yarchoan, R. L. Levine, *Arch. Biochem. Biophys.* **1995**, *322*, 127–134.

[48] F. Lebon, N. Boggetto, M. Ledecq, F. Durant, Z. Benatallah, S. Sicsic, R. Lapouyade, O. Kahn, A. Mouithys-Mickalad, G. Deby-Dupont, M. Reboud-Ravaux, *Biochem. Pharmacol.* **2002**, *63*, 1863–1873.

[49] J. L. Sagripanti, L. B. Routson, C. D. Lytle, *Appl. Environ. Microbiol.* **1993**, *59*, 4374–4376.

[50] J. L. Sagripanti, L. B. Routson, A. C. Bonifacino, C. D. Lytle, *Antimicrob. Agents Chemother.* **1997**, *41*, 812–817.

[51] S. Bradford, J. A. Cowan, *Chem. Commun.* **2012**, *48*, 3118–3120.

[52] W. L. M. Alencar, T. da Silva Arouche, A. F. G. Neto, T. de Castro Ramalho, R. N. de Carvalho Júnior, A. M. de Jesus Chaves Neto, *Sci. Rep.* **2022**, *12*, 3316.

[53] S. Kumar, M. Choudhary, *New J. Chem.* **2022**, *46*, 7128–7143.

[54] A. Andreou, S. Trantza, D. Filippou, N. Sipsas, S. Tsiodras, *In Vivo (Athens, Greece)* **2020**, *34*, 1567–1588.

[55] I. Rani, A. Goyal, M. Bhatnagar, S. Manhas, P. Goel, A. Pal, R. Prasad, *Nutr. Res.* **2021**, *92*, 109–128.

[56] A. L. Wani, N. Parveen, M. O. Ansari, M. F. Ahmad, S. Jameel, G. Shadab, *Curr. Med. Res. Pract.* **2017**, *7*, 90–98.

[57] S. A. Read, S. Obeid, C. Ahlenstiel, G. Ahlenstiel, *Adv. Nutr.* **2019**, *10*, 696–710.

[58] T. Ishida, *AJBSR* **2019**, *2*, 28–37.

[59] A. V. Skalny, L. Rink, O. P. Ajsuvakova, M. Aschner, V. A. Gritsenko, S. I. Alekseenko, A. A. Svistunov, D. Petrakis, D. A. Spandidos, J. Aaseth, A. Tsatsakis, A. A. Tinkov, *Int. J. Mol. Med.* **2020**, *46*, 17–26.

[60] Y. J. Gordon, Y. Asher, Y. Becker, *Antimicrob. Agents Chemother.* **1975**, *8*, 377–380.

[61] P. Gupta, F. Rapp, *SEBM* **1976**, *152*, 455–458.

[62] B. Fridlender, N. Chejanovsky, Y. Becker, *Virology* **1978**, *84*, 551–554.

[63] G. Kümel, S. Schrader, H. Zentgraf, H. Daus, M. Brendel, *J. Gen. Virol.* **1990**, *71* (Pt 12), 2989–2997.

[64] N. Bourne, R. Stegall, R. Montano, M. Meador, L. R. Stanberry, G. N. Milligan, *Antimicrob. Agents Chemother.* **2005**, *49*, 1181–1183.

[65] J. A. Fernández-Romero, C. J. Abraham, A. Rodriguez, L. Kizima, N. Jean-Pierre, R. Menon, O. Begay, S. Seidor, B. E. Ford, P. I. Gil, J. Peters, D. Katz, M. Robbiani, T. M. Zydowsky, *Antimicrob. Agents Chemother.* **2012**, *56*, 358–368.

[66] J. Kenney, A. Rodríguez, L. Kizima, S. Seidor, R. Menon, N. Jean-Pierre, P. Pugach, K. Levendosky, N. Derby, A. Gettie, J. Blanchard, M. Piatak, J. D. Lifson, G. Paglini, T. M. Zydowsky, M. Robbiani, J. A. Fernández Romero, *Antimicrob. Agents Chemother.* **2013**, *57*, 4001–4009.

[67] Z. Y. Zhang, I. M. Reardon, J. O. Hui, K. L. O'Connell, R. A. Poorman, A. G. Tomaselli, R. L. Heinrikson, *Biochemistry* **1991**, *30*, 8717–8721.

[68] Y. Haraguchi, H. Sakurai, S. Hussain, B. M. Anner, H. Hoshino, *Antiviral Res.* **1999**, *43*, 123–133.

[69] K. J. Fenstermacher, J. J. DeStefano, *J. Biol. Chem.* **2011**, *286*, 40433–40442.

[70] S. N. Bae, K. H. Lee, J. H. Kim, S. J. Lee, L. O. Park, *Biochem. Biophys. Res. Commun.* **2017**, *484*, 218–223.

[71] A. B. Sravani, V. Ghate, S. Lewis, *Biol. Trace Elem. Res.* **2022**. https://doi.org/10.1007/s12011-022-03226-2

[72] J. H. Kim, S. N. Bae, C. W. Lee, M. J. Song, S. J. Lee, J. H. Yoon, K. H. Lee, S. Y. Hur, T. C. Park, J. S. Park, *Gynecol. Oncol.* **2011**, *122*, 303–306.

[73] J.-H. Mun, S.-H. Kim, D.-S. Jung, H.-C. Ko, B.-S. Kim, K.-S. Kwon, M.-B. Kim, J. *Dermatol.* **2011**, *38*, 541–545.

[74] R. S. Mboumba Bouassa, B. Gombert, G. Mwande-Maguene, A. Mannarini, L. Bélec, *Heliyon* **2021**, *7*, e07232.

[75] K. Yuasa, A. Naganuma, K. Sato, M. Ikeda, N. Kato, H. Takagi, M. Mori, *Liver Int.* **2006**, *26*, 1111–1118.

[76] S. A. Read, G. Parnell, D. Booth, M. W. Douglas, J. George, G. Ahlenstiel, *J. Viral Hepat.* **2018**, *25*, 491–501.

[77] J. Corver, R. Bron, H. Snippe, C. Kraaijeveld, J. Wilschut, *Virology* **1997**, *238*, 14–21.

[78] C. Y. Liu, M. Kielian, *J. Virol.* **2012**, *86*, 3588–3594.

[79] B. D. Korant, J. C. Kauer, B. E. Butterworth, *Nature* **1974**, *248*, 588–590.

[80] B. D. Korant, B. E. Butterworth, *J. Virol.* **1976**, *18*, 298–306.

[81] F. C. Geist, J. A. Bateman, F. G. Hayden, *Antimicrob. Agents Chemother.* **1987**, *31*, 622–624.

[82] G. A. Eby, *Med. Hypotheses* **2010**, *74*, 482–492.

Antiviral Agents Against SARS-CoV-2 and Other Pathogenic Viruses 135

[83] R. O. Suara, J. E. Crowe, *Antimicrob. Agents Chemother.* **2004**, *48*, 783–790.

[84] A. J. W. te Velthuis, S. H. E. van den Worm, A. C. Sims, R. S. Baric, E. J. Snijder, M. J. van Hemert, *PLoS Pathog.* **2010**, *6*, e1001176.

[85] J. T.-A. Hsu, C.-J. Kuo, H.-P. Hsieh, Y.-C. Wang, K.-K. Huang, C. P.-C. Lin, P.-F. Huang, X. Chen, P.-H. Liang, *FEBS Lett.* **2004**, *574*, 116–120.

[86] C.-C. Lee, C.-J. Kuo, M.-F. Hsu, P.-H. Liang, J.-M. Fang, J.-J. Shie, A. H.-J. Wang, *FEBS Lett.* **2007**, *581*, 5454–5458.

[87] D. Grifagni, V. Calderone, S. Giuntini, F. Cantini, M. Fragai, L. Banci, *Chem. Commun.* **2021**, *57*, 7910–7913.

[88] L. Panchariya, W. A. Khan, S. Kuila, K. Sonkar, S. Sahoo, A. Ghoshal, A. Kumar, D. K. Verma, A. Hasan, M. A. Khan, N. Jain, A. K. Mohapatra, S. Das, J. K. Thakur, S. Maiti, R. K. Nanda, R. Halder, S. Sunil, A. Arockiasamy, *Chem. Commun.* **2021**, *57*, 10083–10086.

[89] X. Tao, L. Zhang, L. Du, K. Lu, Z. Zhao, Y. Xie, X. Li, S. Huang, P.-H. Wang, J.-A. Pan, W. Xia, J. Dai, Z.-W. Mao, *J. Inorg. Biochem.* **2022**, *231*, 111777.

[90] M. A. Synowiecki, L. R. Perk, J. F. W. Nijsen, *EJNMMI Radiopharm. Chem.* **2018**, *3*, 3.

[91] M. Jelikić-Stankov, S. Uskoković-Marković, I. Holclajtner-Antunović, M. Todorović, P. Djurdjević, *J. Trace. Elem. Med. Biol.* **2007**, *21*, 8–16.

[92] D.-L. Ma, M. Wang, Z. Mao, C. Yang, C.-T. Ng, C.-H. Leung, *Dalton Trans.* **2016**, *45*, 2762–2771.

[93] A.-C. Munteanu, V. Uivarosi, *Pharmaceutics* **2021**, *13*(6), 874. https://doi.org/10.3390/pharmaceutics13060874

[94] L. Mishra, H. Itokawa, K. F. Bastow, Y. Tachibana, Y. Nakanishi, N. Kilgore, K.-H. Lee, R. Sinha, *Bioorg. Med. Chem.* **2001**, *9*, 1667–1671.

[95] E. L.-M. Wong, R. W.-Y. Sun, N. P.-Y. Chung, C.-L. S. Lin, N. Zhu, C.-M. Che, *J. Am. Chem. Soc.* **2006**, *128*, 4938–4939.

[96] M. Carcelli, A. Bacchi, P. Pelagatti, G. Rispoli, D. Rogolino, T. W. Sanchez, M. Sechi, N. Neamati, *J. Inorg. Biochem.* **2013**, *118*, 74–82.

[97] L. Cardo, I. Nawroth, P. J. Cail, J. A. McKeating, M. J. Hannon, *Sci. Rep.* **2018**, *8*, 13342.

[98] C. S. Allardyce, P. J. Dyson, D. J. Ellis, P. A. Salter, R. Scopelliti, *J. Organomet. Chem.* **2003**, *668*, 35–42.

[99] E. L. Menon, R. Perera, M. Navarro, R. J. Kuhn, H. Morrison, *Inorg. Chem.* **2004**, *43*, 5373–5381.

[100] C. Chuong, C. M. DuChane, E. M. Webb, P. Rai, J. M. Marano, C. M. Bernier, J. S. Merola, J. Weger-Lucarelli, *Viruses* **2021**, *13*(6), 980. doi: 10.3390/v13060980

[101] A. Garoufis, S. K. Hadjikakou, N. Hadjiliadis, *Coord. Chem. Rev.* **2009**, *253*, 1384–1397.

[102] P. Genova, T. Varadinova, A. I. Matesanz, D. Marinova, P. Souza, *Toxicol. Appl. Pharmacol.* **2004**, *197*, 107–112.

[103] J. Gómez-Segura, S. Caballero, V. Moreno, M. J. Prieto, A. Bosch, *J. Inorg. Biochem.* **2009**, *103*, 128–134.

[104] S. Chernousova, M. Epple, *Angew. Chem. Int. Ed.* **2013**, *52*, 1636–1653.

[105] H. D. Betts, C. Whitehead, H. H. Harris, *Metallomics* **2021**, *13*. https://doi.org/10.1093/mtomcs/mfaa001

[106] S. S. Jeremiah, K. Miyakawa, T. Morita, Y. Yamaoka, A. Ryo, *Biochem. Biophys. Res. Commun.* **2020**, *533*, 195–200.

[107] U. Ghosh, K. Sayef Ahammed, S. Mishra, A. Bhaumik, *Chem. As. J.* **2022**, *17*, e202101149.

[108] V. R. Coleman, J. Wilkie, W. E. Levinson, T. Stevens, E. Jawetz, *Antimicrob. Agents Chemother.* **1973**, *4*, 259–262.

[109] W. Levinson, V. Coleman, B. Woodson, A. Rabson, J. Lanier, J. Whitcher, C. Dawson, *Antimicrob. Agents Chemother.* **1974**, *5*, 398–402.

[110] F. Shimizu, Y. Shimizu, K. Kumagai, *Antimicrob. Agents Chemother.* **1976**, *10*, 57–63.

[111] T. Tokumaru, Y. Shimizu, C. L. Fox, *Res. Commun. Chem. Pathol. Pharmacol.* **1974**, *8*, 151–158.

[112] P. G. Esquezaro, C. M. Manzano, D. H. Nakahata, I. A. Santos, U. E. A. Ruiz, M. B. Santiago, N. B. S. Silva, C. H. G. Martins, D. H. Pereira, F. R. G. Bergamini, A. C. G. Jardim, P. P. Corbi, *J. Mol. Struct.* **2021**, *1246*, 131261.

[113] P. C. Zachariadis, S. K. Hadjikakou, N. Hadjiliadis, A. Michaelides, S. Skoulika, Y. Ming, Y. Xiaolin, *Inorg. Chim. Acta* **2003**, *343*, 361–365.

[114] P. C. Zachariadis, S. K. Hadjikakou, N. Hadjiliadis, S. Skoulika, A. Michaelides, J. Balzarini, E. de Clercq, *Eur. J. Inorg. Chem.* **2004**, *2004*, 1420–1426.

[115] D. E. Bergstrom, X. Lin, T. D. Wood, M. Witvrouw, S. Ikeda, G. Andrei, R. Snoeck, D. Schols, E. de Clercq, *Antivir. Chem. Chemother.* **2002**, *13*, 185–195.

[116] O. Sánchez, S. González, Á. R. Higuera-Padilla, Y. León, D. Coll, M. Fernández, P. Taylor, I. Urdanibia, H. R. Rangel, J. T. Ortega, W. Castro, M. C. Goite, *Polyhedron* **2016**, *110*, 14–23.

[117] I. I. Seifullina, E. É. Martsinko, T. L. Gridina, E. A. Chebanenko, L. M. Mudrik, A. S. Fedchuk, *Pharm. Chem. J.* **2019**, *53*, 318–321.

[118] J. S. M. Rodrigues, A. M. Rodrigues, D. do Nascimento Souza, E. R. P. de Novais, A. M. Rodrigues, G. C. A. de Oliveira, A. de Lima Ferreira Novais, *J. Mol. Model.* **2021**, *27*, 323.

[119] E. Üstün, N. Özdemir, N. Şahin, *J. Coord. Chem.* **2021**, *74*, 3109–3126.

[120] N. Mahmood, A. Burke, S. Hussain, R. M. Anner, B. M. Anner, *Antivir. Chem. Chemother.* **1995**, *6*, 187–189.

[121] Y. Haraguchi, H. Sakurai, S. Hussain, B. M. Anner, H. Hoshino, *Antivir. Res.* **1999**, *43*, 123–133.

[122] A. Shulman, D. O. White, *Chem.-Biol. Interact.* **1973**, *6*, 407–413.

[123] A. Koschinski, G. Wengler, G. Wengler, H. Repp, *J. Gen. Virol.* **2005**, *86*, 3311–3320.

[124] G. Wengler, G. Wengler, A. Koschinski, *J. Gen. Virol.* **2007**, *88*, 3018–3026.

[125] E. Dadachova, M. C. Patel, S. Toussi, C. Apostolidis, A. Morgenstern, M. W. Brechbiel, M. K. Gorny, S. Zolla-Pazner, A. Casadevall, H. Goldstein, *PLoS Med.* **2006**, *3*, e427.

[126] J. Karges, M. Kalaj, M. Bembicky, S. M. Cohen, *Angew. Chem. Int. Ed.* **2021**, *60*, 10716–10723.

[127] C. Wu, K.-J. Wu, J.-B. Liu, X.-M. Zhou, C.-H. Leung, D.-L. Ma, *Chem. Commun.* **2019**, *55*, 6353–6356.

[128] D. Bai, Y. Tian, K. Chen, X. Zhang, F. Wang, Y. Cheng, X. Zheng, K. Xiao, X. Dong, *Dyes Pigm.* **2020**, *182*, 108635.

[129] F. de Castro, E. de Luca, M. Benedetti, F. P. Fanizzi, *Coord. Chem. Rev.* **2022**, *451*, 214276.

[130] H. S. Allaudeen, R. M. Snyder, M. H. Whitman, S. T. Crooke, *Biochem. Pharmacol.* **1985**, *34*, 3243–3250.

[131] T. Okada, B. K. Patterson, S. Q. Ye, M. E. Gurney, *Virology* **1993**, *192*, 631–642.

[132] K. Reiser, K. O. François, D. Schols, T. Bergman, H. Jörnvall, J. Balzarini, A. Karlsson, M. Lundberg, *Int. J. Biochem. Cell Biol.* **2012**, *44*, 556–562.

[133] K. E. Traber, H. Okamoto, C. Kurono, M. Baba, C. Saliou, T. Soji, L. Packer, T. Okamoto, *Int. Immunol.* **1999**, *11*, 143–150.

[134] K. Yamaguchi, H. Ushijima, M. Hisano, Y. Inoue, T. Shimamura, T. Hirano, W. E. Müller, *Microbiol. Immunol.* **2001**, *45*, 549–555.

[135] D. L. Shapiro, J. R. Masci, *J. Rheumatol.* **1996**, *23*, 1818–1820.

[136] M. G. Lewis, S. DaFonseca, N. Chomont, A. T. Palamara, M. Tardugno, A. Mai, M. Collins, W. L. Wagner, J. Yalley-Ogunro, J. Greenhouse, B. Chirullo, S. Norelli, E. Garaci, A. Savarino, *AIDS* **2011**, *25*, 1347–1356.

Antiviral Agents Against SARS-CoV-2 and Other Pathogenic Viruses 137

[137] I. L. Shytaj, B. Chirullo, W. Wagner, M. G. Ferrari, R. Sgarbanti, A. Della Corte, C. LaBranche, L. Lopalco, A. T. Palamara, D. Montefiori, M. G. Lewis, E. Garaci, A. Savarino, *Retrovirol.* **2013**, *10*, 71.

[138] B. Chirullo, R. Sgarbanti, D. Limongi, I. L. Shytaj, D. Alvarez, B. Das, A. Boe, S. DaFonseca, N. Chomont, L. Liotta, E. Petricoin, III, S. Norelli, E. Pelosi, E. Garaci, A. Savarino, A. T. Palamara, *Cell Death Dis.* **2013**, *4*, e944.

[139] M. Benhar, I. L. Shytaj, J. S. Stamler, A. Savarino, *J. Clin. Invest.* **2016**, 126, 1630–1639.

[140] R. S. Diaz, I. L. Shytaj, L. B. Giron, B. Obermaier, E. Della Libera, J. Galinskas, D. Dias, J. Hunter, M. Janini, G. Gosuen, P. A. Ferreira, M. C. Sucupira, J. Maricato, O. Fackler, M. Lusic, A. Savarino, *Int. J. Antimicrob. Ag.* **2019**, *54*, 592–600.

[141] M. V. de Almeida Baptista, L. T. Da Silva, S. Samer, T. M. Oshiro, I. L. Shytaj, L. B. Giron, N. M. Pena, N. Cruz, G. C. Gosuen, P. R. A. Ferreira, E. Cunha-Neto, J. Galinskas, D. Dias, M. C. A. Sucupira, C. de Almeida-Neto, R. Salomão, A. J. Da Silva Duarte, L. M. Janini, J. R. Hunter, A. Savarino, M. A. Juliano, R. S. Diaz, *AIDS Res. Ther.* **2022**, *19*, 2.

[142] K. Tepperman, Y. Zhang, P. W. Roy, R. Floyd, Z. Zhao, J. G. Dorsey, R. C. Elder, *Met.-Based Drugs.* **1994**, *1*, 433–443.

[143] P. N. Fonteh, F. K. Keter, D. Meyer, *Biometals* **2010**, *23*, 185–196.

[144] P. N. Fonteh, F. K. Keter, D. Meyer, *J. Inorg. Biochem.* **2011**, *105*, 1173–1180.

[145] P. Fonteh, D. Meyer, *BMC Inf. Dis.* **2014**, *14*, 680.

[146] N. J. Barrows, R. K. Campos, S. T. Powell, K. R. Prasanth, G. Schott-Lerner, R. Soto-Acosta, G. Galarza-Muñoz, E. L. McGrath, R. Urrabaz-Garza, J. Gao, P. Wu, R. Menon, G. Saade, I. Fernandez-Salas, S. L. Rossi, N. Vasilakis, A. Routh, S. S. Bradrick, M. A. Garcia-Blanco, *Cell Host & Microbe* **2016**, *20*, 259–270.

[147] J. Wu, Q. Liu, H. Xie, R. Chen, W. Huang, C. Liang, X. Xiao, Y. Yu, Y. Wang, *J. Med. Virol.* **2019**, *91*, 2016–2024.

[148] R. W.-Y. Sun, W.-Y. Yu, H. Sun, C.-M. Che, *Chembiochem* **2004**, *5*, 1293–1298.

[149] P. Fonteh, D. Meyer, *Metallomics* **2009**, *1*, 427–433.

[150] T. Marzo, L. Messori, *ACS Med. Chem. Lett.* **2020**, *11*, 1067–1068.

[151] H. A. Rothan, S. Stone, J. Natekar, P. Kumari, K. Arora, M. Kumar, *Virology* **2020**, *547*, 7–11.

[152] M. Gil-Moles, U. Basu, R. Büssing, H. Hoffmeister, S. Türck, A. Varchmin, I. Ott, *Chem. Eur. J.* **2020**, *26*, 15140–15144.

[153] M. Manček-Keber, I. Hafner-Bratkovič, D. Lainšček, M. Benčina, T. Govednik, S. Orehek, T. Plaper, V. Jazbec, V. Bergant, V. Grass, A. Pichlmair, R. Jerala, *FASEB J.* **2021**, *35*, e21651.

[154] R. Kasprzyk, T. J. Spiewla, M. Smietanski, S. Golojuch, L. Vangeel, S. de Jonghe, D. Jochmans, J. Neyts, J. Kowalska, J. Jemielity, *Antivir. Res.* **2021**, *193*, 105142.

[155] H.-L. Xiong, J.-L. Cao, C.-G. Shen, J. Ma, X.-Y. Qiao, T.-S. Shi, S.-X. Ge, H.-M. Ye, J. Zhang, Q. Yuan, T.-Y. Zhang, N.-S. Xia, *Front. Pharmacol.* **2020**, *11*, 609592.

[156] T. R. Malla, A. Tumber, T. John, L. Brewitz, C. Strain-Damerell, C. D. Owen, P. Lukacik, H. T. H. Chan, P. Maheswaran, E. Salah, F. Duarte, H. Yang, Z. Rao, M. A. Walsh, C. J. Schofield, *Chem. Commun.* **2021**, *57*, 1430–1433.

[157] S. Günther, P. Y. A. Reinke, Y. Fernández-García, J. Lieske, T. J. Lane, H. M. Ginn, F. H. M. Koua, C. Ehrt, W. Ewert, D. Oberthuer, O. Yefanov, S. Meier, K. Lorenzen, B. Krichel, J.-D. Kopicki, L. Gelisio, W. Brehm, I. Dunkel, B. Seychell, H. Gieseler, B. Norton-Baker, B. Escudero-Pérez, M. Domaracky, S. Saouane, A. Tolstikova, T. A. White, A. Hänle, M. Groessler, H. Fleckenstein, F. Trost, M. Galchenkova, Y. Gevorkov, C. Li, S. Awel, A. Peck, M. Barthelmess, F. Schlünzen, P. Lourdu Xavier, N. Werner, H. Andaleeb, N. Ullah, S. Falke, V. Srinivasan, B. A. França,

M. Schwinzer, H. Brognaro, C. Rogers, D. Melo, J. J. Zaitseva-Doyle, J. Knoska, G. E. Peña-Murillo, A. R. Mashhour, V. Hennicke, P. Fischer, J. Hakanpää, J. Meyer, P. Gribbon, B. Ellinger, M. Kuzikov, M. Wolf, A. R. Beccari, G. Bourenkov, D. von Stetten, G. Pompidor, I. Bento, S. Panneerselvam, I. Karpics, T. R. Schneider, M. M. Garcia-Alai, S. Niebling, C. Günther, C. Schmidt, R. Schubert, H. Han, J. Boger, D. C. F. Monteiro, L. Zhang, X. Sun, J. Pletzer-Zelgert, J. Wollenhaupt, C. G. Feiler, M. S. Weiss, E.-C. Schulz, P. Mehrabi, K. Karničar, A. Usenik, J. Loboda, H. Tidow, A. Chari, R. Hilgenfeld, C. Uetrecht, R. Cox, A. Zaliani, T. Beck, M. Rarey, S. Günther, D. Turk, W. Hinrichs, H. N. Chapman, A. R. Pearson, C. Betzel, A. Meents, *Science* **2021**, *372*, 642–646.

[158] A. Biji, O. Khatun, S. Swaraj, R. Narayan, R. S. Rajmani, R. Sardar, D. Satish, S. Mehta, H. Bindhu, M. Jeevan, D. K. Saini, A. Singh, D. Gupta, S. Tripathi, *EBioMedicine* **2021**, *70*, 103525.

[159] N. G. Ilbäck, L. Wesslén, J. Fohlman, G. Friman, *Tox. Lett.* **1996**, *89*, 19–28.

[160] L. Josset, J. Textoris, B. Loriod, O. Ferraris, V. Moules, B. Lina, C. N'guyen, J.-J. Diaz, M. Rosa-Calatrava, *PloS One* **2010**, *5*, e13169.

[161] S. Alkhashrom, J. Kicuntod, S. Häge, J. Schweininger, Y. A. Muller, P. Lischka, M. Marschall, J. Eichler, *Viruses* **2021**, *13*, 471.

[162] C. Coelho, G. Gallo, C. B. Campos, L. Hardy, M. Würtele, *PloS One* **2020**, *15*, e0240079.

[163] M. Y. Zakharova, A. A. Kuznetsova, V. I. Uvarova, A. D. Fomina, L. I. Kozlovskaya, E. N. Kaliberda, I. N. Kurbatskaia, I. V. Smirnov, A. A. Bulygin, V. D. Knorre, O. S. Fedorova, A. Varnek, D. I. Osolodkin, A. A. Ishmukhametov, A. M. Egorov, A. G. Gabibov, N. A. Kuznetsov, *Front. Pharmacol.* **2021**, *12*, 773198.

[164] J. D. Baker, R. L. Uhrich, G. C. Kraemer, J. E. Love, B. C. Kraemer, *PloS One* **2021**, *16*, e0245962.

[165] J. Chen, Y. Zhang, D. Zeng, B. Zhang, X. Ye, Z. Zeng, X.-K. Zhang, Z. Wang, H. Zhou, *Biochem. Biophys. Res. Commun.* **2022**, *591*, 118–123.

5 Exploiting the Chemical Diversity of Metal Compounds as a Source of Novel Anti-COVID-19 Drugs

Damiano Cirri, Carlo Marotta
*and Alessandro Pratesi**
Department of Chemistry and Industrial Chemistry
Via Giuseppe Moruzzi 13, I-56124 Pisa, Italy
alessandro.pratesi@unipi.it

Tiziano Marzo
Department of Pharmacy
University of Pisa, Via Bonanno Pisano 6, 56126 Pisa, Italy

*Luigi Messori**
Department of Chemistry 'Ugo Schiff'
University of Florence, Via della Lastruccia
3-13, I-50019 Sesto Fiorentino, Italy
luigi.messori@unifi.it

CONTENTS

1 Metal Substances as a Rich Source of Drugs... 140
2 The COVID-19 Disease: Some General Remarks 144
3 Metal Compounds as Potential Anti-COVID-19 Agents:
  A Few Remarkable Examples...147
   3.1   Auranofin... 148
   3.2   Silver Sulfadiazine 148
   3.3   [Co(acacen)(NH$_3$)$_2$]Cl 149
   3.4   Bismuth Compounds.. 150

---

*Corresponding authors

DOI: 10.1201/9781003272250-5

4 Toward a More Systematic Approach in the Search for Metal-Based Drugs for COVID-19 Disease 152
    4.1 Selection of Metallo-Drugs for the Screening 153
    4.2 Assessment of Metal Compounds as Inhibitors of the Interaction between the S Protein and the ACE2 Receptor 154
    4.3 Assessment of Metal Compounds as Inhibitors of the Papain-Like Protease 154
    4.4 Assessment of Metal Compounds as Anti-SARS-Cov-2 Agents 155
5 Conclusions 156
Acknowledgements 157
Abbreviations 157
References 158

ABSTRACT

The outbreak of the COVID-19 pandemic has triggered the strong and urgent need of finding new effective drugs against the SARS-CoV-2 virus. Despite the intense efforts made by the international scientific community in the course of the last two years and some initial success, this issue remains absolutely open. Metal-based agents form a class of substances possessing a large variety of chemical structures and reactivities that may result in innovative and unprecedented modes of action. This class of substances merits to be explored in the search of effective antiviral agents. In this short review, we offer some examples of the possible role of metal-based drugs as prospective anti-COVID-19 agents. Particular attention is paid to a few established gold and bismuth compounds that looked very promising in some preliminary tests of antiviral efficacy. In addition, we illustrate a systematic strategy proposed very recently by Ott *et al.* for the rational discovery of promising antiviral drug candidates within relatively large libraries of metal compounds. Notably, implementation of this strategy has already resulted in the identification of a few metal compounds endowed with interesting features suitable for further pharmacologic development. Overall, we aim to underscore the valuable role that medicinal inorganic chemistry may play in the search and discovery of new anti-COVID-19 drugs.

KEYWORDS

Metal-Based Drugs; COVID-19; SARS-CoV-2; Gold; Bismuth; POMs

1 METAL SUBSTANCES AS A RICH SOURCE OF DRUGS

Metals and inorganic compounds have been used for medicinal purposes for centuries [1]; this mostly occurred on an empirical basis until the end of the 19th and the beginning of the 20th century. This latter period coincides, indeed, with the first steps of modern pharmacology. At that time, metal salts and some metal- or metalloid-based substances, which were already part of the available therapeutic arsenal, started to be systematically investigated for potential application against various diseases, in particular bacterial and parasitic ones [2–6]. As a result of

Diversity of Metal Compounds as a Source of Novel Anti-COVID-19 Drugs   141

those pioneering studies, many inorganic molecules entered therapeutic protocols and have played afterward, at least for a few decades, a pivotal role in the medical treatment of infections. It is emblematic and historically important the case of the discovery of Salvarsan® by the Nobel laureate Paul Ehrlich (1910) for the treatment of syphilis and, two years later, of the more soluble Neosalvarsan® (1912). Until this discovery, syphilis often represented a deadly infection that was mainly treated with mercury and potassium salts (e.g. KI), with quite poor clinical results [5]. Alongside, bismuth-based molecules were also used for the treatment of syphilis because of the lower toxicity of bismuth compounds compared with arsenicals. Similarly, in more recent times, a few infections caused by *Entamoeba histolytica* (amebiasis) or *Trichomonas vaginalis* have been treated with organoarsenical compounds [5]. These observations altogether underline the significant role of metal compounds in the early times of modern pharmacology.

Later on, in 1965, the discovery and the subsequent FDA approval (1978) of cisplatin represented the beginning of a new era in the treatment and management of cancer where metal compounds still play a central role [7–9]. Indeed, following the huge clinical success of this small platinum inorganic drug, the international research community started to investigate several different transition metals for the synthesis and evaluation of novel and improved drug candidates for the treatment of various types of cancers [6, 10, 11]. In fact, despite the large clinical success of cisplatin-based treatment protocols, anticancer Pt compounds are generally accompanied by the occurrence of severe side effects for the patients as well as the frequent insurgence of resistance phenomena [12]. Nephrotoxicity, hepatotoxicity, ototoxicity, cardiotoxicity, nausea and vomiting, diarrhea, and alopecia are only some of the negative side effects which often emerge after cisplatin administration; similarly, the treatment, especially when prolonged, can become ineffective due to acquired resistance [12]. In this frame, the second- and third-generation platinum anticancer drugs, i.e., carboplatin and oxaliplatin, were developed with subsequent worldwide approval in 1989 and 2001, respectively (Figure 1) [13].

The two latter drugs were basically developed as cisplatin analogues, but are characterized by a greater tolerability owing to their relatively small but functionally relevant structural differences [13, 14]. While cisplatin and carboplatin possess pharmacological profiles that are substantially superimposable, oxaliplatin is instead used, almost exclusively, to treat colorectal cancer for which it is far more efficacious than cisplatin and carboplatin [13, 15]. This significant difference in terms of therapeutic actions is unlikely to depend on the interaction with a single biological target. At variance, most probably, while DNA remains a biologically relevant target for the anticancer profiles of all three Pt drugs, in the case of oxaliplatin, additional mechanisms and additional targets are most likely operative. Notably, a recent paper by Lippard and coworkers pointed out that in this latter case, induction of ribosome biogenesis stress is functionally relevant for oxaliplatin, but not for cisplatin, in order to trigger cancer cell death [16]. In this context, it can be affirmed that even small changes in the ligands coordinated to the metal ions may have a large impact on the mechanism of anticancer platinum

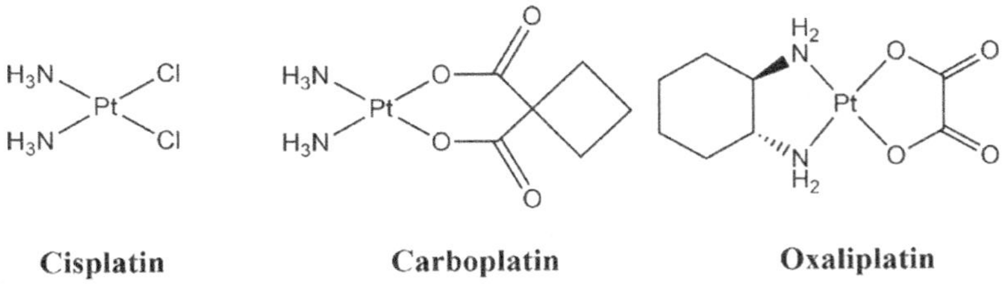

142 Pratesi, Messori, et al.

Cisplatin **Carboplatin** **Oxaliplatin**

FIGURE 1 Chemical structures of the three worldwide-approved platinum drugs.

metallo-drugs [17]. Beyond platinum, several transition metals and metalloids have been exploited in the last decades in an attempt to obtain improved inorganic drugs. Among them, some ruthenium, gold, titanium, copper, iridium, bismuth, arsenic, or tellurium compounds revealed promising medicinal properties and are the subject of further studies [6, 11, 16, 18]. Figure 2 reports some of these important inorganic drugs that are currently used to treat a variety of diseases, additional ones can be seen, e.g., in Chapters 1 and 4 in this book.

In the last years, a number of reasons have prompted a renewed interest in inorganic medicinal chemistry. Prior to then, the development of modern synthetic techniques in organic chemistry during the 20th century, and the discovery of important organic drugs (e.g. Penicillins, Zidovudine) had impacted significantly and positively the clinical treatment of diseases, contributing to a substantial decrease in the overall interest for inorganic drugs. However, in some therapeutic areas such as that of antibacterial agents, quite rapidly, the reduced rate of discovery of new organic drugs and the insurgence of bacterial resistance determined the need for novel drugs and triggered the development of innovative drug discovery strategies [1, 2, 19]. Among the various strategies that have been developed, a reliable and effective one is represented by the reappraisal of approved or established inorganic drugs [1, 20, 21]. This trend has been further spurred in recent times by the emergence of modern omics technologies capable of providing in-depth insights into the mechanism of action of new metal-based compounds [22–25]. In turn, these innovative methods have allowed researchers to approach the drug design issue using a mechanism-oriented strategy. Similarly, this increasing knowledge concerning the relevant pathways for the pharmacological activity of inorganic drugs can be conveniently applied in the frame of the "drug repurposing" strategy [1].

The latter approach, which relies on the use of established/already approved drugs for a therapeutic indication different from the original one, is suitable in all the fields of medicine but may become fundamental in a few selected cases. Specifically, it may be conveniently exploited for the implementation of treatments against neglected diseases (see also Chapter 7 which describes advances in metal-based agents to treat neglected diseases) as well as diseases for which new drugs are highly needed owing to their huge social and economic impact at a global level. Examples of the first case are tropical or endemic diseases that represent a major health problem in some countries (Africa, Asia, and Latin America

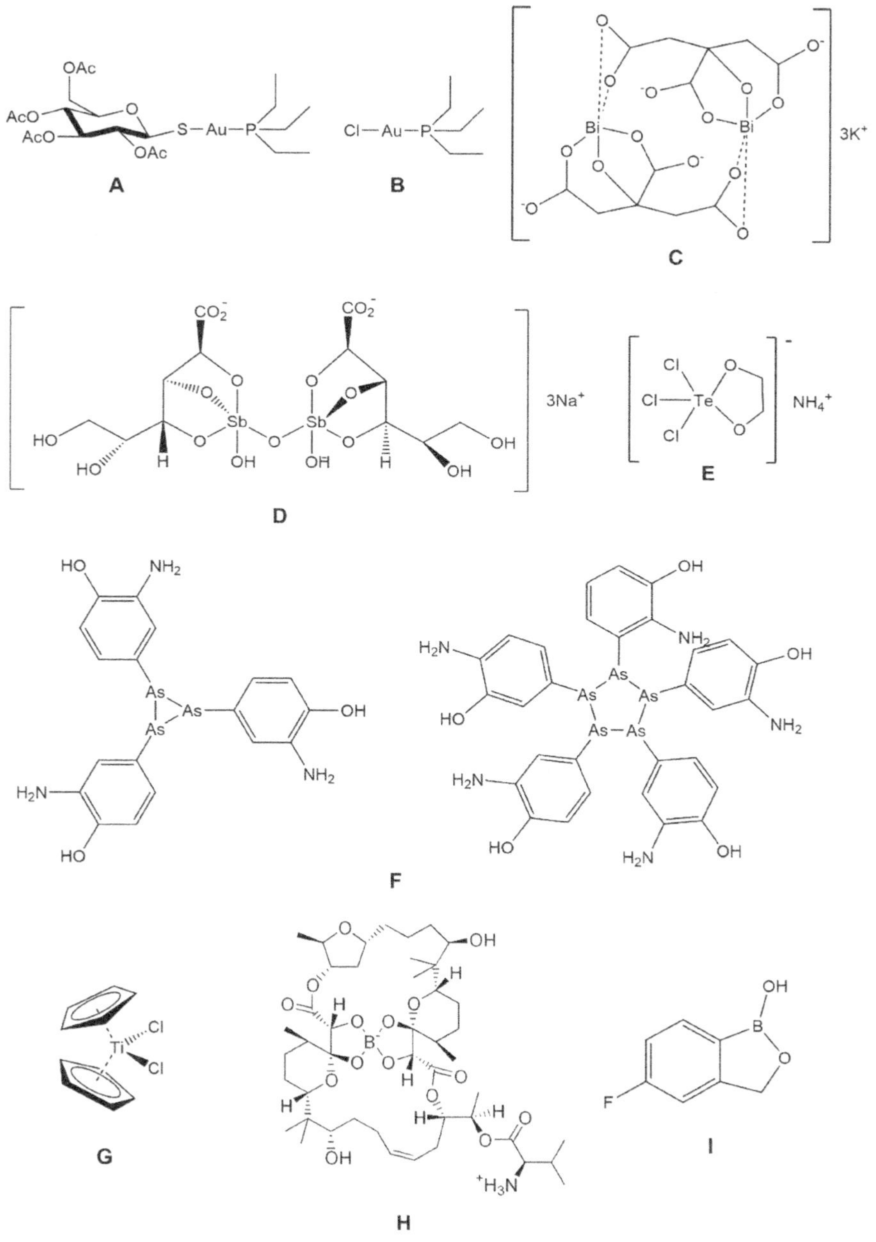

Diversity of Metal Compounds as a Source of Novel Anti-COVID-19 Drugs   143

FIGURE 2 Chemical structures of some relevant inorganic drugs: (**A**) Auranofin; (**B**) Chloro(triethylphosphine)gold(I); (**C**) Bismuth(III) potassium subcitrate; (**D**) Sodium stibogluconate; (**E**) AS101 (Ammonium trichloro(dioxoethylene-O,O′)tellurate); (**F**) Mixture of 3-amino-4-hydroxyphenyl-As(III) compounds containing acyclic As_3 and As_5 species, known as Salvarsan; (**G**) Titanocene dichloride; (**H**) Boromycine; (**I**) Tavaborole.

in particular). In this frame, the use of already FDA-approved drugs represents a suitable option, because of the need for drugs that are quickly available and at a low cost. Moreover, the repurposed drugs are safe since they have already been extensively studied and approved for different clinical applications. The second case typically refers to diseases that have a high impact worldwide and are among the first causes of death, such as cancer. Additionally, drug repurposing may turn extremely important in the case of sudden and unexpected sanitary emergencies where the fast introduction of effective drugs in clinical settings is absolutely needed [20, 26].

This latter situation is clearly exemplified by the COVID-19 pandemic as discussed below. This chapter, which builds on the comprehensive findings showcased in Chapter 4, is specifically aimed at demonstrating how the field of metal-based drugs may offer a valid contribution to the search and identification of novel and effective substances capable of fighting this sudden, unexpected, and severe viral disease.

2 THE COVID-19 DISEASE: SOME GENERAL REMARKS

Between the end of 2019 and the beginning of 2020, in Wuhan, China, a new virus belonging to the coronavirus family suddenly appeared and rapidly began to spread worldwide. The associated disease was soon qualified as a global pandemic health emergency. The causative pathogen was described by the International Committee on Taxonomy of Viruses as the severe acute respiratory syndrome coronavirus-2 (SARS-CoV-2). SARS-CoV-2 caused an outbreak of unprecedented viral pneumonia in the Hubei area. Despite many attempts to contain its spreading, this novel coronavirus, due to the very high transmission rate, broke the borders of that area rapidly. In February 2020, the disease was announced as COVID-2019 by the World Health Organization (WHO) [26]. Looking at the WHO reports (see for further details https://www.who.int/), the dramatic impact of COVID-19 is evident. For instance, estimates suggest that the number of global deaths attributable to the COVID-19 pandemic by the end of 2020 was already, at least, 3 million. Nowadays, with the development of successful vaccines, we have effective weapons against SARS-CoV-2; yet, the virus is continuing to significantly impact health systems in several countries worldwide. In addition, the continuous spreading of the virus causes its mutation in new variants for which the vaccines, based on the original SARS-CoV-2 virus that emerged in Wuhan (China), may be less effective (e.g. Omicron) [27].

Fever, cough, headache, exhaustion, breathing difficulty, loss of smell, and loss of taste are some of the symptoms of COVID-19. Symptoms may appear 1–14 days following the viral contact. However, around a third of the infected people show no signs or symptoms. The majority (81%) of those who manifest symptoms noticeable enough to be classified as patients have mild to moderate symptoms (up to mild pneumonia), whereas 14% have severe symptoms (dyspnea, hypoxia, or more than 50% lung involvement on imaging), and 5% have critical symptoms (respiratory failure, shock, or multiorgan dysfunction) [28]. Older and

Diversity of Metal Compounds as a Source of Novel Anti-COVID-19 Drugs **145**

immune-compromised people are at a greater risk of developing severe forms of this disease. Some people continue to experience a range of effects for months after recovery (the so-called "long COVID"), and significant damage to organs has been observed. Multi-year studies are underway to further investigate the long-term effects of the disease.

The SARS-CoV-2 virus is spread through the air when droplets and minute airborne particles harboring the virus are inhaled. When people are close together, the risk of transmission is greatest; nonetheless, transmission can occur across longer distances, especially indoors. Transmission also occurs if contaminated fluids are splashed or sprayed into an individual's eyes, nose, or mouth, or via contaminated surfaces. Even if they do not exhibit symptoms, people might be contagious for up to 20 days and spread the virus.

Various COVID-19 testing methods are available to diagnose the disease. The standard diagnostic method directly detects the virus's nucleic acid by real-time reverse transcription polymerase chain reaction (rRT-PCR).

Several effective COVID-19 vaccines have been licensed and disseminated in nations where major immunization campaigns have taken place. Physical or social separation, quarantining, ventilation of indoor spaces, covering coughs and sneezes, hand washing, and keeping unclean hands away from the face are some more preventive strategies. In public places, the use of face masks or coverings has been advocated to reduce the risk of transmission. While medications to suppress the virus are being developed, the primary treatment remains symptomatic. Treatment of symptoms, supportive care, isolation, and experimental techniques are all part of disease management.

Already a lot of information has been garnered concerning the SARS-CoV-2 virus, the causative agent of COVID-19 disease. The SARS-CoV-2 virus is a single-stranded RNA virus. It belongs to a family of so-called coronaviruses, being part of the Coronaviridae family (order Nidovirales). The four genera of this subfamily are Alpha, Beta, Delta, and Gamma-Coronaviruses (CoVs). The sequence of SARS-CoV-2 is 96% identical to that of the bats' coronavirus. This evidence is the basis of the assumption that bats are the main reservoir for this virus. SARS-CoV-2 may cause a severe respiratory tract disease that, especially in the presence of comorbidities, may lead to critical symptoms and a poor prognosis [26, 29].

As also outlined in Chapter 4, the infection process of SARS-CoV-2 toward human cells (host) occurs through virus binding to the cell surface protein angiotensin-converting enzyme 2 (ACE2) that is mediated by the Receptor Binding Domain (RBD) of its spike (S) glycoprotein (Figure 3). Furthermore, the cellular transmembrane serine protease 2 (TMPRSS2) is essential for triggering the S glycoprotein. Virus entry in the host cell may also depend on the endosomal/lysosomal cysteine proteases cathepsin B and L (CTSB, CTSL), though their activity seems not to be indispensable. Recently, it was found that furin protease plays a role in the infection process. Indeed, SARS-CoV-2 contains a furin cleavage site in the S protein that is unusual for coronaviruses, and the cellular receptor neuropilin-1 (NRP1, which binds furin-cleaved substrates) potentiates SARS-CoV-2

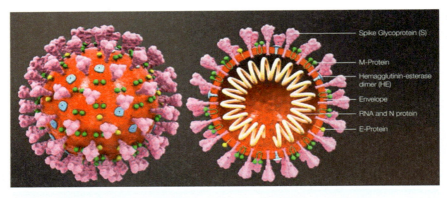

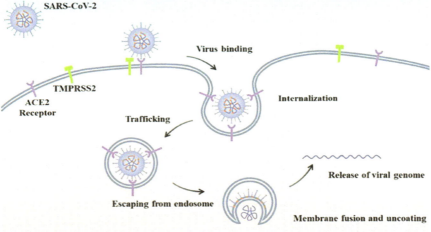

FIGURE 3 Representation of the SARS-CoV-2 cross-section with key proteins (top) and schematic pathway of SARS-CoV-2 viral life cycle. The initial attachment of SARS-CoV-2 to the host cells involves the binding of the viral S glycoprotein on the cellular receptor, ACE2 proteins. Adapted from reference [30] under the terms of the Creative Commons Attribution License (CC BY).

infectivity toward the central nervous system. Additionally, SARS-CoV-2 is capable of exploiting the putative alternative receptor CD147 (expressed in high levels in the brain) to infect the central nervous system [30–33].

Retrospectively, one can assess that other coronaviruses have earlier caused outbreaks of fatal human pneumonia. Examples are the severe acute respiratory syndrome coronavirus (SARS-CoV) and the Middle East Respiratory Syndrome Coronavirus (MERS-CoV). The SARS-CoV infection emerged in the Chinese province of Guangdong in 2003 spreading to other countries and infecting more than 8,000 people with more than 700 deaths [34]. At variance, the so-called MERS-CoV spread from the Middle East in 2012, reaching other countries.

Based on official data, MERS-CoV infected about 2,500 people, making more than 800 victims [34]. The fatality rate for SARS-CoV was lower compared with MERS-CoV being, respectively, estimated to be 10 and 35% [35]. The viral components of the coronaviruses, even in the case of SARS-CoV-2, represent suitable druggable targets for virus inactivation and for the development of effective therapies against the COVID-19 disease [36].

Notably, no effective drugs were available to treat COVID-19 at the time of its appearance. However, based on the information at the molecular level concerning the mechanisms involved in the viral infection that was quickly obtained, it was possible to identify a few viral proteins that are validated druggable targets. Thanks to this information since the very beginning of the pandemic, several approved drugs were screened and evaluated. Some of them entered clinical trials and were immediately tested in COVID-19 patients [37]. In any case, as suggested by WHO, curative drugs have not been discovered yet and novel and effective antiviral agents are absolutely needed worldwide [38]. We are convinced that inorganic drugs may offer important opportunities to reach this goal. Accordingly, some of the efforts sustained by the medicinal inorganic chemistry community in this direction are illustrated in the following sections.

3 METAL COMPOUNDS AS POTENTIAL ANTI-COVID-19 AGENTS: A FEW REMARKABLE EXAMPLES

As previously noted, medication repurposing, i.e., the use of pharmaceuticals that are already in clinical use for a different therapeutic indication, is a straightforward strategy to make active drugs safely and easily available to clinicians for COVID-19 treatment. Accordingly, at the onset of the pandemic, intensive research was conducted on libraries of FDA-approved medications, and a few potential candidates for drug repurposing against COVID-19 were identified (e.g. Tocilizumab, Chloroquine, Remdesivir) [39–41]. We believe that important opportunities for the discovery of new and effective anti-COVID-19 agents may also arise from the repurposing as well as *de novo* testing of metal-based compounds. Indeed, metal-based compounds offer advantages over organic compounds in terms of their structural diversity and wide ranging reactivities that may well translate into drugs with innovative and unprecedented modes of antiviral action. Already, a number of studies, though not systematic, have been conducted on metal-based compounds as potential agents against SARS-CoV-2 and other viruses; these studies are comprehensively summarized in Chapter 4. In this chapter, we highlight a systematic strategy for the rational discovery of promising antiviral drug candidates within relatively large libraries of metal compounds. We include reference, in particular, to the following metal compounds: auranofin, silver sulfadiazine, the cobalt compound $[Co(acacen)(NH_3)_2]$ Cl, and a few related bismuth compounds. While the first three complexes are also reviewed in Chapter 4, we refer to them here also to emphasize the merits of exploiting metal-based drugs as an alternative source to organic drugs for COVID-19 treatment.

3.1 Auranofin

Undoubtedly, one of the most promising candidates for COVID-19 treatment is auranofin, a linear gold(I) complex containing triethylphosphine and tetracetylthioglucose as coordinating ligands (its chemical structure is shown in Figure 2A). Auranofin is a gold drug approved by the FDA in 1985 for the treatment of severe forms of rheumatoid arthritis [37]. This drug was soon proposed for screening against SARS-CoV-2 owing to its intriguing pharmacological features [42]. First of all, regarding its therapeutic profile as an anti-arthritic agent, it displays a high tolerance and a relatively low systemic toxicity [43, 44]. It is well accepted that its mechanism of action mainly involves the inhibition of the key redox enzyme thioredoxin reductase (TrxR), a selenoenzyme that is responsible for the entire cellular redox balance [45]. This feature, likewise, plays a key role for auranofin's activity against the SARS-CoV-2 infection. In fact, Kumar and co-workers recently demonstrated that TrxR inhibition in cells infected with virions of the CoV family downregulates, in turn, the synthesis of key proteins of SARS-CoV-2 [46–48]. Hence, auranofin could indeed be considered as a promising candidate to treat this infection. Furthermore, regarding its general antiviral properties as outlined in Chapter 4, auranofin has previously displayed efficacy against the HIV [49], being tested in clinical trials as an antiretroviral agent [50].

Notably, the potential activity of auranofin toward the SARS-CoV-2 virus was rapidly confirmed in a study conducted on human hepatocellular carcinoma-derived cell line (Huh7) [51]. In this study, auranofin was found to inhibit the replication of the virus by 95% after 48 h at low µM concentration, while it was well tolerated by the tested cells. In addition, auranofin proved to be able to reduce the inflammation in the same panel of cells by decreasing the expression, promoted by the SARS-CoV-2 infection, of the cytokine IL-6. This occurrence is important because the infection typically promotes an over-expression of the mRNA of IL-6 which results in diffuse lung inflammation [51]. Noteworthy, in a different study, auranofin also proved to inhibit the interaction between the active center of the ACE2 enzyme and the spike protein of the virus, which, as mentioned above, is a central pivot for the access of the virus into the cell [52]. In addition, auranofin was also reported to potently inhibit the papain-like protein (PL^{pro}) of SARS-CoV-1 and SARS-CoV-2, a key enzyme for the replication of the virus [52]. In summary, these results, also taking into account the additional anti-viral properties associated with auranofin outlined in Chapter 4, strongly support the potential role of auranofin in the treatment of COVID-19 infection [37] and therefore warrant further experimentation.

3.2 Silver Sulfadiazine

In the frame of metal-based drug repositioning, some attempts have also been made to assess the potential of silver in the treatment of SARS-CoV-2 infection. Indeed, the antibacterial properties of silver have been known for a long time [53]. For example, the commercially available drug silver sulfadiazine (brand

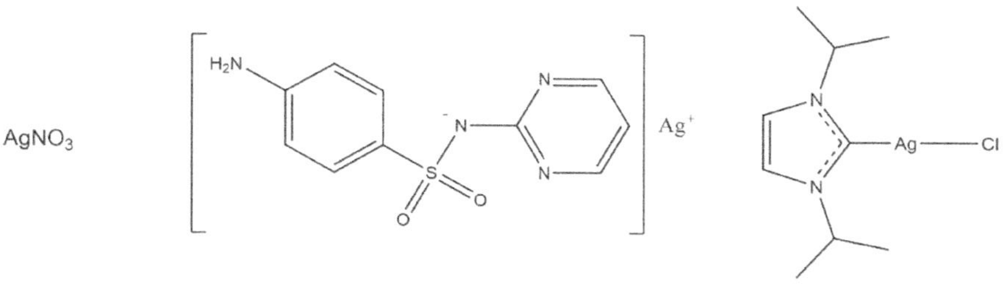

Diversity of Metal Compounds as a Source of Novel Anti-COVID-19 Drugs 149

AgNO₃

Silver Nitrate   **Silver Sulfadiazine**   **Ag-3**

FIGURE 4   Structures of silver nitrate, silver sulfadiazine, and Ag-3, as reported in Ref. [58].

name SOFARGEN®) associates the activity of the silver ion with the antibacterial activity of the sulfadiazine drug and this combination is commonly used as a topical antimicrobial [54]. In contrast, the antiviral activity of this class of compounds has not been studied as much as their antimicrobial properties. However, silver sulfadiazine had been previously demonstrated to manifest antiviral activity against HIV and the herpesvirus [55, 56]. As for the SARS-CoV-2 infection, silver nanoparticles were confirmed to have antiviral activity against this virus [57]. Moreover, research demonstrated the ability of three silver-based compounds (namely silver nitrate, silver sulfadiazine, and Ag-3) (Figure 4) to inhibit PL^{pro} at μM concentration. In particular, all the three species displayed IC$_{50}$ values in the μM range against SARS-CoV-2 PL^{pro}, whereas their activity was lower against SARS-CoV PL^{pro}, proving the selectivity of these compounds for the SARS-CoV-2 PL^{pro} enzyme. Noteworthy, Ag-3 displayed a strong inhibitory activity (in the μM range) against SARS-CoV-2. For these three compounds it has been postulated that their activity might be directly linked to the presence of the silver(I) ion itself, as suggested by the fact that silver nitrate has a similar activity to the other two compounds [58].

3.3   [CO(ACACEN)(NH₃)₂]Cl

Another druggable target of the virus is the SARS-CoV-2 main protease (M^{pro}) (also called 3CL^{pro}) [59–65], against which cobalt-containing compounds have been explored. Indeed, reports have suggested that some regions of this protein might be blocked through the interaction of cobalt(III)-cations with its histidine and cysteine residues, ultimately deactivating the protease [59]. In particular, among all the histidine residues of the protein, His41 represents an interesting target as metal-ion binding to its imidazole side chain might disrupt the H-bonds of the protein, thus deactivating the enzyme [65]. One candidate that was proposed for this purpose is [Co(acacen)(NH₃)₂]Cl (Figure 5), which was also reported to be able to inhibit other proteases by targeting the imidazole ring on the His side chain [66, 67]. In fact, if an excess of [Co(acacen)(NH₃)₂]Cl is used, the binding to at least three histidine residues could be observed [65]. Consequently, similarly

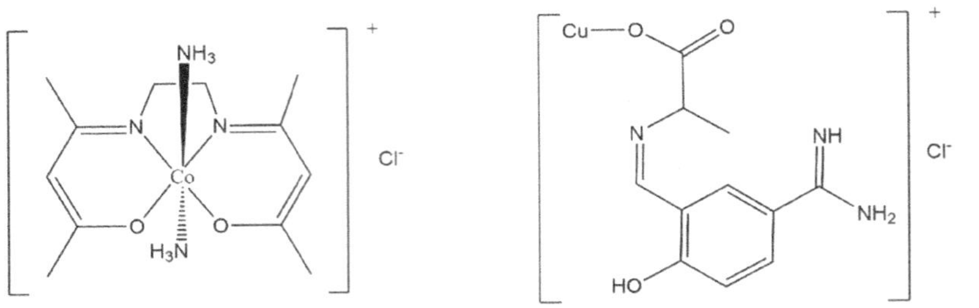

[Co(acacen)(NH₃)₂]Cl   [(meta-amidinosalicylidene-l-alaninato)copper(II)]Cl

FIGURE 5 Molecular structures of [Co(acacen)(NH₃)₂]Cl and [(meta-amidinosalicylidene-l-alaninato)copper(II)]Cl.

to another study of Co(III) binding to the myoglobin protein [68], the binding of the metal compound to this large number of histidines might render the surface of the protein more hydrophilic, thus resulting in its unfolding. In the same way, copper(II) chelates, due to their ability to inhibit a thrombin protease, have also been explored for this purpose [69]. Indeed, some complexes were proved to be able to dock to His41 and Cys145 amino acid residues of the M^{pro} protein [65]. In particular, [(meta-amidinosalicylidene-l-alaninato)copper(II)]Cl (Figure 5) was successfully docked near His41 and it is possible that little motions of the protein might allow the binding of Cu(II) to the Cys145 thiolate, thus disrupting the protein functionality. Other less bulky analogues were also docked into the Cys145 site and the results led to similar consideration [65].

3.4 BISMUTH COMPOUNDS

Bismuth compounds form another class of drugs with promising properties against the SARS-CoV-2 virus. Indeed, in studies conducted against SARS-CoV, some of them proved to be able to inhibit the protease and helicase catalytic activities of the virus, which are vital for its life [70–72]. Noteworthy, a panel of compounds endowed with N,O-containing polydentate ligands showed potent inhibitory activity against helicase ATPase (IC$_{50}$ in the range of μM) (Figure 6) [71]. By comparing the activity of these compounds, it was possible to conclude that the bismuth center plays a crucial role in their activity. Notably, among all the tested complexes, the porphyrin ones turned out to be the most potent in inhibiting the activity of helicase [71]. Regarding the SARS-CoV-2 infection, some bismuth complexes that are currently used in clinical practice, i.e., bismuth citrate, ranitidine bismuth citrate, and bismuth potassium citrate (their chemical structures, together with additional bismuth-based compounds), are shown in Figure 6. Also, Figure 2 shows the chemical structure of the stable dinuclear unit of the so-called bismuth potassium subcitrate, which was evaluated for their inhibitory capabilities against the NTPase and RNA helicase activities of non-structural nsp13 protein, a fundamental protein for the replication of SARS-CoV-2 [73].

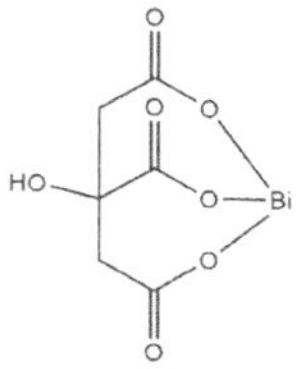

Diversity of Metal Compounds as a Source of Novel Anti-COVID-19 Drugs   151

Bismuth citrate

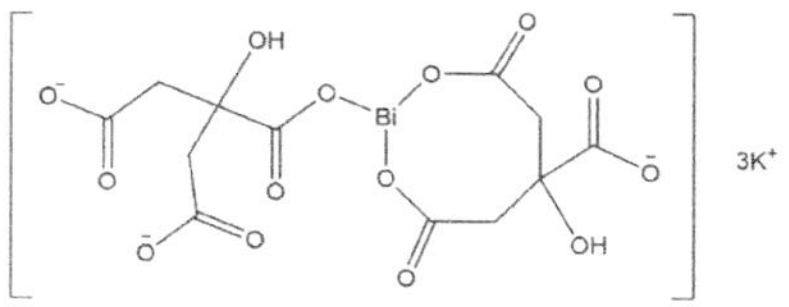

Bismuth potassium citrate

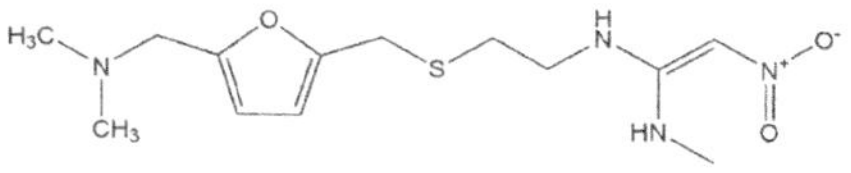

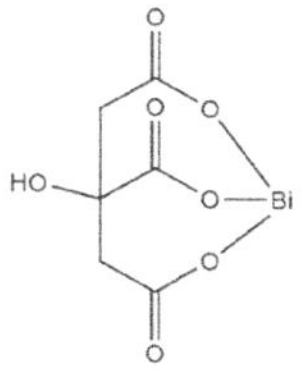

Ranitidine bismuth citrate

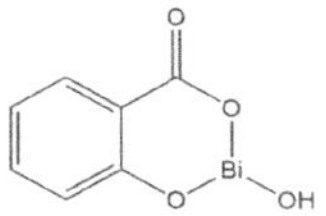

Bismuth subsalicylate

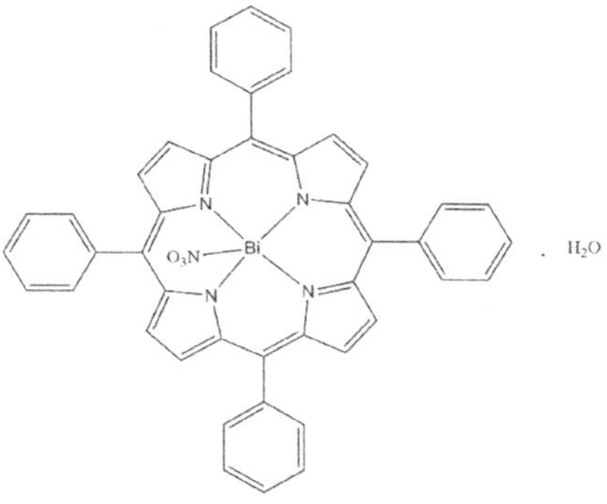

[Bi(5,10,15,20-tetraphenyl-21H,23H-porphine)(NO₃)]·H₂O

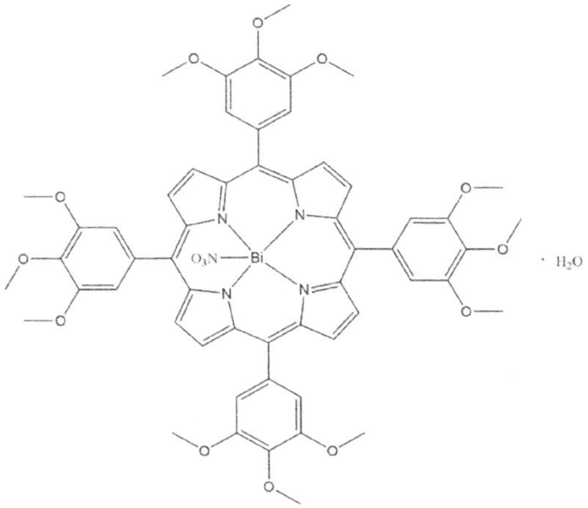

[Bi(5,10,15,20-tetra(1,2,3-trimethoxyphenyl)-21H,23H-porphine)(NO₃)]·H₂O

FIGURE 6   Molecular structures of some relevant Bi-based compounds studied as anti-SARS-CoV-2 agents.

In addition, the activity of ranitidine bismuth citrate, Figure 6, was investigated both *in vitro* and *in vivo*, with very promising results in both cases. On the one hand, in the *in vitro* tests, not only did it display a low toxicity and high selectivity, but also turned able to inhibit the viral helicases [74]. This finding validated previous reports on the relevance of this protein as a target for the virus and on the capability of this complex to target it [43, 75]. On the other hand, in the animal model investigated, it drastically reduced the replication of the virus, which ultimately results in a diminished viral load on the pulmonary system of the tested animals [74]. Furthermore, although these complexes haven't been studied in clinical trials so far, a report showed that administration of bismuth subsalicylate was able to improve the conditions of a patient with Crohn's disease whose conditions had been worsened by the SARS-CoV-2 infection. In particular, this therapy markedly diminished the cough and diarrhea of the patient and improved their appetite [76].

Recently published results presented noticeable preclinical anti-SARS-CoV-2 efficacy of a cocktail therapy consisting of clinically used bismuth-based drugs, e.g., colloidal bismuth subcitrate or bismuth subsalicylate, and *N*-acetyl-L-cysteine [77].

4 TOWARD A MORE SYSTEMATIC APPROACH IN THE SEARCH FOR METAL-BASED DRUGS FOR COVID-19 DISEASE

The examples described above provide solid evidence that metal compounds may play an important role in the medical treatment of COVID-19 and, as such, should be intensely investigated in the search for new antiviral agents. However, more systematic and more effective drug discovery strategies in the field of metal-based drugs need to be implemented.

In this regard, we highlight a seminal study by Ott *et al.* in an attempt to define a more rational approach for the identification of metal-based substances that might manifest important antiviral actions and might be suitable for further pharmaceutical development [58].

Notably, the strategy proposed by Ott and coworkers includes the following steps:

    i. selection of metallo-drugs for the screening;
    ii. assessment of metal compounds as inhibitors of the interaction between the S protein and the ACE2 receptor;
    iii. assessment of metal compounds as inhibitors of the papain-like protease;
    iv. assessment of metal compounds as anti-SARS-Cov-2 agents.

It is evident that this strategy is grounded on the concept that the spike protein and the papain-like protease are primary druggable targets for the development of new antiviral substances. The details of each step of this strategy are illustrated below.

Diversity of Metal Compounds as a Source of Novel Anti-COVID-19 Drugs 153

4.1 SELECTION OF METALLO-DRUGS FOR THE SCREENING

Ott *et al.* exploited an extensive library of metal compounds, featuring large chemical diversity, in their study, supported by the participation of many European laboratories with specific expertise in the field of inorganic synthesis and metal-based drugs. Indeed, about ten distinct laboratories took part in this effort. More specifically, the panel of studied metal compounds included 93 mononuclear compounds and 11 polyoxometalates (POMs). The mononuclear complexes contained many different transition metals, mainly Au, Ru, and Fe, but also Rh, Ag, Pt, Pd, Ti, and others, as already discussed in Chapter 4. Some of the compounds included in the panel as potential anti-SARS-CoV-2 agents were polyoxometalates (POMs) bearing metal or metalloid centers such as As, Co, Pb, Sn, W, and Ge among others. Basically, this family of metal-oxide cluster compounds is featured by a wide range of structures that have been reported to provide effective anticancer, antiviral, and antibacterial agents (see Figure 7) [78–83]. Specifically, their proven ability to inhibit viral replication is relevant for our purposes here [84–86]. Indeed, the possible recognition of the S protein of coronavirus by polyoxometalates has been recently highlighted [87].

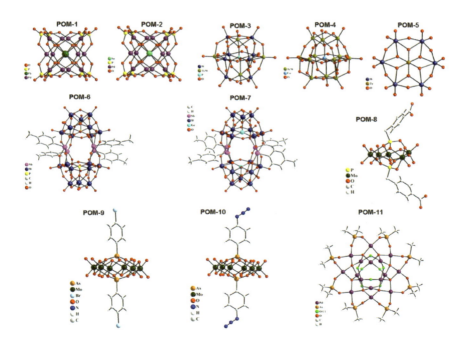

FIGURE 7 Some relevant examples for polyoxometalate compounds with biological activity. (Reproduced from reference [58] under the terms of the Creative Commons Attribution License (CC BY).)

4.2 Assessment of Metal Compounds as Inhibitors of the Interaction between the S Protein and the ACE2 Receptor

This step concerns the screening of the panel compounds for their ability to inhibit the interaction of the spike protein with the Angiotensin-Converting Enzyme-2 (ACE2) receptor; the observation of a strong inhibition may well be predictive of potent antiviral activity. As described in detail in Section 2, the S protein plays a key role in the early phases of infection; it primarily mediates virus entry into the host. This viral protein is capable of binding toward the ACE2 on the cell membrane of the host. These considerations clearly delineate the S protein as an exploitable druggable target to block the entry of the virus and, as a consequence, the infection cascade [88–91]. Furthermore, the S1 subunit of the S protein is featured by the presence of the so-called receptor-binding domain (RBD). This domain is capable of tightly binding the N-terminal helix of ACE2 in turn allowing the viral attachment. Noteworthy, the receptor-binding domain contains nine cysteine residues forming four disulfide bonds [92] representing exploitable targets for metallodrugs or metal fragments, preventing the cellular entry of SARS-CoV-2.

The ELISA test was the reference method by which the panel of inorganic drugs was assessed for their ability to impair the S/ACE2 recognition and the associated binding process. Overall, the mononuclear complexes were inactive or only scarcely active in these tests. Indeed, an inhibition ranging from 25 to 50% was reported only in a small number of tested molecules including some gold, ruthenium, iron, and platinum-based complexes (e.g., cisplatin). In this frame, the only exception was titanocene dichloride, characterized by an inhibition percentage of about 69%.

At variance, better results were obtained with POMs; in seven cases, an inhibitory activity >50% of the S/ACE2 recognition process was observed. Based on these results, four compounds were selected for further studies as the best performers including titanocene dichloride (its chemical structure is shown in Figure 2G) and three POMs (POM-6, POM-7, POM-11 in Figure 7).

4.3 Assessment of Metal Compounds as Inhibitors of the Papain-Like Protease

Proteases are exploitable targets for the design and implementation of new antiviral agents. In fact, their impairment may lead to the blockade of the viral life and of the replication cycle without affecting the host. With a view to developing effective inorganic anti-SARS-CoV-2 agents, given the fact that the papain-like protease (PL^{pro}) and the 3-chymotrypsin-like protease (3CL^{pro}, even known as M^{pro}) are crucial for viral replication, these proteases are suitable targets for the design and testing of specific antiviral drugs against SARS-CoV-2 [93–95]. Interestingly, the sequence of SARS-CoV-2 PL^{pro} is very similar (about 83%) to that of SARS-CoV which was responsible for the sudden outbreak of the SARS epidemic in 2003. The two viruses share domains of the papain-like protease that are very similar. Specifically, the two domains are known as the putative

Diversity of Metal Compounds as a Source of Novel Anti-COVID-19 Drugs   **155**

labile zinc-binding domain and the catalytic cysteine cleavage domain, which bear druggable cysteines [52, 94, 96]. Notably, a number of panel compounds, in particular auranofin, aurothiomalate, a few triphenylphosphine gold compounds, and many POMs, produced potent inhibition of this viral protease [52, 58, 97].

4.4 ASSESSMENT OF METAL COMPOUNDS AS ANTI-SARS-COV-2 AGENTS

For the selection of suitable drug candidates against SARS-CoV-2, an important feature of the drug is that it is well tolerated by the host cells. In other words, the drug should possess a certain degree of selectivity toward the virus, so that the treatment impairs the viral infection and virus replication without causing undesirable side reactions and associated side effects. Accordingly, before the evaluation of the efficacy of a selected drug in SARS-CoV-2 infected cells, it is necessary to assess the effects (and toxic effects) of the selected molecule in suitable cell models such as Caco-2 and CaLu-3 cell lines [98]. Indeed, the best candidates for further drug development should be metallo-drugs characterized by high tolerability and no significant toxic effects. Ott and coworkers reported that, among the investigated complexes, some mononuclear gold and titanium-based drugs, including aurothiomalate and titanocene dichloride, showed a suitable antiviral profile featured by good tolerability even at the highest tested doses (500 µM). Among POMs, some compounds were very toxic in the above cell models and, accordingly, were not suitable for further assessment, while other POMs were tolerated up to tested doses of 200 µM. Beyond the tolerability in cell lines, other aspects were evaluated including solubility. Putting together all these preliminary evaluations, some compounds showing no or reasonable toxic effects, a good capability to bind the viral targets and a suitable solubility profile were selected for the evaluation in SARS-CoV-2 infected Caco-2 cells. Upon combining all the results obtained, a small panel of drug candidates emerged containing titanocene dichloride (Figure 2C), one silver-based complex (Ag-3 in Figure 4), and a POM (POM-11 in Figure 7) as well as aurothiomalate and three additional gold-based agents (Figure 8).

For comparative purposes, Remdesivir was used as a reference in these tests because of its ability to impair viral replication at low micromolar doses. It is important to highlight the strategy delineated by Ott *et al.* features a smart and systematic approach for screening structurally diverse metal-based compounds. As a matter of fact, the screening of large panels of metallo-drugs with established and reliable methods may conveniently support the selection of inorganic drugs endowed with both strong inhibitory profile toward the S/ACE2 recognition process and satisfactory tolerability and chemico-physical profile. Overall, at the end of the in-cell screening, it was possible to recognize three compounds as the most promising candidates, i.e., Au-12, Ag-3, and POM-11. All three featured antiviral activity falling in the range of µM. Beyond the selection of the above drug candidates, this investigation pointed out that, through systematic screening of a large panel of inorganic drugs featured by a wide chemical diversity, it is possible, using reliable methods, to select promising drug candidates against SARS-CoV-2 infection. This also makes clear that metallo-drugs and, more in general,

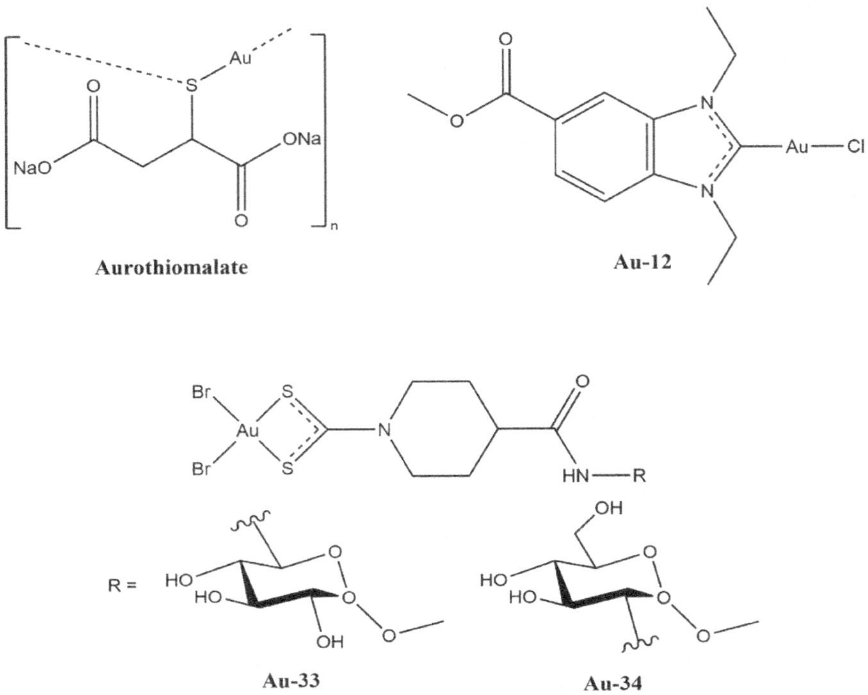

FIGURE 8 Structures of aurothiomalate (Au-2), Au-12, Au-33, Au-34.

inorganic molecules may well be considered for the development of novel and effective agents against the virus, hopefully leading to novel and improved treatments for COVID-19 disease.

5 CONCLUSIONS

Metal-based drugs form an intriguing class of potential therapeutic agents with very interesting and attractive chemical and biological properties. Here we have tried to delineate the role that metal-based drugs may play against COVID-19 on the grounds of the available literature evidence from the very first empirical attempts to the design of more systematic drug discovery strategies. We have shown that metallo-drugs, and inorganic drugs in general, offer the chance to finely tune, through an appropriate molecular design approach, their chemico-physical profiles, their reactivity, and thus their pharmacological profile. For instance, by varying the metal center it is possible to drive the reactivity toward selected biological substrates bearing residues with a greater affinity for that metal center. Similarly, it is possible to control the stability and the reactivity of the same metal center through the choice of proper ligands.

Thus, the proposal to screen a panel of inorganic drugs in the search of candidates against SARS-CoV-2 appears to be well supported, allowing to conveniently expand the "chemical space" for novel and improved antiviral agents. Accordingly, it is highly recommended that inorganic drugs are included in new drug discovery screening programs.

In this frame, both the strategies relying on drug reprofiling or on the assessment of newly synthesized inorganic drugs are exploitable. From the first strategy, some interesting results have already emerged for the gold(I)-based compound auranofin. Similarly, bismuth-based drugs have been evaluated against SARS-CoV-2 with promising results. The design and the testing of newly synthesized molecules are inherently more complex. However, it may offer the interesting opportunity of synthesizing compounds in a rational manner because of the increasing information on the virus, available at the molecular level. Additionally, the inclusion of novel metallo-drugs in large screening programs may offer the opportunity to further expand the chemical libraries, providing further opportunities for drug discovery. Noteworthy, even the problems associated with the systemic toxicity of metals and metalloids may be overcome through the drug repurposing approach, thus using approved inorganic drugs, as well as through selecting newly synthesized compounds featured by the accomplishment of specific requirements in terms of selective reactivity toward the desired biological substrates and stability. Finally, considering that drugs for the treatment of COVID-19 patients are not for chronic use, it is reasonable to assess that long-term side effects might be avoided. This further contributes to the chance of widening the range of clinical applications for inorganic drugs [37].

ACKNOWLEDGEMENTS

AP gratefully acknowledges funding by the University of Pisa under the "PRA–Progetti di Ricerca di Ateneo" (Institutional Research Grants)–Project no. PRA_2022-2023_12. TM thanks University of Pisa for financial support through Fondi di Ateneo "PRA – Progetti di Ricerca di Ateneo" Institutional Research Grants – Project no. PRA_2020_58.

ABBREVIATIONS

3CL^{pro}	3-chymotrypsin-like protease
ACE2	angiotensin-converting enzyme 2
Caco-2	immortalized human colorectal adenocarcinoma cells
CaLu-3	non-small-cell lung cancer cell line
CoVs	alpha, beta, delta, and gamma-coronaviruses
CTSB	cysteine proteases cathepsin B
CTSL	cysteine proteases cathepsin L
ELISA	enzyme-linked immunosorbent assay
MERS-CoV	Middle East respiratory syndrome coronavirus
M^{pro}	SARS-CoV-2 main protease
NRP1	cellular receptor neuropilin-1
PL^{pro}	papain-like protein
POMs	polyoxometalates

RBD	receptor binding domain
rRT-PCR	real-time reverse transcription polymerase chain reaction
S	spike
SARS-CoV	severe acute respiratory syndrome coronavirus
SARS-CoV-2	severe acute respiratory syndrome coronavirus-2
TMPRSS2	cellular transmembrane serine protease 2
TrxR	thioredoxin reductase
WHO	World Health Organization

REFERENCES

[1] D. Cirri, F. Bartoli, A. Pratesi, E. Baglini, E. Barresi, T. Marzo, *Biomedicines* **2021**, *9*, 504.

[2] J. A. Lemire, J. J. Harrison, R. J. Turner, *Nat. Rev. Microbiol.* **2013**, *11*, 371–384.

[3] N. P. E. Barry, P. J. Sadler, *Chem. Commun.* **2013**, *49*, 5106–5131.

[4] N. P. E. Barry, P. J. Sadler, *Pure Appl. Chem.* **2014**, *86*, 1897–1910.

[5] M. Patra, G. Gasser, N. Metzler-Nolte, *Dalt. Trans.* **2012**, *41*, 6350–6358.

[6] E. J. Anthony, E. M. Bolitho, H. E. Bridgewater, O. W. L. Carter, J. M. Donnelly, C. Imberti, E. C. Lant, F. Lermyte, R. J. Needham, M. Palau, P. J. Sadler, H. Shi, F. X. Wang, W. Y. Zhang, Z. Zhang, *Chem. Sci.* **2020**, *11*, 12888–12917.

[7] T. Marzo, G. Ferraro, A. Merlino, L. Messori, in *Encyclopedia of Inorganic and Bioinorganic Chemistry*, Wiley, **2020**, pp. 1–17.

[8] B. Rosenberg, L. VanCamp, J. E. Trosko, V. H. Mansour, *Nature* **1969**, *222*, 385–386.

[9] S. M. Cohen, S. J. Lippard, *Prog. Nucleic Acid Res. Mol. Biol.*, **2001**, *67*, 93–130.

[10] K. D. Mjos, C. Orvig, *Chem. Rev.* **2014**, *114*, 4540–4563.

[11] T. Marzo, D. La Mendola, *Inorganics* **2021**, *9*, 46.

[12] R. Oun, Y. E. Moussa, N. J. Wheate, *Dalt. Trans.* **2018**, *47*, 6645–6653.

[13] T. Marzo, L. Messori, D. La Mendola, *Curr. Top. Med. Chem.* **2021**, *21*, 2435–2438.

[14] T. C. Johnstone, K. Suntharalingam, S. J. Lippard, *Chem. Rev.* **2016**, *116*, 3436–3486.

[15] D. Cirri, S. Pillozzi, C. Gabbiani, J. Tricomi, G. Bartoli, M. Stefanini, E. Michelucci, A. Arcangeli, L. Messori, T. Marzo, *Dalt. Trans.* **2017**, *46*, 3311–3317.

[16] P. M. Bruno, Y. Liu, G. Y. Park, J. Murai, C. E. Koch, T. J. Eisen, J. R. Pritchard, Y. Pommier, S. J. Lippard, M. T. Hemann, *Nat. Med.* **2017**, *23*, 461–471.

[17] T. Marzo, A. Pratesi, D. Cirri, S. Pillozzi, G. Petroni, A. Guerri, A. Arcangeli, L. Messori, C. Gabbiani, *Inorganica Chim. Acta* **2018**, *470*, 318–324.

[18] Y. Gothe, T. Marzo, L. Messori, N. Metzler-Nolte, *Chem. Commun.* **2015**, *51*, 3151–3153.

[19] L. Chiaverini, A. Pratesi, D. Cirri, A. Nardinocchi, I. Tolbatov, A. Marrone, M. Di Luca, T. Marzo, D. La Mendola, *Molecules* **2022**, *27*, DOI: 10.3390/molecules27082578

[20] T. Marzo, S. Taliani, S. Salerno, F. Da Settimo, E. Barresi, D. La Mendola, *Curr. Top. Med. Chem.* **2021**, *21*, 2767–2770.

[21] T. Marzo, D. Cirri, S. Pollini, M. Prato, S. Fallani, M. I. Cassetta, A. Novelli, G. M. Rossolini, L. Messori, *ChemMedChem* **2018**, *13*, 2448–2454.

[22] J. Sharma, L. Balakrishnan, S. Kaushik, M. K. Kashyap, *Front. Bioeng. Biotechnol.* **2020**, *8*, 829.

[23] F. Magherini, T. Fiaschi, E. Valocchia, M. Becatti, A. Pratesi, T. Marzo, L. Massai, C. Gabbiani, I. Landini, E. Nobili, E. Mini, L. Messori, A. Modesti, T. Gamberi, *Oncotarget* **2018**, *9*, 28042–28068.

[24] T. Gamberi, A. Pratesi, L. Messori, L. Massai, *Coord. Chem. Rev.* **2021**, *438*, 213905.

[25] G. Scalese, K. Kostenkova, D. C. Crans, D. Gambino, *Curr. Opin. Chem. Biol.* **2022**, *67*, 102127.

Diversity of Metal Compounds as a Source of Novel Anti-COVID-19 Drugs 159

[26] P. Tarighi, S. Eftekhari, M. Chizari, M. Sabernavaei, D. Jafari, P. Mirzabeigi, *Eur. J. Pharmacol.* **2021**, *895*, 173890.

[27] E. Callaway, *Nature* **2022**, *607*, 18–19.

[28] NIH, "Clinical Spectrum | COVID-19 Treatment Guidelines," can be found under https://www.covid19treatmentguidelines.nih.gov/overview/clinical-spectrum/, **2021**.

[29] X. Li, T. Li, H. Wang, *Exp. Ther. Med.* **2021**, *21*, 3.

[30] Y. Wang, Y. Hao, S. Fa, W. Zheng, C. Yuan, W. Wang, *Front. Bioeng. Biotechnol.* **2021**, *9*, 849.

[31] I. P. Trougakos, K. Stamatelopoulos, E. Terpos, O. E. Tsitsilonis, E. Aivalioti, D. Paraskevis, E. Kastritis, G. N. Pavlakis, M. A. Dimopoulos, *J. Biomed. Sci.* **2021**, *28*, 1–18.

[32] M. Hoffmann, H. Kleine-Weber, S. Pöhlmann, *Mol. Cell* **2020**, *78*, 779–784.e5.

[33] L. Cantuti-Castelvetri, R. Ojha, L. D. Pedro, M. Djannatian, J. Franz, S. Kuivanen, F. van der Meer, K. Kallio, T. Kaya, M. Anastasina, T. Smura, L. Levanov, L. Szirovicza, A. Tobi, H. Kallio-Kokko, P. Österlund, M. Joensuu, F. A. Meunier, S. J. Butcher, M. S. Winkler, B. Mollenhauer, A. Helenius, O. Gokce, T. Teesalu, J. Hepojoki, O. Vapalahti, C. Stadelmann, G. Balistreri, M. Simons, *Science* **2020**, *370*, 856–860.

[34] Y. Yang, F. Peng, R. Wang, K. Guan, T. Jiang, G. Xu, J. Sun, C. Chang, *J. Autoimmun.* **2020**, *109*, 102434.

[35] T. M. Abdelghany, M. Ganash, M. M. Bakri, H. Qanash, A. M. H. Al-Rajhi, N. I. Elhussieny, *Biomed. J.* **2021**, *44*, 86–93.

[36] G. Kanimozhi, B. Pradhapsingh, C. Singh Pawar, H. A. Khan, S. H. Alrokayan, N. R. Prasad, *Front. Pharmacol.* **2021**, *12*, 638334.

[37] D. Cirri, A. Pratesi, T. Marzo, L. Messori, *Expert Opin. Drug Discov.* **2021**, *16*, 39–46.

[38] C. T. R. Vegivinti, K. W. Evanson, H. Lyons, I. Akosman, A. Barrett, N. Hardy, B. Kane, P. R. Keesari, Y. S. Pulakurthi, E. Sheffels, P. Balasubramanian, R. Chibbar, S. Chittajallu, K. Cowie, J. Karon, L. Siegel, R. Tarchand, C. Zinn, N. Gupta, K. M. Kallmes, K. Saravu, J. Touchette, *BMC Infect. Dis.* **2022**, *22*, 107.

[39] I. O. Rosas, N. Bräu, M. Waters, R. C. Go, B. D. Hunter, S. Bhagani, D. Skiest, M. S. Aziz, N. Cooper, I. S. Douglas, S. Savic, T. Youngstein, L. Del Sorbo, A. Cubillo Gracian, D. J. De La Zerda, A. Ustianowski, M. Bao, S. Dimonaco, E. Graham, B. Matharu, H. Spotswood, L. Tsai, A. Malhotra, *N. Engl. J. Med.* **2021**, *384*, 1503–1516.

[40] A. Cortegiani, G. Ingoglia, M. Ippolito, A. Giarratano, S. Einav, *J. Crit. Care* **2020**, *57*, 279–283.

[41] R. L. Gottlieb, C. E. Vaca, R. Paredes, J. Mera, B. J. Webb, G. Perez, G. Oguchi, P. Ryan, B. U. Nielsen, M. Brown, A. Hidalgo, Y. Sachdeva, S. Mittal, O. Osiyemi, J. Skarbinski, K. Juneja, R. H. Hyland, A. Osinusi, S. Chen, G. Camus, M. Abdelghany, S. Davies, N. Behenna-Renton, F. Duff, F. M. Marty, M. J. Katz, A. A. Ginde, S. M. Brown, J. T. Schiffer, J. A. Hill, *N. Engl. J. Med.* **2022**, *386*, 305–315.

[42] T. Marzo, L. Messori, *ACS Med. Chem. Lett.* **2020**, *11*, 1067–1068.

[43] K. Ioannou, M. C. Vlasiou, *BioMetals* **2022**, DOI: 10.1007/s10534-022-00386-5

[44] W. F. Kean, L. Hart, W. W. Buchanan, *Rheumatology* **1997**, *36*, 560–572.

[45] M. B. Harbut, C. Vilchèze, X. Luo, M. E. Hensler, H. Guo, B. Yang, A. K. Chatterjee, V. Nizet, W. R. Jacobs, P. G. Schultz, F. Wang, *Proc. Natl. Acad. Sci. U. S. A.* **2015**, *112*, 4453–4458.

[46] T. S. Fung, D. X. Liu, *Front. Microbiol.* **2014**, *5*, 296.

[47] K. L. Siu, C. P. Chan, K. H. Kok, P. C. Y. Woo, D. Y. Jin, *Cell Biosci.* **2014**, *4*, 1–9.

[48] H. A. Rothan, M. Kumar, *Pathogens* **2019**, *8*, 148.

[49] R. S. Diaz, I. L. Shytaj, L. B. Giron, B. Obermaier, E. della Libera, J. Galinskas, D. Dias, J. Hunter, M. Janini, G. Gosuen, P. A. Ferreira, M. C. Sucupira, J. Maricato, O. Fackler, M. Lusic, A. Savarino, *Int. J. Antimicrob. Agents* **2019**, *54*, 592–600.

[50] "Multi Interventional Study Exploring HIV-1 Residual Replication: A Step Towards HIV-1 Eradication and Sterilizing Cure – Full Text View – ClinicalTrials.gov," can be found under https://clinicaltrials.gov/ct2/show/NCT02961829?cond=Multi+Inte rventional+Study+Exploring+HIV-1+Residual+Replication%3A+a+Step+Towards +HIV-1+Eradication+and+Sterilizing+Cure&draw=2&rank=1, **n.d.**

[51] H. A. Rothan, S. Stone, J. Natekar, P. Kumari, K. Arora, M. Kumar, *Virology* **2020**, *547*, 7–11.

[52] M. Gil-Moles, U. Basu, R. Büssing, H. Hoffmeister, S. Türck, A. Varchmin, I. Ott, *Chem. – A Eur. J.* **2020**, *26*, 15140–15144.

[53] H. D. Betts, C. Whitehead, H. H. Harris, *Metallomics* **2021**, *13*, 1.

[54] L. C. Cancio, *Surg. Infect. (Larchmt).* **2021**, *22*, 103–112.

[55] T. W. Chang, L. Weinstein, *J. Infect. Dis.* **1975**, *132*, 79–81.

[56] R. E. F. De Paiva, A. Marçal Neto, I. A. Santos, A. C. G. Jardim, P. P. Corbi, F. R. G. Bergamini, *Dalt. Trans.* **2020**, *49*, 16004–16033.

[57] F. Pilaquinga, J. Morey, M. Torres, R. Seqqat, M. de las N. Piña, *Wiley Interdiscip. Rev. Nanomed. Nanobiotechnol.* **2021**, *13*, e1707.

[58] M. Gil-Moles, S. Türck, U. Basu, A. Pettenuzzo, S. Bhattacharya, A. Rajan, X. Ma, R. Büssing, J. Wölker, H. Burmeister, H. Hoffmeister, P. Schneeberg, A. Prause, P. Lippmann, J. Kusi-Nimarko, S. Hassell-Hart, A. McGown, D. Guest, Y. Lin, A. Notaro, R. Vinck, J. Karges, K. Cariou, K. Peng, X. Qin, X. Wang, J. Skiba, Ł. Szczupak, K. Kowalski, U. Schatzschneider, C. Hemmert, H. Gornitzka, E. R. Milaeva, A. A. Nazarov, G. Gasser, J. Spencer, L. Ronconi, U. Kortz, J. Cinatl, D. Bojkova, I. Ott, *Chem. – A Eur. J.* **2021**, *27*, 17928–17940.

[59] J. J. Kozak, H. B. Gray, R. A. Garza-López, *J. Inorg. Biochem.* **2020**, *211*, 111179.

[60] A. Belhassan, S. Chtita, H. Zaki, T. Lakhlifi and M. Bouachrine, *Bioinformation* **2020**, *16*, 404–410.

[61] S. Das, S. Sarmah, S. Lyndem, A. Singha Roy, *J. Biomol. Struct. Dyn.* **2021**, *39*, 3347–3357.

[62] R. Islam, M. R. Parves, A. S. Paul, N. Uddin, M. S. Rahman, A. Al Mamun, M. N. Hossain, M. A. Ali, M. A. Halim, *J. Biomol. Struct. Dyn.* **2021**, *39*, 3213–3224.

[63] R. S. Joshi, S. S. Jagdale, S. B. Bansode, S. S. Shankar, M. B. Tellis, V. K. Pandya, A. Chugh, A. P. Giri, M. J. Kulkarni, *J. Biomol. Struct. Dyn.* **2021**, *39*, 1–16.

[64] N. Lobo-Galo, M. Terrazas-López, A. Martínez-Martínez, Á. G. Díaz-Sánchez, *J. Biomol. Struct. Dyn.* **2021**, *39*, 3419–3427.

[65] R. Garza-Lopez, J. Kozak, H. Gray, *ChemRxiv* **2020**, 1–13. doi: 10.26434/chemrxiv.12673436.

[66] A. Böttcher, T. Takeuchi, K. I. Hardcastle, T. J. Meade, H. B. Gray, D. Cwikel, M. Kapon, Z. Dori, *Inorg. Chem.* **1997**, *36*, 2498–2504.

[67] T. Takeuchi, A. Bottcher, C. M. Quezada, M. I. Simon, T. J. Meade, H. B. Gray, *J. Am. Chem. Soc.* **1998**, *120*, 8555–8556.

[68] O. Blum, A. Haiek, D. Cwikel, Z. Dori, T. J. Meade, H. B. Gray, *Proc. Natl. Acad. Sci. U. S. A.* **1998**, *95*, 6659–6662.

[69] E. Toyota, K. K. S. Ng, H. Sekizaki, K. Itoh, K. Tanizawa, M. N. G. James, *J. Mol. Biol.* **2001**, *305*, 471–479.

[70] W. Li, L. Jin, N. Zhu, X. Hou, F. Deng, H. Sun, *J. Am. Chem. Soc.* **2003**, *125*, 12408–12409.

[71] N. Yang, J. A. Tanner, Z. Wang, J. D. Huang, B. J. Zheng, N. Zhu, H. Sun, *Chem. Commun.* **2007**, 4413–4415.

[72] N. Yang, J. A. Tanner, B. J. Zheng, R. M. Watt, M. L. He, L. Y. Lu, J. Q. Jiang, K. T. Shum, Y. P. Lin, K. L. Wong, M. C. M. Lin, H. F. Kung, H. Sun, J. D. Huang, *Angew. Chemie - Int. Ed.* **2007**, *46*, 6464–6468.

Diversity of Metal Compounds as a Source of Novel Anti-COVID-19 Drugs 161

[73] T. Shu, M. Huang, D. Wu, Y. Ren, X. Zhang, Y. Han, J. Mu, R. Wang, Y. Qiu, D. Y. Zhang, X. Zhou, *Virol. Sin.* **2020**, *35*, 321–329.

[74] S. Yuan, R. Wang, J. F.-W. Chan, A. J. Zhang, T. Cheng, K. K.-H. Chik, Z.-W. Ye, S. Wang, A. C.-Y. Lee, L. Jin, H. Li, D.-Y. Jin, K.-Y. Yuen, H. Sun, *Nat. Microbiol.* **2020**, *5*, 1439–1448.

[75] D. N. Frick, *Drug News Perspect.* **2003**, *16*, 355–362.

[76] D. C. Wolf, C. H. Wolf, D. T. Rubin, *Am. J. Gastroenterol.* **2020**, *115*, 1298.

[77] R. Wang, J. F.-W. Chan, S. Wang, H. Li, J. Zhao, T. K.-Y. Ip, Z. Zuo, K.-Y. Yuen, S. Yuan, H. Sun, *Chem. Sci.* **2022**, *13*, 2238–2248.

[78] M. Aureliano, N. I. Gumerova, G. Sciortino, E. Garribba, A. Rompel, D. C. Crans, *Coord. Chem. Rev.* **2021**, *447*, 214143.

[79] A. Bijelic, M. Aureliano, A. Rompel, *Chem. Commun.* **2018**, *54*, 1153–1169.

[80] P. Yang, U. Kortz, *Acc. Chem. Res.* **2018**, *51*, 1599–1608.

[81] N. V. Izarova, M. T. Pope, U. Kortz, *Angew. Chemie Int. Ed.* **2012**, *51*, 9492–9510.

[82] J. T. Rhule, C. L. Hill, D. A. Judd, R. F. Schinazi, *Chem. Rev.* **1998**, *98*, 327–357.

[83] M. B. Čolović, M. Lacković, J. Lalatović, A. S. Mougharbel, U. Kortz, D. Z. Krstić, *Curr. Med. Chem.* **2020**, *27*, 362–379.

[84] J. Wang, Y. Liu, K. Xu, Y. Qi, J. Zhong, K. Zhang, J. Li, E. Wang, Z. Wu, Z. Kang, *ACS Appl. Mater. Interfaces* **2014**, *6*, 9785–9789.

[85] S. G. Sarafianos, U. Kortz, M. T. Pope, M. J. Modak, *Biochem. J.* **1996**, *319*, 619–626.

[86] R. Francese, A. Civra, M. Rittà, M. Donalisio, M. Argenziano, R. Cavalli, A. S. Mougharbel, U. Kortz, D. Lembo, *Antiviral Res.* **2019**, *163*, 29–33.

[87] O. W. L. Carter, Y. Xu, P. J. Sadler, *RSC Adv.* **2021**, *11*, 1939–1951.

[88] S. Xiu, A. Dick, H. Ju, S. Mirzaie, F. Abdi, S. Cocklin, P. Zhan, X. Liu, *J. Med. Chem.* **2020**, *63*, 12256–12274.

[89] S. K. Nayak, *Mini Rev. Med. Chem.* **2021**, *21*, 689–703.

[90] F. Li, *Annu. Rev. Virol.* **2016**, *3*, 237–261.

[91] K. Al Adem, A. Shanti, C. Stefanini, S. Lee, *Pharmaceuticals* **2020**, *13*, 447.

[92] J. Lan, J. Ge, J. Yu, S. Shan, H. Zhou, S. Fan, Q. Zhang, X. Shi, Q. Wang, L. Zhang, X. Wang, *Nature* **2020**, *581*, 215–220.

[93] R. Cannalire, C. Cerchia, A. R. Beccari, F. S. Di Leva, V. Summa, *J. Med. Chem.* **2022**, *65*, 2716–2746.

[94] B. K. Maiti, *ACS Pharmacol. Transl. Sci.* **2020**, *3*, 1017–1019.

[95] C. Gil, T. Ginex, I. Maestro, V. Nozal, L. Barrado-Gil, M. Á. Cuesta-Geijo, J. Urquiza, D. Ramírez, C. Alonso, N. E. Campillo, A. Martinez, *J. Med. Chem.* **2020**, *63*, 12359–12386.

[96] K. Sargsyan, C. C. Lin, T. Chen, C. Grauffel, Y. P. Chen, W. Z. Yang, H. S. Yuan, C. Lim, *Chem. Sci.* **2020**, *11*, 9904–9909.

[97] M. Aureliano, *BioChem* **2022**, *2*, 8–26.

[98] D. Cirri, T. Marzo, I. Tolbatov, A. Marrone, F. Saladini, I. Vicenti, F. Dragoni, A. Boccuto, L. Messori, *Biomolecules* **2021**, *11*, 1858.

6 Evaluating the Potential of Novel Metal-Based Drugs for Treating Drug-Resistant Bacteria

Andris Evans
Department of Microbiology and Immunology
The University of Western Ontario,
London, Ontario, Canada

*Kevin Kavanagh**
SSPC Pharma Research Centre
Department of Biology, Maynooth
University, Co. Kildare, Ireland
Kevin.Kavanagh@mu.ie

CONTENTS

1 Introduction 165
   1.1 Overview of Conventional Antibiotics 166
2 MRSA: An Antibiotic-Resistant Pathogen with a Significant
   Clinical Burden 167
   2.1 Treatment 168
3 Metal-Based Drugs as Antibacterial Agents 168
   3.1 Copper 169
      3.1.1 Copper Antibacterial Mode of Action 171
      3.1.2 Copper-Based Antibacterial Compounds 171
      3.1.3 Safety and Toxicology of Copper-Based
            Antibacterial Compounds 173
   3.2 Silver 174
      3.2.1 Silver Antibacterial Mode of Action 174
      3.2.2 Silver-Based Antibacterial Compounds 174
      3.2.3 Safety and Toxicology of Silver-Based
            Antibacterial Compounds 175

---

*Corresponding author

DOI: 10.1201/9781003272250-6

3.3	Gold		176
	3.3.1	Gold Antibacterial Mode of Action	176
	3.3.2	Gold-Based Antibacterial Compounds	176
	3.3.3	Safety and Toxicology of Gold-Based Antibacterial Compounds	178
3.4	Gallium		178
	3.4.1	Gallium Antibacterial Mode of Action	178
	3.4.2	Gallium-Based Antibacterial Compounds	179
	3.4.3	Safety and Toxicology of Gallium-Based Antibacterial Drugs	180
3.5	Tellurium		180
	3.5.1	Tellurium Antibacterial Mode of Action	181
	3.5.2	Tellurium-Based Antibacterial Compounds	181
	3.5.3	Safety and Toxicology of Tellurium-Based Antibacterial Compounds	182
3.6	Zinc Chelators		182
	3.6.1	Zinc Chelators Combined with β-Lactams Antibacterial Mode of Action	183
	3.6.2	Zinc Chelator-Based Antibacterial Compounds	183
	3.6.3	Safety and Toxicology of Zinc Chelators Combined with β-Lactams	183
4	General Conclusion		185
Abbreviations			186
References			187

ABSTRACT

As a consequence of rising antimicrobial resistance, we may now be entering a "post-antibiotic" area where conventional antibiotics will no longer be effective. For the effective treatment of resistant bacterial infections, it is essential to look to developing novel antimicrobial agents with distinct modes of action from conventional antibiotics. Metal-based antibacterial compounds have novel and diverse modes of action compared to conventional antibiotics, conveying an advantage for the treatment of resistant bacterial infections. The antibacterial effects of certain metals have been known for thousands of years and the rise in antimicrobial resistance has reignited interest and research into developing and evaluating metal-based compounds for antibacterial purposes. This chapter will review some metal-based compounds that show promise as antibacterial agents, their antibacterial mode of action, and toxicology and safety for topical and/or systemic use.

KEYWORDS

Bacterial Pathogens; Resistance; Metal-Based Compounds; Infection; Antibiotics

1 INTRODUCTION

Bacterial pathogens cause significant levels of disease in susceptible populations and can produce high mortality rates [1, 2]. Prior to the advent of the antibiotic era, bacterial infections could not be treated effectively and deaths from simple infections, such as skin infections, were not uncommon. The discovery and use of antibiotics transformed the treatment of bacterial infections and have saved the lives of millions of people [3]. However, the beneficial effects of antibiotics have been compromised by their over-use and misuse leading to the emergence of bacteria that exhibit resistance to a broad range of agents. Bacteria in the environment naturally encounter toxic compounds and have developed resistance mechanisms to allow continued growth and development in the presence of these compounds [2]. Many of these mechanisms confer resistance to antibiotics (Figure 1). As bacteria can rapidly exchange genes encoding resistance mechanisms, resistance rapidly spreads within populations and between unrelated bacteria [4]. Consequently, we are at risk of entering the "post-antibiotic era" when conventional antibiotics will no longer be effective.

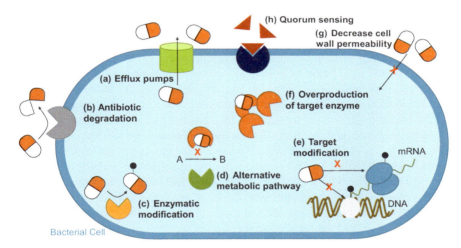

FIGURE 1 Mechanisms of antibiotic resistance. Bacteria can acquire resistance to certain antibiotics through a variety of different mechanisms. (a) Upregulation of efflux pumps allows bacteria to remove the antibiotic from the intracellular space before it can attack its target site. (b) Enzymes can be expressed to degrade the antibiotic before it is able to attack its target site. (c) Enzymes can modify the antibiotic so it cannot interact with its target. (d) Alternative metabolic pathways can be used that do not require the proteins targeted by the antibiotic. (e) Antibiotic targets can be modified to prevent interaction with the antibiotic. (f) The target enzyme or protein can be made in excess so only some are inhibited by the antibiotic. (g) Cell wall permeability can be decreased to prevent the antibiotic from entering the intracellular space. (h) Quorum sensing between members of a biofilm consortium can be used to transfer antimicrobial resistance genes.

To tackle antibiotic-resistant bacteria, it is essential to develop novel antimicrobial agents with distinct modes of action compared to conventional antibiotics. The antibacterial effects of selected metals have been known for thousands of years [5]. In recent years, research programmes have been initiated to evaluate the potential of metal-based compounds as safe and effective agents for the treatment of drug-resistant bacterial pathogens. Metal-based compounds may provide a novel weapon in our war against resistant bacteria.

1.1 OVERVIEW OF CONVENTIONAL ANTIBIOTICS

Traditionally, antibiotics are used for the treatment of bacterial infections, and have several major mechanisms of antibacterial activity [6]. The first mechanism is to interfere with cell wall synthesis. Antibiotic classes that function through this mechanism include β-lactams such as penicillin, and monobactams such as vancomycin. β-lactams inhibit cell wall synthesis by preventing transpeptidation between the N-acetylglucosamine and N-acetylmuramic acid chains. This inhibition weakens the cell wall, resulting in cell lysis. Monobactams function in a similar way to β-lactams, but bind the terminal D-alanine residue on the peptidoglycan chain to prevent cross-linking instead (Figure 1) [6].

Antibiotics such as aminoglycosides, tetracyclines, and fluoroquinolones can inhibit bacterial protein synthesis. These antibiotics bind bacterial ribosomes to prevent the translation of mRNA to protein, thus preventing the synthesis of essential proteins and killing the bacteria (Figure 1). As human and bacterial ribosomes are structurally distinct, the antibiotics selectively target bacteria while human cells remain undamaged [6]. Antibiotics can also block the metabolic pathways critical for DNA synthesis, so the bacteria are unable to propagate. This method is used by antibiotics such as fluoroquinolones, sulfonamides, and trimethoprim (Figure 1). An example of a critical metabolic pathway is the folic acid pathway, which is blocked by trimethoprim and sulfamethoxazole [6].

Diverse classes of antibiotics with different modes of action are required to treat bacteria with antimicrobial resistance (Figure 1). In cases where certain bacterial strains have inherent or acquired resistance to a specific antibiotic, a different antibiotic with an alternative mode of action will be used to treat the infection. However, if a bacterial strain has multidrug resistance, alternative modes of action may not be available [7]. Consequently, novel antibacterial drugs with differing modes of action are required for the effective treatment of antibiotic-resistant bacteria.

Since the World Health Organization first analysed the clinical antibacterial pipeline in 2017, 12 new antibacterial drugs have been approved, only one of which has a new antibacterial drug-related pharmacophore [8]. Of the 43 antibiotic drugs currently in clinical development, only 11 have novel structural classes, while the rest are modified versions or derivatives of current antibiotics. Furthermore, none of these are potentially active against WHO critical threat pathogens or Gram-negative ESKAPE pathogens [9]. Without novel structures and modes of action, the resistance mechanisms presented by bacteria cannot be avoided, and antibiotics will continue to become increasingly ineffective.

Novel Metal-Based Drugs for Treating Drug-Resistant Bacteria   **167**

2 MRSA: AN ANTIBIOTIC-RESISTANT PATHOGEN WITH A SIGNIFICANT CLINICAL BURDEN

Staphylococcus aureus is a Gram-positive bacterium that is frequently found colonising the skin and mucosal surfaces (e.g. nasal passages) of healthy individuals. It is estimated that approximately 30% of the population is colonised by *S. aureus* but colonisation is mostly asymptomatic [10]. Although frequently encountered as a commensal, *S. aureus* can induce a number of skin infections (e.g. impetigo, cellulitis, wound infections) and systemic infections (e.g. pneumonia, sinusitis, osteomyelitis) in susceptible patients [11].

S. aureus can grow in a wide variety of *in vitro* and *in vivo* environments, partly due to its production of diverse enzymes and toxins that facilitate growth as well as host immune system suppression and evasion. The most studied toxins produced by *S. aureus* are exfoliative toxin, enterotoxins, and toxic shock syndrome toxin-1 (TSST-1) [12]. Staphylococcal scalded skin syndrome (SSSS) is caused by the production of exfoliative toxin and results in inflammation, tissue degradation, and blistering [13]. *S. aureus* is also one of the leading causes of food poisoning through enterotoxin production, which leads to diarrhoea and vomiting. As enterotoxins are heat stable (up to 100°C) and resistant to degradation in the gastrointestinal tract, low temperature cooking does not inactivate them [13]. TSST-1 causes toxic shock syndrome and was first implicated following severe cases of illness in women using hyper-absorbent tampons [14]. Also, it binds MHC class II, activating T cells and resulting in extensive inflammation and tissue damage [15].

Antibiotic treatment of *S. aureus* infections has become increasingly difficult due to the rapid development of resistance. *S. aureus* is a member of the ESKAPE pathogen species, a group of bacteria with a propensity to develop resistance at higher rates and as a result, have an increased threat of morbidity and mortality [7]. Resistance to β-lactams, the first antibiotics against *S. aureus*, began to appear within a few years, with the emergence of methicillin-resistant *S. aureus* (MRSA) confirmed in 1959 [16]. In the EU, an estimated 150,000 patients are affected by MRSA and up to 7,000 deaths are directly attributable to this pathogen annually [17]. Key risk factors for MRSA infection are surgery, long-term hospitalisation, urinary catheterisation, and intensive care [14]. The resistance phenotype in MRSA is caused by the presence of a mobile genetic element, or plasmid, which codes for mecA to produce the penicillin-binding protein 2a (PBP2a) [14]. This plasmid was likely acquired from another bacterial species by conjugation, a common mechanism for transferring resistance genes across mixed bacterial populations [18]. Penicillin-resistant *S. aureus* isolates can produce β-lactamase enzymes, inactivating the antibiotics before they can exert their effect [19]. Antibiotics such as methicillin disrupt the cross-linking domain of penicillin-binding proteins. In the absence of cross-linking of the peptidoglycan layer, the bacterial cell wall is weakened leading to leakage of the cell contents and cell death. PBP2a is not inhibited by β-lactam antibiotics and continues cross-linking the peptidoglycan layer in the presence of the antibiotic thus ensuring cell division and population growth [19].

MRSA infections are classified as either community-acquired (CA) or health care-acquired (HA) and have differing phenotypes depending on their classification. HA-MRSA infections are almost exclusively nosocomial, while CA-MRSA infections can be contracted among people in the community, prisoners, creche/play school attendees, athletes, and people who use drugs [20]. Poor hygiene and crowded accommodation can accelerate person-to-person transmission of CA-MRSA. CA- and HA-MRSA isolates have genetic differences and altered patterns of resistance phenotypes [21]. HA-MRSA isolates contain the type I–III Staphylococcal Cassette Chromosome *mec* (SCCmec) providing resistance to many antibiotics. In comparison, CA-MRSA possesses type IV or V SCCmec elements [22]. CA-MRSA also contains the panton-valentine leukocidin toxin (PVL) which destroys human leukocytes and causes necrosis of epithelial cells [23]. As a result of the reduced immune cell population caused by PVL, the CA-MRSA strain can utilise human tissue for nutrition and development [24]. CA-MRSA may be more virulent than HA-MRSA due to the presence of virulence determinants including phenol soluble modulin (PSM) cytolysins and α-toxin [14]. Phenol soluble modulins are a group of peptides with cytolytic properties towards human neutrophils. The cytolysin α-toxin has no effect on neutrophils but does cause lysis of erythrocytes [14]. The differences between CA- and HA-MRSA isolates and their resistance phenotypes have implications in the choice of treatment options for MRSA infections.

2.1 TREATMENT

Due to the inherent resistance of MRSA isolates, control of infection in patients is difficult but not impossible. To prevent infections, clinical settings implement stringent measures to reduce transmission and ensure sterility during surgery. For instance, susceptible patients may be decolonised prior to surgery by topical antimicrobial agents. MRSA-infected patients can be treated intravenously with vancomycin or daptomycin [25]. For localised skin or sub-cutaneous infections, clindamycin can be administered. Due to the rapid acquisition of resistance, many MRSA isolates now show resistance to vancomycin [26] necessitating the use of alternative antimicrobials for patient therapy. Metal-based antibiotics offer a promising avenue for the treatment of resistant bacteria such as MRSA as they offer differing and diverse modes of action compared to conventional organic antibiotics [27] and can be complexed to current antibiotic drugs to enhance their antibacterial function [28].

3 METAL-BASED DRUGS AS ANTIBACTERIAL AGENTS

Metal ions have a long history of use for their antibacterial properties [5]. For instance, Persian kings would use silver to carry water and keep it fresh, particularly during military conflicts when it was difficult to acquire fresh water from natural resources [5]. The arsenic-containing compound Salvarsan,

Novel Metal-Based Drugs for Treating Drug-Resistant Bacteria   **169**

discovered at the beginning of the 20th century, served as the first effective treatment of syphilis, a bacterial infection caused by *Treponema pallidum* [28]. The discovery of penicillin, and the antibiotics that followed, ultimately stopped the clinical use of metal-compounds for their antibacterial properties. However, rising antibiotic resistance has reignited interest in the use of metal-based pharmaceuticals as antibacterial agents due to their multiple and varied modes of action compared to conventional antibiotics [27, 29].

To increase their antibacterial efficacy, metal ions can be complexed to biomolecules or antibiotics, or can be used in conjunction with antibiotics, potentially leading to new metallo-drug candidates with different antibacterial mechanisms that can bypass bacterial resistance mechanisms. The metal ion and antibiotic can also work synergistically, increasing the compound's antibacterial activity and reducing the therapeutic dose [28]. Biomolecules are compounds commonly taken into specific areas of a bacterial cell, and can mediate entry of the biomolecule-metal complex, allowing for targeted antibacterial effects [30].

Different metal-based compounds, targeting antibiotic-resistant bacterial infections, are currently at various stages of research and development. This chapter will discuss some metals and their respective metal-based complexes at the forefront of this field: copper, silver, gold, gallium, and tellurium. Zinc chelators are also discussed, as they target zinc ions to circumvent bacterial resistance and are a promising therapy against antibiotic-resistant bacteria. These metals demonstrate promising antibacterial activity, as well as toxicity data that indicate potential for topical and/or systemic use. Metals not discussed in detail in this chapter that also demonstrate antibacterial potential are outlined in Table 1.

3.1 COPPER

Copper has a long history of antibacterial use [48] and was recognised as the first metal with antimicrobial properties by the United States Environmental Protection Agency in 2008 [49]. Currently, its antimicrobial properties are widely used for external purposes, such as in face masks and stain-resistant fabrics to prevent bacterial growth [50]. Furthermore, numerous studies have examined the use of copper-coated surfaces in clinical settings to reduce hospital-acquired infections [49]. In comparison to the other metals discussed, copper is less expensive. Copper ions also exhibit a high inhibitory potential for Gram-positive bacteria, increased physical and chemical stability, and a higher ability to bind amine and carboxyl groups on the surface of Gram-positive bacteria allowing it to target these bacteria with increased efficacy in physiological conditions [51]. Although its antibacterial activity is often lower than that of the other metals discussed, copper ions have demonstrated synergistic effects with antibiotics for increased activity against drug-resistant bacteria [52].

TABLE 1
Additional Metals with Antibacterial Potential

Metal	Observed Activities
Bismuth	• Bi(III) exhibits low toxicity in humans with potent toxicity against bacteria • *Helicobacter pylori* particularly susceptible to three bismuth drugs: colloidal bismuth subcitrate (CBS, De-Nol), bismuth subsalicylate (Pepto-Bismol), and ranitidine bismuth citrate (Pylorid) • Bi(III) and colloidal bismuth subcitrate demonstrate potential as broad-spectrum MBL inhibitors [31, 32]
Iridium	• Ir(III) complexes show antibacterial activity as well as autophagy and apoptosis, proposed as both antimicrobial and anticancer treatment • Limited by cost and high dose required for antibacterial effect [31, 33, 34]
Iron	• Iron-based antibiotics have moderate antibacterial activity against *S. aureus* • Iron-based metal organic frameworks delivered through inhalable system show potential against *M. tuberculosis* • Iron chelators (e.g. DIBI) show potential for use as antibacterial agents, particularly in combination with existing antibiotics [35, 36] • More research required to determine efficacy, toxicity, and mode of action of iron-based antibacterial compounds *in vitro* and *in vivo*
Manganese	• Mn(I) tricarbonyl complexes with clotrimazole ligand show improved antibacterial activity against Gram-positive bacteria compared to antimicrobial alone *in vitro* • Mn(II) complexes containing 1,10-phenanthroline and dicarboxylate ligands demonstrate high antibacterial activity against (multi)drug-resistant strains of *M. tuberculosis in vitro* • Mn(III) Schiff base complexes demonstrate some antibacterial activity *in vitro*, although limited research exists on these compounds [37–39]
Palladium	• Antibacterial activity observed against *P. aeruginosa* and *E. faecalis*, varying activity against *S. aureus*, *E. coli*, and *K. pneumonia* • Antibacterial activity likely caused by binding DNA and protein • More research required to determine efficacy, toxicity, and mode of action of palladium-based antibacterial compounds *in vitro* and *in vivo* [40, 41]
Platinum	• Bactericidal activity, inducing bacterial filamentation and lysis in lysogenic bacteria • Antibacterial activity observed against Gram-positive bacteria, including vancomycin and methicillin-resistant *S. aureus* • Proposed antibacterial activity caused by interaction with DNA • Low efficacy *in vivo* indicate compounds may require alternative administration routes (e.g. topical administration) [42, 43]
Rhenium	• Antimicrobial activity not well researched • Preliminary studies show promising activity against MRSA and colistin-resistant *E. coli* • Lack of *in vivo* data requires further research [31, 44]

(Continued)

Novel Metal-Based Drugs for Treating Drug-Resistant Bacteria 171

TABLE 1 (*Continued*)
Additional Metals with Antibacterial Potential

Metal	Observed Activities
Rhodium	• Bacteriostatic effect *in vitro* against *S. pneumoniae* without significant cytotoxic side effect on host cell • Interferes with bacterial metal ion binding and metabolic pathways • Some Rh(II) compounds show both antibacterial and anticancer activity *in vitro* • More research required to determine efficacy, toxicity, and mode of action of rhodium-based antibacterial compounds *in vitro* and *in vivo* [45, 46]
Ruthenium	• Bactericidal activity • Antibacterial activity caused by binding nucleic acids and proteins • Strong bactericidal activity shown *in vitro* and *in vivo* against *Bacillus subtilis* and *S. aureus* strains, including several methicillin-resistant strains • Treatment with Ru(II)-based compounds increased *S. aureus* susceptibility to aminoglycoside antibiotics • Rapid clearance following IV administration reduces *in vivo* efficacy, likely better for topical administration • Lower propensity to induce resistance in *Streptococcus pyogenes* and *S. aureus* than conventional antibiotics • More research required to determine efficacy, toxicity, and mode of action of ruthenium-based antibacterial compounds *in vivo* [31, 47]

3.1.1 Copper Antibacterial Mode of Action

Although not fully understood, the antimicrobial activity of copper is often attributed to the release of its ions in an aqueous environment [53]. Copper ions such as Cu(I) and Cu(II) are involved in genotoxicity, the disruption of metalloproteins, disruption of membrane integrity, generation of reactive oxygen species (ROS), and as a carrier of charged antibiotic compounds which lead to bacterial cell death [54]. The ability of copper ions to attack essential proteins within the bacterial cell membrane has been predominantly observed in *Escherichia coli* [54], indicating that copper-based compounds may be particularly useful for the treatment of antibiotic-resistant strains of *E. coli*. Taking advantage of these antimicrobial properties, macrophages use elevated Cu(I) levels in the phagosome as a defence mechanism against pathogens [55]. Copper is also essential for the bacterial cell cycle and can be found both inside and outside the cell, allowing copper complexes to serve as a delivery method through the bacterial cell envelope to target internal organelles and the DNA [56, 57].

3.1.2 Copper-Based Antibacterial Compounds

Copper(II) is the most well-studied ion in copper complexes and has proven effective for the treatment of bacterial infections, rheumatoid diseases, tuberculosis (TB), cancers, and gastric ulcers [58, 59]. The current focus on Cu(II)-based compounds is to increase their antibacterial activity and safety *in vivo* through addition and modification of their ligands.

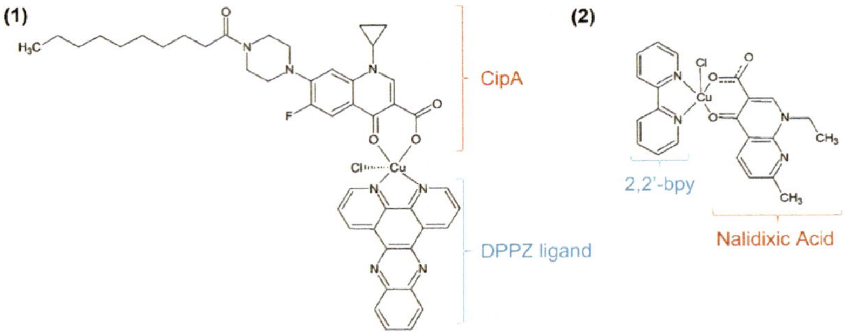

FIGURE 2 Molecular structures of copper-based compounds. CipA and nalidixic acid (highlighted in red) are derivatives of quinolone antibiotics with antiproliferative and antimicrobial activities. The co-ligands (highlighted in blue) are phen = 1,10-phenanthroline and DPPZ = dipyridophenazine in complexes (1) and (2), respectively.

Cu(II) is frequently examined in complexes with antibiotics such as quinolones to increase the antibacterial activity of these compounds [57, 60]. Quinolone-based copper complexes are known to interfere with DNA replication by damaging bacterial DNA [60]. Recently, a family of metal-based antibiotics containing a phenanthrene ligand to act as a photosensitiser and the antibiotic ciprofloxacin (CipA) was developed for prophylactic use in immunocompromised cancer patients [61]. These Cu(II)-antibiotic compounds, particularly compound (1) (Figure 2), inhibited Gram-positive bacteria and MRSA with greater potency than free CipA. In the Gram-negative strains, these complexes exhibited moderate to poor antibacterial activity, suggesting selective targeting of Gram-positive bacteria [61]. Proteomic analysis of the response of *S. aureus* and MRSA to Cu(II)-CipA derivatives revealed an increase in proteins associated with the cellular stress response and altered abundance of proteins associated with virulence and DNA repair [62]. Another recent study by Masram *et al.* reported a ternary Cu(II) complex with nalidixic acid and 2,2′-bipyridine (2,2′-bpy), compound (2) (Figure 2), which showed higher clearance with broad-spectrum antibacterial activity in both Gram-positive and -negative bacteria compared to nalidixic acid alone [63]. However, when compared to neomycin and streptomycin, compound (2) had lower antibacterial activity [63]. These studies highlight how a clinically used fluoroquinolone could be complexed with a metal ion to provide novel anti-MRSA activities.

Another recent study expanded upon the phenanthroline-based ligand family by lengthening the alkyl-chain moiety of the L-tyrosine ester to alter the lipophilicity of the ligands [56]. The best antibacterial activity was achieved by the Cu(II) complexes containing hexyl- and octyl-alkyl-chain derivatives, which showed strong antibacterial activity against both *S. aureus* and MRSA ($MIC_{50} = 1\,\mu M$) (Figure 2) [56]. These compounds had lower MIC values than all tested antibiotics (ampicillin, doxycycline, streptomycin, tetracycline, and vancomycin) and were twice as effective as the most effective antibiotic, vancomycin [56]. These data indicate that this class of Cu(II)-based antibacterial agents may be greatly beneficial in the treatment of antibiotic-resistant Gram-positive bacteria, such as MRSA.

Novel Metal-Based Drugs for Treating Drug-Resistant Bacteria

One advantage of copper-based antibacterial agents over conventional antibiotics is the low level of resistance to copper among clinically relevant bacteria. Bacteria with copper-resistant mechanisms are primarily found as environmental microorganisms living in copper-rich niches, such as marine sediments and mines [64]. In studies attempting to promote the development of tolerance with low dosages of copper and antibiotic, no adaptive evolution to the treatments was observed [65].

3.1.3 Safety and Toxicology of Copper-Based Antibacterial Compounds

After zinc and iron, copper is the third most abundant trace element and is essential for the proper function of several processes in the human body [66]. Following copper ingestion, it is incorporated into copper-dependent proteins in the liver and is regulated through biliary excretion to maintain homeostasis. Copper is used by the innate immune response to increase the phagocytic and bactericidal activity of neutrophils and the antimicrobial function of macrophages [67]. As copper is essential for processes in the human body and regulated by the liver, copper toxicity due to excess ingestion is rare. If copper toxicity occurs, it can lead to nausea, vomiting, hematemesis, hypotension, melena, diarrhoea, and jaundice [68]. Although uncommon, chronic excess copper exposure can damage the liver and kidneys [50].

High internal concentrations of copper ions can be toxic, but its exogenous application is considered safe to humans. Copper-impregnated textiles are commonly used and for almost half a century, long-term copper intrauterine devices have been used safely with no reported adverse effects [69]. This safety is because human skin cells are able to metabolise and use copper ions, while microbes cannot and are more sensitive to excess concentrations of copper ions, allowing for an effective therapeutic range [70]. Different ligands or structures of copper-based antibacterial compounds may further increase the antibacterial activity of copper at lower doses, allowing for safe and effective use of copper-based antibiotics.

The Cu(II) compounds with phenanthroline-based ligands and CipA, such as compound (1), were well tolerated by *Galleria mellonella* larvae when administered via direct injection into the haemocoel through the last pro-leg [61]. *G. mellonella* larvae are a valuable and commonly used infection model for evaluating the *in vivo* toxicity and mode of action of novel drug candidates due to their low cost, ease of handling, and high degree of structural and functional similarities to the human immune response [71–73]. *In vivo* toxicity studies with the hexyl- and alkyl-chain derivatives of Cu(II)-phenanthroline-oxazine complexes in a *G. mellonella* model also showed that these compounds were well tolerated by the larvae and that all compounds are likely non-toxic to mammalian models at the studied concentrations [56]. When left at 37°C for a further 2 weeks, all *G. mellonella* larvae developed into adult moths, demonstrating that the injected compounds did not disrupt their life cycle [56]. The high tolerability of these Cu(II) antibacterial complexes in *in vivo* larvae models suggests that they hold promise for safe systemic administration, although further research is required in more advanced models to determine their safety for use in humans.

3.2 SILVER

Silver is one of the most well-known metals for its antibacterial properties. There are many historical accounts of using the antimicrobial properties of silver prior to the introduction of antibiotics in the 1940s [5, 31, 74] and the metal and its complexes currently have many applications for these properties [5, 74–78]. For example, silver sulfadiazine is a broad-spectrum topical antibiotic currently approved by the Food and Drug Administration (FDA) to treat burn wounds [76, 77].

3.2.1 Silver Antibacterial Mode of Action

Silver is inert in its metallic form, but in an aqueous environment releases small amounts of ions with antibacterial activity [74]. Silver interacts rapidly with the sulfhydryl groups on the surface of microorganisms, replacing the hydrogen atoms and forming an S-Ag bond. This interaction completely blocks respiration and electron transfer, damaging vital cellular mechanisms [79]. This activity also collapses the proton motive force within cells, de-energising the membrane and causing cell death [80]. Disruption of the cell membrane allows silver ions to enter the cytoplasm, where they target bacterial nucleic acids, proteins, and membranes and can produce ROS [79, 81–83]. This strong, multifaceted antibacterial activity demonstrates promise for the development of silver-based antibacterial compounds.

3.2.2 Silver-Based Antibacterial Compounds

Currently only topical silver-based antimicrobials, such as silver sulfadiazine, are on the market [76, 77]. However, a range of silver-based antibiotic agents that demonstrate promising antimicrobial activity against resistant strains of bacteria are currently in development. For instance, recent work has shown how silver-impregnated glutaraldehyde hydrogels, which can be used in place of sutures to seal wounds, display strong activity against MRSA [84], offering a possibility of controlling wound infection.

N-heterocyclic carbene (NHC) complexes of Ag(I) are strong nucleophiles that bind metals with high stability, leading to increased bioavailability of the metal in physiological conditions. These compounds demonstrate both antibacterial activity [76] and clinical level antifungal activity [85]. One of the most promising NHC-Ag(I) complexes investigated is 1,3-dibenzyl-4,5-diphenyl-imidazol-2-ylidene Ag(I) acetate (SBC3) (Figure 3) [86]. SBC3 demonstrates effective MIC values against several bacterial strains including MRSA [87], and shows antibacterial activity against MRSA growth in *in vivo* studies in *G. mellonella* larvae, without any stimulation of the immune response [88].

Other NHC-Ag complexes are currently in development with differing antibiotic potential and targets depending on their structure. NHC*-Ag(I) benzoate complexes (4) to (7) (Figure 3) show activity against both MRSA and *E. coli* comparable to that of SBC3 [85]. Although lower than the tetracycline and ciprofloxacin antibiotic controls, their observed antibacterial activity is high enough to warrant further research into their use as antibacterial agents.

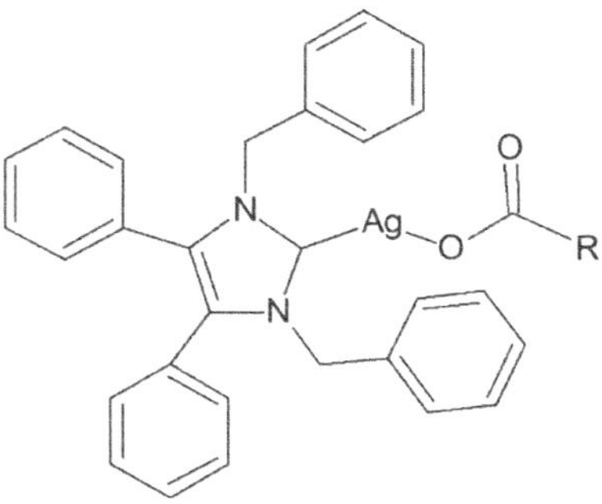

Novel Metal-Based Drugs for Treating Drug-Resistant Bacteria

(3) R = CH$_3$
(4) R = Ph
(5) R = (CH)$_2$F(CH)$_4$
(6) R = (CH)$_3$F(CH)$_3$
(7) R = (CH)$_4$F(CH)$_2$
(8) R = CF$_3$

FIGURE 3 Molecular structures of silver-based compounds. **(3)** is SBC3 and **(4–8)** are other NHC-Ag(I) complexes.

NHC*-Ag carboxylate derivatives of SBC3 have recently been synthesised and tested, leading to the identification of compound **(8)** (Figure 3). Compound **(8)** has been changed structurally to include a more lipophilic trifluoroacetate group, and shows increased efficacy compared to SBC3 at clearing both MRSA and *C. parapsilosis* biofilms *in vitro* as well as *in vivo* efficacy in a murine thigh infection model [89]. These data suggest that structural modifications of this compound class to target key virulence factors in resistant pathogens has the potential to improve their efficacy against antibiotic-resistant pathogens.

3.2.3 Safety and Toxicology of Silver-Based Antibacterial Compounds

Low doses of silver ions can be effectively removed from the body and do not have significant adverse effects, whereas acute or chronic overexposure to silver has an increased risk of toxicity. Silver ions can be absorbed into the body and enter the systemic circulation as a protein complex that is eliminated by the liver and kidneys [90]. Cases of clinical exposure to silver ions through ingestion, inhalation, dermal application, or haematogenous or urological entry show low toxicity with minimal risk [90]. However, symptoms of acute overexposure to silver ions can include hypotension, diarrhoea, bradypnea, and stomach irritation. Chronic silver ingestion or inhalation through common clinical silver preparations, such as silver nitrate or colloidal silver, can cause deposits of silver metal or silver sulphide in the eye (argyosis), skin (argyria), or other organs. Although not life threatening, these silver deposits are cosmetically undesirable [90]. Furthermore, soluble silver compounds have greater potential for adverse effects due to their increased bioavailability [91]. Although these possible toxicities may limit the use of silver-based antibacterial complexes, there is decade-long experience and information in the application of colloidal silver providing a wealth of toxicologically relevant data with few reported adverse effects [75–77].

Preclinical studies investigating the toxicity of SBC3 *in vivo* in *G. mellonella* larvae demonstrate low toxicity at effective antimicrobial concentrations with no indications of acute toxicity [88]. Although further research is required in more advanced animal models, this study shows that SBC3 may be safe for use as an antibacterial agent. *In vivo* assessment of the antibacterial activity of SBC3 and its derivative compound **(8)** at lower doses demonstrate inhibition of MRSA proliferation with minimal toxicity in a murine thigh infection model [89]. The high antibacterial activity demonstrated by these NHC*-Ag(I) complexes makes them promising antibiotic candidates for additional research to understand their safety and efficacy in the systemic or topical treatment of antibiotic-resistant bacteria.

3.3 GOLD

Gold complexes also have a long history in medical and antimicrobial applications including the use of sodium tetrachloroaurate ($Na[AuCl_4]$) for the treatment of syphilis, and potassium dicyanidooaurate(I) ($K[Au(CN)_2]$) against *Mycobacterium tuberculosis*, both used in the 19th century [92]. Since the discovery of conventional antibiotics such as penicillin, there have not been significant advances in exploiting gold as an antibacterial agent. Furthermore, use of gold is limited by its high cost relative to other metals. Notably, several gold-based drugs that demonstrate antimicrobial activity are currently in clinical use for other purposes, providing several ideal candidates for repurposing as antibacterial agents [93].

3.3.1 Gold Antibacterial Mode of Action

Several identified molecular targets of gold-based drugs may help to confer its antimicrobial activity, although their exact antibacterial mode of action is not fully understood [94]. The Au(I) and Au(III) ions are particularly attractive for biological and medicinal applications due to their stability and biological activity [94, 95]. Mitochondrial oxidative phosphorylation pathways are likely important intracellular targets of Au(I) and Au(III) ions [96]. They inhibit thioredoxin reductases (TrxR), enzymes required for the reduction and activation of thioredoxin to form reduced disulphide bonds [97]. Thioredoxin is involved in numerous other essential cellular functions, such as DNA replication and responses to oxidative stress [98, 99]. As many Gram-positive pathogenic bacteria, such as *S. aureus*, lack sufficient levels of glutathione, their metabolism is highly dependent on the activity of TrxR [100]. As a result, strong inhibition of TrxR by Au-based compounds is likely to have bactericidal effects. Long exploited for their anticancer and other therapeutic effects, recent literature investigating the antimicrobial potential of Au(I) and Au(III) complexes has demonstrated their potential for use as novel antibiotics as well.

3.3.2 Gold-Based Antibacterial Compounds

Auranofin is an Au(I)-phosphine derivative that targets and disrupts TrxR, leading to cellular oxidative stress and intrinsic apoptosis in bacterial cells [101] (Figure 4). Approved for the treatment of rheumatoid arthritis in the 1980s, this drug has a long history of medical use and a well-characterised toxicity profile, making it an ideal candidate for repurposing as an antibacterial agent [93].

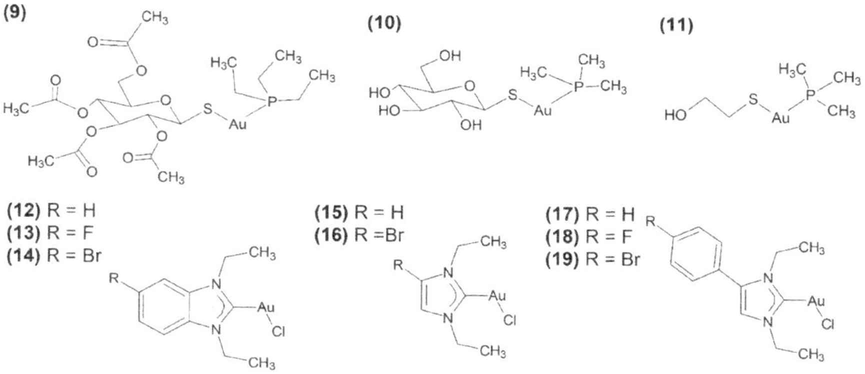

Novel Metal-Based Drugs for Treating Drug-Resistant Bacteria

FIGURE 4 Molecular structures of gold-based compounds. **(9)** is Auranofin, **(10–11)** are auranofin analogues, and **(12–19)** are NHC-Au(I) complexes.

Auranofin has shown antibacterial activity against drug-resistant Gram-positive bacteria, including *S. aureus*, MRSA, *Enterococcus faecium*, and *Enterococcus faecalis*, as well as *M. tuberculosis* [100]. Auranofin has also demonstrated effective antibacterial activity leading to increased survival in a murine systemic MRSA infection model [102]. As it can suppress bacterial protein synthesis, auranofin significantly reduces toxin production by MRSA [102]. Topical administration has also shown superior antimicrobial activity compared to the topical antimicrobials fusidic acid and mupirocin [103]. A lack of observed antibacterial activity of auranofin against Gram-negative bacteria is likely due to the outer membrane of these bacteria creating a barrier [102].

Auranofin has also demonstrated potent anti-biofilm activity and synergistic antibacterial effects against *S. aureus* and MRSA with linezolid, fosfomycin, and chloramphenicol both *in vitro* and *in vivo* [104]. This compound also shows significant disruption against established *S. aureus* and *Staphylococcus epidermidis* biofilms, which is more effective than that of the traditional antimicrobials linezolid and vancomycin [103]. Furthermore, a recent study found no detectable resistance in an *S. aureus* strain following 25 days of auranofin exposure [105]. These properties reduce the likelihood of the development of bacterial resistance against auranofin.

To improve the efficacy and therapeutic index of auranofin, analogues have been developed and tested against both Gram-positive and -negative bacteria [106]. Two analogues in particular, compounds **(10)** and **(11)** (Figure 4), demonstrate broad-spectrum activity against both strains of bacteria and up to 65-fold higher bactericidal activities compared to auranofin [106]. This activity, combined with the extensive clinical history of its use, provides a strong foundation for the use of auranofin and its analogues as antibacterial agents.

Although research into gold-based compounds primarily focuses on those with phosphine ligands, such as auranofin, interest is rising in novel ligands for Au-based antibiotic candidates. An example are the NHC ligands, which have more stable and versatile steric, electronic, and physical properties with thermodynamically stronger bonds to the metal in comparison to phosphine ligands [107]. The antibacterial modes of action of these drugs are similar to that of gold ions, although they may differ slightly depending on the oxidation state of the metal and the nature of the NHC ligand. Targets of NHC-Au drugs include TrxR enzymes, the zinc-finger enzyme PARP-1, mitochondrial respiration, and G-quadruplexes to provide antimicrobial activity [108–111].

Several NHC-Au(I) complexes (12) to (19) and their Au(III) analogues (Figure 4) demonstrate effective inhibition of bacterial TrxR and highly effective antibacterial activity against the Gram-positive bacteria *E. faecium* and MRSA, although their activity was found to be lower than that of auranofin [110, 111]. Many of the tested compounds were more effective at treating the bacteria compared to conventional antibiotic controls, with lower MIC values [111]. Similar to studies with auranofin, all NHC-Au(I) complexes demonstrated low activity against the Gram-negative bacteria *Acinetobacter baumannii*, *E. cloacae*, *E. coli*, *Klebsiella pneumoniae*, and *Pseudomonas aeruginosa* [110, 111]. The Au(I) and Au(III) analogues were comparable in most assays [110, 111]. Further research is required to determine the efficacy of NHC-Au(I) complexes with different structures both *in vitro* and *in vivo* to greater understand their antibacterial potential.

3.3.3 Safety and Toxicology of Gold-Based Antibacterial Compounds

Given auranofin's long history of medical use and known safety profile, it is an attractive drug candidate for repurposing as an antimicrobial [112]. Auranofin is considered safe for systemic administration [100], with no cumulative toxicity observed with long-term use as an antirheumatic drug [113]. A clinical trial investigating short-term auranofin use as an antiparasitic agent observed that it is generally well tolerated in healthy subject populations [114]. As auranofin is currently approved as an antirheumatic drug, its approval for antibacterial use could be accelerated.

Little research has been conducted to date on the toxicity of NHC-Au(I) complexes or auranofin analogues on mammalian cells and *in vivo*. This lack of research is a limitation as these compounds will take longer to progress to the clinic as antibacterial agents for either systemic or topical use.

3.4 Gallium

The antimicrobial properties of gallium compounds were identified almost a century ago for the treatment of syphilis and trypanosomiasis [115], but they have not been considered as antimicrobial agents until recently. However, gallium-based radiopharmaceuticals and gallium-based anticancer drugs have been used clinically for over three decades [116, 117].

3.4.1 Gallium Antibacterial Mode of Action

Both bacteria and humans require iron for essential physiological processes including the metabolic processes associated with respiration, redox homeostasis, DNA synthesis and repair, and transcription [118]. Although iron is sequestered by the host to protect against infection [119], some pathogenic bacteria can still

Novel Metal-Based Drugs for Treating Drug-Resistant Bacteria

acquire iron through the use of siderophores. Siderophores possess a high binding affinity for Fe(III) and binding can vary significantly, often being unique to each bacterial species [120]. Interestingly, bacterial iron uptake systems cannot differentiate between Fe(III) and Ga(III) [121].

Galium(III) ions can replace Fe(III) ions in key chemical reactions required for bacterial cell survival, ultimately killing the bacteria [121]. Unlike Fe(III), Ga(III) is redox inert and cannot be reduced to Ga(II) by bacterial ferric reductases [122]. As a result, Ga(III) ions cannot be incorporated into iron-dependent enzymes. These enzymes are essential for survival of the bacterium and their inhibition through Ga(III) uptake has potent antibacterial activity [123–125]. Galium(III) is commonly delivered as a salt, such as gallium nitrate ($Ga(NO_3)_3$), or as complexes like gallium maltolate and gallium citrate (Figure 5) [124–126].

3.4.2 Gallium-Based Antibacterial Compounds

The $Ga(NO_3)_3$ salt demonstrates promise in the treatment of pathogenic drug-resistant bacteria. As a result of its success and observed safety in preclinical studies [124–126], clinical trials have investigated its antimicrobial activity for various applications including the treatment of cystic fibrosis (CF) patients who commonly experience antibiotic-resistant bacterial infections [127]. A phase Ib non-randomised clinical trial of CF patients with chronic *P. aeruginosa* infections observed that micromolar concentrations of $Ga(NO_3)_3$ added to patient sputum samples inhibited bacterial growth and increased its sensitivity to oxidants [125]. Systemic $Ga(NO_3)_3$ treatment also improved lung function [125]. A phase II multicentre, randomised, placebo-controlled study observed that intravenous $Ga(NO_3)_3$ treatment in patients with CF and chronic *P. aeruginosa* infections decreased sputum *P. aeruginosa* density compared to the control group [NCT02354859]. As an alternative mode of delivery, a phase I/IIa randomised, double-blind, multicentre study tested the antibacterial activity of an inhaled formulation of gallium citrate (AR-501) both alone and in combination with other conventional antibiotics (Figure 5) [NCT03669614]. Preliminary data from this study show efficacy against Gram-positive, Gram-negative, and several species of mycobacterial clinical isolates [128]. The ability of gallium compounds to effectively control clinically relevant ESKAPE pathogens that are highly prone

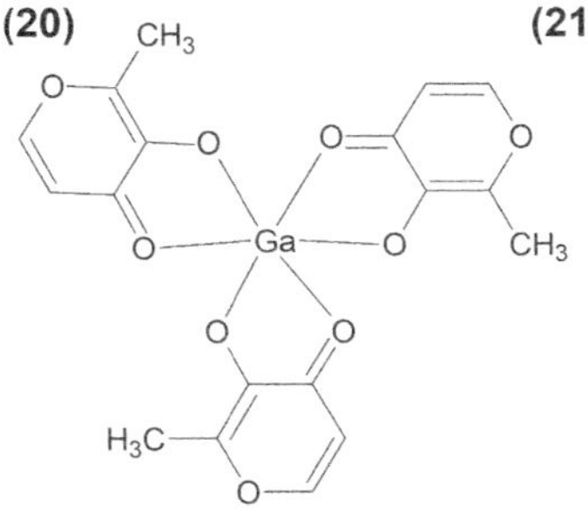

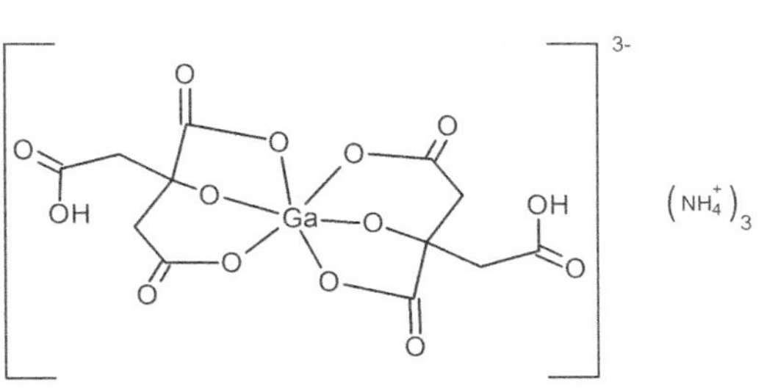

FIGURE 5 Molecular structures of gallium-based compounds. (**20**) is Gallium maltolate and (**21**) is gallium citrate.

to resistance make $Ga(NO_3)_3$ a promising candidate for treatment of antibiotic-resistant bacterial infections [123, 124].

Phase I/IIa clinical trial data also show that patients administered $Ga(NO_3)_3$ salt treatment have a lower propensity to develop resistance than the conventional antibiotics tested [128]. Other studies have shown that spontaneous resistance to $Ga(NO_3)_3$ is comparable to that of successful anti-*Pseudomonal* antibiotics [125] and appears to not quickly lead to resistance [129]. These data indicate that this treatment may be particularly effective against bacteria with high propensities to develop resistance.

Gallium-based drugs are especially effective against biofilm-living bacteria, which are more resistant to antibiotics and often cause chronic infections [130, 131]. Several Ga(III) compounds strongly inhibit *P. aeruginosa* biofilm formation at sub-micron concentrations, and kill bacterial cells deeply embedded in the biofilm matrix at higher concentrations [124, 132]. Most antibiotic activity is lost deep within the biofilm matrix and *P. aeruginosa* biofilms are relatively difficult to eradicate by using antibiotics [131, 133]. The unique and potent anti-biofilm activity of gallium-based drugs may be a significant advantage in the treatment of biofilm-producing bacteria that are resistant to conventional antibiotics. Indeed, administration of a gallium porphyrin complex and $Ga(NO_3)_3$ followed by relatively low concentrations of vancomycin effectively eliminated mature MRSA biofilms and eradicated biofilm-enclosed bacteria within 1 week. This treatment was found to work by reducing the antibiotic tolerance of the mature biofilms [134]. This anti-biofilm activity is an advantage for gallium-based drugs as they may have greater efficacy against infections caused by *P. aeruginosa* or other biofilm-producing bacteria that are resistant to conventional antibiotics.

3.4.3 Safety and Toxicology of Gallium-Based Antibacterial Drugs

Gallium nitrate has been used medically for other applications and is currently in clinical trials as an antibacterial agent [135, 136]. Therefore, extensive data exist on its safety for both local and systemic administration. No adverse effects were observed upon systemic $Ga(NO_3)_3$ treatment in patients with CF. In addition, kidney function, blood counts, sputum levels, and electrolyte levels all appeared unaffected, leading to the conclusion that $Ga(NO_3)_3$ appears safe for systemic use [125]. Gallium nitrate is the active component in Ganite®, a bone resorption inhibitor, approved by the FDA, for the treatment of hypercalcaemia in cancer patients. As Ganite®, gallium demonstrates a potent, site-specific effect, concentrating in inflamed tissues, macrophages, neutrophils, and bacteria [135, 136].

3.5 TELLURIUM

Prior to the discovery of antibiotics, tellurium complexes were also used in the treatment of microbial infections [137]. For instance, a Te-glucose complex was once used as a treatment for syphilis in humans. Furthermore, diseases such as leprosy and TB were treated with tellurium compounds [138]. With the rise in antibiotic resistance and reduced efficacy of conventional antibiotics, tellurium has recently gained interest for its antibacterial properties.

Novel Metal-Based Drugs for Treating Drug-Resistant Bacteria 181

3.5.1 Tellurium Antibacterial Mode of Action

The relationship between the biological properties of tellurium and its method of antibacterial activity is poorly understood. Some bacteria and fungi are known to take up Te(IV) ions as if they are amino acids and replace the sulphur atom to form telluro-cysteine and telluro-methionine amino acid complexes [139]. Depending on the oxidation state of tellurium, its biological activity may vary.

An oxidation state of +4 is the most stable form of tellurium with interesting biological applications. Complexes of Te(IV) and organotellurium compounds demonstrated stability in aqueous solution with potential roles in protease inhibition and integrin inactivation [140–143]. As proteases and integrins play a key role in bacterial pathogenicity [144], their inhibition may have antibacterial effects. Specifically, bacterial integrins have a key role in bacterial adhesion, migration, and mediation of metalloproteinase secretion. These functions are also important for the development of antibiotic resistance mechanisms, and their inhibition may prevent the development of resistance in addition to antibacterial effects.

3.5.2 Tellurium-Based Antibacterial Compounds

The antibacterial activity of Te(IV) species, including both nanoparticles and metal-based complexes, has been demonstrated against a variety of bacteria, including *E. coli*, *E. cloacae*, and *P. aeruginosa* [145, 146]. Ammonium trichloro(dioxoethylene-O,O')tellurate (AS-101) (Figure 6) is a tellurium-based compound developed by Albeck and colleagues that has been considered for several protective therapeutic applications due to its effective inhibition of cysteine protease [140–143]. *In vivo* preclinical and clinical studies have since been conducted using AS-101 against a variety of diseases, such as human papillomavirus, human immunodeficiency virus, and acute myeloid leukaemia [78]. AS-101 may also have antibacterial activity, leading to its investigation as a potential metal-based antibiotic.

The AS-101 complex exhibits a positive effect on the immune system as well as strong antibacterial activity [146]. This complex can stimulate the production of lymphokines that regulate lymphopoiesis and myelopoiesis to increase the proliferation of lymphoid cells and augment the patient's immune response against pathogens [147]. Moreover, it has exhibited strong antibacterial activity against the Gram-negative bacterium *E. cloacae* (MIC = 9.4 µg mL^{-1}) [146]. The immune-modulating and antibacterial activity of AS-101 makes it a promising candidate as a metal-based antibiotic. However, AS-101 is not stable in physiological conditions and undergoes hydrolysis where the

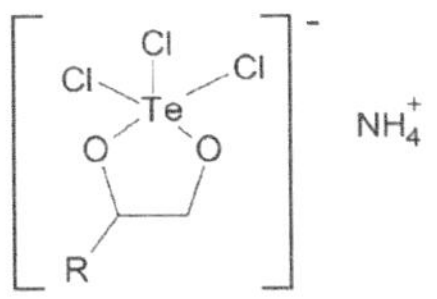

(22) R = H (AS-101)   **(26)** R = CH$_2$CH$_2$CH$_2$CH$_3$

(23) R = CH$_3$ **(27)** R = CH$_2$CH$_2$CH$_2$CH$_2$CH$_2$CH$_3$

(24) R = CH$_2$CH$_3$ **(28)** R = CH$_2$Cl

(25) R = CH$_2$CH$_2$CH$_3$ **(29)** R = Ph

FIGURE 6 Molecular structures of tellurium-based compounds. **(22)** is AS-101 and **(23–29)** are analogues.

diol ligand is displaced by the formation of $NH_4[Te(IV)OCl_3]$, which is likely the bioactive species involved in its antibacterial and immune-modulating properties [148, 149]. This instability may reduce the efficacy of AS-101 in physiological conditions.

In an attempt to overcome this limitation, D'Arcy *et al.* designed, synthesised, and characterised a series of AS-101 analogues with different ligands to evaluate their stability in an aqueous environment (Figure 6). Unlike AS-101, some analogues were considered stable enough to perform biological studies in physiological conditions. The study demonstrated a direct relationship between complex stability and the diol alkyl chain, where increased chain length corresponded to increased stability [150]. The antimicrobial activity of each compound was also evaluated *in vitro* in *E. coli*, *S. aureus*, MRSA, and *P. aeruginosa*. In *E. coli*, the MIC_{50} values ranged from 15 to $20\,\mu M$ and the compounds were less active or inactive against the other bacteria. The similar antibacterial activity between the complexes may be because the compounds act as prodrugs, releasing the bioactive hydrolysed product $NH_4[Cl_3OTe]$ [148–150]. Although the AS-101 analogues showed lower antibacterial activity compared to other metal-based antibacterial compounds, the observation of the relationship between ligand length and stability in physiological conditions provides insight for the development of other potential Te(IV)-based antibacterial complexes.

3.5.3 Safety and Toxicology of Tellurium-Based Antibacterial Compounds

The AS-101 compound has undergone multiple clinical trials for its systemic toxicity. These include a phase II/III clinical trials for the prevention of chemotherapy-induced bone marrow toxicity [151], a phase I clinical trial for patients with AIDS-related complex [NCT00001006], and phase I/II clinical trials for topical treatment of genital warts [NCT01555112] [78]. If AS-101 is approved as a systemic treatment for other applications, gaining approval for its use as an antibacterial agent may be more efficient.

3.6 ZINC CHELATORS

Although they do not contain metals, zinc chelators directly interact with zinc to re-sensitise some bacteria resistant to β-lactam antibiotics. A key method of antibiotic resistance in both Gram-positive and -negative bacteria is the production of metallo-β-lactamases (MBL) which prevent the activity of β-lactam antibiotics with the exception of monobactams [152]. Due to the frequent co-presence of other resistance mechanisms, bacteria with acquired MBL production are often also resistant to aminoglycosides, sulfonamides, and fluoroquinolones [153]. Zinc chelators used in combination with β-lactams can inhibit MBLs, re-sensitising MBL-producing bacteria to β-lactam antibiotics. The increasing prevalence of MBL-producing bacteria has raised interest into the use of zinc chelators to prevent the activity of MBLs and re-sensitise the bacteria to β-lactam antibiotics [154, 155].

3.6.1 Zinc Chelators Combined with β-Lactams
Antibacterial Mode of Action

β-lactam antibiotics are the most broadly used antibiotics worldwide [156, 157] and exhibit their antibacterial functions by acylating a serine active site in penicillin-binding proteins (PBP) [158]. These PBP enzymes are essential in the final stages of cell wall biosynthesis, by mediating the cross-linking of peptide chains to form peptidoglycan. The change induced in the PBPs by β-lactams prevents proper cell wall biosynthesis, resulting in cell death [159]. Resistance to β-lactams has increased through several different mechanisms, including the production of β-lactamases, particularly in Gram-negative bacteria [160]. These enzymes catalyse the hydrolysis of the amide bond in the β-lactam ring to render the drugs ineffective. β-lactamases are classified into two broad divisions based on the method by which they hydrolyse their substrate. Hydrolysis can occur either by forming an acyl enzyme with an active-site serine or through a hydrolytic reaction facilitated by essential zinc ions that exist in the active sites of MBLs [160]. Zinc chelators remove zinc ions required for the biological activity of MBL enzymes through competitive binding, depriving the MBLs of their anti-β-lactam activity [161]. As a result, recent literature has investigated the antibacterial activity of zinc chelators used in combination with β-lactams against MBL-producing bacteria.

3.6.2 Zinc Chelator-Based Antibacterial Compounds

A study conducted by Principe *et al.* evaluated the efficacy of six zinc chelators (Figure 7) in restoring meropenem activity against MBL-producing Gram-negative bacteria [162]. These bacteria included New Delhi MBL-producing *K. pneumoniae*, *Chryseobacterium indologenes*, *Elizabethkingia meningoseptica*, and *Stenotrophomonas maltophilia* isolates. Two of the six chelators, compounds (**33**) and (**32**) (Figure 7), demonstrated intrinsic antibacterial activity *in vitro*, thus warranting further *in vivo* studies [162].

The *in vivo* antibacterial activity of (**33**) and (**32**), combined with meropenem, was evaluated in infected *G. mellonella* larvae and compared to the activity of meropenem alone. *G. mellonella* larvae infected with *K. pneumoniae* and treated with meropenem alone had a 10% survival rate, whereas meropenem combined with either (**33**) or (**32**) had a 66% survival rate 48 h post-infection. The use of these chelators in combination with meropenem also increased the survival of *G. mellonella* larvae infected with *E. meningoseptica* and *S. maltophilia* [162]. Therefore, the combination of (**33**) or (**32**) with meropenem may be an effective antibacterial therapy against MBL-producing bacteria. These data suggest that zinc chelators may be effective as carbapenem adjuvants to increase the antibacterial efficacy of β-lactam antibiotics in clearing sustained MBL-producing bacterial infections.

3.6.3 Safety and Toxicology of Zinc Chelators Combined with β-Lactams

Of the zinc chelators listed above (Figure 7), many are currently in use for other applications, which provides extensive knowledge on the toxicities associated

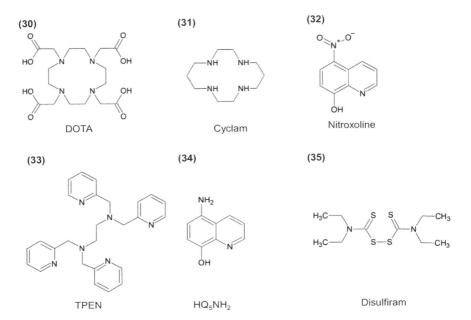

FIGURE 7 Molecular structures of the zinc chelators. The six zinc chelators include (**30**) 1,4,7,10-tetraazacyclododecane-1,4,7-tetraacetic acid (DOTA), (**31**) 1,4,8,11-tetraazacyclotradecane (cyclam), (**32**) HQ₅NO₂ (5-nitro-8-hydroxyquinoline, nitroxoline), (**33**) *N,N,N′,N′*-tetrakis(2-pyridinylmethyl)-1,2-ethanediamine (TPEN), (**34**) 5-amino-8-hydroxyquinoline (HQ₅NH₂), and (**35**) disulfiram.

with their systemic use. These include applications as anticancer agents, contrast agents, the treatment of UTIs, and in chelation therapy for the removal of toxic metals from the body [163–166].

Inoculation of *G. mellonella* larvae with compounds (**30**) to (**35**) did not reduce survival over 72 hours and did not cause any observed melanisation of the cuticle. As melanisation can indicate stress or activation of the host immune response, a lack of melanisation indicates that the compounds did not have this effect. After 2 weeks, some larvae formed pupae, indicating that the compounds had no adverse effect on larval development and supporting the hypothesis that they could be used to treat bacterial infections in humans [162].

Overall, zinc chelators provide great promise when used in combination with β-lactams for the re-sensitisation of MBL-producing bacteria. Nitroxoline (**32**) demonstrates promise, as it effectively inhibited all bacterial strains in the study conducted by Principe *et al.* and is considered safe for systemic administration [162]. As the zinc chelators described are used clinically for other forms of treatment, the process of repurposing these as antibacterial agents and garnering their approval for human clinical use may be more efficient.

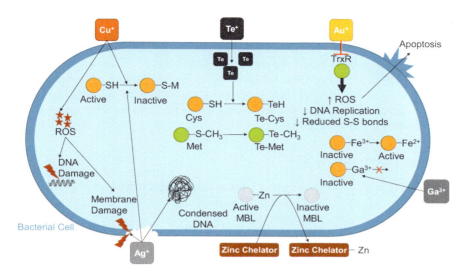

FIGURE 8 Mode of antibacterial activity of selected metals. M=metal. Silver releases ions which can target bacterial membranes, increasing permeability. Disruption of the cell membrane allows silver ions to enter the cytoplasm where they can interact with the sulfhydryl groups within cysteine residues on enzymes, inhibiting enzymatic activity. Silver can also bind to and condense DNA, preventing replication and increasing susceptibility to mutations. Ga(III) is an iron mimetic, incorporating itself into iron-dependent bacterial enzymes. Ga(III) cannot be reduced to Ga(II), inhibiting enzymatic activity. Gold inhibits TrxR and its reducing activity, promoting ROS formation and reducing DNA replication and disulphide bond formation. Tellurium ions are taken up as amino acids and replace the sulphur atom to form telluro-cysteine and telluro-methionine. Copper promotes the production of ROS, which can cause bacterial DNA and membrane damage. Zinc chelators remove the zinc ions required for the biological activity of MBL enzymes through competitive binding.

4 GENERAL CONCLUSION

Antimicrobial drug resistance is one of the most significant issues facing our global society and will lead to large-scale loss of life by mid-century if not addressed. It is predicted that by 2050, most conventional antibiotics will no longer be clinically effective due to the widespread presence of antibiotic resistance in bacteria [2]. Bacteria rapidly exchange DNA encoding resistance genes with related and unrelated bacteria and as a result, the development of resistance in one population rapidly leads to the dispersal of resistance genes into other bacterial species with consequent implications for the treatment of infected patients [4].

Although their antimicrobial properties have been well known for many years, there has recently been a reawakening of interest in the use of metal-based compounds as novel antimicrobial agents for the treatment of drug-resistant bacterial infections. Their ability to provide novel and distinct modes of action to the conventional antibiotics with a lower propensity for the development of resistance make metal-containing compounds a promising candidate for the treatment of infections either alone, or in combination with existing antibiotics (Figure 8). The combination of metal-based and conventional antibiotics can cause a "double hit" to the bacterial cell and allow for lower doses of the antibiotic for a therapeutic effect. As a result, despite their long, and often unappreciated, history, metal-based antibacterial compounds may have a bright future in the fight against drug-resistant bacterial pathogens.

ABBREVIATIONS

AIDS	acquired immunodeficiency syndrome
CDC	Centre for Disease Control
CA	community acquired
CF	cystic fibrosis
CipA	ciprofloxacin
DIBI	3-hydroxypyridin-4-one
DOTA	1,4,7,10-tetraazacyclododecane-1,4,7-tetraacetic acid
ESKAPE pathogens	*Enterococcus faecium, Staphylococcus aureus, Klebsiella pneumoniae, Acinetobacter baumannii, Pseudomonas aeruginosa,* and *Enterobacter* pathogens
FDA	Food and Drug Administration
HA	healthcare acquired
IC	Inhibitory Concentration
MBL	metallo-β lactamase
MIC	minimum inhibitory concentration
MRSA	methicillin-resistant *Staphylococcus aureus*
NHC	*N*-heterocyclic carbene
PBP	penicillin-binding protein
PBP2a	penicillin-binding protein 2a
PVL	Panton-Valentine ieukocidin toxin
PSM	phenol soluble modulin
SCCmec	staphylococcal cassette chromosome *mec*
SBC3	1,3-dibenzyl-4,5-diphenyl-imidazol-2-ylidene Ag(I) acetate
TPEN	*N,N,N',N'*-tetrakis(2-pyridymethylethylenediamine)
TrxR	thioredoxin reductase
TSST-1	toxic shock syndrome toxin-1
SSSS	staphylococcal scalded skin syndrome
TB	tuberculosis
ROS	reactive oxygen species

REFERENCES

[1] ECDPC, in *Surveillance of Antimicrobial Resistance in Europe 2018*, European Centre for Disease Prevention and Control, Stockholm, **2019**.

[2] WHO, in *Antimicrobial Resistance: Global Report on Surveillance*, WHO, **2014**.

[3] R. Aminov, *Front. Microbiol.* **2010**, *1*. https://doi.org/10.3389/fmicb.2010.00134

[4] J. M. A. Blair, M. A. Webber, A. J. Baylay, D. O. Ogbolu, L. J. V. Piddock, *Nat. Rev. Microbiol.* **2015**, *13*, 42–51.

[5] J. W. Alexander, *Surg. Infect.* **2009**, *10*, 289–292.

[6] F. C. Tenover, *Am. J. Infect. Control* **2006**, *34*, S3–S10.

[7] CDC, **2019**. Centers for Disease Control and Prevention (U.S.), National Center for Emerging Zoonotic and Infectious Diseases (U.S.), Division of Healthcare Quality Promotion and Antibiotic Resistance Coordination and Strategy Unit in *Antibiotic resistance threats in the United States, 2019*, Atlanta, GA, **2019**. https://stacks.cdc.gov/view/cdc/82532

[8] T. Sato, K. Yamawaki, *Clin. Infect. Dis.* **2019**, *69*, S538–S543.

[9] PEW Trusts, in *Antibiotics Currently in Global Clinical Development*, Vol. **2021**. https://www.pewtrusts.org/en/research-and-analysis/data-visualizations/2014/antibiotics-currently-in-clinical-development

[10] H. F. L. Wertheim, D. C. Melles, M. C. Vos, W. van Leeuwen, A. van Belkum, H. A. Verbrugh, J. L. Nouwen, *Lancet Infect. Dis.* **2005**, *5*, 751–762.

[11] S. Lakhundi, K. Zhang, *Clin. Microbiol. Rev.* **2018**, *31*, e00020–00018.

[12] C. Kong, H.-M. Neoh, S. Nathan, *Toxins* **2016**, *8*, 72.

[13] P. Murray, K.Rosenthal, M. Pfaller, *Medical Microbiology, 9th Ed.*, Elsevier Health Sciences, **2021**. https://www.elsevier.com/books/medical-microbiology/murray/978-0-323-67322-8

[14] M. Otto, *Cell. Microbiol.* **2012**, *14*, 1513–1521.

[15] P. M. Schlievert, C. C. Davis, *Clin. Microbiol. Rev.* **2020**, *33*, e00032–00019.

[16] M. P. Jevons, A. W. Coe, M. T. Parker, *The Lancet* **1963**, *281*, 904–907.

[17] C. Gagliotti, L. D. Högberg, H. Billström, T. Eckmanns, C. G. Giske, O. E. Heuer, V. Jarlier, G. Kahlmeter, D. L. F. Wong, J. Monen, *Eurosurveillance* **2021**, *26*, 2002094.

[18] P. D. Stapleton, P. W. Taylor, *Sci. Prog.* **2002**, *85*, 57–72.

[19] J. Fishovitz, J. Hermoso, M. Chang, S. Mobashery, *IUBMB Life* **2014**, *66*, 572–577.

[20] M. Z. David, R. S. Daum, *Clin. Microbiol. Rev.* **2010**, *23*, 616–687.

[21] H. Peng, D. Liu, Y. Ma, W. Gao, *Sci. Rep.* **2018**, *8*, 17916.

[22] M. Z. David, D. Glikman, S. E. Crawford, J. Peng, K. J. King, M. A. Hostetler, S. Boyle-Vavra, R. S. Daum, *J. Infect. Dis.* **2008**, *197*, 1235–1243.

[23] A. Pantosti, M. Venditti, *Eur. Respir. J.* **2009**, *34*, 1190–1196.

[24] N. Tsouklidis, R. Kumar, S. E. Heindl, R. Soni, S. Khan, *Cureus* **2020**, 12(6):e8867. doi: 10.7759/cureus.8867.

[25] A. S. Lee, H. de Lencastre, J. Garau, J. Kluytmans, S. Malhotra-Kumar, A. Peschel, S. Harbarth, *Nat. Rev. Dis. Primers* **2018**, *4*, 18033.

[26] M. Lambert, *Am. Fam. Physician* **2011**, *84*, 455–463.

[27] P. Simpson, N. Desai, I. Casari, M. Massi, M. Falasca, *Future Med. Chem.* **2019**, *11*, 119–135.

[28] G. Gasser, *CHIMIA* **2015**, *7*, 442–446.

[29] A. Evans, K. A. Kavanagh, *J. Med. Microbiol.* **2021**, 70(5):001363. doi: 10.1099/jmm.0.001363.

[30] S. Domingos, V. André, S. Quaresma, I. Martins, M. Minas da Piedade, M. Duarte, *J. Pharm. Pharmacol.* **2015**, *67*, 830–846.

[31] A. Frei, *Antibiotics* **2020**, *9*, 90.

[32] P. Nazari, R. Dowlatabadi-Bazaz, M. Mofid, M. Pourmand, N. Daryani, M. Faramarzi, Z. Sepehrizadeh, A. Shahverdi, *Appl. Biochem. Biotechnol.* **2014**, *172*, 570–579.

[33] F. Chen, J. Moat, D. McFeely, G. Clarkson, I. J. Hands-Portman, J. P. Furner-Pardoe, F. Harrison, C. G. Dowson, P. J. Sadler, *J. Med. Chem.* **2018**, *61*, 7330–7344.

[34] B.-B. Chen, N.-L. Pan, J.-X. Liao, M.-Y. Huang, D.-C. Jiang, J.-J. Wang, H.-J. Qiu, J.-X. Chen, L. Li, J. Sun, *J. Inorg. Biochem.* **2021**, *219*, 111450.

[35] M. Patra, G. Gasser, M. Wenzel, K. Merz, J. E. Bandow, N. Metzler-Nolte, *Organometallics* **2010**, *29*, 4312–4319.

[36] G. Wyszogrodzka, P. Dorożyński, B. Gil, W. J. Roth, M. Strzempek, B. Marszałek, W. P. Węglarz, E. Menaszek, W. Strzempek, P. Kulinowski, *Pharm. Res.* **2018**, *35*, 144.

[37] P. Simpson, C. Nagel, H. Bruhn, U. Schatzschneider, *Organometallics* **2015**, *34*, 3809–3815.

[38] P. McCarron, M. McCann, M. Devereux, K. Kavanagh, C. Skerry, P. Karakousis, A. Aor, T. Mello, A. Santos, D. Campos, F. Pavan, *Front. Microbiol.* **2018**, *9*. https://doi.org/10.3389/fmicb.2018.01432

[39] P. Paul, K. R. N. Bhowmik, S. Roy, D. Deb, N. Das, M. Bhattacharjee, R. N. Dutta Purkayastha, L. Male, V. McKee, R. Pallepogu, D. Maiti, A. Bauza, A. Fontera, A. M. Kirillov, *Polyhedron* **2018**, *151*, 407–416.

[40] P. Kalaivani, R. Prabhakaran, E. Ramachandran, F. Dallemer, G. Paramaguru, R. Renganathan, P. Poornima, V. Padma, K. Natarajan, *Dalton Trans.* **2012**, *41*, 2486–2499.

[41] P. Kalaivani, R. Prabhakaran, F. Dallemer, P. Poornima, E. Vaishnavi, E. Ramachandran, V. Padma, R. Renganathan, K. Natarajan, *Metallomics* **2011**, *4*, 101–113.

[42] A. Frei, S. Ramu, G. Lowe, H. Dinh, L. Semenec, A. Elliott, J. Zuegg, A. Deckers, N. Jung, S. Bräse, A. Cain, M. Blaskovich, *ChemMedChem* **2021**, *16*, 3165–3171.

[43] T. Johnstone, S. Alexander, W. Lin, S. Lippard, *JACS* **2014**, *136*, 116–118.

[44] A. Frei, M. Amado, M. Cooper, M. Blaskovich, *Chemistry* **2020**, *26*, 2852–2858.

[45] M. Fandzloch, A. W. Augustyniak, L. Dobrzańska, T. Jędrzejewski, J. Sitkowski, M. Wypij, P. Golińska, *J. Inorg. Biochem.* **2020**, *210*, 111072.

[46] X. Yang, J. Xu, M. Meng, N. Li, C. Liu, Q. He, *J. Prot.* **2019**, *194*, 160–167.

[47] S. Bu, G. Jiang, G. Jiang, J. Liu, X. Lin, J. Shen, Y. Xiong, X. Duan, J. Wang, X. Liao, *JBIC J. Biol. Inorg. Chem.* **2020**, *25*, 747–757.

[48] G. Borkow, J. Gabbay, *Curr. Chem. Biol.* **2009**, *3*, 272–278.

[49] D. Montero, C. Arellano, M. Pardo, R. Vera, R. Gálvez, M. Cifuentes, M. Berasain, M. Gómez, C. Ramírez, R. Vidal, *Antimicrob. Resist. Infect. Control* **2019**, *8*, 3.

[50] L. Arendsen, R. Thakar, A. Sultan, *Clin. Microbiol. Rev.* **2019**, *32*, e00125–00118.

[51] A. J. Huh, Y. J. Kwon, *JCR* **2011**, *156*, 128–145.

[52] J. A. Drewry, P. T. Gunning, *Coord. Chem. Rev.* **2011**, *255*, 459–472.

[53] J. Imlay, S. Chin, S. Linn, *Science* **1988**, *240*, 640–642.

[54] R. Thurman, C. Gerba, G. Bitton, *Crit. Rev. Environ. Control* **1989**, *18*, 295–315.

[55] N. German, D. Doyscher, C. Rensing, *Future Microbiol.* **2013**, *8*, 1257–1264.

[56] M. Ahmed, S. Ward, M. McCann, K. Kavanagh, F. Heaney, M. Devereux, B. Twamley, D. Rooney, *BioMetals* **2022**, *35*, 173–185.

[57] E. Chalkidou, F. Perdih, I. Turel, D. P. Kessissoglou, G. Psomas, *J. Inorg. Biochem.* **2012**, *113*, 55–65.

[58] L. Ruiz-Ramírez, M. de la Rosa, I. Gracia-Mora, A. Mendoza, G. Pérez, G. Ferrer-Sueta, A. Tovar, M. Breña, P. Gutierrez, M. Cruces Martínez, E. Pimentel, A. Natarajan, *J. Inorg. Biochem.* **1995**, *59*, 207.

[59] D. Brown, W. Smith, J. Teape, A. Lewis, *J. Med. Chem.* **1980**, *23*, 729–734.

Novel Metal-Based Drugs for Treating Drug-Resistant Bacteria 189

[60] V. Uivarosi, *Molecules* **2013**, *18*, 11153–11197.
[61] Z. Ude, K. Kavanagh, B. Twamley, M. Pour, N. Gathergood, A. Kellett, C. Marmion, *Dalton Trans.* **2019**, *48*, 8578–8593.
[62] Z. Ude, N. Flothkötter, G. Sheehan, M. Brennan, K. Kavanagh, C. J. Marmion, *Int. J. Antimicrob. Agents* **2021**, *58*, 106449.
[63] M. Kumar, N. K. Mogha, G. Kumar, F. Hussain, D. T. Masram, *Inorg. Chim. Acta* **2019**, *490*, 144–154.
[64] L. Besaury, J. Bodilis, F. Delgas, S. Andrade, R. De la Iglesia, B. Ouddane, L. Quillet, *Mar. Pollut. Bull.* **2013**, *67*, 16–25.
[65] T. Forman, in *Synergistic Relationship Between Copper and Ribosome-Targeting Antibiotics in Close Relatives of B. subtilis ssp. spizizenii*, Vol. *Biology*, Wesleyan U., Masters Theses, **2019**.
[66] G. Crisponi, V. M. Nurchi, D. Fanni, C. Gerosa, S. Nemolato, G. Faa, *Coord. Chem. Rev.* **2010**, *254*, 876–889.
[67] K. Djoko, C.-L. Ong, M. Walker, A. McEwan, *JBC* **2015**, *290*, 18954–18961.
[68] C. D. Klaassen, *Casarett and Doull's Toxicology: The Basic Science of Poisons*, McGraw-Hill, New York, **2013**.
[69] D. R. Mishell, Jr., in *Intrauterine Devices*, Eds.: T. M. Goodwin, M. N. Montoro, L. I. Muderspach, R. J., Paulson, S. Roy, Blackwell Publishing Ltd Wiley, **2010**, pp. 494–499. https://doi.org/10.1002/9781444323030.ch110.
[70] L. Macomber, J. A. Imlay, *Proc. Natl. Acad. Sci.* **2009**, *106*, 8344–8349.
[71] M. O'Shaughnessy, M. Piatek, P. McCarron, M. McCann, M. Devereux, K. Kavanagh, O. Howe, *Biomedicines* **2022**, *10*, 222.
[72] N. Browne, M. Heelan, K. Kavanagh, *Virulence* **2013**, *4*, 597–603.
[73] C. J.-Y. Tsai, J. M. S. Loh, T. Proft, *Virulence* **2016**, *7*, 214–229.
[74] S. Chernousova, M. Epple, *Angew. Chem., Int. Ed.* **2013**, *52*, 1636–1653.
[75] B. Nowack, H. F. Krug, M. Height, *ES&T* **2011**, *45*, 1177–1183.
[76] M. A. Sierra, L. Casarrubios, M. C. de la Torre, *Eur. J. Chem.* **2019**, *25*, 7232–7242.
[77] Z. Aziz, S. F. Abu, N. J. Chong, *Burns* **2012**, *38*, 307–318.
[78] U.S. National Library of Medicine in *ClinicalTrials.gov*. https://clinicaltrials.gov/
[79] O. Gordon, T. V. Slenters, P. S. Brunetto, A. E. Villaruz, D. E. Sturdevant, M. Otto, R. Landmann, K. M. Fromm, *Antimicrob. Agents Chemother.* **2010**, *54*, 4208–4218.
[80] P. Dibrov, J. Dzioba, K. K. Gosink, C. C. Häse, *Antimicrob. Agents Chemother.* **2002**, *46*, 2668–2670.
[81] J. Morones-Ramirez, J. Winkler, C. Spina, J. Collins, *Sci. Transl. Med.* **2013**, *5*, 190ra181.
[82] H. Wang, A. Yan, Z. Liu, X. Yang, Z. Xu, Y. Wang, R. Wang, M. Koohi-Moghadam, L. Hu, W. Xia, H. Tang, Y. Wang, H. Li, H. Sun, *PLOS Biolo.* **2019**, *17*, e3000292.
[83] H. Wang, M. Wang, X. Yang, X. Xu, Q. Hao, A. Yan, M. Hu, R. Lobinski, H. Li, H. Sun, *Chem. Sci.* **2019**, *10*, 7193–7199.
[84] L. Gallagher, A. Smith, K. Kavanagh, M. Devereux, J. Colleran, C. Breslin, K. G. Richards, M. McCann, A. D. Rooney, *Chemistry* **2021**, *3*, 672–686..
[85] C. O'Beirne, N. F. Alhamad, Q. Ma, H. Müller-Bunz, K. Kavanagh, G. Butler, X. Zhu, M. Tacke, *Inorganica. Chimica. Acta* **2019**, *486*, 294–303.
[86] S. Patil, A. Deally, B. Gleeson, H. Müller-Bunz, F. Paradisi, M. Tacke, *Metallomics* **2011**, *3*, 74–88.
[87] M. A. Sharkey, J. P. Gara, S. V. Gordon, F. Hackenberg, C. Healy, F. Paradisi, S. Patil, B. Schaible, M. Tacke, *Antibiotics* **2012**, *1*, 25–28.
[88] N. Browne, F. Hackenberg, W. Streciwilk, M. Tacke, K. Kavanagh, *BioMetals* **2014**, *27*, 745–752.

[89] C. O'Beirne, M. E. Piatek, J. Fossen, H. Müller-Bunz, D. R. Andes, K. Kavanagh, S. A. Patil, M. Baumann, M. Tacke, *Metallomics* **2021**, *13*. mfaa011, https://doi.org/10.1093/mtomcs/mfaa011

[90] A. Lansdown, *Karger* **2006**, *33*, 17–34.

[91] F. W. Weir, *Am. Ind. Hyg. Assoc. J.* **1979**, *40*, 245–247.

[92] S. P. Pricker, *Gold Bulletin* **1996**, *29*, 53–60.

[93] C. Roder, M. J. Thomson, *Drugs in R&D* **2015**, *15*, 13–20.

[94] B. Bertrand, A. Casini, *Dalton Trans.* **2014**, *43*, 4209–4219.

[95] W. Liu, R. Gust, *Coord. Chem. Rev.* **2016**, *329*, 191–213.

[96] O. Rackham, A. Shearwood, R. Thyer, E. McNamara, S. Davies, B. Callus, A. Miranda-Vizuete, S. Berners-Price, Q. Cheng, E. Arnér, A. Filipovska, *Free Radic. Biol. Med.* **2011**, *50*, 689–699.

[97] A. Bindoli, M. P. Rigobello, G. Scutari, C. Gabbiani, A. Casini, L. Messori, *Coord. Chem. Rev.* **2009**, *253*, 1692–1707.

[98] T. Gustafsson, M. Sahlin, J. Lu, B. Sjöberg, A. Holmgren, *JBC* **2012**, *287*, 39686–39697.

[99] E. R. Rocha, A. O. Tzianabos, C. J. Smith, *J. Bac.* **2007**, *189*, 8015–8023.

[100] M. Harbut, C. Vilchèze, X. Luo, M. Hensler, H. Guo, B. Yang, A. Chatterjee, V. Nizet, W. Jacobs, P. Schultz, F. Wang, *Proc. Natl. Acad. Sci.* **2015**, *112*, 4453–4458.

[101] J. Madeira, D. Gibson, W. Kean, A. Klegeris, *Inflammopharmacology* **2012**, *20*, 297–306.

[102] S. Thangamani, H. Mohammad, M. Abushahba, T. Sobreira, V. Hedrick, L. Paul, M. Seleem, *Sci. Rep.* **2016**, *6*, 22571.

[103] S. Thangamani, H. Mohammad, M. Abushahba, T. Sobreira, M. Seleem, *Int. J. Antimicrob. Agents* **2016**, *47*, 195–201.

[104] P. She, L. Zhou, S. Li, Y. Liu, L. Xu, L. Chen, Z. Luo, Y. Wu, *Front. Microbiol.* **2019**, *10*. https://doi.org/10.3389/fmicb.2019.02453

[105] N. Tharmalingam, N. Ribeiro, D. D. Silva, M. Naik, L. Cruz, W. Kim, S. Shen, J. D. Santos, K. Ezikovich, E. D'Agata, E. Mylonakis, B. Fuchs, *Future Med. Chem.* **2019**, *11*, 1417–1425.

[106] B. Wu, X. Yang, M. Yan, *J. Med. Chem.* **2019**, *62*, 7751–7768.

[107] M. N. Hopkinson, C. Richter, M. Schedler, F. Glorius, *Nature* **2014**, *510*, 485–496.

[108] P. Holenya, S. Can, R. Rubbiani, H. Alborzinia, A. Jünger, X. Cheng, I. Ott, S. Wölfl, *Metallomics* **2014**, *6*, 1591–1601.

[109] M. Baker, P. Barnard, S. Berners-Price, S. Brayshaw, J. Hickey, B. Skelton, A. White, *Dalton Trans.* **2006**, 3708–3715.

[110] C. Schmidt, B. Karge, R. Misgeld, A. Prokop, R. Franke, M. Brönstrup, I. Ott, *Eur. J. Chem.* **2017**, *23*, 1869–1880.

[111] R. Büssing, B. Karge, P. Lippmann, P. G. Jones, M. Brönstrup, I. Ott, *ChemMedChem* **2021**, *16*, 3402–3409.

[112] N. S. Saba, M. Ghias, R. Manepalli, K. Schorno, S. Weir, C. Austin, K. Maddocks, J. C. Byrd, S. Kambhampati, K. Bhalla, A. Wiestner, *Blood* **2013**, *122*, 3819.

[113] J. R. Blodgett, R. Pietrusko, *Scand. J. Rheumatol. Suppl.* **1986**, *63*, 67–78.

[114] E. V. Capparelli, R. Bricker-Ford, M. J. Rogers, J. H. McKerrow, S. L. Reed, *Antimicrob. Agents Chemother.* **2016**, *61*, e01947–01916.

[115] C. Levaditi, J. Bardet, A. Tchakirian, A. Vaisman, *CR Hebd. Seances. Acad. Sci. Ser. D. Sci. Nat.* **1931**, *192*, 1142–1143.

[116] C. Chitambar, *Future Med. Chem.* **2012**, *4*, 1257–1272.

[117] C. L. Edwards, R. L. Hayes, *J. Nucl. Med.* **1969**, *10*, 103–105.

[118] M. Caza, J. Kronstad, *Front. Cell. Infect. Microbiol.* **2013**, *3*. https://doi.org/10.3389/fcimb.2013.00080

Novel Metal-Based Drugs for Treating Drug-Resistant Bacteria

[119] E. D. Weinberg, *Biometals* **2000**, *13*, 85–89.

[120] J. E. Cassat, E. P. Skaar, *Cell Host Microbe* **2013**, *13*, 509–519.

[121] C. Chitambar, *Pharm. Res.* **2017**, *115*, 56–64.

[122] I. Schröder, E. Johnson, S. de Vries, *FEMS Micro. Rev.* **2003**, *27*, 427–447.

[123] C. Bonchi, F. Imperi, F. Minandri, P. Visca, E. Frangipani, *BioFactors* **2014**, *40*, 303–312.

[124] Y. Kaneko, M. Thoendel, O. Olakanmi, B. E. Britigan, P. K. Singh, *J. Clin. Investig.* **2007**, *117*, 877–888.

[125] C. Goss, Y. Kaneko, L. Khuu, G. Anderson, S. Ravishankar, M. Aitken, N. Lechtzin, G. Zhou, D. Czyz, K. McLean, O. Olakanmi, H. Shuman, M. Teresi, E. Wilhelm, E. Caldwell, S. Salipante, D. Hornick, R. Siehnel, L. Becker, B. Britigan, P. Singh, *Sci. Trans. Med.* **2018**, *10*, eaat7520.

[126] L. C. S. Antunes, F. Imperi, F. Minandri, P. Visca, *Antimicrob. Agents Chemother.* **2012**, *56*, 5961–5970.

[127] E. P. Price, D. S. Sarovich, *Trends Microbiol.* **2019**, *27*, 289–291.

[128] J. Woo, K. Hearne, A. Kelson, L. Yee, C. Espadas, V. Truong, *OFID* **2019**, *6*, S322–S322.

[129] J. Zeng, L. Wu, Z. Liu, Y. Lv, J. Feng, W. Wang, Y. Xue, D. Wang, J. Li, K. Drlica, X. Zhao, *Antimicrob. Agents Chemother.* **2021**, *65*, e01595–01520.

[130] L. Yang, Y. Liu, H. Wu, Z. Song, N. Høiby, S. Molin, M. Givskov, *FEMS Immunol. Medical Microbiol.* **2012**, *65*, 146–157.

[131] N. Høiby, O. Ciofu, H. K. Johansen, Z. J. Song, C. Moser, P. Jensen, S. Molin, M. Givskov, T. Tolker-Nielsen, T. Bjarnsholt, *Int. J. Oral. Sci.* **2011**, *3*, 55–65.

[132] O. Rzhepishevska, B. Ekstrand-Hammarström, M. Popp, E. Björn, A. Bucht, A. Sjöstedt, H. Antti, M. Ramstedt, *Antimicrob. Agents Chemother.* **2011**, *55*, 5568–5580.

[133] J. Fothergill, C. Winstanley, C. James, *Expert Rev. Anti. Infect. Ther.* **2012**, *10*, 219–235.

[134] W. Xia, N. Li, H. Shan, Y. Lin, F. Yin, X. Yu, Z. Zhou, *ACS Infect. Dis.* **2021**, *7*, 2565–2582.

[135] L. R. Bernstein, *Pharm. Res.* **1998**, *50*, 665–682.

[136] A. Hopkins, in *Determination That GANITE (Gallium Nitrate) Injectable and Five Other Drug Products Were Not Withdrawn from Sale for Reasons of Safety or Effectiveness*, Vol. 79 *Office of the Federal Register*, NARA, **2014**, p. 9225.

[137] R. K. Matharu, Z. Charani, L. Ciric, U. E. Illangakoon, M. Edirisinghe, *J. App. Polym. Sci.* **2018**, *135*, 46368.

[138] R. DeMeio, F. Henriques, Jr., *JBC* **1947**, *169*, 609–623.

[139] S. Ramadan, A. Razak, A. Ragab, M. El-Meleigy, *Biol. Trace Elem. Res.* **1989**, *20*, 225.

[140] H.-L. Seng, E. R. T. Tiekink, *Appl. Organomet. Chem.* **2012**, *26*, 655–662.

[141] E. Okun, T. V. Arumugam, S.-C. Tang, M. Gleichmann, M. Albeck, B. Sredni, M. P. Mattson, *J. Neurochem.* **2007**, *102*, 1232–1241.

[142] H. Rosenblatt-Bin, Y. Kalechman, A. Vonsover, R. Xu, J. Da, F. Shalit, M. Huberman, A. Klein, G. Strassmann, M. Albeck, B. Sredni, *Cell. Immunol.* **1998**, *184*, 12–25.

[143] S. Yosef, M. Brodsky, B. Sredni, A. Albeck, M. Albeck, *ChemMedChem* **2007**, *2*, 1601–1606.

[144] A. Scibelli, S. Roperto, L. Manna, L. M. Pavone, S. Tafuri, R. D. Morte, N. Staiano, *Vet* **2007**, *173*, 482–491.

[145] Z.-H. Lin, C.-H. Lee, H.-Y. Chang, H.-T. Chang, *Chem. Asian J.* **2012**, *7*, 930–934.

[146] M. Daniel-Hoffmann, B. Sredni, Y. Nitzan, *J. Antimicrob. Chemother.* **2012**, *67*, 2165–2172.

[147] B. Sredni, R. Caspi, A. Klein, Y. Kalechman, Y. Danziger, M. Benya'Akov, T. Tamari, F. Shalit, M. Albeck, *Nature* **1987**, *330*, 173–176.

[148] A. Silberman, M. Albeck, B. Sredni, A. Albeck, *Inorg. Chem.* **2016**, *55*, 10847–10850.

[149] C. Princival, M. Archilha, A. Dos Santos, M. Franco, A. Braga, A. Rodrigues-Oliveira, T. Correra, R. Cunha, J. Comasseto, *ACS Omega* **2017**, *2*, 4431–4439.

[150] K. D'Arcy, A. P. Doyle, K. Kavanagh, L. Ronconi, B. Fresch, D. Montagner, *J. Inorg. Biochem.* **2019**, *198*, 110719.

[151] B. Sredni, M. Albeck, T. Tichler, A. Shani, J. Shapira, I. Bruderman, R. Catane, B. Kaufman, Y. Kalechman, *J. Clin. Oncol.* **1995**, *13*, 2342–2353.

[152] D. Giacobbe, M. Mikulska, C. Viscoli, *Expert Rev. Clin. Pharmacol.* **2018**, *11*, 1219–1236.

[153] P. Nordmann, T. Naas, L. Poirel, *Emerg. Infect. Dis.* **2011**, *17*, 1791–1798.

[154] A. M. King, S. A. Reid-Yu, W. Wang, D. T. King, G. De Pascale, N. C. Strynadka, T. R. Walsh, B. K. Coombes, G. D. Wright, *Nature* **2014**, *510*, 503–506.

[155] C. Schnaars, G. Kildahl-Andersen, A. Prandina, R. Popal, S. Radix, M. Le Borgne, T. Gjøen, A. M. S. Andresen, A. Heikal, O. A. Økstad, C. Fröhlich, Ø. Samuelsen, S. Lauksund, L. P. Jordheim, P. Rongved, O. A. H. Åstrand, *ACS Infect. Dis.* **2018**, *4*, 1407–1422.

[156] D. M. Livermore, N. Woodford, *Trends Microbiol.* **2006**, *14*, 413–420.

[157] D. M. Livermore, *Int. J. Antimicrob. Agents* **2012**, *39*, 283–294.

[158] J. Frère, C. Duez, J. Ghuysen, J. Vandekerkhove, *FEBS Lett.* **1976**, *70*, 257–260.

[159] D. J. Tipper, J. L. Strominger, *Proc. Natl. Acad. Sci. USA* **1965**, *54*, 1133–1141.

[160] T. Palzkill, *Ann. N. Y. Acad. Sci.* **2013**, *1277*, 91–104.

[161] P. Linciano, L. Cendron, E. Gianquinto, F. Spyrakis, D. Tondi, *ACS Infect. Dis.* **2019**, *5*, 9–34.

[162] L. Principe, G. Vecchio, G. Sheehan, K. Kavanagh, G. Morroni, V. Viaggi, A. Masi, D. Giacobbe, F. Luzzaro, R. Luzzati, S. Bella, *Microb. Drug Resist.* **2020**, *26*, 1133–1143.

[163] A. Sobke, M. Klinger, B. Hermann, S. Sachse, S. Nietzsche, O. Makarewicz, P. M. Keller, W. Pfister, E. Straube, *Antimicrob. Agents Chemother.* **2012**, *56*, 6021–6025.

[164] E. Ekinci, S. Rohondia, R. Khan, Q. P. Dou, *Rec. Pat. Anti-Cancer Drug Disc.* **2019**, *14*, 113–132.

[165] W. Breeman, E. de Blois, H. Sze Chan, M. Konijnenberg, D. Kwekkeboom, E. Krenning, *Semin. Nucl. Med.* **2011**, *41*, 314–321.

[166] R. J. Radford, S. J. Lippard, *Curr. Opinion Chem. Biol.* **2013**, *17*, 129–136.

7 Prospective Metallo-Drugs Including Bioactive Compounds:
Selection of Co-Ligands to Tune Biological Activity Against Neglected Tropical Diseases

Dinorah Gambino* and Lucía Otero*
Área Química Inorgánica, Departamento Estrella Campos
Facultad de Química, Universidad de la
República, Montevideo, Uruguay
dgambino@fq.edu.uy
luotero@fq.edu.uy

CONTENTS

1 Introduction 194
    1.1   Neglected Tropical Diseases 194
2 Rational Design of Prospective Metallo-Drugs 197
3 Selection of Co-Ligands 199
    3.1   Non-Active Co-Ligands: Improving Relevant Physicochemical
         Properties 199
    3.2   Bioactive Co-Ligands: Development of Multifunctional
         Compounds 205
4 General Conclusions 209
Acknowledgments 209
Abbreviations and Definitions 210
References 210

---

*Corresponding authors

DOI: 10.1201/9781003272250-7

193

ABSTRACT

Metal complexes have demonstrated to be a promising alternative in the search of new drugs for the treatment of neglected tropical diseases and, particularly, those caused by trypanosomatid parasites. Although random screening has been a useful weapon in metal-based drug discovery of antiparasitic compounds, current research and development (R&D) in this field should be guided by rational design. The precise selection of the metal ion and the nature of the coordinated ligands are crucial in tuning the chemical and biological properties of the metal complex. In fact, the complexation of bioactive ligands has been extensively used as a strategy to improve the pharmacological properties of metal-based drugs. Additionally, ancillary ligands or co-ligands could also be included in the metal ion coordination sphere. On the one hand, properties like stability, water solubility, or lipophilicity of the metal compound can be tuned through the correct selection of the co-ligand. On the other hand, co-ligands could have an intrinsic biological activity leading to multifunctional metal compounds. In this chapter, some examples of these approaches in the design of prospective antiparasitic metal-based compounds will be discussed.

KEYWORDS

Neglected Diseases; Trypanosomatids; Metallo-Drugs; Co-Ligands

1   INTRODUCTION

1.1   NEGLECTED TROPICAL DISEASES

According to the World Health Organization (WHO), Neglected Tropical Diseases (NTDs) currently include 20 illnesses that are mainly prevalent in tropical areas, where they affect people who live mostly in impoverished communities. As a whole, they cause devastating health, social, and economic consequences to more than 1 billion people, within 149 countries. More than half a million deaths per year are caused by NTDs. They are considered "neglected" because they are not included in the global health agenda. Even today, NTDs get very limited resources and are almost ignored by global funding agencies and pharmaceutical companies developing new drugs. These diseases affect significantly rural areas, where access to clean water and sanitation is scarce. They severely affect regions without quality healthcare, like several countries in Africa, Asia, and Latin America. They are caused by a variety of pathogens including viruses, bacteria, parasites, fungi, or toxins. NTDs category includes the following diseases: buruli ulcer, Chagas disease (American trypanosomiasis), cysticercosis, dengue fever, dracunculiasis, equinococcosis, fascioliasis, human African trypanosomiasis (African sleeping sickness), leishmaniasis, leprosy, lymphatic filariasis, mycetoma, onchocerciasis, rabies, schistosomiasis, soil-transmitted helminthiasis (Ascaris, Hookworm, and Whipworm), and trachoma [1–3].

Due to the limited available resources to afford the development of new drugs, the drugs currently in clinic use for the treatment of NTDs are quite old. Many of them show clinical disadvantages, like high toxicity and side effects, development of resistance, inadequate route of administration, and prolonged therapeutic schedules. Therefore, new chemotherapeutics are urgently needed.

Approaches undertaken in the field of Medicinal Inorganic Chemistry have led to bioactive metal-based compounds for the treatment of some of these diseases. In particular, classical coordination compounds and organometallics have been designed against the NTDs Chagas disease, human African trypanosomiasis, leishmaniasis, and schistosomiasis, with particular emphasis on the three first diseases, caused by genomically related trypanosomatid parasites. Although eight NTDs of the list are infections by worm-like organisms, only in recent years have efforts been made on developing metallo-drugs but with the approach of generating organometallic analogues of commercial drugs [4–7].

In this work, the importance of the selection of co-ligands in the process of rational design of prospective metallo-drugs will be exemplified by metal-based compounds developed for the treatment of Chagas disease, human African trypanosomiasis (HAT), and leishmaniasis. Therefore, only these NTD diseases will be briefly described.

These are infections produced by trypanosomatid protozoan parasites belonging to the kinetoplastid order that are among the most important NTDs and constitute an urgent health problem in developing countries. Kinetoplastids are a group of flagellated protozoans that have a DNA-containing region, called kinetoplast, in their single large mitochondrion. Although the different kinetoplastid pathogens have a similar genomic organization, similar cellular structures, and undergo related morphological changes during their life cycles, these protozoan parasites are transmitted by different insect vectors causing different human diseases. These diseases are co-endemic in certain regions: Leishmaniasis and Chagas' disease in South America and Leishmaniasis and HAT in Africa [8–10].

Chagas' disease (American trypanosomiasis) is endemic in Latin America. There are around 8 million infected people, 10,000 annual deaths, and 25 million people at risk of infection [11]. In the last decades, the disease has spread to non-endemic countries outside Latin America due to immigration of unknowingly infected people that transmit the disease through blood transfusion, organ transplant or congenital transmission. The disease is caused by the parasite *Trypanosoma cruzi* (*T. cruzi*), which is mainly transmitted to the mammalian hosts by infected blood-sucking bugs. Acute infections can be lethal, but usually the disease evolves into a chronic stage that may result in death. The available chemotherapy options include two drugs developed more than 50 years ago, benznidazole and nifurtimox, which are highly toxic, require long treatments, are not effective in the chronic stage of the disease, and often develop resistance [10, 11].

Leishmaniasis affects 350 million people in 98 countries, in four continents [12]. It is a group of diseases caused by different *Leishmania* species. There are three main forms of the disease, with different levels of severity, i.e., visceral leishmaniasis, cutaneous leishmaniasis, and mucocutaneous leishmaniasis. Leishmania–HIV co-infection has been reported as the most difficult to treat. An infected female phlebotomine sandfly transmits the disease through its bite.

Some current drugs for the treatment of this disease include pentavalent antimonials (meglumine antimoniate and sodium stibogluconate), pentamidine, sitamaquine, amphotericin B, miltefosine, and paromomycin [12–16].

Human African tripanosomiasis (HAT, sleeping sickness) mainly occurs in the sub-Saharan regions of Africa. It is transmitted through the bite of an infected tsetse fly. Control efforts have reduced the number of cases, but the lack of surveillance and new drugs and the emergence of resistance to the old ones have contributed to the resurgence of the disease. It is caused by the protozoan parasite *Trypanosoma brucei* (*T. brucei*). The disease has a first stage in which the parasites remain in the bloodstream and a second stage in which they enter the central nervous system with a fatal course if untreated. Five drugs are currently recommended: pentamidine, melarsoprol, eflornithine, suramin, and fexinidazole. Nifurtimox-eflornithine combination therapy is currently a first-line treatment [9, 14, 17].

As previously mentioned, only a small number of drugs exist for the treatment of diseases caused by trypanosomatids, with poor safety, efficacy, and pharmacokinetic profiles. Even though in the last years public-private efforts have pushed forward the drug discovery process, no new drugs to treat these diseases have entered the clinic in the last decades [18, 19].

Although these trypanosomatid protozoan parasites are transmitted by different insect vectors and are responsible for clinically different human diseases, it has been demonstrated that they show similar biological features. The genome of these parasites has been sequenced and is available in TriTrypDB (http://tritrypdb.org), an integrated genomic and functional genomic database for pathogenic parasites of the family Trypanosomatidae, which includes leishmania and trypanosoma protozoa [20, 21]. Particularly, they show around 6,000 closely related genes codifying proteins of a total of 8,000–12,000 genes. This could lead to the development of broad-spectrum drugs that affect common targets in the different parasites [22, 23].

For the drug discovery process it is important to consider that all these parasites exhibit complicated lifecycles alternating between stages in the insect vector gut and stages in the mammalian host. These different stages or forms show different biological properties and, most importantly, different susceptibility to drugs. The epimastigote form of *T. cruzi* is a non-infective stage that only exists inside the gut of the triatome insect vector. In the host blood, the infective trypomastigote form invades the tissues and inside the host cells it converts into the replicative amastigote form. A similar lifecycle is observed for *T. brucei* that includes four main stages, some present in the infected insect and others present in the mammalian host: epimastigotes and procyclic forms, slender metacyclic trypomastigotes, and stumpy bloodstream proliferative metacyclic trypomastigotes. The last stage is the most relevant form in the development of therapeutic agents against *T. brucei*. It is important to note that, in contrast to other trypanosomatids, the part of the life cycle of *T. brucei* in the mammalian host occurs extracellularly. During the lifecycle of *Leishmania* sp. the parasite alternates between the infective promastigote form generated in the intestine of the insect vector and the replicative amastigote form inside the host macrophages [9].

2 RATIONAL DESIGN OF PROSPECTIVE METALLO-DRUGS

Metal complexes have found many applications in medicine since ancient times. An increasing number of novel inorganic and organometallic complexes are under development as therapeutic agents with several of them currently in clinical trials or already approved for clinical use. Even though the basis for their use has often been empirical without detailed understanding of structure–activity relationships, the more recent and major development of platinum-based anticancer drugs has helped to establish metal complexes as viable treatments [24, 25].

Metal complexes as prospective drugs have been widely investigated in the field of cancer therapy. Despite their high potential in such diseases, less attention has been paid to their application as antiparasitic compounds. However, compounds including metals have been used in therapy of these diseases since a long time ago. For example, the first treatment for leishmaniasis, antimony(III) potassium tartrate (tartar emetic), was introduced in 1912. Tartar emetic was effective but very toxic. Therefore, pentavalent antimonials were introduced as alternatives. Although these pentavalent antimonial compounds have been clinically used worldwide for more than 70 years, their exact chemical structure and composition remain still unknown [6].

Although random screening has been a useful weapon in metal-based drug discovery of antiparasitic compounds, current R&D in this field should be guided largely by rational design [25]. In fact, the systematic research and development of metal complexes as prospective drugs for treating these diseases started only some decades ago with the leading work of Sánchez Delgado [26, 27].

The search of metal complexes as an alternative for the antiparasitic existing therapies is based on the need to develop new species with improved pharmacological activity and that were able to bypass resistance mechanisms acting via more than one mode of action and/or inhibiting more than one target enzyme [6].

The vast diversity of metals, types of ligands, and geometries makes metal-based coordination complexes very useful in accomplishing these goals and accessing an underexplored chemical space for drug development, and especially for the design of new antiparasitic drugs.

Some of these unique properties of metal complexes, quite distinct from those for purely organic drugs, are stated below:

- can generate cationic, anionic, or neutral species, depending on the oxidation state of the metal ion and the coordination environment. This could be used to target them to charged biomolecules like parasitic DNA. In addition, for charged species, different counterions could modulate complexes' solubility, and consequently their activity.
- can adopt a variety of coordination numbers and geometries leading to three-dimensional structures that can be shaped to defined molecular targets like specific parasitic enzymes.
- can provide unique modes of action by exchange or release of ligands that need to be controlled under biological conditions. The thermodynamic and

kinetic properties of metal–ligand interactions influence ligand exchange reactions and hence, the ability of metal compounds to undergo coordinative interactions with biological molecules. These reactions should also be controlled to avoid unspecific toxicity for the mammalian host.

- can undergo oxidation and reduction reactions participating in redox activation and catalytic generation of toxic species (reactive oxygen species, ROS). These toxic species might be more deleterious for parasites than for mammal cells due to the absence in parasites of complex free radical detoxification systems.
- can act by depleting essential substrates leading, for example, to abolish enzymatic activities [28–31].

Based on the statements above, in designing a new antiparasitic agent, several structural features can be strategically selected [32]. On the one hand, the selection of the metal ion is crucial in turning the chemical and biological properties of the metal complex. From the chemical point of view, the metal ion should be selected considering the nature of the prospective ligands in the sense of Pearson's acid-base principle, to obtain complexes with adequate stability. Redox properties of the selected metal ion should be considered as well to avoid or facilitate redox reactions *in vivo*. In addition, as previously stated, different metal ions could also lead to different geometrical features and different coordination numbers. This last aspect is very relevant to the possibility of including co-ligands that could modulate the physicochemical and biological properties of the metal-containing species (see below).

From the biological or pharmacological point of view, the selection of the metal ion should also be based on its role in the complex species. The metal ion could act as a chaperone of an active ligand delivering it to the biological target or could have an intrinsic biological activity by itself summing up additional mechanisms of action for the metal complex. In this sense, essential metal ions (Cu, Fe, Mn, V, Ni, Zn) could be selected to potentially avoid toxicity problems or the so-called metals of the "platinum group" (Pt, Pd, Ru, Os, Rh, Ir) and other heavy metals like gold, which are pharmacologically active [33].

On the other hand, the selection of ligands is a key aspect in the rational design of a biologically active metal complex. One of the most used strategies for obtaining metal complexes with antiparasitic activity is to coordinate with a suitable metal ion, an organic compound that has proven to have this activity: a bioactive ligand. This includes not only those drugs in clinical use for the different parasitosis but also other organic compounds bearing the desired biological activity. Metal complexation of a bioactive ligand leads to modifications in some of its physicochemical properties like stability, solubility, or lipophilicity which would influence its biological properties modifying its bioavailability, activity, or toxicity. In addition, being included in a different species, the metal complex could help to bypass parasitic resistance mechanisms to the organic compound. Finally, depending on the nature of the metal ion, dual or multiple mechanisms of action could be obtained [6, 27, 33–36].

Prospective Metallo-Drugs Against Neglected Tropical Diseases **199**

Finally, different co-ligands could be selected in order to tune the physico-chemical and biological properties of the metal-containing species. In this chapter, examples showing the different aspects of the selection of co-ligands in the rational design of metal complexes with antiparasitic activity will be discussed.

3 SELECTION OF CO-LIGANDS

One of the main advantages of metal complexes as prospective metal-based drugs is the possibility of including in the metal ion's coordination sphere, various ligands with different properties. In the previously described approach for the rational design of antiparasitic metal complexes, at least one of these ligands should be a bioactive one. Depending on the denticity of this bioactive ligand, as well as on the coordination number of the selected metal ion, ancillary ligands or co-ligands could be included. These co-ligands could be selected to modulate both the physicochemical and the biological properties of the metal complex. In fact, depending on their nature, co-ligands could be innocent, not having an intrinsic biological activity or they could constitute a second bioactive ligand.

3.1 NON-ACTIVE CO-LIGANDS: IMPROVING RELEVANT PHYSICOCHEMICAL PROPERTIES

The inclusion of non-active co-ligands in the design of a prospective antiparasitic metal-based compound is a useful strategy to modify some of the physicochemical properties that may affect the biological and pharmacological behavior of the final compound. Properties like stability, water solubility, or lipophilicity can be tuned through the correct selection of the co-ligand.

Stability in solution of potential therapeutic agents is a very important physicochemical property because speciation chemistry affects the drug's interaction with enzymes, other biomolecules, receptors, and molecular targets in general. This is particularly relevant for metal-based drugs since, in solution, chemical changes modify speciation and, consequently, biological activity [37].

Water solubility is also a desired property for new drugs favoring oral uptake and/or transport in blood. Metallo-drugs usually show low solubility in aqueous media. Inclusion of adequate co-ligands can favorably modify water solubility.

Lipophilicity is a very important physicochemical property that controls biological behavior of a drug, particularly, transmembrane transport and interaction with biological receptors. Therefore, modifying lipophilicity of a prospective drug will probably modify the observed biological activity [38].

Sánchez-Delgado et al. used this concept in designing a series of organoruthenium compounds of the formula $[Ru[(\eta^6\text{-}p\text{-cymene})L_x(CTZ)]^{n+}$ with CTZ=clotrimazole and L=chloride, ethylenediamine (en), acetylacetonate (acac), or bipyridine (bipy) (Figure 1). The bioactive ligand CTZ, a well-known antifungal agent, also displays anti-*T. cruzi* activity by inhibiting parasitic sterol biosynthesis. In an early work, the same authors had reported $[RuCl_2(CTZ)_2]$ (Figure 1) that produced a 10-fold increase in activity when compared to free CTZ as well

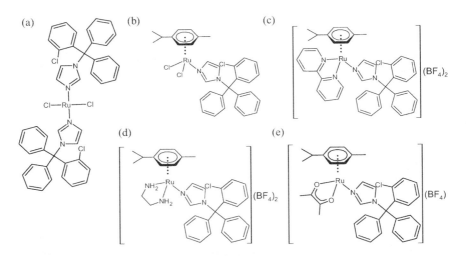

FIGURE 1 Developed Ru-CTZ compounds. (a) [RuCl$_2$(CTZ)$_2$], (b) [Ru[(η^6-p-cymene)Cl$_2$(CTZ)], (c) [Ru[(η^6-p-cymene)(bipy)(CTZ)](BF$_4$)$_2$, (d) [Ru[(η^6-p-cymene)(en)(CTZ)](BF$_4$)$_2$. (e) [Ru[(η^6-p-cymene)(acac)(CTZ)](BF$_4$).

as 10-fold decrease in toxicity against normal mammalian cells. Nevertheless, the low water solubility of this compound leads to poor *in vivo* activity. The designed organometallic "piano stool" arene-Ru–CTZ compounds including the selected bidentate co-ligands were selected to improve the compounds' stability and by leading to charged species, also the desired water solubility.

Compounds were evaluated against promastigotes of *L. major* and epimastigotes of *T. cruzi* and compared to that of CTZ. The effect of the different co-ligands on the antiparasitic activity was evident. All compounds showed an increased activity against both parasites, compared to the bioactive ligand CTZ and a decrease in toxicity; [Ru[(η^6-p-cymene)Cl$_2$(CTZ)] presented the most outstanding results. This last compound enhances the activity of CTZ by a factor of 58 against *T. cruzi*, which represents almost a 6-fold increase with reference to [RuCl$_2$(CTZ)$_2$]. It should be noted that, for this series of complexes, no clear correlations emerged between antiparasitic activity and solubility alone. However, according to the proposed hypothesis, soluble [Ru[(η^6-p-cymene)Cl$_2$(CTZ)] and [Ru[(η^6-p-cymene)(acac)(CTZ)](BF$_4$) complexes demonstrated to be efficient for the treatment of cutaneous leishmaniasis in a murine model, with imperceptible toxicity to the experimental animals [39, 40].

A clear example of the strategy of including co-ligands to improve the stability of a designed metal-based potential drug has been performed by part of our group. In the last two decades, we have developed vanadium-based compounds with different bioactive ligands and co-ligands as antiproliferative agents against *T. cruzi* [41, 42].

It is well known that vanadium is a biologically relevant bioelement and many vanadium-based therapeutic drugs have been proposed for the treatment of different diseases [42–46].

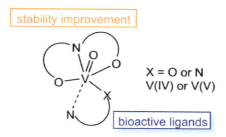

FIGURE 2 General structure of the heteroleptic oxidovanadium compounds rationally designed.

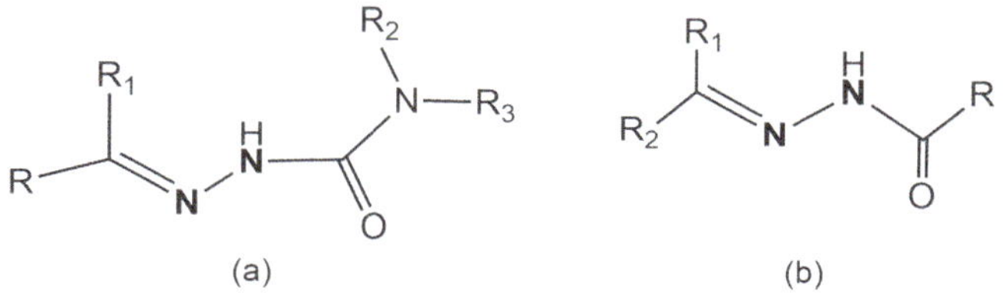

FIGURE 3 General structure of (a) semicarbazones and (b) acid hydrazones. R, R_1, R_2, and R_3 = alkyl or aryl groups.

In this context, different series of structurally related oxidovanadium compounds were rationally designed by changing the bidentate bioactive ligand and including tridentate innocent co-ligands with a ONO donor set in the general structure shown in Figure 2.

The coordination of a tridentate ligand to the oxidovanadium(IV) or (V) center, together with the bidentate bioactive ligand, would increase the stability of the final complex for thermodynamic reasons. Selected ONO tridentate ligands for this purpose were Schiff bases, particularly semicarbazones and hydrazones. Schiff bases are an important class of ligands that have been extensively studied in the field of coordination chemistry mainly because of their facile syntheses, easy availability, and broad range of biological activities and pharmacological applications [47–51]. If R_1 contains a donor ligand such as N or O, tridentate binding is possible (Figure 3).

Initially, different series of $V^{IV}O$-based heteroleptic compounds bearing activity against *T. cruzi* were developed by including polypyridyl ligands having DNA intercalating capacity and a tridentate ONO ligand. It was demonstrated that most of these 1,10-phenanthroline derivatives acting as ligands show *in vitro* activity against the parasite by themselves. Their activity was improved by coordination to the vanadium center. In particular, heteroleptic compounds including dideprotonated tridentate salicylaldehyde semicarbazones as co-ligands showed promising results (Figure 4) [52–54].

A hit compound, including the $V(O)^{2+}$ $(VO)^{2+}$ moiety and 5-bromosalicylaldehyde semicarbazone as well as aminophen as ligands, was identified and further omic studies were performed to unravel its mechanism of action [55].

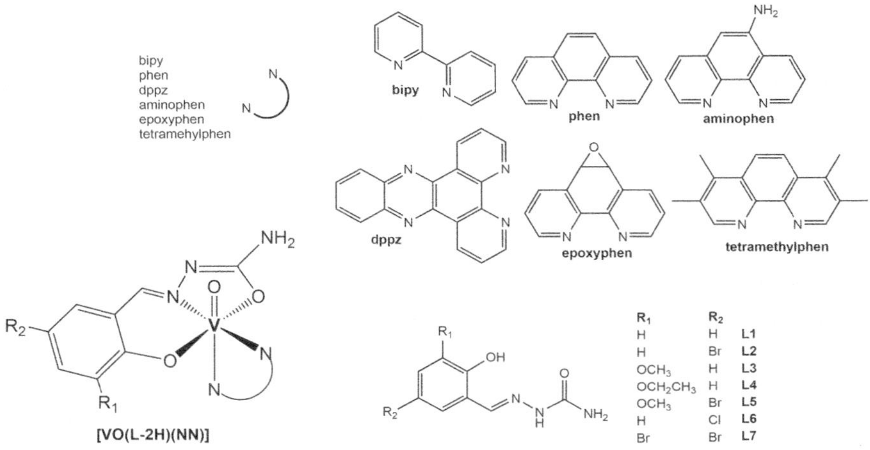

FIGURE 4 Structurally related oxidovanadium(IV) compounds [VO(L-2H)(NN)].

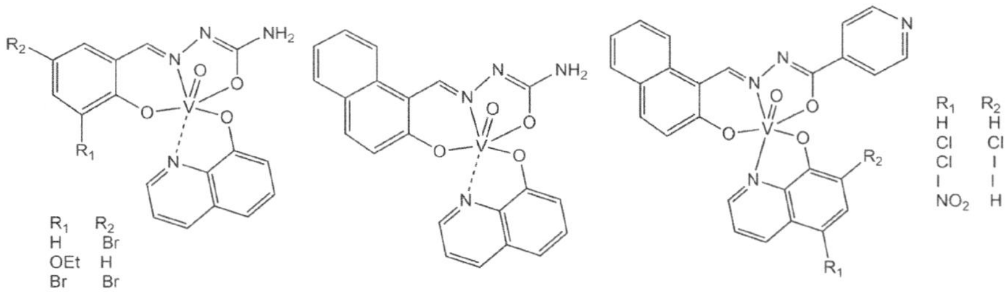

FIGURE 5 [V(V)O(L-2H)(8HQ-H)] complexes. L=tridentate co-ligand.

Based on these results, the hit compound was structurally modified to further optimize its activity by changing not only the vanadium oxidation state and the bioactive ligand but also the tridentate co-ligand. For instance, the N,N bioactive ligand was substituted by the bidentate 8-hydroxyquinoline (8HQ) scaffold, an important heterocyclic pharmacophore that possesses a diversity of biological properties. In particular, our group demonstrated that 8HQ and some of its derivatives show activity against *T. cruzi* [56].

A different series of heteroleptic oxidovanadium(V) compounds, including 8HQ derivatives, were therefore developed and their biological behavior on *T. cruzi* studied in detail (Figure 5) [56, 57].

In addition, two homoleptic series $[V^{IV}O(L-H)_2]$ and $[V^VO(OCH_3)(L-H)_2]$, with L=8HQ derivatives, were studied in depth to shed light into the significance of the presence of the tridentate co-ligand on the biological behavior of the vanadium compounds [58].

All this research led to the conclusion that the tridentate co-ligand provides stability to the whole entity without a significant effect on biological activity. In

Prospective Metallo-Drugs Against Neglected Tropical Diseases

the case of the 8HQ complexes, the most stable compound was that with the naphtylsemicarbazone as co-ligand (Figure 5). Globally, these results demonstrated the importance of the presence and nature of the tridentate co-ligand.

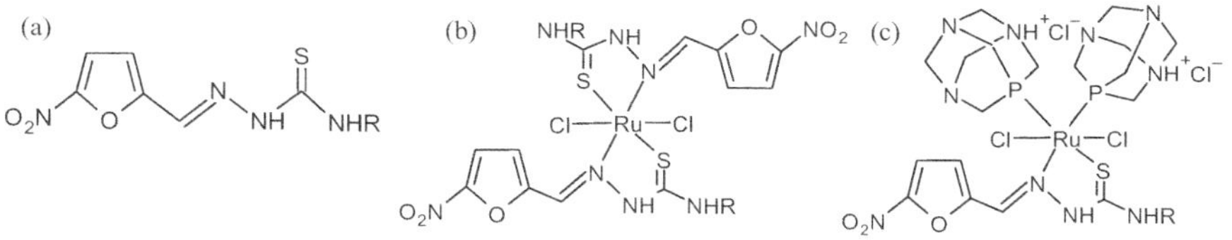

FIGURE 6 (a) 5-Nitrofuryl containing thiosemicarbazones, (b) [RuCl$_2$(HL)$_2$], (c) [Ru^{II}Cl$_2$(HL)(HPTA)$_2$]Cl$_2$ with HL = the 5-nitrofuryl containing thiosemicarbazones, HPTA = protonated PTA and R = H, methyl, ethyl, phenyl.

Additionally, our group has been also working for a long time in developing metal complexes bearing anti *T. cruzi* activity with 5-nitro-2-furaldehyde thiosemicarbazones as bioactive ligands (Figure 6). These ligands, designed based on the pharmacophore of the drug Nifurtimox, showed very good activity against trypanosomatid parasites, and they were also able to produce toxic ROS by redox cycling as the commercial drug does as part of its mode of action [59–61].

Almost 100 complexes, including both organometallic and classical coordination compounds, have been obtained. The rational design of these compounds included modifications on the bioactive ligand (substitutions at the N^4 level of the thiosemicarbazone moiety), on the metal ions (Pd(II), Pt(II), Ru(II), Ru(III)) and also on the co-ligands that completed the coordination sphere. In particular, co-ligands were selected with the aim of modulating the compounds' stability, water solubility, lipophilicity, or more than one of these physicochemical properties at the same time [34–36].

As an example, ruthenium complexes [RuCl$_2$(HL)$_2$] with HL = the 5-nitrofuryl containing thiosemicarbazones presented in Figure 6, showed a poor anti-*T. cruzi* activity that was related to their very low solubility in water that could lead to their partial precipitation from the aqueous culture medium [62].

As a way of improving the water solubility of the designed metal compounds, PTA (1,3,5-triaza-7-phosphaadamantane) was selected as co-ligand. PTA is a hydrophilic phosphine that has been used as an ancillary ligand for medicinal chemistry purposes, as it is known to endow metal complexes with aqueous solubility and solubility in polar organic solvents. In fact, ruthenium complexes of the formula [Ru^{II}Cl$_2$(HL)(HPTA)$_2$]Cl$_2$, where HL = the 5-nitrofuryl containing thiosemicarbazones and HPTA = the protonated form of PTA, were obtained (Figure 6). All of them resulted in being very soluble in water (solubility >10 mM) but the anti *T. cruzi* activity did not increase accordingly. It should be noted that lipophilicity was also modified as a consequence of the inclusion of the hydrophilic phosphine [63].

In order to study the effect of different co-ligands on the lipophilicity of the metal compounds and the consequences of this effect on their biological activity,

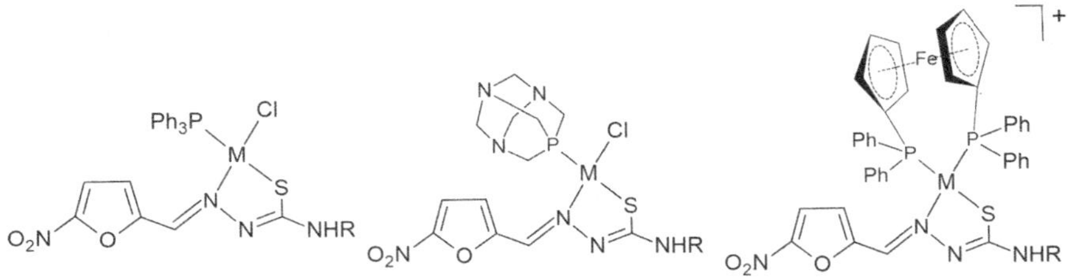

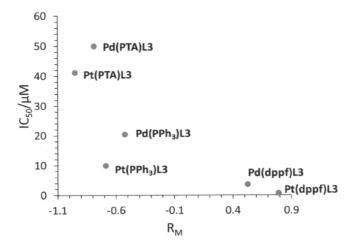

FIGURE 7 [MCl(PPh$_3$)L], [MCl(PTA)L] and [M(dppf)L](PF$_6$) complexes, where M=Pd or Pt, L=deprotonated form of 5-nitrofuryl containing thiosemicarbazones and R=H, methyl, ethyl, phenyl.

R_M = log[(1/R_f) − 1], elution mixture DMSO/water 70:30 (v/v).

FIGURE 8 Correlation between the IC$_{50}$ (activity against trypomastigote form of *T. cruzi*) and lipophilicity. L3 = N_4-methyl-5-nitrofuraldeyde thiosemicarbazone.

three series of palladium and platinum compounds with three different phosphine derivatives as co-ligands were compared. Selected co-ligands were PTA, dppf = 1,1'-bis(diphenylphosphino) ferrocene, and PPh$_3$ = triphenylphosphine (Figure 7). Lipophilicity of [MCl(PTA)L], [M(dppf)L](PF$_6$) and [MCl(PPh$_3$)L] complexes, where M = Pd or Pt and L = deprotonated form of 5-nitrofuryl containing thiosemicarbazones, was determined by TLC using C18 reverse phase precoated plates. Obtained R$_M$ values (R$_M$ = log (1/R$_F$) − 1)) showed a very good correlation between lipophilicity and the anti-*T. cruzi* activity of the compounds. The [M(dppf)L](PF$_6$) compounds were the most lipophilic and also the most biologically active ones (Figure 8) [64, 65].

More recently, the effect of modifying the halide co-ligand in some of the above series of compounds, most notably complexes of the formula [MCl(PTA)L] and [MCl(PPh$_3$)L], was studied (unpublished results). Therefore, complexes of the formula [MI(PTA)L] and [MI(PPh$_3$)L] were obtained. The aim of changing between chloride and iodide ligands was to modulate the stability of the compounds toward hydrolysis in the biological media. In fact, substitution of labile ligands, like halides, by water has been described as one of the key points in the mode of action of anticancer platinum drugs. In this sense, the low anticancer activity of iodido compounds in comparison to that of their chlorido analogues had been historically ascribed to the greater stability and lower reactivity of Pt-I bonds as compared to Pt-Cl bonds in aqueous solution, disfavoring the hydrolysis process. However, more recent studies have described very good antiproliferative properties *in vitro* for iodido Pt(II) and Pt(IV) complexes and high reactivity toward some biomolecular targets like serum albumin and glutathione. In addition, iodido compounds used to be more lipophilic than the chlorido analogues [66–68].

As expected, the [MI(PTA)L] and [MI(PPh$_3$)L] complexes were more lipophilic than the analogous chlorido compounds. The first ones also showed higher activities *in vitro* against the trypomastigote form of *T. cruzi* than their chlorido analogues.

3.2 BIOACTIVE CO-LIGANDS: DEVELOPMENT OF MULTIFUNCTIONAL COMPOUNDS

Molecular hybridization is an established concept in drug design based on the combination of pharmacophoric moieties of different bioactive substances to produce a hybrid compound with improved efficacy, when compared to the parent drugs or organic moieties. This design strategy could lead to multifunctional compounds showing dual or multiple modes of action and, additionally, to reduced undesired side effects and modified selectivity profile. The new molecule impacts separate biological targets to create a combination effect that could be additive or even synergistic. A multifunctional compound derived from two or more different pharmacophores exerts its activity by interacting with respective receptors of its constituent pharmacophores. It may also exhibit additional binding interactions with other receptor sites that may be responsible for significantly improved or additional activities. This hybridization strategy could overcome drawbacks and limitations of combination chemotherapies; each drug in a combination will have its own pharmacokinetic profile and so the treatment regimen could be hard to control. A single drug designed to affect multiple biological targets may overcome this shortcoming [69–72].

The multi-target drug design strategy has been proposed several years ago to overcome the challenges in the development of metal-based drugs against NTDs [73].

Although multi-action metal compounds were described as antitumorals, this strategy has not been widely used yet for the development of metallo-drugs against NTDs [74, 75].

Designing multifunctional metal-based drugs involves, in many cases, the inclusion in a single chemical entity of a bioactive or pharmacologically relevant metal center, a bioactive ligand, and a bioactive co-ligand. Some examples applied to the development of antitrypanosomal metal-based drugs will clarify this topic.

Bisphosphonates are the most commonly prescribed drugs for the treatment of osteoporosis and other bone illnesses. Nitrogen-containing bisphosphonates (NBPs), like alendronate and pamidronate, inhibit a key enzyme in the mevalonate pathway, farnesyl pyrophosphate synthase (FPPS) [76]. NBPs are also potent inhibitors of the proliferation of trypanosomatid (*Trypanosoma cruzi*, *Trypanosoma brucei rhodesiense*, and *Leishmania donovani*) and apicomplexan (*Toxoplasma gondii* and *Plasmodium falciparum*) parasites [77]. Our group has developed with success several coordination compounds of these commercial drugs bearing activity against *T. cruzi* [78–80].

Recently and according to the explained rational design strategy, four new multifunctional palladium heteroleptic complexes including two bioactive ligands, *N*-containing commercial NBPs alendronate or pamidronate and DNA intercalating polypyridyl co-ligands phen or bipy, were developed (Figure 9). Complexes displayed anti-*T. cruzi* activity which could be related to the inhibition of the parasitic farnesyl diphosphate synthase enzyme, the molecular target of NBPs, but mainly to their ability to interact with DNA. In addition, the phen complexes showed a slight increase in the activity against *Toxoplasma gondii*, the causative parasite of toxoplasmosis, when compared to the selected free NBPs [81].

A similar example of the generation of multifunctional compounds by including bioactive co-ligands involves a series of five Re^I-tricarbonyl compounds explored as antitrypanosomal agents (Figure 10) [82].

The designed *fac*-[Re^I(CO)$_3$(NN)(CTZ)](PF$_6$) compounds, with NN=five different polypyridyl phenanthroline derivatives and CTZ=clotrimazole, showed improved activity in respect to the free CTZ and NN ligands in *Trypanosoma cruzi* epimastigotes and trypomatigotes. The evaluation of their multi-target nature was accomplished by studying their effect on the free ligands molecular targets: DNA and lanosterol 14 α-demethylase [82].

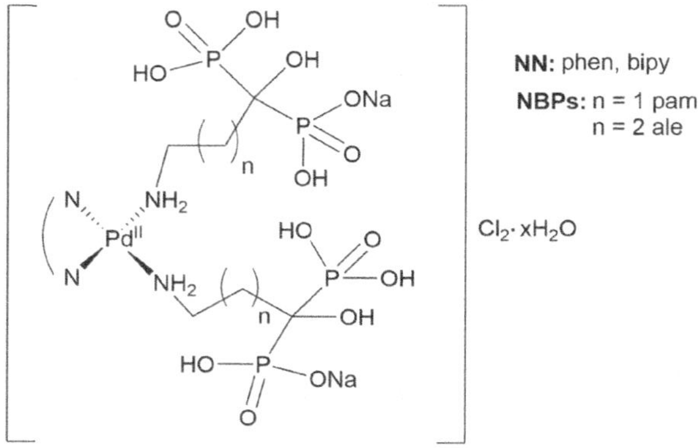

FIGURE 9   Pamidronate (pam) and alendronate (ale) multifunctional Pd(II) compounds.

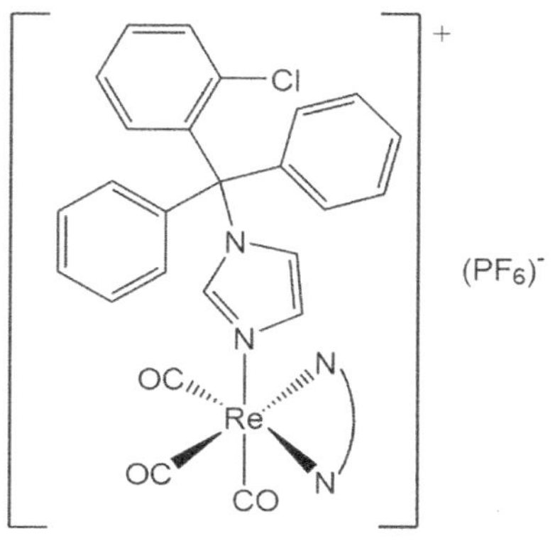

FIGURE 10 General structure of the fac-[Re^I(CO)$_3$(NN)(CTZ)](PF$_6$) compounds. NN = phen, aminophen, dimethylbipy, tetramethylphen and bipy.

Another example of a sequential rational design of metal-based drugs involves pyridine-2-thiol N-oxide (2-mercaptopyridine N-oxide, Hmpo) as a bioactive ligand (Figure 11). This ligand shows high anti-$T.$ $cruzi$ activity against all forms of the parasite and no unspecific toxicity on mammalian cells. The action of Hmpo is mainly mediated by the inhibition of NADH fumarate reductase enzyme [83–85].

In the first stage, homoleptic [Pd(mpo)$_2$] and [Pt(mpo)$_2$] compounds were synthesized and fully characterized. The compounds were 39–115 times more active than the trypanocidal drug Nifurtimox and showed low unspecific cytotoxicity on mammalian macrophages. In the assayed conditions, both complexes show an inhibitory effect on NADH fumarate reductase, which strongly suggests the involvement of this enzyme in the mode of action of these complexes [86].

Further rational design lead to the development of organometallic M-dppf-mpo compounds of Pt(II), Pd(II) and Ru(II) centers, where dppf is included as co-ligand (Figure 11).

As previously stated, dppf provides adequate lipophilicity to the final compounds which could favor their biological behavior. In addition, the "sandwich type" ferrocene moiety has demonstrated high potentiality for the development of organometallic drugs improving the activity and unspecific toxicity [24, 87].

Additionally, ferrocenes are able to undergo one electron oxidation leading to the generation of radicals in a Fenton-like manner. $T.$ $cruzi$ and other trypanosomatid parasites possess a very primitive system of radical species detoxification. Therefore, the inclusion of a ferrocenyl moiety in the new structure could provide this additional mode of action on the parasite (Figure 11).

Therefore, structural modifications were done on the homoleptic Pd and Pt mpo compounds to include this organometallic co-ligand derived from ferrocene. Our synthetic strategy was to include the ferrocene fragment as a co-ligand in the Pt or Pd coordination sphere, instead of the traditional coupling of the ferrocene

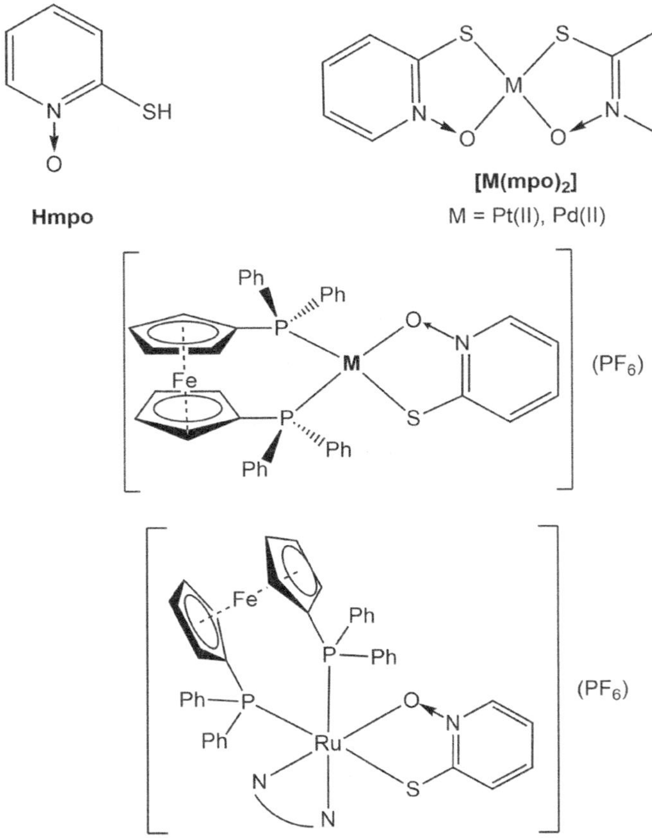

FIGURE 11 Pyridine-2-thiol *N*-oxide (Hmpo) and rationally designed mpo metal complexes: [M^{II}(mpo)$_2$], [M^{II}dppf(mpo)](PF$_6$) and [Ru^{II}dppf(mpo)(NN)](PF$_6$). M=Pt or Pd, NN=bidentate polypyridyl 1,10-phenanthroline derivatives.

moiety to an organic skeleton as in the antimalarial drug ferroquine. In this sense, 1,1′-bis(diphenylphosphino) ferrocene (dppf) was selected as co-ligand. The obtained [M(dppf)(mpo)](PF$_6$) compounds showed IC$_{50}$ values in the nanomolar range on *T. cruzi* epimastigotes (Dm28c strain) as well as low cytotoxicity on VERO epithelial cells (ATCC CCL81) selected as mammalian cell model. The complexes were about 10–20 times more active than the antitrypanosomal drug Nifurtimox. Molecular docking studies conducted on the model structure of the *T. cruzi* NADH fumarate reductase, together with experimental *in vitro* studies on *T. cruzi* protein extracts, demonstrated the inhibitory effect of the compounds on the enzyme. The generation of radical species inside the parasite cells by the action of M-dppf-mpo compounds was confirmed through EPR (electron paramagnetic resonance) experiments (unpublished results) [88].

Prospective Metallo-Drugs Against Neglected Tropical Diseases   **209**

Moreover, a high-throughput omic analysis of the *Trypanosoma cruzi* response to both organometallic compounds confirmed a wider multi-target mechanism of action of the compounds [89].

Taking into account all of these highly promising results, the structure of the compounds was further modified to generate multifunctional and, hopefully, multi-target Ru[II] compounds. Ru compounds have been widely studied for medicinal chemistry purposes due to their low toxicity and suitable chemical and biological properties for the development of drugs. From a chemical point of view, Ru in its more common oxidation states +2 and +3 usually form complexes with a coordination number of six. Related to the inclusion of different co-ligands, this constitutes an advantage of this metal ion in comparison to Pd(II) or Pt(II) which form four coordinated complexes [24, 34].

Based on this advantage, Pd[II] and Pt[II] metal centers were changed by Ru[II]. New heterobimetallic Ru-Fe compounds were developed including dppf co-ligand and mpo as bioactive ligand together with an additional polypyridyl bioactive ligand. These multifunctional compounds could act on molecular targets of the two bioactive ligands and dppf, leading to an improvement in biological activity. In our attempts to follow this design strategy, we recently developed Ru[II]-dppf-mpo-L compounds, [Ru[II]dppf(mpo)(NN)](PF$_6$), with NN = bioactive polypyridyl derivatives that showed promising activity on *T. cruzi* and *T. brucei* (Figure 11) (unpublished results).

4   GENERAL CONCLUSIONS

Many efforts have focused on developing metal complexes as treatments for neglected parasitic diseases. The rational design of new prospective drugs is currently a relevant area of research. In particular, very promising results have been obtained through coordinating bioactive ligands.

On the other hand, the accurate and rational selection of different co-ligands to be included in the metal ion coordination sphere has proved to be a powerful tool to modulate the physicochemical and biological properties of prospective antiparasitic metallo-drugs. In addition, the design of multifunctional metal-based compounds can be developed in the context of this strategy.

However, further efforts should be made for antiparasitic metallo-drugs to reach clinical trials. Exhaustive studies to identify parasitic targets and elucidate the mode of action in more detail, testing against additional stages of the appropriate parasite, *in vivo* studies, and quantitative structure–activity relationships for a rational drug design are still lacking in this field.

ACKNOWLEDGMENTS

DG and LO thank Universidad de la República, National Agency of Investigation and Innovation (ANII) and Program for the Development of Basic Sciences (PEDECIBA), Uruguay for financial support.

ABBREVIATIONS AND DEFINITIONS

8HQ	8-hydroxyquinoline
acac	acetylacetonate
aminophen	5-amino-1,10-phenantroline
bipy	2,2′-bipyridine
CTZ	clotrimazole
dimethylbipy	4,4′-dimethyl bipyridine
DNA	deoxyribonucleic acid
dppf	1,1′-bis(diphenylphosphino)ferrocene
dppz	dipyrido[3,2-a:2′,3′-c]phenazine
en	ethylenediamine
epoxyphen	5,6-epoxy-5,6-dihydro-1,10-phenanthroline
EPR	electron paramagnetic resonance
FPPS	farnesyl diphosphate synthase
HAT	human African trypanosomiasis
HIV	human immunodeficiency virus
Hmpo	pyridine-2-thiol N-oxide
NADH	reduced form of nicotinamide adenine dinucleotide
NBP	nitrogen-containing bisphosphonate
NTDs	neglected tropical diseases
η^6-p-cymene	*para* cymene with an η^6 coordination mode
phen	1,10-phenanthroline
PF$_6$	hexafluorophosphate anion
PPh$_3$	triphenylphosphine
PTA	1,3,5-triaza-7-phosphaadamantane
R$_F$	retardation factor
ROS	reactive oxygen species
R&D	research and development
L. major	*Leishmania major*
***Leishmania* sp**	*Leishmania* species
T. brucei	*Trypanosoma brucei*
T. cruzi	*Trypanosoma cruzi*
tetramethylphen	3,4,7,8-tetramethyl-1,10-phenantroline
TLC	thin layer chromatography
TriTrypDB	a functional genomic resource for the Trypanosomatidae
***Vero* cells**	kidney epithelial cells extracted from *Chlorocebus* sp monkey
WHO	World Health Organization

REFERENCES

[1] https://www.who.int/news-room/questions-and-answers/item/neglected-tropical-diseases#:~:text=Neglected%20tropical%20diseases%20(NTDs)%20are, %2C%20 parasites%2C%20fungi%20and%20toxins (Accessed 14 April 2022).

[2] V. Jayaprakash, D. Castagnolo, Y. Özkay, *Medicinal Chemistry of Neglected and Tropical Diseases: Advances in the Design and Synthesis of Antimicrobial Agents*, CRC Press Taylor and Francis Group, London, 2019.

Prospective Metallo-Drugs Against Neglected Tropical Diseases   211

[3] A. B. Caballero, J. M. Salas, M. Sánchez-Moreno, in *Leishmaniasis – Trends in Epidemiology, Diagnosis and Treatment*, Ed D. M. Claborn, IntechOpen, London, 2014.

[4] M. Navarro, R. M. S. Justo, G. Y. S. Delgado, G. Visbal, *Curr. Pharm. Design*, **2021**, *27*, 1763–1789.

[5] R. W. Brown, C. J. T. Hyland, *MedChemComm* **2015**, *6*, 1230–1243.

[6] Y. C. Ong, S. Roy, P. C. Andrews, G. Gasser, *Chem. Rev.* **2019**, *119*, 730–796.

[7] Y. Lin, Y. Ching Ong, S. Keller, J. Karges, R. Bouchene, E. Manoury, O. Blacque, J. Müller, N. Anghel, A. Hemphill, C. Häberli, A. C. Taki, R. B. Gasser, K. Cariou, J. Keiser, G. Gasser, *Dalton Trans.* **2020**, *49*, 6616–6626.

[8] M. De Rycker, B. Baragaña, S.L. Duce, I.H. Gilbert, *Nature* **2018**, *559*, 498–506.

[9] V. Kourbeli, E. Chontzopoulou, K. Moschovou, D. Pavlos, T. Mavromoustakos, I. P. Papanastasiou, *Molecules* **2021**, *26*, 4629.

[10] S. S. Santos, R. V. de Araujo, J. Giarolla, O. E. Seoud, E. I. Ferreira, *Int. J. Antimicrob. Agents* **2020**, *55*, 105906.

[11] World Health Organization. Chagas disease (American trypanosomiasis). https://www.who.int/health-topics/chagas-disease#tab=tab_1 (Accessed March 2022).

[12] World Health Organization. https://www.who.int/es/news-room/fact-sheets/detail/leishmaniasis (Accessed March 2022).

[13] J. Brindha, M. Balamurali, K. Chanda, *Front. Chem.* **2021**, *9*, 1–19.

[14] A. S. Nagle, S. Khare, A. B. Kumar, F. Supek, A. Buchynskyy, A. Mathison, C. J. N. Chennamaneni, N. K. Pendem N. Buckner, F. S. Gelb, M. H. Molteni, *Chem. Rev.* **2014**, *114*, 11305–11347.

[15] S. Burza, S. L. Croft, M. Boelaert, *The Lancet* **2018**, *392*, 951–970.

[16] S.K. Kwofie, E. Broni, B. Dankwa, K. S. Enninful, G. B. Kwarko, L. Darko, R. Durvasula, P. Kempaiah, B. Rathi, W. A. Miller, III, A. Yaya, M. D. Wilson, *Curr. Top. Med. Chem.* **2020**, *20*, 349–366.

[17] World Health Organization. http://www.who.int/trypanosomiasis_african/ (Accessed March 2022.

[18] O. T. Kayode, C. K. Lele, A. A. A. Kayode, *Glob. J. Infect. Dis. Clin. Res.* **2020**, *6*, 37–41.

[19] S. P. S. Rao, M. P. Barrett, G. Dranoff, C. J. Faraday, C. R. Gimpelewicz, A. C. Hailu, L. Jones, J. M. Kelly, J. K. Lazdins-Helds, P. Mäser, J. Mengel, J. C. Mottram, C. E. Mowbray, D. L. Sacks, P. Scott, G. F. Späth, R. L. Tarleton, J. M. Spector, T. T. Diagana, *ACS Infect. Dis.* **2019**, *5*, 152–157.

[20] N. M. El-Sayed, P. J. Myler, G. Blandin, M. Berriman, J. Crabtree, G. Aggarwal, E. Caler, H. Renauld, E. A. Worthey, C. Hertz-Fowler, E. Ghedin, C. Peacock, D. C. Bartholomeu, B. J. Haas, A.-N. Tran, J. R. Wortman, U. C. M. Alsmark, S. Angiuoli, A. Anupama, J. Badger, F. Bringaud, E. Cadag, J. M. Carlton, G. C. Cerqueira, T. Creasy, A. L. Delcher, A. Djikeng, T. M. Embley, C. Hauser, A. C. Ivens, S. K. Kummerfeld, J. B. Pereira-Leal, D. Nilsson, J. Peterson, S. L. Salzberg, J. Shallom, J. C. Silva, J. Sundaram, S. Westenberger, O. White, S. E. Melville, J. E. Donelson, B. Andersson, K. D. Stuart, N. Hall, *Science* **2005**, *309*, 404–409.

[21] M. Aslett, C. Aurrecoechea, M. Berriman, J. Brestelli, B.P. Brunk, M. Carrington, D. P. Depledge, S. Fischer, B..Gajria, X. Gao, M. J. Gardner, A. Gingle, G. Grant, O. S. Harb, M. Heiges, C. Hertz-Fowler, R. Houston, F. Innamorato, J. Iodice, J.C. Kissinger, E. Kraemer, W. Li, F.J. Logan, J.A. Miller, S. Mitra, P.J. Myler, V. Nayak, C. Pennington, I. Phan, D.F. Pinney, G. Ramasamy, M.B. Rogers, D.S. Roos, C. Ross, D. Sivam, D.F. Smith, G. Srinivasamoorthy, C.J. Stoeckert, S. Jr, Subramanian, R. Thibodeau, A. Tivey, C. Treatman, G.Velarde, H. Wang, *Nucleic Acids Res.* **2010**, *38*, D457–D462.

[22] A. Ilari, I. Genovese, F. Fiorillo, T. Battista, I. De Ionna, A. Fiorillo, G. Colotti, *Mol. Pharmaceutics* **2018**, *15*(8), 3069–3078.

[23] K. Stuart, R. Brun, S. Croft, A. Fairlamb, R. E. Gurtler, J. McKerrow, S. Reed, R. Tarleton, *J. Clin. Invest.* **2008**, *118*,1301–1310.

[24] P. Chellan, P. J. Sadler, *Chem. Eur. J.* **2020**, *26*, 8676–8688.

[25] N. P. E. Barry, P. J. Sadler, *Chem. Commun.* **2013**, *49*, 5106–5131.

[26] R.A. Sánchez-Delgado, A. Anzellotti, *Mini-Rev. Med. Chem.* **2004**, *4*, 159–165.

[27] R. A. Sánchez-Delgado, A. Anzellotti, L. Suárez, in *Metal Ions in Biological Systems 41: Metal Ions and Their Complexes in Medication*, Eds. H. Sigel, A. Sigel, Marcel Dekker, New York, **2004**, p. 379.

[28] M. Claudel, J. V. Schwarte, K. M. Fromm, *Chemistry* **2020**, *2*, 849–899.

[29] R. Kour Sodhi, S. Paul, *Canc. Therapy Oncol. Int J.* **2019**, *14*, 555883.

[30] J. Karges, *ChemBioChem.* **2020**, *21*, 1–4.

[31] J. F. Turrens, *Mol. Asp. Med.* **2004**, *25*, 211–220.

[32] J. J. Wilson, S. J. Lippard, *Chem. Rev.* **2013**, *114*, 4470–4495.

[33] Metal compounds in the development of antiparasitic agents: rational design from basic chemistry to the clinic. D. Gambino, L. Otero, in *Metal Ions in Life Sciences*, Volume 19. *Essential Metals in Medicine: Therapeutic Use and Toxicity of Metal Ions in the Clinic.* Guest-edited by P. L. Carver. Series Editors: A. Sigel, E. Freisinger, R. K. Sigel, Walter De Gruyter Verlag, Berlin, Germany, **2019**. eISSN: 1868-0402. *Met. Ions Life Sci.* **2019**, *19*, 331–357.

[34] D. Gambino, L. Otero, *Inorganica Chim. Acta* **2012**, *393*, 103–114.

[35] D. Gambino, L. Otero, *Inorganica Chim. Acta* **2018**, *472*, 58–75.

[36] D. Gambino, L. Otero, *Front. Chem.* **2022**, *9*, 816266.

[37] K. Kostenkova, G. Scalese, D. Gambino, D. C. Crans, Highlighting the roles of transition metals and speciation in chemical biology. *Curr. Op. Chem. Biol.* Accepted 5 April 2022.

[38] E. H. Kerns, L. Di, *Drug-Like Properties: Concepts, Structure Design and Methods from ADME to Toxicity Optimization*, Academic Press, Amsterdam, **2008**.

[39] A. Martínez, T. Carreon, E. Iniguez, A. Anzellotti, A. Sánchez, M. Tyan, A. Sattler, L. Herrera, R. A. Maldonado, R. A. Sánchez-Delgado, *J. Med. Chem.* **2012**, *55*, 3867–3877.

[40] E. Iniguez, A. Varela-Ramirez, A. Martínez, C. L. Torres, R. A. Sánchez-Delgado, R. A. Maldonado, *Acta Tropica.* **2016**, *164*, 402–410.

[41] D. Gambino, *Coord. Chem. Rev.* **2011**, *255*, 2193–2203.

[42] J. C. Pessoa, S. Etcheverry, D. Gambino, *Coord. Chem. Rev.* **2015**, *301*, 24–48.

[43] A. Bijelic, M. Aureliano, A. Rompel, *Angew. Chem. Int. Ed. Engl.* **2019**, *58*, 2980–2999.

[44] D. C. Crans, L. Henry, G. Cardiff, B. I. Posner, in *Essential Metals in Medicine: Therapeutic Use and Toxicity of Metal Ions in the Clinic*, Ed P. Carver, De Gruyter, *Met. Ions Life Sci.* **2019**, *19*, 203–230.

[45] S. Kowalski, D. Wyrzykowski, I. Inkielewicz-Stepniak, *Molecules* **2020**, *25*, 1–25; T. Scior, J. A. Guevara-Garcia, Q. T. Do, H. Bernard, S. Laufer, *Curr. Med. Chem.* **2016**, *23*, 2874–2891.

[46] K. H. Thompson, J. Lichter, C. LeBel, M. C. Scaife, J. H. McNeill, C. Orvig, *J. Inorg. Biochem.* **2009**, *103*, 554–558.

[47] J. de Oliveira Carneiro Brum, T. C. Costa França, S. R. LaPlante, J. D. Figueroa Villar, *Mini Rev. Med. Chem.* **2020**, *20*, 342–368.

[48] S. N. Mali, B. R. Thorat, D. R. Gupta, A. Pandey, *Eng. Proc.* **2021**, *11*, 21.

[49] G. Verma, A. Marella, M. Shaquiquzzaman, M. Akhtar, M. Rahmat Ali, M. Mumtaz Alam, *J. Pharm. Bioallied Sci.* **2014**, *6*, 69–80.

[50] H. Beraldo, D. Gambino, *Mini Rev. Med. Chem.* **2004**, *4*, 159–165.

[51] R. P. Vieira, H. Beraldo, in *Ligand Design in Medicinal Inorganic Chemistry*, Ed T. Storr, John Wiley & Sons, Ltd., Chichester, UK, **2014**, 175–204.

Prospective Metallo-Drugs Against Neglected Tropical Diseases 213

[52] M. Fernández, L. Becco, I. Correia, J. Benítez, O. E. Piro, G. A. Echeverria, A. Medeiros, M. Comini, M. L. Lavaggi, M. González, H. Cerecetto, V. Moreno, J. Costa Pessoa, B. Garat, D. Gambino, *J. Inorg. Biochem.* **2013**, *127*, 150–160.

[53] M. Fernández, J. Varela, I. Correia, E. Birriel, J. Castiglioni, V. Moreno, J. Costa Pessoa, H. Cerecetto, M. González, D. Gambino, *Dalton Trans.* **2013**, *42*, 11900–11911.

[54] G. Scalese, J. Benítez, S. Rostan, I. Correia, L. Bradford, M. Vieites, L. Minini, A. Merlino, E.L. Coitino, E. Birriel, J. Varela, H. Cerecetto, M. González, J. Costa Pessoa, D. Gambino, *J. Inorg. Biochem.* **2015**, *147*, 116–125.

[55] M. F. Mosquillo, P. Smircich, A. Lima, S. A. Gehrke, G. Scalese, I. Machado, D. Gambino, B. Garat, L. Perez-Diaz, *Bioinorg. Chem. Appl.* **2020**, *2020*, 1–10.

[56] G. Scalese, I. Machado, C. Fontana, G. Risi, G. Salinas, L. Perez-Diaz, D. Gambino, *J. Biol. Inorg. Chem.* **2018**, *23*, 1265–1281.

[57] G. Scalese, I. Machado, G. Salinas, L. Pérez-Díaz, D. Gambino, *Molecules* **2021**, *26*, 5375.

[58] G. Scalese, I. Machado, I. Correia, J. Costa Pessoa, L. Bilbao, L. Pérez-Diaz, D. Gambino, *New J. Chem.* **2019**, *43*, 17756–17773.

[59] C. Rigol, C. Olea-Azar, F. Mendizábal, L. Otero, D. Gambino, M. González, H. Cerecetto, *Spectrochim. Acta Part A Mol. Biomol. Spectroscopy* **2005**, *61*, 2933–2938.

[60] L. Otero, J. D. Maya, A. Morello, C. Rigol, G. Barriga, J. Rodriguez, C. Folch, E. Norambuena, M. González, C. Olea Azar, H. Cerecetto, D. Gambino, *Med. Chem.* **2008**, *4*, 11–17.

[61] G. Aguirre, L. Boiani, H. Cerecetto, M. González, A. Denicola, L. Otero, D. Gambino, C. Rigol, C. Olea-Azar, M. Faundez, *Bioorg. Med. Chem.* **2004**, *12*, 4885–4893.

[62] M. Pagano, B. Demoro, J. Toloza, L. Boiani, M. González, H. Cerecetto, C. Olea-Azar, E. Norambuena, D. Gambino, L. Otero L, *Eur. J. Med. Chem.* **2009**, *44*, 4937–4943.

[63] C. Sarniguet, J. Toloza, M. Cipriani, M., M. Vieites, Y. Toledano-Magaña, J. C. García-Ramos, L. Ruiz-Azuara, V. Moreno, J. D. Maya, C. Olea Azar, D. Gambino, L. Otero, *Biol. Trace Elem. Res.* **2014**, *159*, 379–392.

[64] M. Cipriani, J. Toloza, L. Bradford, E. Putzu, M. Vieites, E. Curbelo, A. I. Tomaz, B. Garat, J. Guerrero, J. S. Gancheff, J. D. Maya, C. Olea Azar, D. Gambino, L. Otero, *Eur. J. Inorg. Chem.* **2014**, *27*, 4677–4689.

[65] E. Rodríguez Arce, E. Putzu, M. Lapier, J. D. Maya, C. Olea Azar, G. A. Echeverría, O. E. Piro, A. Medeiros, F. Sardi, M. Comini, G. Risi, G. Salinas, I. Correia, J. Costa Pessoa, L. Otero, D. Gambino, *Dalton Trans.* **2019**, *48*, 7644–7658.

[66] T. Marzo, S. Pillozzi, O. Hrabina, J. Kasparkova, V. Brabec, A. Arcangeli, G. Bartoli, M. Severi, A. Lunghi, F. Totti, C. Gabbiani, A. G. Quiroga, L. Messori, *Dalton Trans.* **2015**, *44*, 14896–14905.

[67] D. Cirri, S. Pillozzi, C. Gabbiani, J. Tricomi, G. Bartoli, M. Stefanini, E. Michelucci, A. Arcangeli, L. Messori, T. Marzo, *Dalton Trans.* **2017**, *46*, 3311–3317.

[68] L. Messori, L. Cubo, C. Gabbiani, A. Alvarez-Valdes, E. Michelucci, G. Pieraccini, C. Rios-Luci, L. G. León, J. M. Padrón, C. Navarro Ranninger, A. Cassini, A. G. Quiroga, *Inorg. Chem.* **2012**, *51*, 1717–1726.

[69] C. Viegas-Junior, A. Danuello, V. da Silva Bolzani, E. J. Barreiro, C. A. Manssour Fraga, *Cur. Med. Chem.* **2007**, *14*, 1829–1852.

[70] G. R. Zimmermann, J. Lehár, C. T. Keith. *Drug Discov. Today*, **2007**, *12*, 34–42.

[71] Y. Bansal, O. Silakari. *Eur. J. Med. Chem.* **2014**, *76*, 31–42.

[72] M. L. Bolognesi, *ACS Med. Chem. Lett.* **2019**, *10*, 273–275.

[73] A. Cavalli, M. L. Bolognesi, *J. Med. Chem.* **2009**, *52*, 7339–7359.

[74] D. Gibson, *J. Inorg. Biochem.* **2019**, *191*, 77–84.

[75] R. G. Kenny, C. J. Marmion, *Chem. Rev.* **2019**, *119*, 1058–1137.

[76] M. J. Rogers, J. C. Crockett, F. P. Coxon, J. Mönkkönen, *Bone* **2011**, *49*, 34–41.

[77] R. Docampo, S. N. J. Moreno, *Curr. Drug Targ.* **2001**, *1*, 51–61.

[78] B. Demoro, F. Caruso, M. Rossi, D. Benítez, M. González, H. Cerecetto, B. Parajón-Costa, J. Castiglioni, M. Gallizi, R. Docampo, L. Otero, D. Gambino, *J. Inorg. Biochem.* **2010**, *104*, 1252–1258.

[79] B. Demoro, F. Caruso, M. Rossi, D. Benítez, M. González, H. Cerecetto, M. Galizzi, L. Malayil, R. Docampo, R. Faccio, A.W. Mombrú, D. Gambino, L. Otero, *Dalton Trans.* **2012**, *41*, 6468–6476.

[80] B. Demoro, S. Rostán, M. Moncada, Z. H. Li, R. Docampo, C. Olea Azar, J. D. Maya, J. Torres, D. Gambino, L. Otero, *J. Biol. Inorg. Chem.* **2018**, *23*, 303–312.

[81] M. Cipriani, S. Rostán, I. León, Z.H. Li, J. S. Gancheff, U. Kemmerling, C. Olea-Azar, S. Etcheverry, R. Docampo, D. Gambino, L. Otero, *J. Biol. Inorg. Chem.* **2020**, *25*, 509–519.

[82] M. Soba, G. Scalese, F. Casuriaga, N. Pérez, N. Veiga, G. A. Echeverría, O. E. Piro, R. Faccio, L. Pérez-Díaz, G. Gasser, I. Machado, D. Gambino, *Dalton Tran.* **2023**, *52*, 1623–1641.

[83] J. F. Turrens, C. L. Newton, L. Zhong, F. R. Hernández, J. Whitfield, R. Docampo, *FEMS Microbiol. Lett.* **1999**, *175*, 217–221.

[84] D. Tobin, M. Arvanitidis, R. H. Bisby, *Biochem. Biophys. Res. Commun.* **2002**, *299*, 155–159.

[85] G. F. dos Santos Fernandes, A. R. Pavan, J. L. dos Santos, *Curr. Pharm. Design* **2018**, *24*, 1–16.

[86] M. Vieites, P. Smircich, B. Parajón-Costa, J. Rodríguez, V. Galaz, C. Olea-Azar, L. Otero, G. Aguirre, H. Cerecetto, M. González, A. Gómez-Barrio, B. Garat, D. Gambino, *J. Biol. Inorg. Chem.* **2008**, *13*, 723–735.

[87] C. G. Hartinger, P. J. Dyson, *Chem. Soc. Rev.* **2009**, *38*, 391–401.

[88] E. R. Rodríguez Arce, M. F. Mosquillo, L. Pérez-Díaz, G. A. Echeverría, O. E. Piro, A. Merlino, E. L. Coitiño, C. M. Ribeiro, C. Q. F. Leite, F. R. Pavan, L. Otero, D. Gambino, *Dalton Trans.* **2015**, *44*, 14453–14464.

[89] M. F. Mosquillo, P. Smircich, M. Ciganda, A. Lima, D. Gambino, B. Garat, L. Pérez-Díaz, *Metallomics* **2020**, *12*, 813–828.

8 Challenges in Targeting Cyanide Poisoning: *Advantages in Exploiting Metal Complexes in Its Treatment*

Sigridur G. Suman
Science Institute
University of Iceland, Dunhagi 3, IS-107 Reykjavik, Iceland
sgsuman@hi.is

CONTENTS

1 Introduction 216
2 Cyanide Concentrations *In Vivo* 217
    2.1 Tissue Uptake and Distribution of Cyanide 218
    2.2 Treatment of Cyanide Toxicity with Organic Compounds 220
3 Metal Antidotes 221
    3.1 Methemoglobin 221
    3.2 Cobalt Compounds and Toxicity 224
    3.3 Cobalt Compounds in Clinical Use 225
    3.4 Emerging Cobalt Compounds 225
    3.5 Molybdenum Compounds 228
4 Advantages of Metalloantidotes 230
5 Concluding Remarks 232
Abbreviations and Definitions 232
References 233

ABSTRACT

The identification of novel treatment regimens to address cyanide toxicity in humans has been investigated by many researchers. One important area of clinical focus involves the identification of cyanide biomarkers that may be used to confirm and quantify cyanide poisoning. The clinical setting also necessitates consideration of concurrent CO poisoning since cyanide poisoning often occurs as inhalation injury

DOI: 10.1201/9781003272250-8

in smoke. The reader is referred to Chapter 14 of the *Metal Ions in Life Sciences* series, volume 19, where the chemical and clinical aspects of metal-containing antidotes are discussed. In this chapter, we include an overview of the chemistry of the commercially available metal antidotes, and a brief discussion of emerging approaches relevant to the benefits of using a metallo-drug. In this context we also discuss tissue distribution of cyanide, the organic molecules tested as antidotal treatment and challenges associated with their use and how metal antidotes can avoid some of the physiological pitfalls presented by these organic molecules.

KEYWORDS

Cyanide; Antidotes; Cobalt; Molybdenum; Cobinamide; Cobalamin; Inhalation Injuries; Tissue Distribution; Methemoglobin; Poisoning Treatments

1 INTRODUCTION

The main sources of cyanide poisoning, its clinical manifestations, analytical methods for confirming cyanide poisoning, a summary of commercially available metal-based antidotes, and a brief discussion of emerging approaches to tackle cyanide toxicity have been comprehensively reviewed recently [1]. This chapter builds on this review, providing a brief overview for context, citing relevant literature, and bringing the reader up to date on the latest developments in this important field.

Cyanide poisoning is no doubt an interesting topic for a diverse group of scientists, physicians, and clinical practitioners. It is difficult to detect, challenging to confirm its presence, and almost impossible to confirm if the treatment was a success [2]. Unpredictable, but very deadly. Cyanide is an endogenous molecule that is metabolized by several pathways, the most prominent involving sulfur transferase enzymes, which catalyze the conversion of cyanide to thiocyanate [1]. It is usually present in low concentrations in blood *and* is excreted at a rate sufficiently rapid to prevent build-up under normal circumstances [3]. The cyanide anion hydrolyzes *in vivo* to form hydrogen cyanide (HCN) allowing it to dissipate freely into tissue. Its small size and polarity results in high distribution to all major tissues including lungs, liver, kidneys, heart, and brain [4, 5]. These tissues have received the most attention in literature owing to life-threatening consequences if compromised, and are the ones mostly discussed in this chapter.

Detoxification of cyanide with a single compound has not been entirely successful since most compounds that have been employed and tested simply do not have comparable biological availability and distribution as cyanide [6]. To date, none of the commercial antidotes have been proven to reverse cyanide inhibition of cytochrome c oxidase (CcO) *in vivo*. Its inhibition of CcO is non-competitive, not irreversible, although the enzyme's natural substrate, O_2, cannot reverse its inhibition even under hyperbaric conditions [7]. Antidotal treatment has focused on neutralization of cyanide from tissues and blood by either transformation into a less toxic thiocyanate or by binding via a metal ion center [8].

Metal-Based Compounds Targeting Cyanide Poisoning

The challenges in targeting cyanide poisoning become obvious from its physical properties which allow it to travel freely *in vivo*, and the fact that all potential accidental exposure routes (inhalation, oral, and absorption) potentially lead to death [6]. Notwithstanding this, these three entry points of cyanide result in different expressions of cyanide toxicity allowing for consideration of different transport routes for detoxification [7].

Both organic and inorganic compounds to combat cyanide poisoning were screened with various successes [1, 8–23]. Organic compounds selected often have biological relevance but because of their own biological function and metabolic pathways they can become ineffective or the large doses employed to increase efficacy may cause adverse effects [20].

Screened inorganic compounds may be divided into metal complexes and inorganic salts. The salts are divided into "methemoglobin (MetHb) formers" or "sulfur donors" to encompass their intended function *in vivo*. They target specific biological pathway to detoxify cyanide by forming MetHb or donating sulfur to the rhodanese enzyme respectively [1, 24]. The synthetic metal complexes including those of molybdenum and cobalt bind cyanide very effectively are not rendered ineffective by biological functions and have shown superior cyanide-scavenging properties to organic molecules [1, 13, 25]. In contrast, metal centers in MetHb and cobalamine (Cbl) that form strong bonds with cyanide also have important biological functions in their own right but can also be sequestered *in vivo* for use in multiple biological functions [26–30].

2 CYANIDE CONCENTRATIONS *IN VIVO*

As an endogenous molecule cyanide is found in the bloodstream at quantifiable levels of about 78 µg L^{-1} [3]. This concentration is believed to arise from catabolic processes, for example, breakdown and regeneration of neuronal tissue [31]. Double to triple cyanide concentrations are found in the blood of heavy smokers [32], and individuals exposed to cyanides in their daily environment also have higher background concentrations [33]. About 3 mg L^{-1} is considered a lethal blood concentration [34–36]. Sources of cyanide poisoning were covered recently [1] as well as its common distribution in the environment [33].

The main cause of cyanide poisoning arises from inhibition of oxidative phosphorylation in the mitochondria, halting aerobic respiration [37]. The tissues that are most strongly affected are those that are most O_2 dependent e.g. brain and heart. Hydrogen cyanide inhalation has been suggested to retain over half of the HCN in lungs as dissolved gas [38], although experimental methodology and quantification of gas retained *in vivo* is a complex matter [39]. Cyanide blood concentrations are notoriously difficult to generalize and fire victims have been reported with cyanide blood concentrations as low as 0.12 mg L^{-1} [40]. This large range of lethal concentration is believed to be related to the rapid dissipation of cyanide from the bloodstream [2] and concurrent carbon monoxide (CO) poisoning in fire victims [34, 41].

The distribution of cyanide in tissues and known elimination pathways are described briefly in the following two subsections. The sections are by no means complete; rather, they serve to provide a representative overview with relevant literature cited should the reader wish to delve further into the topics.

2.1 Tissue Uptake and Distribution of Cyanide

Cyanide is found in all major tissues, including the lungs, liver, kidneys, brain, and heart muscle [2, 4, 35, 42]. It appears to play a role as a signaling or transport molecule *in vivo* [43], although most researchers believe it is a metabolic product that is transported as waste. It has also been speculated that cyanide has a reduced evolutionary role as a primary molecule [44, 45]. In either case, endogenous cyanide is formed from amide metabolism and is well known as a side product in neuron metabolism [31].

The literature reflects large variances in case reports and toxicity ranges. These may appear as discrepancies but are fully explained upon further examining each case [36]. All administration routes show varied onset of action depending on the form of cyanide exposure [46, 47]. Inhalation of HCN is the most rapid mode of absorption, followed by oral consumption of soluble cyanides such as KCN or NaCN, and finally a much slower dermal absorption [42]. Soluble cyanide salts of transition metals are common in metallurgy as their isolation is a convenient and efficient route to purify metals [48, 49]. These salts have been suggested as a route for dermal poisoning of workers using efficient ventilators during metal purification work [42]. The exact composition and solubility of the cyanide salt in question affects significantly the onset of toxicity [36].

Furthermore, tissue distribution of cyanide is species-dependent [50, 51]. Species-based tolerance toward cyanide is not size related, since dogs have much lower tolerance than mice, and mice and humans have comparable tolerance [52, 53]. This tolerance has been related specifically to the amount and bioavailability of the rhodanese enzyme which is significantly deficient in dogs compared to mice or humans [42].

As a representative example, Ballantyne investigated the distribution of cyanide in the liver, kidney, brain, heart, and lungs of rabbits, after lethal cyanide exposure, and focused on variations according to the chosen administration route [50]. Administration routes employed were intraperitoneal (IP), intramuscular (IM), percutaneous (PC), transocular (TO), and inhalation (INH). Brain and heart tissues have high demand for O_2. As such, O_2 deprivation influences these tissues strongly. Comparable cyanide concentration profiles were found in these tissues for all routes. In contrast, lung and liver tissues showed administration-dependent differences in cyanide concentrations [50]. Kidneys showed the lowest cyanide tissue concentrations regardless of the administration route apart from INH which gave undetectable cyanide concentrations in the kidney and liver [50].

The IP route gave two to three times higher cyanide concentrations in the liver compared to the INH route [50] and, of note, higher concentrations than any other tissue for all routes. The INH route gave low cyanide concentrations for all tissues, respectively [5]. The variance in cyanide uptake in the tissue samples investigated was attributed to the property of each tissue. Interestingly but perhaps not surprisingly, a parallel study by the same group showed variance in cyanide concentrations in tissues, following IM administration, across species (sheep, rat, monkey, pig, and rabbit). More comprehensive details may be found in the paper by Ballantyne who conducted this study [50].

Cyanide is classified as a neurotoxin, exerting most of its significant influence on the brain (encephalopathy) and the central nervous system (CNS). Not surprisingly, tremors and headaches are symptoms arising from mild cyanide poisoning, progressing to severe Parkinson-like symptoms after acute poisoning from oral exposure [42]. More comprehensive details regarding toxic doses may be found in Chapter 14 of MILS-19 [1].

Anaerobic metabolism is an inevitable outcome of cyanide toxicity, and it is accompanied by a rise in lactate plasma concentrations [54, 55]. Lactic acidosis is now a useful diagnostic tool for poisoning by cyanide in both smoke inhalation injury victims and pure cyanide poisoning cases [55]. A study of data from pure cyanide poisoning cases from 1988 to 2015 revealed its significant correlation as a primary marker [55]. Emerging analytical methods for rapid cyanide blood concentration are hoped to greatly improve emergency care [56].

Neurotoxic effects of cyanide poisoning have been reported to influence dopaminergic, GABAergic, and glutamatergic pathways through changes in ion regulation [3, 57]. Pathological changes during acute exposure may complicate recovery where changes in ion regulation and neurotransmitter release, nitric oxide, and possibly peroxide/ROS formation take place [3, 57, 58]. Myelin degeneration was observed via both dietary and inhalation exposure [42]. Elimination routes of cyanide (Figure 1) are few, with a minor route in sweat, but its major elimination pathway accounting for 80% of total cyanide metabolism is carried out by converting it to thiocyanate by the rhodanese enzyme and excreting it with urine through the kidneys [5, 59]. A second important elimination pathway, accounting for 15% of its metabolism, is a reaction with cysteine [60] in the synthesis of 2-amino-2-thiazoline-4-carboxylic acid and its tautomer [36]. Other elimination routes form formate, CO_2, and binding by vitamin-B_{12} [60].

Cyanide amelioration may require treatment with a highly bioavailable compound, yet reactive and selective to cyanide, with very low cytotoxicity to cells

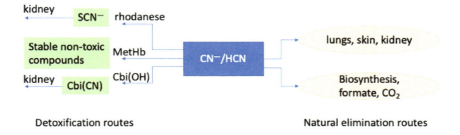

FIGURE 1 Elimination routes of cyanide *in vivo*.

and with a high safety profile. Since thiocyanate elimination is a major metabolic pathway, it is attractive to connect that into an amelioration approach. Many researchers have exploited this route, where thiosulfate has been particularly successful as a sulfur donor [1, 8, 9, 14, 61].

2.2 TREATMENT OF CYANIDE TOXICITY WITH ORGANIC COMPOUNDS

As described, cyanide effects its toxicity through different routes and can spread widely *in vivo*, affecting many different enzymes and cell functions [36]. It has been suggested that a cyanide antidote should not be a single compound because of its widespread activity and partially unknown mode of action.

Treatment methods focus on trapping and converting cyanide before it can do permanent tissue damage [1]. Despite the simplicity of Table 1 (Section 3), describing commercial antidotes, numerous organic compounds were screened and studied with respect to efficacy to ameliorate specific cyanide-induced inhibition and toxicity [3, 20, 31, 58, 62].

In an eloquent study, Borowitz et al. identified a series of six major biomarkers indicative of cyanide toxicity in cultured rat pheochromocytoma (PC 12) cells: CcO activity, superoxide dismutase activity (SOD), catalase activity, cytosolic-free Ca levels, peroxide formation [62], and dopamine release [36]. These biomarkers were employed to screen 39 substances, mainly organic, as anti-cyanide compounds. The compounds screened included anti-convulsants, adrenergic blockers, antioxidants, and anti-psychotics. Of the compounds tested and based on a composite scoring across all six biological assays, four compounds, namely carbamazepine, mannitol, allopurinol, and phenytoin, were ranked highest in terms of their potential to act as potent anti-cyanide poisoning compounds. Established cyanide antidotes, namely pyruvate, mercaptopyruvate, a-ketoglutarate, naloxone, and flunarizine, were also ranked highly in this study. As the focus of this chapter is related to metal-based cyanide antidotes, the reader is directed to this study by Borowitz et al. which also includes a comprehensive table listing the 39 compounds and their relative activities against CcO, SOD, catalase, cytosolic-free Ca levels, peroxide formation and dopamine release in PC 12 cells [62]. Since 1993, the development of organic compounds has focused on sulfur-containing molecules. Of particular note are dimethyltrisulfide and mercaptopyruvate (sulfanegen), both are substrates for sulfur transferases and act as sulfur donors [11, 63]. Of the many organic compounds screened, only mercaptopyruvate progressed further and into *in vivo* studies [10–12, 63–65].

Mercaptopyruvate can easily transport into tissue and has high bioavailability [10, 11, 63, 64]. It showed high promise as a small efficacious molecule for treatment against cyanide poisoning but metabolized quickly and proved unstable *in vivo* and with a problematic shelf life [10]. As a potential intramuscular administered drug, its low molecular weight and low toxicity suggested it would be superior to all other efforts [64, 65].

Metal-Based Compounds Targeting Cyanide Poisoning

TABLE 1

Content of Commercial Antidote Kits and Types of Compounds

Antidote Kit	Content	Mode of Action	Antidote
Cyanokit™	Hydroxocobalamin	Coordination	Metallo-drug
Nithiodote™	$NaNO_3$	MetHb former	Inorganic salts
	$Na_2S_2O_3$	Sulfur donor	
Kelocyanor™	$[Co_2(EDTA)(H_2O)_4]$	Coordination	Metallo-drug
CAK™	$Na_2S_2O_3$	Sulfur donor	Inorganic
	$NaNO_3$/amyl nitrite	MetHb former	NO release
4-DMAP	$4\text{-HO-}C_6H_4\text{-NMe}_2$	MetHb former	Organic compound
Thiosulfate	$Na_2S_2O_3$	Sulfur donor	Inorganic salt

CAK, cyanide antidote kit; 4-DMAP, 4-dimethylaminophenol; $C_5H_{11}ONO$, amyl nitrite.

3 METAL ANTIDOTES

Commercially, seven antidotes are available either as single compounds or as kits. They are: Cyanokit™, Nithiodote™, and Kelocyanor™, Cyanide Antidote Kit (CAK™), 4-DMAP, and thiosulfate. Their specific composition is given in Table 1. A striking discovery looking at the table is that out of seven treatments, five aim to use a metal complex and one is a sulfur donor for the rhodanese enzyme.

As Table 1 shows, thiosulfate poses as an efficient sulfur donor, but it has a challenge *in vivo* where it needs to donate sulfur to rhodanese enzyme in the liver under conditions where its solubility is low, and a large excess is administered to increase its concentration in the liver [61]. (Rhodanese is an enzyme with a modest turnover and its bioavailability is highest in the liver in humans [66, 67].) Despite these hurdles, thiosulfate was widely used as an antidote off-label [1]. Of note, two metal centers, cobalt and iron, are incorporated into antidotes as presented in Table 1. Cobalt is administered as Co(II) as an antidote to yield Co(III) cyano products. MetHb is accessed by oxidizing hemoglobin (Hb) Fe(II) center to Fe(III) *in vivo*. The following sections will describe these compounds, their bioavailability, and their abilities as treatment agents for cyanide poisoning. New metal complexes incorporating cobalt and molybdenum are in development and their reported abilities to combat cyanide poisoning are also described.

3.1 METHEMOGLOBIN

Our previous review in MILS-19 discussed the use of nitrates to form MetHb as an antidote. This section focuses on the antidotal properties of MetHb as a metallo-drug [1].

Hemoglobin (Hb) is a metalloprotein incorporating Fe(II) which binds and transports O_2 from the lungs to tissues as oxyhemoglobin (Figure 2). It returns, in its

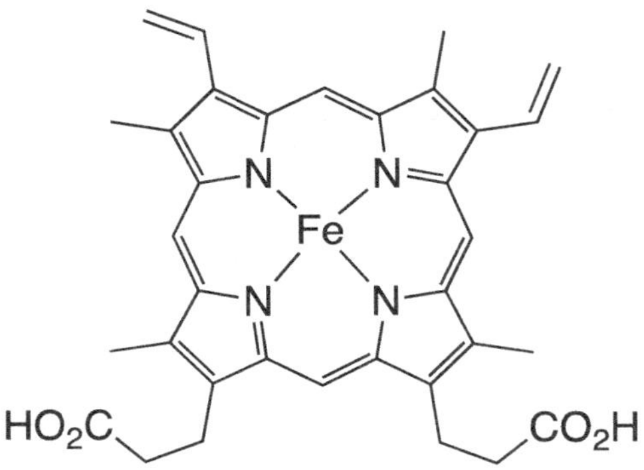

FIGURE 2 Heme A porphyrin with Fe center.

deoxygenated state, from tissues to the lungs to excrete CO_2 as carbaminohemoglobin [68–70]. The CO_2 transport is supplementary to other CO_2 release mechanisms *in vivo* [71, 72]. The Fe(II) center in Hb binds competitively to small molecules such as CO, H_2S, CN^-, SO, and S^{2-} [69]. It can also carry a NO molecule, bound via a protein side chain thiol group, which is released in parallel with O_2 release. The NO carried in such a way is believed to have a regulatory function [73]. Administered NO in the form of nitrate is able to oxidize the Fe in Hb partially to Fe(III) or fully to form methemoglobin (MetHb) [1]. When MetHb is formed *in vivo* under oxidative stress, its main physiological reduction route is by NADH cytochrome b5 reductase [74]. In the clinic, methylene blue is able to reduce it back to Fe(II) [19, 20]. MetHb does not bind O_2; rather, its Fe(III) center binds the small molecules above (except CO) better than the Hb Fe(II) center [70].

MetHb formation has been used to treat cyanide poisoning because of its natural presence *in vivo*, and its facile route of reduction back to Hb, although it requires careful consideration due to loss of O_2 transport in parallel with cyanide binding. Methemoglobin has two key properties that play an important role in the coordination of cyanide. Firstly, the coordination of cyanide is not cooperative suggesting that cyanide binding is not dependent on the cyanide concentration present. Secondly, despite rapid cyanide binding to MetHb, the cyanide-binding mode is non-linear leading to facile dissociation of the cyanide anion from MetHb *in vivo* [75]. The therapeutic MetHb ratio to total Hb has been reported as a range of 25–40% because of individual hematocrit variations [17, 76]. The % volume of Hb in blood, or hematocrit, makes up 36–50% of the total content of red blood cells in humans. The following text describes the coordination chemistry of cyanide with MetHb in more detail.

Oxidation of Fe(II) in Hb, generating the Fe(III)-containing MetHb, significantly increases the binding affinity of cyanide to the metalloprotein [70], The few equilibrium constants for the formation of the complex cyanMetHb [73, 77, 78] (taking the effect of the H^+ competition in the cases of conditional constants determined at pH = 7.4 [77, 78]) are around or somewhat higher than 10^8, much higher compared to the value for the CcO-cyanide complex ($\sim 10^5$ M^{-1}) [77]. Consequently,

Metal-Based Compounds Targeting Cyanide Poisoning

coordination of cyanide to MetHb in the bloodstream occurs, which induces a rebalancing of the cyanide concentration between the cells and the bloodstream.

The reaction mechanism and kinetic aspects of cyanide binding to MetHb have been discussed in several papers [66, 77–80]. It was found that cyanide binding is at least a two-step process that appears to be non-cooperative, contrary to what is well known for Hb O_2 binding [69]. This property is favorable for intentional binding of cyanide with MetHb. Cyanide binding is expected to result in a low spin Fe(III) complex where a spin conversion step from high spin Fe(II) is necessary to complete the binding [78]. Kinetic reaction of MetHb A and cyanide was found to take place via a *pseudo*-first-order time dependence [78]. However, both the thermodynamic and kinetic behaviors show heterogeneity and at least two steps are required to describe its binding, presumably arising from the dissimilar high-low spin states of the four iron centers in the protein [79, 80], suggesting cyanide coordination is indiscriminate of the spin state of the Fe center.

Concurrent cyanide and CO poisoning [7] encountered in smoke inhalation injuries leads to a competition of O_2 and CO for the Fe(II) in Hb which compromises both the O_2-carrying capacity of Hb and disrupts aerobic cellular respiration [20]. CO poisoning is primarily caused by the formation of carboxyhemoglobin and severely reduced O_2 transport ability [81]. MetHb formation treatment is a risky approach for smoke inhalation victims mostly because of its influence on the O_2-carrying capabilities of Hb [82]. Hyperbaric oxygen therapy (HBO) is a standard treatment for CO poisoning [83], although use of 100% O_2 has also been claimed as sufficiently effective [83].

In the clinic, MetHb is formed by oxidizing the iron center with "methemoglobin formers" (see Table 1) [17, 82, 84]. To prevent latent cyanide poisoning, thiosulfate is administered as a co-treatment to provide a sulfur donor into the bloodstream and liver to capture the cyanide when released and convert it to thiocyanate for excretion as a non-toxic product [17, 76]. This treatment is dependent on confirmation of cyanide poisoning before treatment by determining the actual concentration of cyanide in blood, and confirmation of efficacious MetHb generation in terms of hematocrit values [20].

The "Cyanide Antidote kit" (CAK™) contains sodium nitrite, amyl nitrite, and sodium thiosulfate (Table 1). It has been suggested that nitrites have therapeutic effects as vasodilators that can become severe and lead to cardiovascular collapse in the absence of cyanide poisoning [7]. The uncertainty of the outcomes from nitrite use has led some researchers to recommend its suspension [20, 85, 86]. Fear of loss of O_2 transport capacity in victims of smoke inhalation injuries and concurrent CO poisoning lead to case study reports of elimination of its use in the commercial antidote kit [76, 82, 84].

Confirmation of cyanide poisoning and quantification of MetHb present after nitrite administration is an important step in the safe use of nitrite antidotes. Its quantification requires determination of its concentration by subtracting all other Hb, including any cyanMetHb present [87]. Both the traditional Evelyn-Malloy method and the most used CO-oxymetric method [87] lead to a potential judgment error in the level of MetHb formed. High MetHb concentrations should discourage use of additional nitrites, but low MetHb levels certainly do not suggest it is safe to administer more nitrites. Blood analysis for cyanide concentrations via acid digestion and the König reaction [88] is also problematic because of acid stability of the cyanocobalamin in the *in vitro* media [7].

Use of MetHb is selective and safe at carefully controlled conditions. The chemistry involved is based on physiologically favorable metal binding constants to effectively compete with CcO for cyanide binding, and the following physiological reduction of the cyanMetHb does not give rise to latent cyanide poisoning [75, 78, 84, 89]. The downside is the requirement for carefully controlled conditions rendering MetHb as a non-option for concurrent cyanide and CO poisoning [7]. Analytical methods for quantification of MetHb and for cyanide blood concentration determination are both few and need to be interpreted with caution [7, 87].

3.2 COBALT COMPOUNDS AND TOXICITY

Early cobalt compounds tested for antidotal efficacy against cyanide toxicity were chloride, nitrite, and acetate salts of Co(II) [90]. Cobalt nitrite and ethylenediaminetetraacetic acid (EDTA) compounds showed promising results [90], although only $[Co_2(EDTA)(H_2O)_4]$ was further developed as the Kelocyanor™ antidote [16]. Table 2 showcases the cobalt compounds discussed in this chapter with key references.

Cobalt toxicity presents itself in the absence of cyanide intoxication [91] requiring confirmation of poisoning prior to treatment due to possible adverse effects [8, 92]. The antidotal mechanism associated with Co complexes relies on the stability and relatively non-toxic $[Co(CN)_6]^{3-/4-}$ formed for both the salts and Kelocyanor™ [93]. A recent meta-analysis of the literature provides a substantial summary of the antidotal efficacy data of Kelocyanor™ [92]. Glucose is included in the Kelocyanor™ kit for intravenous administration to provide an open chain keto (oxo) compound for Co to chelate in the absence of sufficient cyanide [92]. Co(II) also interferes with Fe and Cu homeostasis, and ion channels [91].

TABLE 2
Cobalt Compounds Studied for Cyanide Toxicity Amelioration

Compound	See Section	Key References	Brand Name
Cbl	MLS-19 Chapter 14	[15, 54, 109]	Cyanokit™
Cbi and salts of Cbi; bis (sulfate, sulfite, nitrate, nitrite) or with aqua or hydroxy co-ligand	This chapter	[12, 113, 115]	n/a
$[Co_2(EDTA)(H_2O)_4]$	MILS-19 Chapter 14	[1, 92]	Kelocyanor™
CoTMPyP	This chapter	[25, 116]	n/a
$CoN_4[11.3.1]$	This chapter	[25, 117]	n/a

n/a, not applicable.

Metal-Based Compounds Targeting Cyanide Poisoning

The salts $CoCl_2$ and $Co(NO_3)_2$ are able to enter cells, although the free metal ions cause toxicity *in vivo* by direct reactions with biomolecules in the Krebs cycle that contain oxo or keto groups like α-ketoglutarate, pyruvate, and dihydroxyacetone as well as many compounds that can form cyanohydrins (see Section 2) [91, 92]. They showed efficacy but without sufficient cyanide, Co reacts with other available compounds [90].

The only endogenous form of Co is in vitamin B12, and the free ions, especially Co(II), are considered harmful to humans at blood concentrations over 100 $\mu g\ L^{-1}$ [91, 94]. Free Co is mainly found in serum, whole blood, liver, kidneys, heart, and spleen [94]. Free Co that is administered orally is mainly excreted in feces and does not appear to accumulate *in vivo* [91].

3.3 COBALT COMPOUNDS IN CLINICAL USE

Cobalt compounds were the first metal-based compounds used to combat cyanide poisoning [95]. Chapter 14 in MILS-19 discusses two commercial cobalt antidotes, marketed under brand names Kelocyanor™ and Cyanokit™ (Table 2) [16, 96] and their use [1].

Vitamin B12 (a hydroxocobalamin) is an endogenous organometallic cobalt cofactor *in vivo* [97]. Cobalamins (Cbls) carry different common names according to their function where Vitamin B12 is cyanocobalamin derived from the commercial Cbl isolation process [93], and coenzyme B12 is 5'-deoxyadenosylcobalamin or Ado-Cbl [69]. Cobinamide (Cbi), a derivative of Cbl, has been more recently investigated as a cyanide antagonist [13]. It is isolated as Co(III) with two axially coordinated water molecules, where the nucleotide side chain has been hydrolyzed leaving an amide terminal group.

3.4 EMERGING COBALT COMPOUNDS

Several cobalt compounds (summarized in Table 2) have been studied as emerging treatments [13, 16, 25, 96, 98]. Cobalamin (Cbl) is a 15-membered tetra-aza corrole ring that has a pendant nucleotide benzimidazole (BenzIm) side chain that coordinates in an axial position to the Co center leaving a single coordination site vacant to bind cyanide. It is found as an intracellular compound where it is present as methyl-Cbl or Ado-Cbl. It is metabolized in the liver and excreted in urine and feces [99]. The two axial ligands carry two negative charges, and a corrin ring nitrogen atom carries the third charge. The hydroxo, cyano, and Ado ligands have high second-order ligand substitution rates of the order of $10^3\ M^{-1}s^{-1}$ [100]. The ligand exchange takes place via a dissociative interchange mechanism [100–102]. The corrin ring is partially conjugated resulting in a butterfly conformation with the Co(III) center in a tetragonally distorted octahedral geometry [69]. It is also well known that the BenzIm ligand plays an important role in the kinetic and thermodynamic stability of the Co bond with the other axial ligand [103–105]. Cbl antidotal efficacy is directly related to the Co(III) center binding of cyanide.

Exchanging the BenzIm ligand was for a long time considered inaccessible except toward HCN [103]. Modeling of the mechanism revealed that it was highly pH and ligand concentration dependent [101] where the base dissociates at high pH. Cyanide coordinates irreversibly to both axial sites at a pH of 11.7, forming $[Cbl(CN)_2]^-$ with the pendant deprotonated BenzIm [102]. $[Cbl(CN)_2]^-$ was described as a purple solid formed at a pH of 9.5 from a dilute KCN solution [106]. Enhanced *trans*-influence of cyanide increased the rate of the base-off ring opening reaction [102]. The difficulty in forming a base-off bis-cyanide coordinated Cbl left Cbl(OH) as the best Cbl antidote choice that was later developed into Cyanokit™. Chapter 14 in MILS-19 provides data for this antidote dose requirements [1]. The Cyanokit™ contains added thiosulfate for co-administration to serve as a sulfur donor to capture cyanide that dissociates from Cbl(CN) to prevent latent cyanide toxicity [54]. Thiosulfate and Cbl(OH) have been reported to react [98], and therefore they need to be administered separately intravenously [54].

If the nucleotide side chain of Cbl is hydrolyzed, then Cbi is formed. The Cbi derivative was first studied as a potential cyanide antagonist in 1964 [98]. It has a lower molecular weight than Cbl and slightly different physical properties [12]. Aqueous solubility of cobinamide sulfite and hydroxocobalamin were reported as 350 and 70 mM, respectively [12]. Safe dose of cobinamide sulfite was reported as 300 and 800 mg kg^{-1} for rats and mice, respectively [12]. It is isolated as the bis-aqua, aquahydroxo, and bis-hydroxo complexes, and is a dianion, a monoanion or neutral complex, respectively. The tetragonal distortion of the octahedral low spin Co(III) geometry renders the Co center very reactive [69]. The ligand exchange rates for Cbi have been studied in detail with cyanide for all three common versions [98, 100, 107], and the stepwise equilibrium constants for the cyanide binding were determined as at least $K_{CN(1)} \sim 10^{14}$ M^{-1} [105] for formation of $[Cbi(H_2O)(CN)]^+$, and $K_{CN(2)} \sim 10^8$ M^{-1} for the bis-cyanocobinamide, $Cbi(CN)_2$ [108]. The overall stability constant (β_2) for the two steps has been reported as $\sim 10^{19}$ M^{-1} [107]. As an antidote, this is a favorable modification of Vitamin B12a where it is possible to bind twice the amount of cyanide compared to the hydroxocobalamin. Aquahydroxo-cobinamide, $[Cbi(H_2O)(OH)]^+$, received a lot of attention and has been extensively studied as a potential antidote [12, 13, 109, 110], while $[Cbi(H_2O)(CN)]^+$ received more attention as a potential colorimetric indicator for blood cyanide concentrations [111, 112]. A study of the cyanide binding of $[Cbi(H_2O)(OH)]^+$ revealed it to be very fast. Interestingly, the $Cbi(CN)_2$ is formed first as the kinetic product, followed by $[Cbi(H_2O)(CN)]^+$ upon dissociation of one cyanide anion [113]. Detailed calculations of the equilibrium constants of Cbi with OH$^-$, CN$^-$, and H$_2$O ligands revealed $[Cbi(H_2O)(OH)]^+$ as superior to Cbl(OH) in *in vitro* studies and more efficacious in inhalation and ingestion models with fruit flies [110, 113]. The Cbi molecule has a charge of +2 after the BenzIm ligand is displaced via hydrolysis and therefore the formulations studied to enhance performance and solubility have led to multiple anion combinations for the Cbi^{2+} cation.

A Cbi sulfite complex was developed to improve aqueous solubility and to double the cyanide-binding ability compared to Cbl [10, 13]. This was likely

Metal-Based Compounds Targeting Cyanide Poisoning

successful since the efficacious dose of Cbi(OH)(SO$_3$) in mmol/kg is about half that of Cbl, although the exact formulation of Cbi was not reported but referred to as sulfitohydroxocobinamide [10, 13]. Sulfitocyanocobinamide and thiosulfatocobalamin are both known coordination compounds with reported formation constants as ~2.2×10^4 M^{-1} and 7.9×10^4 M^{-1}, respectively [114], demonstrating active interaction of these anions with the Co(III) center in Cbi and Cbl. The stable coordination of sulfite and thiosulfate ligands with Cbi were considered as likely explanation for why thiosulfate does not show enhanced antidotal efficacy when co-administered with Cbi [98]. The Cbi(OH)(SO$_3$) complex showed no clinical toxicity at high doses in mice [13]. Inhalation, IP, and IM studies in a mouse models showed promising results with increased survival compared to Cbl(OH). It also outperformed other commercial antidotes such as sodium thiosulfate, sodium nitrite, and the CAK™ treatment (Table 1) in experiments with IM administration, aqueous solubility, and absorption studies [13]. The Cbi(OH)(SO$_3$) complex showed improved survival up to 100% in a co-administration with sulfanegen (see Section 2) at HCN concentrations that gave about 40% survival for either compound by itself, and these promising results show additive effects rather than synergy due to their different mechanisms of action [10]. The downsides reported for Cbi(OH)(SO$_3$) and Cbi(OH)(H$_2$O) compounds were lack of stability in solution, and for the latter poor absorption after intramuscular injection [115]. Sulfitocobinamide showed improved shelf life but improved stability in solution was achieved by exchanging the axial ligands to the nitrite: (Cbi(NO$_2$)$_2$) and revealed improved absorption in intramuscular administration [115]. Pharmacokinetic properties of the *bis*-nitrite formulation were also reported [115]. A formulation with four equivalents of nitrite was used since nitrite appeared to dissociate from a stoichiometric Cbi(NO$_2$)$_2$ complex during the experiments. This compound showed performance parameters that could be satisfactory for antidote development [115]. Metabolism of Vitamin B12 takes place in the liver, and its major elimination route is in feces [98]. Presumably Cbi compounds may take the same route.

Two macrocyclic Co complexes, [CoTMPyP] and [Co-N$_4$[11.3.1]], were reported recently as potential cyanide-binding agents [25, 116]. Animal study data shows they are efficacious and promising in combating cyanide toxicity [25, 116, 117]. The importance of aqueous solubility has been considered in their choice, and similarly the lesson learned from the Co salts is reflected in that the compounds are macrocycles (Figure 3) rendering free Co presence *in vivo* as unlikely. Studies of the physiological properties of the compounds are at an early stage where their biological properties such as cytotoxicity, cell uptake, or tissue distribution and their aqueous solubility remain unreported.

The TMPyP ligand exhibits good water solubility as the perchlorate, iodide, chloride, and PF$_6^-$ salts [118]. The Co complex has been studied in ligand exchange reactions with cyanide and thiocyanate [119, 120] and absence of ligand aggregation was demonstrated in solution; an important property known to reduce solubility and solution properties of porphyrin compounds [120]. Interaction of [CoTMPyP] with BSA showed minor reduction in cyanide-binding

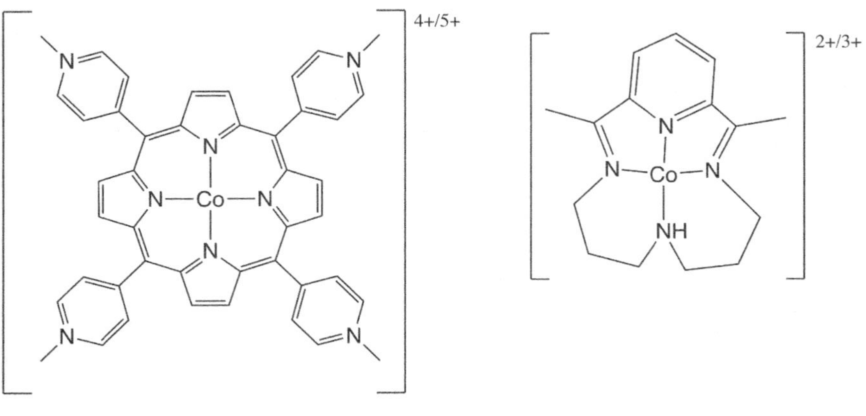

FIGURE 3 Recent cobalt compounds investigated as antidotes. Left: [CoTMPyP], where TMPyP is meso-tetra(4-*N*-methylpyridyl)porphyrin, right: [CoN$_4$[11.3.1]], where N$_4$[11.3.1] is 2,12-dimethyl-3,7,11,17-tetraazabicyclo[11.3.1] heptadeca-1,17-2,11,13,15-pentaene.

ability *in vitro* [116]. The [CoN$_4$[11.3.1]] complex was initially reported in 1970 but has regained interest recently for electrocatalytic reduction of CO$_2$ and cyanide toxicity treatment [117, 121, 122]. The Co center in this complex has a complicated oxidation state related to the proton on the secondary amine [122]. The crystal structure of the Co(II) complex is five coordinate with an acetonitrile axial ligand in *pseudo* square pyramidal geometry. For the animal studies, the bromide analog was used [117]. Both complexes appear well tolerated in mice and appear to prevent neurological damage according to a Rota-Rod test after therapeutic treatment [25].

3.5 MOLYBDENUM COMPOUNDS

Molybdenum compounds can affect many chemical transformations [123–126]. It is an essential metal for humans usually present in molybdoenzymes [125, 127, 128] and often non-toxic *in vivo* [129]. Biological studies have shown that in *vivo* Mo compound distribution and influence is largely dependent on the specific compound structure [130]. Minimal neurological influence or DNA damage was reported, but the general lack of data prevents specific conclusions [130].

Organometallic complexes of Mo have been studied as potential cancer therapy with biological studies focusing on cytotoxicity as a primary screen for potential efficacy [131]. Biological studies and DNA binding were reported for the Cp$_2$MoX$_2$ compounds (X=halogen) [132, 133], MoO$_2$(acac)$_2$ [134], and Mo-salophen complexes [135]. DNA binding was concluded as most likely a result of π-stacking since compounds lacking aromatic ligands did not exhibit

Metal-Based Compounds Targeting Cyanide Poisoning

DNA binding while other complexes showed concentration-dependent behavior [133, 135, 136].

The Mo=S moiety in $[MoS_4]^{2-}$ resembles the active site in xanthine oxidase and is a primary functional group present in many transformations by Mo compounds [137]. Another important ligand is the S_2^{2-} ligand which is polar and readily disproportionates into S^{2-} and S atom [138]. A reaction of cyanide and "MoS$_2$" results in formation of the thiocyanate and Mo=S moiety, which then further reacts with a sulfur donor and cyanide in a rapid reaction to form thiocyanate [29, 30, 139]. Interestingly, the thiocyanate formed does not coordinate and deactivate the metal center [126]. The reaction with the S_2^{2-} is a ligand-based reaction and the Mo remains in the +V oxidation state [126]. Employing the Mo(V) center is an advantage *in vivo* for applications looking to extend cell survival. Owing to its redox inertness, metal-based ROS generation that contributes to apoptosis and cell death is avoided [131]. Binuclear Mo complexes $[(L-L)Mo_2O_2(\mu-S)_2(S_2)]^-$, an example is shown in Figure 4, have been reported as potential cyanide detoxification agents [126, 140].

The binuclear Mo complex shown in Figure 4 combines the advantages of both small molecules and metal complexes: high aqueous solubility, biocompatibility, and ability to enter cells [140, 141]. It is non-toxic and likely enters mitochondria [141, 142]. The mechanism of action is catalyst activation via an initiation step that is a reaction of the compound with cyanide to form thiocyanate, followed by catalysis of the active species of the reaction of cyanide and a sulfur donor that could be thiosulfate or *in vivo* sulfur donor [1, 140, 143]. The compound is a stoichiometric sulfur donor by itself, offering alternatives in its use [140]. This class of compounds exhibits low cytotoxicity, stability in air, water, and acidic solutions [140, 141]. An interesting feature of this system is that it mimics the rhodanese enzyme (E) activity (Figure 5) where the sulfur donor reacts with the E to form a perthiol (E-S), which then reacts with cyanide to form thiocyanate [144].

Since rhodanese bioavailability is mostly in the liver, a synthetic non-toxic functional model with high bioavailability may show enhanced efficacy. These studies involving binuclear Mo compounds are at an earlier stage compared to those of Cbi compounds. Notwithstanding this, investigations into the biological and physiological effects of these Mo compounds demonstrated ability to enter cells and partitioning into cytosol, mitochondria, and nucleus [142].

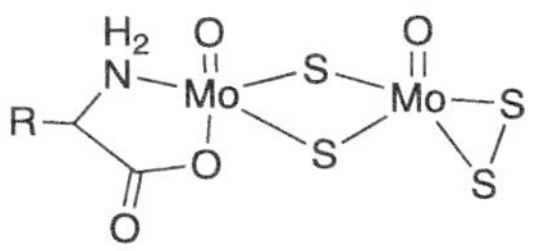

FIGURE 4 Structure of a binuclear molybdenum complex anion with S_2^{2-} ligands and deprotonated amino acid (R = amino acid side chain).

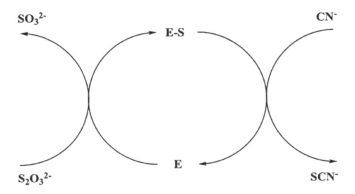

FIGURE 5 Detoxification of cyanide by rhodanese. (Reproduced from ref [1].)

4 ADVANTAGES OF METALLOANTIDOTES

Methods to target cyanide toxicity necessitate high bioavailability, high aqueous solubility, and negligible reaction chemistry *in vivo*. The main tissue targets are the brain and heart tissue necessitating the antidote to cross the blood-brain barrier, and preferably to enter cells. It should be pointed out that commercial amelioration approaches do not attempt to reactivate CcO but focus on rapidly coordinating cyanide to remove it from the bloodstream and tissues in the shortest time possible. The ultimate therapeutic goal in this field is to restore CcO activity requiring the antidote to enter mitochondria as well as crossing the blood-brain barrier. Another important aspect is the elimination of the antidote cyanide product. The metal complexes are eliminated in urine and feces (see Section 3).

For cyanide elimination, the chemical bond between the metal center and cyanide, and the reaction rate of the Co-CN bond formation is the largest advantage of using cobalt metallo-drugs. The properties of cyanide as a strong sigma donor, combined with the strong π acceptor properties associated with metal ions, drive this reaction. It results in compounds that are low spin metal centers and stable toward ligand exchange reactions in chance encounters *in vivo*. The metal ion oxidation state is important since cyanide, as an anionic ligand, forms a stronger bond with higher oxidation states. The $[Co_2(EDTA)(H_2O)_4]$ complex has two Co(II) ions but the analyzed excreted cyano complex is Co(III) [1]. The Cbi, Cbl, and all versions thereof employ Co(III). A stronger M-C bond with Fe(III) compared to Fe(II) is the reason why cyanide is less harmful to metalloenzymes other than CcO heme a3 [1]. Infrared frequencies of the cyanide stretching band of selected Fe(II)/Fe(III), Co(II/III), and Mo(V) cyano compounds show that cyanide exhibits strong π-bonding to the metal while Co(II) revealed significantly less π acceptor character with cyanide ν(CN) stretching energy higher than in the free cyanide [123, 142–144]. Metal ion size, electron configuration, and effective nuclear charge also play a role in the bond energies excluding detailed comparison here [145]. *In vivo* cyanide is mostly present as HCN and protonation of a neighboring proton acceptor most likely takes place simultaneously to coordination. The [CoN₄[11.3.1]] complex has been shown effective in hydrogen evolution reactions (HER) and CO_2 reduction in parallel with redox reactions and protonation/deprotonation where a secondary amine on the ligand was protonated/deprotonated in the process [122]. It follows that even if the Co(II) complex is administered as treatment, one expects the Co(III)cyano compound to form in the reaction with HCN.

In MetHb the alignment of the cyanide ligand is not linear [75] leading to less π-bonding and easier dissociation of the cyanide as a result of the weaker M-C bond. One cyanide ligand in $Cbi(CN)_2$ dissociates presumably promoted by *trans*-effects to form the thermodynamic product $[Cbi(CN)(H_2O)]$ [113]. Property comparison is a challenge, although important properties of the metalloantidotes that are directly comparable are molecular weights, aqueous solubility, bioavailability, and cyanide-binding ability. Table 3 summarizes selected data for the compounds discussed.

The molecular weights and solubility are important because when combined they determine the possible route of antidote administration. Intramuscular administration is the best approach for uncooperative victims and requires the least training of first responders. This requires balancing a high-performing compound with the lowest molecular weight possible. The three last entries in Table 3 are a potentially significant advancement in this direction where emerging compounds possess lower molecular weights and bind more cyanide compared to MetHb and Cbi/Cbl. MetHb(CN) and Cbl(CN) are naturally reduced back to Hb

TABLE 3
Molecular Weights, Water Solubility, and Cyanide-Binding Ability per Mol of Metalloantidotes for Cyanide Toxicity

Compound	MW, g mol⁻¹	s, g L⁻¹	Enters Mitochondria?	Crosses BBB?	#CN/mol
MetHb	~ 64,500	Soluble[a]	No	Yes	1
Cbl	1355	12.5	Yes	Yes	1
Cbi(SO₃)(OH)	1015	355	[b]	[b]	2
[Co₂(EDTA)(H₂O)₄]	482	Soluble[a]	Yes	Yes	4–6
CoTMPyP	736	Soluble[a]	[b]	[b]	2
CoN₄[11.3.1]	477	Soluble[a]	[b]	[b]	2
[Mo₂O₂(μ-S)₂(L-L)]	492[c]	103[c]	[b]	[b]	~8

BBB, blood-brain barrier.
[a] Measured values were not found.
[b] Presumably yes.
[c] Representative for a series of compounds, where L-L is: amino acid [140].

and Cbl; the cyanide further dissociates to be metabolized by natural routes (see Sections 2.1 and 3). Latent cyanide toxicity is possible under these conditions, and co-administration of compounds like thiosulfate acting as sulfur donors acts as a preventive measure forming thiocyanate that is excreted through the kidneys. Metalloantidotes have the advantage of forming stable compounds with cyanide inducing rapid reduction of cyanide toxicity.

5 CONCLUDING REMARKS

Numerous valiant efforts and many creative ideas have been presented by different researchers, spanning over a century, to tackle cyanide poisoning in humans. Metal complexes appear to offer superior advantages over alternative approaches to tackle this difficult problem. This is validated by the available commercial treatments for cyanide poisoning that all rely on a metal complex for efficacy. Use of small molecules has demonstrated less efficacy than expected with conclusions that these small molecules, if endogenous, are metabolized or incorporated into physiological catabolism before they perform their intended work. Treatment of cyanide poisoning with a non-toxic metal complex therefore appears to be the preferred approach.

ABBREVIATIONS AND DEFINITIONS

Ado-Cbl	5′-deoxyadenosyl-cobalamin
acac	acetylacetonate
BenzIm	benzimidazole
BSA	bovine serum albumin
Cbl	cobalamin
Cbi	cobinamide
Cbl(OH)	cobalamin hydroxide
Cbl(CN)	cobalamin cyanide
Cbi(OH)(H$_2$O)	aquahydroxocobinamide
cyanMetHb	cyanmethemoglobin
3-MP	3-mercaptopyruvate
3-MST	3-mercaptopyruvate sulfurtransferase
4-DMAP	dimethylaminophenol
CAK	Cyanide Antidote Kit
CcO	cytochrome c oxidase
CcO-CN	cyano-cytochrome c oxidase
CN⁻	cyanide anion
CNS	central nervous system
CO	carbon monoxide
CobCN	cyanohydroxocobalamin
CobOH	hydroxocobalamin
COHb	carboxyhemoglobin
Cp	cyclopentadienyl

EDTA	ethylenediaminetetraacetic acid
Hb	hemoglobin
HCN	hydrogen cyanide, prussic acid
IP	intraperitoneal
IM	intramuscular
PC	percutaneous
TO	transocular
INH	inhalation
MRL	minimum risk level
N_4**[11.3.1.]**	2,12-dimethyl-3,7,11,17-tetraazabicyclo-[11.3.1]-heptadeca-1,17-2,11,13,15-pentaenyl
LC$_{50}$	50% lethal concentration
MetHb	methemoglobin
3-MP	3-mercaptopyruvate
DMTS	dimethyltrisulfide
ELA cells	Ehrlich-Lettré ascites tumor cells
GSH	glutathione
NO	nitric oxide
RBC	red blood cells
ROS	reactive oxygen species
salophen	o-phenylenediaminebis(salicylidenaminato)
SOD	superoxide dismutase
TMPyP	tetramethylpyridineporhyrin
US FDA	United States Food and Drug Administration
WHO	World Health Organization

REFERENCES

[1] S. G. Suman, J. M. Gretarsdottir, in *Chemical and Clinical Aspects of Metal-Containing Antidotes for Poisoning by Cyanide,* Vol. 19 of *Metal Ions in Life Sciences,* Eds P. L. Carver, A. Sigel, E. Freisinger, R. K. O. Sigel, De Gruyter, Berlin/Boston, 2019, pp. 359–391.

[2] M. J. Ellenhorn, *Ellenhorn's Medical Toxicology: Diagnosis and Treatment of Human Poisoning,* Eds M. J. Ellenhorn, S. Schonwald, G. Ordog, J. Wasserberger, Williams & Wilkins, Baltimore, MD, 1997, pp. 1476–1484.

[3] J. L. Borowitz, P. G. Gunasekar, G. E. Isom, *Brain Res.* **1997**, *768*, 294–300.

[4] B. Ballantyne, in *Clinical and Experimental Toxicology of Cyanides,* Eds B. Ballantyne, T. C. Marrs, IOP Publishing, Bristol, UK, **1987**, pp. 41–126.

[5] B. Ballantyne, in *Clinical and Experimental Toxicology of Cyanides,* Eds B. Ballantyne, T. C. Marrs, IOP Publishing, Bristol, UK, **1987**, pp. 248–291.

[6] A. H. Hall, B. H. Rumack, *Ann. Emerg. Med.* **1986**, *15*, 1067–1074.

[7] S. W. Borron, F. J. Baud, *Arh. Rada Toksikol.* **1996**, *47*, 307–322.

[8] A. H. Hall, J. Saiers, F. Baud, *Crit. Rev. Toxicol.* **2009**, *39*, 541–552.

[9] L. K. Cambal, M. R. Swanson, Q. Yuan, A. C. Weitz, H. H. Li, B. R. Pitt, L. L. Pearce, J. Peterson, *Chem. Res. Toxicol.* **2011**, *24*, 1104–1112.

[10] A. Chan, D. L. Crankshaw, A. Monteil, S. E. Patterson, H. T. Nagasawa, J. E. Briggs, J. A. Kozocas, S. B. Mahon, M. Brenner, R. B. Pilz, T. D. Bigby, G. R. Boss, *Clin. Toxicol.* **2011**, *49*, 366–373.

[11] M. Brenner, J. G. Kim, J. Lee, S. B. Mahon, D. Lemor, R. Ahdout, G. R. Boss, W. Blackledge, L. Jann, H. T. Nagasawa, S. E. Patterson, *Toxicol. Appl. Pharmacol.* **2010**, *248*, 269–276.

[12] M. Brenner, J. G. Kim, S. B. Mahon, J. Lee, K. A. Kreuter, W. Blackledge, D. Mukai, S. Patterson, O. Mohammad, V. S. Sharma, G. R. Boss, *Ann. Emerg. Med.* **2010**, *55*, 352–363.

[13] A. Chan, M. Balasubramanian, W. Blackledge, O. M. Mohammad, L. Alvarez, G. R. Boss, T. D. Bigby, *Clin. Toxicol.* **2010**, *48*, 709–717.

[14] A. H. Hall, R. Dart, G. Bogdan, *Ann. Emerg. Med.* **2007**, *49*, 806–813.

[15] S. W. Borron, F. J. Baud, B. Megarbane, C. Bismuth, *Am. J. Emerg. Med.* **2007**, *25*, 551–558.

[16] B. Hillman, K. D. Bardhan, J. T. B. Bain, *Postgrad. Med. J.* **1974**, *50*, 171–174.

[17] M. Kiese, N. Weger, *Eur. J. Pharmacol.* **1969**, *7*, 97–105.

[18] C. J. Clemedson, H. I. Hultman, B. Sorbo, *Acta Phys. Scand.* **1954**, 245–251.

[19] W. B. Wendel, *J. Am. Med. Assoc.* **1933**, *100*, 1054–1055.

[20] J. L. Way, *Annu. Rev. Pharmacol. Toxicol.* **1984**, *24*, 451–481.

[21] A. K. Nath, X. Shi, D. L. Harrison, J. E. Morningstar, S. Mahon, A. Chan, P. Sips, J. Lee, C. A. MacRae, G. R. Boss, M. Brenner, R. E. Gerszten, R. T. Peterson, *Cell. Chem. Biol.* **2017**, *24*, 565–575.e564.

[22] H. Praekunatham, L. L. Pearce, J. Peterson, *Chem. Res. Toxicol.* **2019**, *32*, 1630–1637.

[23] J. Lee, S. B. Mahon, D. Mukai, T. Burney, B. S. Katebian, A. Chan, V. S. Bebarta, D. Yoon, G. R. Boss, M. Brenner, *J. Med. Toxicol.* **2016**, *12*, 370–379.

[24] P. Lawson-Smith, E. C. Jansen, O. Hyldegaard, *Scand. J. Trauma Resusc. Emerg. Med.* **2011**, *19*, 14.

[25] A. A. Cronican, K. L. Frawley, E. P. Straw, E. Lopez-Manzano, H. Praekunatham, J. Peterson, L. L. Pearce, *Chem. Res. Toxicol.* **2018**, *31*, 259–268.

[26] E. C. Thiel, K. N. Raymond, in *Bioinorganic Chemistry*, Eds I. Bertini, H. B. Gray, S. J. Lippard, J. S. Valentine, University Science Books, Mill Valley, CA, 1994, pp. 1–36.

[27] A. Thapper, J. P. Donahue, K. B. Musgrave, M. W. Willer, E. Nordlander, B. Hedman, K. O. Hodgson, R. H. Holm, *Inorg. Chem.* **1999**, *38*, 4101–4114.

[28] P. C. H. Mitchell, *J. Inorg. Biochem.* **1986**, *28*, 107–123.

[29] M. P. Coughlan, J. L. Johnson, K. V. Rajagopalan, *J. Biol. Chem.* **1980**, *255*, 2694–2699.

[30] P. C. H. Mitchell, C. F. Pygall, *J. Inorg. Biochem.* **1979**, *11*, 25–29.

[31] P. G. Gunasekar, J. L. Borowitz, J. J. Turek, D. A. V. Horn, G. E. Isom, *J. Neurosci. Res.* **2000**, *61*, 570–575.

[32] J. C. Forsyth, P. D. Mueller, C. E. Becker, J. Osterloh, N. L. Benowitz, B. H. Rumack, A. H. Hall, *J. Toxicol. Clin. Toxicol.* **1993**, *31*, 277–294.

[33] E. Jaszczak, Z. Polkowska, S. Narkowicz, J. Namiesnik, *Environ. Sci. Pollut. Res. Int.* **2017**, *24*, 15929–15948.

[34] R. A. Anderson, W. A. Harland, *Med. Sci. Law.* **1982**, *22*, 35–40.

[35] J. Taylor, N. Roney, C. Harper, M. E. Fransen, S. Swarts, in *Toxicological Profile for Cyanide*, Department of Health and Human Services, Atlanta, GA, **2006**, pp 25–131.

[36] A. R. Allen, L. Booker, G. A. Rockwood, in *Toxicology of Cyanides and Cyanogens: Experimental, Applied and Clinical Aspects*, Eds. A. H. Hall, G. E. Isom, G. A. Rockwood, John Wiley & Sons, Ltd., **2015**, pp 1–20.

[37] D. L. Nelson, A. L. Lehninger, M. M. Cox, in *Lehninger Principles of Biochemistry*, Ed K. Ahr, W. H. Freeman and Company, New York, **2008**, pp. 708–741.

Metal-Based Compounds Targeting Cyanide Poisoning 235

[38] H. Landahl, R. Herrmann, *Arch. Indust. Hyg. Occup. Med.* **1950**, *1*, 36–45.
[39] A. R. Dahl, *Toxicol. Appl. Pharmacol.* **1990**, *103*, 185–197.
[40] F. Moriya, Y. Hashimoto, *Legal Medicine* **2003**, *5*, S113–S117.
[41] R. A. Anderson, A. A. Watson, W. A. Harland, *Med. Sci. Law* **1981**, *21*, 288–294.
[42] J. G. Ryan, in *Emergency Toxicology*, 2nd edn, Ed E. P. Vicciello, Lippincott-Raven, Philadelphia, USA, **1998**, pp. 678–696.
[43] D. Bordo, P. Bork, *EMBO Reports.* **2002**, *3*, 741–746.
[44] J. Oró, *Space Life Sci.* **1972**, *3*, 507–550.
[45] J. Oró, K. Rewers, D. Odom, *Orig. Life* **1982**, *12*, 285–305.
[46] J. Blake, *Edinburgh Med. Surg. J.* **1840**, *53*, 35–49.
[47] J. Blake, *Edinburgh Med. Surg. J.* **1839**, *51*, 330–345.
[48] B. Sceresini, in *Advances in Gold Ore Processing*, Ed M. D. Adams, Elsevier, Amsterdam, **2005**, *15*, 789–824.
[49] J. Marsden, I. House, *The Chemistry of Gold Extraction*, Society for Mining, Metallurgy, and Exploration, Ellis Horword Limited, *Chichester*, **2006**.
[50] B. Ballantyne, *Fundam. Appl. Toxicol.* **1983**, *3*, 400–408.
[51] B. Ballantyne, *J. Forensic Sci. Soc.* **1975**, *15*, 51–56.
[52] B. P. McNamara, in *Estimates of the Toxicity of Hydrocyanic Acid Vapors in Man*, Ed Department of the Army, Aberdeen Proving Ground, Maryland, **1976**.
[53] F. P. Simeonova, L. Fishbein, *Concise International Chemical Assessment Document (CICAD) 61*, WHO, Geneva, **2004**.
[54] B. Megarbane, A. Delahaye, D. Goldgran-Toledano, F. J. Baud, *J. Chin. Med. Assoc.* **2003**, *66*, 193–203.
[55] F. J. Baud, M. K. Haidar, R. Jouffroy, J.-H. Raphalen, L. Lamhaut, P. Carli, *Crit. Care. Med.* **2018**, 1–7.
[56] C. Männel-Croisé, F. Zelder, *Anal. Met.* **2012**, *4*, 2632–2634.
[57] S. Å. Persson, G. Cassel, Å. Sellström, *Fundam. Appl. Toxicol.* **1985**, *5*, S150–S159.
[58] P. G. Gunasekar, P. W. Sun, A. G. Kanthasamy, J. L. Borowitz, G. E. Isom, *J. Pharmacol. Exp. Ther.* **1996**, *277*, 150.
[59] A. B. Sousa, H. Manzano, B. Soto-Blanco, S. L. Górniak, *Arch. Toxicol.* **2003**, *77*, 330–334.
[60] A. A. Salkowski, D. G. Penney, *Vet. Human Toxiciol.* **1994**, *36*, 455–466.
[61] A. D. Ivankovich, B. Braverman, T. S. Stephens, M. Shulman, H. J. Heyman, *Anesth.* **1980**, *58*, 11–17.
[62] J. L. Borowitz, A. G. Kanthasamy, P. J. Mitchell, G. E. Isom, *Fundam. Appl. Toxicol.* **1993**, *20*, 133–140.
[63] S. E. Patterson, A. R. Monteil, J. F. Cohen, D. L. Crankshaw, R. Vince, H. T. Nagasawa, *J. Med. Chem.* **2013**, *56*, 1346–1349.
[64] S. E. Patterson, B. Moeller, H. T. Nagasawa, R. Vince, D. L. Crankshaw, J. Briggs, M. W. Stutelberg, C. V. Vinnakota, B. A. Logue, *Ann. N. Y. Acad. Sci.* **2016**, *1374*, 202–209.
[65] H. T. Nagasawa, D. J. W. Goon, D. L. Crankshaw, R. Vince, S. E. Patterson, *J. Med. Chem.* **2007**, *50*, 6462–6464.
[66] W. G. J. Hol, L. J. Lijk, K. H. Kalk, *Fundam. Appl. Toxicol.* **1983**, *3*, 370–376.
[67] R. B. Drawbaugh, T. C. Marrs, *Comp. Biochem. Physiol. B: Comp. Biochem.* **1987**, *86*, 307–310.
[68] R. M. Roat-Malone, in *Bioinorganic Chemistry: A Short Course*, Wiley-Interscience, New York, **2007**, pp. 343–342.
[69] W. Kaim, B. Schwederski, A. Klein, *Inorganic Elements in the Chemistry of Life*, Eds D. Atwood, B. Crabtree, G. Meyer, D. Woollins, John Wiley and Sons, Ltd., Singapore, 2013, pp. 77–98.

[70] O. Bodansky, *Pharmacol. Rev.* **1951**, *3*, 144–191.

[71] B. J. Krieg, S. M. Taghavi, G. L. Amidon, G. E. Amidon, *J. Pharm Sci.* **2014**, *103*, 3473–3490.

[72] C. Geers, G. Gros, *Physiol. Rev.* **2000**, *80*, 681–715.

[73] P. Sarti, A. Giuffrè, M. C. Barone, E. Forte, D. Mastronicola, M. Brunori, *Free Radical Biol. Med.* **2003**, *34*, 509–520.

[74] D. A. Tanen, M. J. Matteucci, in *Harwood-Nuss' Clinical Practice of Emergency Medicine*, Eds A. B. Wolfson, G. W. Hendey, L. J. Ling, C. L. Rosen, G. Q. Sharieff, Lippincott Williams & Wilkins, Philadelphia, **2009**, pp. 319.

[75] A. C. Anusiem, J. G. Beetlestone, D. H. Irvine, *J. Chem. Soc. A: Inorg. Phys. Theor.* **1968**, 960–969.

[76] J. Jones, M. J. McMullen, J. Dougherty, *Am. J. Emerg. Med.* **1987**, *5*, 317–321.

[77] M. G. Jones, D. Bickar, M. T. Wilson, M. Brunori, A. Colosimo, P. Sarti, *Biochem. J.* **1984**, *220*, 57.

[78] M. H. Klapper, H. Uchida, *J. Biol. Chem.* **1971**, *246*, 6849–6854.

[79] A. Jain, R. J. Kassner, *J. Biol. Chem.* **1984**, *259*, 10309–10314.

[80] Y.-P. Huang, R. J. Kassner, *J. Am. Chem. Soc.* **1979**, *101*, 5807–5810.

[81] C. Locatelli, S. M. Candura, D. Maccarini, R. Butera, L. Manzo, *Indoor Environ.* **1994**, *3*, 16–21.

[82] S. J. Moore, J. C. Norris, A. Walsh, A. S. Hume, *J. Pharm. Exp. Ther.* **1987**, *242*, 70–74.

[83] L. Eichhorn, T. Marcus, B. Jüttner, *Dtsch. Arzebl. Int.* **2018**, *115*, 863–870.

[84] M. A. Kirk, R. Gerace, K. W. Kulig, *Ann. Emerg. Med.* **1993**, *22*, 1413–1418.

[85] F. J. Baud, P. Barriot, V. Troffis, B. Riou, E. Vicaut, Y. Lecarpentier, R. Bourdon, A. Astier, C. Bismuth, *N. Engl. J. Med.* **1991**, *325*, 1761–1766.

[86] A. H. Hall, K. W. Kulig, B. H. Rumack, *J. Clin. Toxicol. Exp.* **1989**, *9*, 3–9.

[87] A. Taulier, P. Levillain, A. Lemonnier, *Clin. Chem.* **1987**, *33*, 1767–1770.

[88] American Society for Testing and Materials, Method D 2036 – 98, in *Standard Test Methods for Cyanides in Water*, Annual Book of ASTM Standards, West Conshohocken, PA, **1998**.

[89] D. C. Blumenthal, R. J. Kassner, *J. Biol. Chem.* **1980**, *255*, 5859–5863.

[90] G. Isom, J. L. Way, *Toxicol. Appl. Pharmacol.* **1973**, *24*, 449–456.

[91] D. J. Paustenbach, B. E. Tvermoes, K. M. Unice, B. L. Finley, B. D. Kerger, *Crit. Rev. Toxicol.* **2013**, *43*, 316–362.

[92] T. C. Marrs, J. P. Thompson, *Clin. Toxicol.* **2016**, *54*, 609–614.

[93] H. Fang, J. Kang, D. Zhang, *Microb. Cell Factories* **2017**, *16*, 15.

[94] L. Leyssens, B. Vinck, C. Van Der Straeten, F. Wuyts, L. Maes, *Toxicol.* **2017**, *387*, 43–56.

[95] J. Antal, *Ungar. Arch. Med.* **1894**, *3*, 117–128.

[96] S. W. Borron, F. J. Baud, P. Barriot, M. Imbert, C. Bismuth, *Ann. Emerg. Med.* **2007**, *49*, 794–801, e791–e792.

[97] N. Metzler-Nolte, in *Comprehensive Organometallic Chemistry III*, Eds D. M. P. Mingos, R. H. Crabtree, Elsevier, Oxford, 2007, pp. 883–920.

[98] C. L. Evans, *Br. J. Pharm.* **1964**, *23*, 455–475.

[99] EGVM, in *Safe Upper Levels for Vitamins and Minerals*, Ed. Expert Group on Vitamins and Minerals, Food Standards Agency, London, **2003**, pp. 91–99.

[100] H. M. Marques, J. C. Bradley, K. L. Brown, H. Brooks, *J. Chem. Soc., Dalton Trans.* **1993**, 3475–3478.

[101] A. G. Cregan, N. E. Brasch, R. van Eldik, *Inorg. Chem.* **2001**, *40*, 1430–1438.

[102] W. W. Reenstra, W. P. Jencks, *J. Am. Chem. Soc.* **1979**, *101*, 5780–5791.

Metal-Based Compounds Targeting Cyanide Poisoning 237

[103] J. M. Pratt, *Inorganic Chemistry of Vitamin B12*, Academic Press, New York, NY, 1972.

[104] H. A. Hill, J. M. Pratt, R. G. Thorp, B. Ward, R. J. P. Williams, *Biochem. J.* **1970**, *120*, 263–269.

[105] G. C. Hayward, H. A. O. Hill, J. M. Pratt, N. J. Vanston, A. R. W. Williams, *J. Chem. Soc.* **1965**, 6485–6493.

[106] G. H. Beaven, E. A. Johnson, *Nature* **1955**, *176*, 1264–1265.

[107] H. M. Marques, J. C. Bradley, K. L. Brown, H. Brooks, *Inorg. Chim. Acta.* **1993**, *209*, 161–169.

[108] P. George, D. H. Irvine, S. C. Glauser, *Ann. New York Acad. Sci.* **1960**, *88*, 393–415.

[109] K. E. Broderick, M. Balasubramanian, A. Chan, P. Potluri, J. Feala, D. D. Belke, A. McCculloch, V. S. Sharma, R. B. Pilz, T. D. Bigby, G. R. Boss, *Exp. Biol. Med.* **2007**, *232*, 789–798.

[110] K. E. Broderick, Prasanth Potluri, S. Zhuang, Immo E. Scheffler, V. S. Sharma, R. B. Pilz, G. R. Boss, *Exp. Biol. Med.* **2006**, *231*, 641–651.

[111] C. Männel-Croisé, B. Probst, F. Zelder, *Anal. Chem.* **2009**, *81*, 9493–9498.

[112] C. Männel-Croisé, F. Zelder, *ACS Appl. Mat. Int.* **2012**, *4*, 725–729.

[113] J. Ma, P. K. Dasgupta, F. H. Zelder, G. R. Boss, *Anal. Chim. Acta.* **2012**, *736*, 78–84.

[114] R. A. Firth, H. A. O. Hill, J. M. Pratt, R. G. Thorp, R. J. P. Williams, *J. Chem. Soc. A: Inorg. Phys. Theor.* **1969**, 381–386.

[115] A. Chan, J. Jiang, A. Fridman, L. T. Guo, G. D. Shelton, M.-T. Liu, C. Green, K. J. Haushalter, H. H. Patel, J. Lee, D. Yoon, T. Burney, D. Mukai, S. B. Mahon, M. Brenner, R. B. Pilz, G. R. Boss, *J. Med. Chem.* **2015**, *58*, 1750–1759.

[116] O. S. Benz, Y. Quan, A. A. Amoscato, L. L. Pearce, J. Peterson, *Chem. Res. Toxicol.* **2012**, *25*, 2678–2686.

[117] E. Lopez-Manzano, A. A. Cronican, K. L. Frawley, J. Peterson, L. L. Pearce, *Chem. Res. Toxicol.* **2016**, *29*, 1011–1019.

[118] P. Hambright, E. B. Fleisher, *Inorg. Chem.* **1970**, *9*, 1757–1761.

[119] R. F. Pasternack, M. A. Cobb, *J. Inorg. Nucl. Chem.* **1973**, *35*, 4327–4339.

[120] R. F. Pasternack, P. R. Huber, P. Boyd, G. Engasser, L. Francesconi, E. Gibbs, P. Fasella, G. Cerio Venturo, L. D. Hinds, *J. Am. Chem. Soc.* **1972**, *94*, 4511–4517.

[121] K. M. Long, D. H. Busch, *Inorg. Chem.* **1970**, *9*, 505–512.

[122] D. C. Lacy, C. C. L. McCrory, J. C. Peters, *Inorg. Chem.* **2014**, *53*, 4980–4988.

[123] F. Montilla, A. Galindo, *Oxidodiperoxidomolybdenum Complexes: Properties and Their Use as Catalysts in Green Oxidations*, Elsevier, New York, 2017.

[124] D. Coucouvanis, *J.Biol. Inorg. Chem.* **1996**, *1*, 594–600.

[125] E. I. Stiefel, *J. Chem. Soc., Dalton Trans.* **1997**, 3915–3923.

[126] S. G. Suman, J. M. Gretarsdottir, P. E. Penwell, J. P. Gunnarsson, S. Frostason, S. Jonsdottir, K. K. Damodaran, A. Hirschon, *Inorg. Chem.* **2020**, *59*, 7644–7656.

[127] A. M. Crawford, J. J. H. Cotelesage, R. C. Prince, G. N. George, in *Metallocofactors that Activate Small Molecules: Structure and Bonding*, Vol. 179, Ed M. W. Ribbe, Springer International Publishing, Cham, **2019**, pp. 63–100.

[128] R. Hille, *Arch. Biochem. Biophys.* **2005**, *433*, 107–116.

[129] R. Hille, *Trends Biochem. Sci.* **2002**, *27*, 360–368.

[130] G. D. Todd, S. Keith, O. Faroon, M. Buser, L. Ingerman, M. Citra, G. L. Diamond, C. Hard, J. M. Klotzbach, A. Nguyen, in *Toxicological Profile for Molybdenum*, Ed ATSDR, SRC, Inc., North Syracuse, NY, 2020.

[131] M. Mohanty, G. Sahu, A. Banerjee, S. Lima, S. A. Patra, A. Crochet, G. Sciortino, D. Sanna, V. Ugone, E. Garribba, R. Dinda, *Inorg. Chem.* **2022**, *61*, 4513–4532.

[132] J. B. Waern, H. H. Harris, B. Lai, Z. Cai, M. M. Harding, C. T. Dillon, *J. Biol. Inorg. Chem.* **2005**, *10*, 443–452.

[133] J. B. Waern, C. T. Dillon, M. M. Harding, *J. Med. Chem.* **2005**, *48*, 2093–2099.

[134] K. Zhang, S. Cui, J. Wang, X. Wang, R. Li, *Med. Chem. Res.* **2012**, *21*, 1071–1076.

[135] S. Majumder, S. Pasayat, A. K. Panda, S. P. Dash, S. Roy, A. Biswas, M. E. Varma, B. N. Joshi, E. Garribba, C. Kausar, S. K. Patra, W. Kaminsky, A. Crochet, R. Dinda, *Inorg. Chem.* **2017**, *56*, 11190–11210.

[136] D. Bandarra, M. Lopes, T. Lopes, J. Almeida, M. S. Saraiva, M. Vasconcellos-Dias, C. D. Nunes, V. Félix, P. Brandão, P. D. Vaz, M. Meireles, M. J. Calhorda, *J. Inorg. Biochem.* **2010**, *104*, 1171–1177.

[137] D. Coucouvanis, A. Toupadakis, S.-M. Koo, A. Hadjikyriacou, *Polyhedron.* **1989**, *8*, 1705–1716.

[138] D. Coucouvanis, in *Advances in Inorganic Chemistry*, Vol. 45, Ed A. G. Sykes, Academic Press, 1998, pp. 1–73.

[139] P. Traill, E. Tiekink, M. Oconnor, M. Snow, A. Wedd, *Aust. J. Chem.* **1986**, *39*, 1287–1295.

[140] J. M. Gretarsdottir, S. Jonsdottir, W. Lewis, T. W. Hambley, S. G. Suman, *Inorg. Chem.* **2020**, *59*, 18190–18204.

[141] J. M. Gretarsdottir, S. Bobersky, N. Metzler-Nolte, S. G. Suman, *J. Inorg. Biochem.* **2016**, *160*, 166–171.

[142] J. M. Gretarsdottir, I. H. Lambert, S. Stürup, S. G. Suman, *ACS Pharmacol. Transl. Sci.*, **2022**, *5*(10), 907–918.

[143] J. M. Gretarsdottir, *Syntheses of New Molybdenum-Sulfur Complexes; Biological Studies Thereof In Vitro and Catalysis of the Transformation of Cyanide to Thiocyanate*, University of Iceland, Reykjavik, Iceland, **2018**, pp. 211.

[144] M. Chaudhary, R. Gupta, *Curr. Biotech.* **2012**, *1*, 327–335.

[145] L. H. Jones, *Inorg. Chem.* **1963**, *2*, 777–780.

9 Advanced Microscopy Methods for Elucidating the Localization of Metal Complexes in Cancer Cells

*Johannes Karges**
Faculty for Chemistry and Biochemistry,
Ruhr University Bochum, Universitätsstrasse 150,
D-44801 Bochum, Germany
johannes.karges@ruhr-uni-bochum.de

*Nils Metzler-Nolte**
Faculty for Chemistry and Biochemistry,
Chair of Inorganic Chemistry I – Bioinorganic Chemistry,
Ruhr University Bochum, Universitätsstrasse 150,
D-44801 Bochum, Germany
nils.metzler-nolte@ruhr-uni-bochum.de

CONTENTS

1 Introduction 240
2 X-Ray Fluorescence Microscopy 241
    2.1 Fundamentals of X-Ray Fluorescence Imaging 241
    2.2 Selected Biomedical Problems Investigated by X-Ray
        Fluorescence Microscopy of Metal Complexes 243
3 Luminescence Lifetime Imaging Microscopy 247
    3.1 Advantages of Luminescence Lifetime Microscopy over
        Confocal Microscopy 247
    3.2 Selected Biomedical Problems Investigated by Luminescence
        Lifetime Microscopy of Metal Complexes 249
        3.2.1 Detection of the Metal Complexes through Elimination of
            Background Fluorescence 249

---

*Corresponding authors

DOI: 10.1201/9781003272250-9

239

	3.2.2	Detection of the Change in Localization of Metal Complexes by Changes in Their Lifetime in Different Cellular Environments	249
	3.2.3	Metal Complexes as Luminescent Lifetime Sensors	250
	3.2.4	Conversion of Metal Complexes Inside Cancer Cells	251
4	Two-Photon Excitation Microscopy		252
	4.1	Advantages of Two-Photon Excitation Over One-Photon Excitation	254
	4.2	Advantages of Metal Complexes as Two-Photon Excited Chromophores	255
	4.3	Selected Biomedical Problems Investigated by Two-Photon Excitation Microscopy of Metal Complexes	256
		4.3.1 Metal Complexes as Two-Photon Excited Cell Organelle Dyes	256
		4.3.2 Metal Complexes as Two-Photon Excited Sensors for Small Molecules	258
		4.3.3 Metal Complexes as Two-Photon Excited Luminophores for Biomolecules	259
5	Conclusions		259
Acknowledgments			260
Abbreviations			260
References			261

ABSTRACT

The localization of a metal complex has a dramatic effect on its biological activity as well as therapeutic or diagnostic efficiency. To rationally design novel compounds with specifically tailored properties, it is crucial to understand the subcellular accumulation of the compound inside human cells. Herein, advanced methods for the detection of metal-based compounds inside cancerous cells are described and their application for the intracellular localization of metal-based anticancer compounds is highlighted based on recent examples from the chemical literature. In particular, this chapter covers X-ray Fluorescence Imaging, and optical microscopy methods that have recently gained popularity, namely Luminescence Lifetime Imaging and Two-Photon Excitation Microscopy.

KEYWORDS

Anticancer; Bioinorganic Chemistry; Imaging; Localization; Luminescence Lifetime Imaging; Metals in Medicine; Two-Photon Excitation Microscopy; X-ray Fluorescence

1 INTRODUCTION

Studies have shown that the localization of a metal complex has a crucial effect on their therapeutic efficiency as well as mode of action. While the metal content in subcellular organelles or human cells can be traditionally analyzed by inductively coupled plasma mass spectrometry or atomic emission spectroscopy,

Elucidating the Localization of Metal Complexes in Cancer Cells

these methods require additional experimental treatments which could change the respective localization of the metal complexes. Capitalizing on this, it would be of high interest to monitor the localization of the metal/metal complex in living biological organisms. In this chapter, recent analytical methods for the localization (i.e., visualizing at one given point in time) or tracking (i.e., following over a time course, either continuously or via individual frames taken during that course) of metal complexes as potential anticancer agents are discussed.

The first section of the chapter thematizes the application of X-ray fluorescence radiation for the selective detection of metals. This technique uses high-intensity, high-energy radiation for the excitation of a core electron of the metal ion which, upon decay of the electron, emits, element-specific radiation, making this method uniquely suitable for the study of metal-based compounds [1]. The second part of this chapter discusses the use of luminescence lifetime microscopy for the detection of luminescent metal complexes upon modification of their photophysical properties through different cellular environments or the conversion of the compound into a new species [2]. The third part utilizes the two-photon absorption properties of metal complexes for selective excitation of the chromophore. Two-photon excitations are associated with a higher spatial and temporal resolution than the corresponding one-photon excitations. While luminescence lifetime and two-photon excitation microscopy have not been specifically designed for metal complexes, these techniques allow for the selective and highly sensitive detection of certain luminescent metal complexes within human cells [3]. Within the chapter, we will introduce the basic concepts and advantages of these respective methods on the basis of recent examples in the chemical literature.

2   X-RAY FLUORESCENCE MICROSCOPY

When an X-ray beam with energy above the absorption edge hits a given element, a core electron can be excited to a photoelectron and a core hole. This hole is filled by decay of an outer electron with concomitant emission of energy either as Auger electron or as X-ray fluorescence photon. The decay follows the usual selection rules for optical transitions, and the emitted photon will have a very specific energy, depending mostly on the element and on the type of transition that is observed. K-lines are observed for transitions into the $1s$ core electron level, and L-lines will result from decay into the $2s$ or $2p$ levels (Figure 1). The high element-specific energy of the emitted photon makes X-ray fluorescence perfectly suited for elemental analysis in complex samples.

2.1   FUNDAMENTALS OF X-RAY FLUORESCENCE IMAGING

Spatial resolution in two dimensions can be achieved by focusing on the incident X-ray beam and stepwise scanning. The foundation and numerous technical details, such as beam focusing, detectors, scanning technique, and quantitative data analysis, have been described from a chemical perspective in a review article by George and colleagues in 2014 [4]. Here, we will just note that spectacular advances have been achieved using synchrotron X-ray radiation, detector technology advancement, and

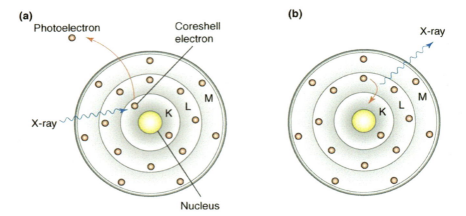

FIGURE 1 Schematic illustration of the concept of X-ray fluorescence using the Bohr atom model. (a) Excitation of a core electron of the metal ion. (b) Decay of the electron upon emission of element-specific radiation. (Reproduced by permission from Ref. [1]; Copyright 2007 Elsevier)

computer analysis software over the last years, making a lateral spatial resolution of 100 nm and even less possible, as well as enabling the operator to scan a whole array of cells two-dimensionally with resolution matching optical fluorescence microscopy within around 1 h. As a logical further development, three-dimensional imaging (also called X-ray fluorescence tomography) is becoming a reality. A number of different acronyms, typically combining a selection of words like synchrotron, X-ray radiation, emission, fluorescence, imaging, and related ones in a descriptive way, are used in the literature. Also, we note that most 2D applications are strictly speaking element mapping rather than imaging, but for convenience we settle for the acronym "X-ray fluorescence imaging" (XRF imaging) here, which seems most commonly used and offers some flexibility in describing variants of the technique [5, 6].

One critical aspect is the sample preparation, especially when individual cells are to be investigated as close as possible to their natural state. Chemical fixation, storage, preservation, or any other sample preparation and handling may lead to unintended redistribution of cellular components, especially of the highly mobile metals that are of particular interest in XRF imaging studies. This situation is akin to the challenges of fixation in optical fluorescence microscopy and has led to a preference for life imaging wherever possible. This, however, is not technically possible for XRF imaging, and as a next-best substitute to life imaging, shock-freezing and cryo-preservation of life samples is currently the technique of choice. By rapidly freezing cells that are grown on suitable sample grids in liquid hydrocarbons below liquid nitrogen temperatures, a close-to-natural frozen-hydrated state is preserved. If a cooled sample stage and additional sophisticated equipment are not available at the synchroton site, freeze-drying the cooled samples may be an option to maintain all cellular features with simplified technical requirements. As with each additional handling step, there is a danger

Elucidating the Localization of Metal Complexes in Cancer Cells   **243**

of (i) re-localization and redistribution of metal ions within the sample, and (ii) changes to or even destruction of cellular morphology, both eventually giving an image that is discrepant from the original cellular state. Capitalizing on this, the obtained results from XRF imaging are often compared with other techniques. The challenges of simultaneously identifying cellular organelles by fluorescence microscopy and elemental distribution by XRF imaging were nicely summarized by Ortega and colleagues, and best practices were described therein [7]. Leary and Ralle give a recent account on advances in visualization of Cu in mammalian cells by XRF imaging which also contains useful technical details [8].

2.2 SELECTED BIOMEDICAL PROBLEMS INVESTIGATED BY X-RAY FLUORESCENCE MICROSCOPY OF METAL COMPLEXES

Given the overwhelming importance of Pt-based anticancer drugs, and cisplatin in particular, it comes as no surprise that Pt-based compounds were among the first and most intensely studied also with XRF imaging. The generally accepted mode of action of cisplatin (Figure 2) is through binding of the metal complex to cellular DNA, crosslinking of neighboring bases, and thereby inhibiting translation of the genetic information. Subsequent events such as futile DNA repair and activation of p53 ultimately lead to cell death [9]. In keeping with this notion, it would be expected that high concentrations of Pt can be detected in the cellular nucleus. The first XRF images of individual human ovarian adenocarcinoma (IGROV1) cells incubated with cisplatin were reported in 1996 with a resolution of $2\,\mu m$. The images indicated an even distribution of Pt in the cancer cell, similar to Cu and Zn. Interestingly, the analogous cisplatin-resistant cancer cell line (IGROV1-DDP) showed a highly reduced amount of Pt inside the cells when compared with Cu and Zn, suggesting the ability of the cancer cell to excrete cisplatin as a resistance mechanism [10]. In 2003, these studies were followed up and the amount of Pt in human ovarian 2008 cells was quantified using XRF imaging. The authors found approximately 20 attograms (2×10^{-17}g or as little as 60,000 atoms) of platinum in a beam spot of 0.2 μm^2 in human ovarian cells. Through stepwise scanning of the cell in increments of 1 μm, the Pt distribution inside the whole cell was mapped (Figure 2) [11].

In an effort to study the integrity and distribution of the Pt(II) complex during the treatment, a 3-bromopyridine derivative was prepared and investigated in human ovarian cancer cells (A2780). The XRF image indicated a similar distribution of Pt and Br, suggesting that the pyridine moiety is not released upon entering the cancer cell (Figure 3) [12].

In theranostic compounds, one moiety serves as the medicinally active ingredient ("therapy"), while the other serves a diagnostic purpose for visualizing the conjugate or tracking its fate intracellularly. One challenge in such theranostics is to ensure that the conjugate remains intact and the two moieties indeed end up in the same location. Especially when the theranostic agent is made up of two different metals (called heterobimetallic theranostics) [13], XRF imaging seems ideally

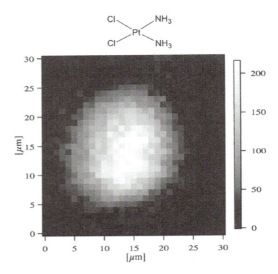

FIGURE 2 *Top*: Structure of the Pt(II) complex cisplatin *cis*-[PtCl$_2$(NH$_3$)$_2$]. *Bottom*: X-ray fluorescence microscopy image showing the distribution of Pt in human ovarian 2008 cells. (Reproduced by permission from Ref. [11]; Copyright 2003 American Association for Cancer Research.)

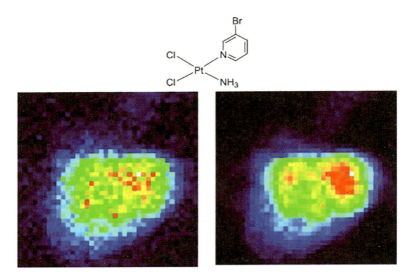

FIGURE 3 *Top*: Structure of the Pt(II) complex *cis*-[PtCl$_2$(NH$_3$)(3-bromopyridine)]. *Bottom*: X-ray fluorescence microscopy images showing the distribution of Br (left) and Pt (right) in human ovarian cancer (A2780) cells. (Reproduced by permission from Ref. [12]; Copyright 2006 Elsevier.)

Elucidating the Localization of Metal Complexes in Cancer Cells   245

suited to proof this co-localization. Following this concept, the localization of a bimetallic Pt-Gd complex was studied by XRF imaging. The Gd moiety was used as a contrast-enhancing group for nuclear magnetic imaging of the conjugate, and the co-localization of Gd and Pt, as shown by XRF imaging, provided ultimate proof that the signal observed from the Gd moiety was indeed equivalent to the Pt localization (Figure 4) [14].

Beyond theranostic applications that involve two metals, the integrity of metal complexes can be further probed by XRF imaging by utilizing clever ligand design. Two recent publications describe the determination of the localization of iodo-functionalized Re(I) complexes by XRF imaging. In both cases, the authors showed an identical distribution of Re and I, indicating the inertness of the complex in the cellular environment (Figure 5) [15, 16]. Wilson's group has also very recently studied the co-localization of Re and Pt metals by XRF imaging in a covalent, photoactivated Re(I)/Pt(IV) bioconjugate [17]. Here also, intracellular

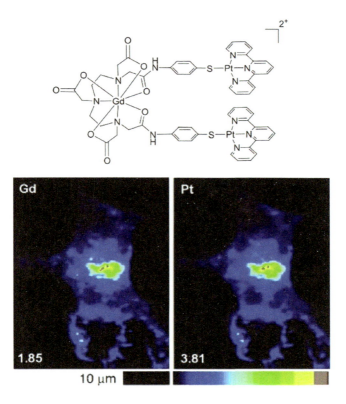

FIGURE 4 *Top*: Structure of the Pt(II)-Gd(III) bimetallic complex. *Bottom*: X-ray fluorescence microscopy images showing the distribution of Gd (left) and Pt (right) in adenocarcinomic human alveolar basal epithelial (A549) cells. (Reproduced by permission from Ref. [14]; Copyright 2010 Wiley.)

metal co-localization indicates excellent stability of the conjugate, with and without irradiation to induce antitumoral activity.

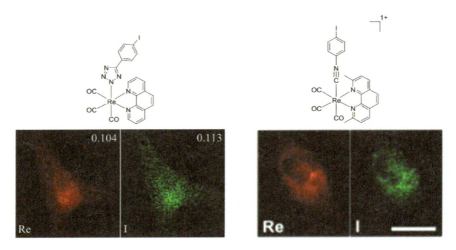

FIGURE 5 *Top*: Structure of an iodine-functionalized Re(I) complex. *Bottom*: X-ray fluorescence microscopy images showing the distribution of Re and I in human prostate epithelial carcinoma cells (left) and in human cervical carcinoma (HeLa) cells (right). (Reproduced by permission from Ref. [15, 16]; Copyright 2017, 2020 The Royal Society of Chemistry.)

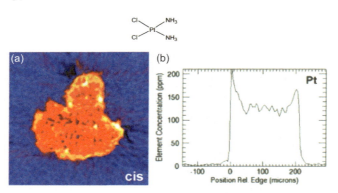

FIGURE 6 *Top*: Structure of the Pt(II) complex cisplatin *cis*-[PtCl$_2$(NH$_3$)$_2$]. *Bottom*: X-ray fluorescence microscopy image (left) and distribution across the spheroid showing the distribution of Pt in human colon carcinoma (CLD-1) multicellular tumor spheroids. (Reproduced by permission from Ref. [18]; Copyright 2007 American Chemical Society.)

Recognizing the limitations of 2D monolayer cell models, increasing interest is being devoted toward 3D tissue culture models, which are believed to better represent the conditions found in clinically treated solid tumors. In an early example, XRF imaging was used to study the penetration of Pt-based drugs in multicellular tumor spheroids. Indeed, all investigated Pt complexes including cisplatin were

Elucidating the Localization of Metal Complexes in Cancer Cells   **247**

able to fully penetrate the 3D cellular architecture (Figure 6) [18]. Using a similar 3D XRF tomographic imaging technique, penetration of an Os-arene anticancer drug candidate into the interior of a 3D tumor spheroid was also established [19]. As discussed above for 2D cell culture and XRF imaging, sample preparation is equally critical for 3D XRF imaging of tumor spheroids, and this aspect has been investigated by Hambley and coworkers [20].

3 LUMINESCENCE LIFETIME IMAGING MICROSCOPY

The fundamental achievements leading toward the development of a luminescence lifetime spectrometer are credited to various scientists. Herein, we would like to highlight Sir George Gabriel Stokes who pioneered fluorescence-based studies and actually coined the term "fluorescence" in 1852. Alexandre-Edmond Becquerel discovered phosphorescence and first designed instrumentation to detect luminescence in 1859 [21]. Robert Williams Wood performed the first fluorescence lifetime measurements using the Kerr cell in 1921 [22]. Enrique Gaviola assembled the first fluorescence lifetime spectrometer in 1926 [23]. Since these discoveries, much research has focused on the development and improvement of luminescence lifetime spectrometers, presenting nowadays an effective and powerful tool to study cellular processes.

3.1 Advantages of Luminescence Lifetime Microscopy over Confocal Microscopy

During the photophysical luminescence mechanism, the chromophore absorbs a photon and migrates into an excited singlet state. During fluorescence a lower excited singlet state is reached through vibrational relaxation and internal conversion. The fluorophore is then able to relax back to the ground state upon emission of a photon. In contrast, during phosphorescence an excited triplet state is populated through intersystem crossing from the excited singlet state. Upon emission of a photon, the ground state of the chromophore is accessed (Figure 7). Typically, the time a chromophore is able to stay within the respective excited state is referred to as the luminescence lifetime. While compounds that interact through fluorescence have relatively short-lived excited states with a lifetime in the order of several nanoseconds, a compound that is relaxing through phosphorescence has a long-lived excited state with a lifetime in the order of several hundred nanoseconds to several microseconds. This difference in luminescence lifetime could be exploited to differentiate between different chromophores. Importantly, the majority of components within a cancerous cell are either nonluminescent or poorly luminescent with a short lifetime. As the vast majority of metal complexes with luminescence properties release their energy by phosphorescence with long lifetimes, this technique presents a powerful method for the specific detection of metal complexes. During luminescence lifetime imaging the emission stemming from short-lived chromophores is filtered out upon using a detection delay, allowing for the specific detection of long-lived luminophores (Figure 8).

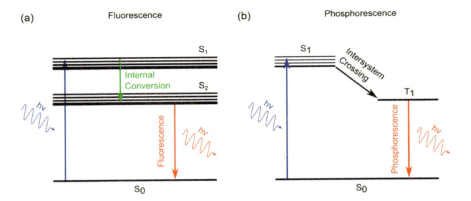

FIGURE 7 Jablonski diagram of (a) fluorescence or (b) phosphorescence. S = Singlet state, T = Triplet state.

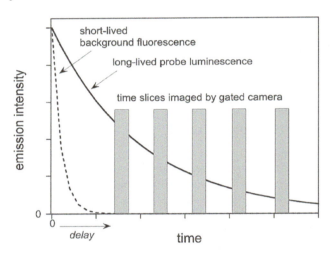

FIGURE 8 Concept of luminescence lifetime imaging to eliminate short-lived background fluorescence. (Reproduced by permission from Ref. [2]; Copyright 2008 United States National Academy of Sciences.)

The ability to detect specifically compounds with a certain luminescence lifetime presents several advantages including

1. Reduction of background fluorescence: As only a specific interval of luminescence lifetime is detected, components with shorter or longer lifetimes are filtered out. This allows for an improved resolution and specific detection (Figure 9).
2. Simultaneous use of several chromophores: Due to the selective detection of a specific window of luminescence lifetimes, several chromophores with different lifetimes could be simultaneously used (Figure 9).

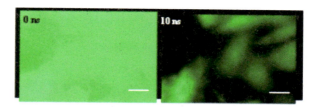

FIGURE 9 Comparison of confocal microscopy (left) and luminescence lifetime microscopy (right) images of Chinese hamster ovary (CHO) cells incubated with a luminescent Pt(II) complex and fluorescein (λ_{ex}=355 nm) with a 10 ns delay. (Reproduced by permission from Ref. [2]; Copyright 2008 United States National Academy of Sciences.)

3. Monitoring of the conversion of the chromophore: Metal complexes could interact within a cellular environment with various biomolecules or reactive species by ligand exchange reactions, metal center reduction/oxidation, or modification of the ligand. As these chemical modifications typically also influence the photophysical properties of the metal complex, including its luminescence lifetime, this technique can be applied for the direct monitoring of chemical conversions in cancer cells.

3.2 Selected Biomedical Problems Investigated by Luminescence Lifetime Microscopy of Metal Complexes

3.2.1 Detection of the Metal Complexes through Elimination of Background Fluorescence

The presence of luminescent biomolecules or the co-incubation with other luminophores could hinder the detection of luminescent metal complexes. To differentiate between the different species, luminescence lifetime microscopy can be applied. To date, this technique has been used for the detection of Pt(II) and Pd(II) porphyrins [24, 25] and cyclometallated Pt(II) complexes [2, 26, 27]. As an exemplary example, herein a cyclometallated Pt(II) complex which preferably interacts with nucleic acid structures at the nucleoli of CHO cancer cells is presented. The metal complex has an exceptionally high long luminescence lifetime in the microsecond range as well as strong emission, offering excellently suitable properties for luminescence lifetime microscopy. Using this technique, the uptake and localization of the metal complex with various luminescence delays in the range from 100 to 2,900 ns was studied (Figure 10) [2].

3.2.2 Detection of the Change in Localization of Metal Complexes by Changes in Their Lifetime in Different Cellular Environments

The photophysical properties of a metal complex can drastically change in different environments. As such, luminescence lifetime microscopy can be applied to study the localization and interaction in cellular compartments within cancerous cells. This technique has been applied for detecting changes in the subcellular

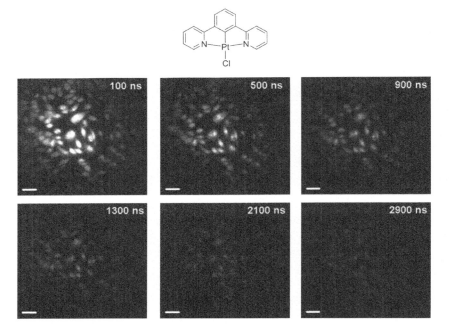

FIGURE 10 *Top*: Structure of a luminescent Pt(II) complex. *Bottom*: Luminescence lifetime microscopy images of CHO cells incubated with the luminescent Pt(II) complex (λ_{ex}=355 nm) and recorded with various luminescence delays. Scale bar=50 μm. (Reproduced by permission from Ref. [2]; Copyright 2008 United States National Academy of Sciences.)

localization of a cyclometallated Pt(II) [27] and a dinuclear Ru(II) complex [28]. Herein, as an example, the nuclear uptake of a dinuclear Ru(II) polypyridine complex is demonstrated. The metal complex showed different photophysical properties and, in particular, a different luminescence lifetime in the cytoplasm and the nucleus. Upon utilizing these properties, the internalization into the cancer cell nucleus can be monitored by luminescence lifetime microscopy (Figure 11) [28].

3.2.3 Metal Complexes as Luminescent Lifetime Sensors

Metal complexes are able to interact with various biomolecules or other important components within the cell. If these interactions change the photophysical properties of the metal complex, such compounds could be applied as luminescent lifetime sensors. The current literature is focused on the application of metal complexes as oxygen sensors [29–31]. As an exemplary example, the use of a luminescent Pt(II) porphyrin complex, which was encapsulated with Eudragit RL100 into nanoparticles, as an oxygen sensor is demonstrated. The lifetime of the chromophore is strongly reduced in the presence of oxygen. The nanomaterial showed to efficiently detect oxygen by luminescence lifetime microscopy under

Elucidating the Localization of Metal Complexes in Cancer Cells

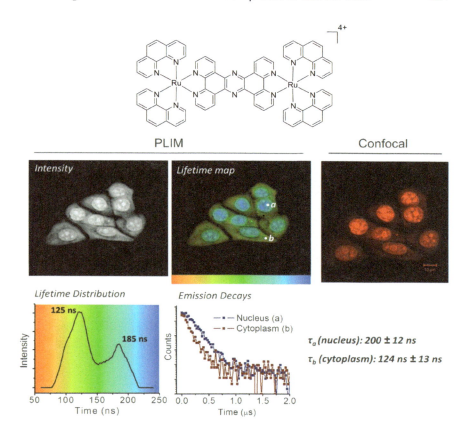

FIGURE 11 *Top*: Structure of a dinuclear luminescent Ru(II) complex. *Bottom*: Luminescence lifetime microscopy image (PLIM, left) and confocal microscopy image (right) of human breast cancer (MCF-7) cells incubated with the dinuclear Ru(II) polypyridine complex. The different cellular environment of the Ru(II) complex results in a different luminescence lifetime, allowing for the monitoring of the changes in localization of the metal complex. (Reproduced by permission from Ref. [26]; Copyright 2014 Wiley.)

normoxic (21% O_2) or hypoxic conditions (3% O_2). This allows for the detection of oxygen over the profile of the neurosphere (Figure 12) [31].

3.2.4 Conversion of Metal Complexes Inside Cancer Cells

Luminescence lifetime microscopy can be used to monitor the reactivity of a metal complex in cancerous cells if the conversion results in a metal complex with a significantly different luminescence lifetime. The application of an endoperoxide Ir(III) prodrug is presented as an exemplary example herein. The metal complex is efficiently taken up into the cancerous A549 cells where it accumulates preferably in the mitochondria. Upon light irradiation, singlet oxygen is released and the endoperoxide Ir(III) prodrug is converted into an anthracene

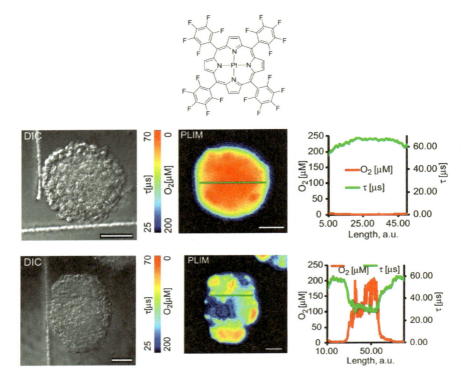

FIGURE 12 *Top*: Structure of a luminescent Pt(II) complex. *Middle*: Luminescence lifetime microscopy image of neurospheres under normoxic conditions (21% O_2) incubated with the Pt(II) complex encapsulated with Eudragit RL100 as an oxygen sensor. *Bottom*: Luminescence lifetime microscopy image of neurospheres under hypoxic conditions (3% O_2) incubated with the Pt(II) complex encapsulated with Eudragit RL100 as an oxygen sensor. (Reproduced by permission from Ref. [31]; Copyright 2013 Elsevier.)

Ir(III) complex as well as an alkoxy radical metal complex (for simplicity this alkoxy radical is not shown). As the prodrug has a long luminescence lifetime of ~850 ns and the generated product has a significantly shorter lifetime of ~450 ns, the light-induced conversion could be monitored in cancerous cells by luminescence lifetime microscopy (Figure 13) [32].

4 TWO-PHOTON EXCITATION MICROSCOPY

The theoretical concept of the simultaneous absorption of two photons by a single chromophore was first described in 1931 by Maria Göppert-Mayer [33]. Despite having presented the theoretical foundation, it was not until three decades later in 1961 that a two-photon excitation was experimentally observed by Kaiser and Garrett [34]. Notably, this discovery was made soon after the invention of the laser,

Elucidating the Localization of Metal Complexes in Cancer Cells   253

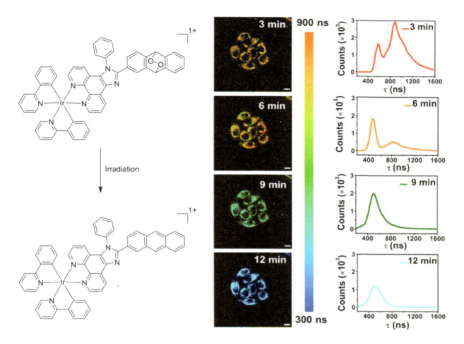

FIGURE 13 *Left*: Simplified conversion of the endoperoxide Ir(III) prodrug into the anthracene Ir(III) complex upon release of singlet oxygen (for simplicity the alkoxy radical which is generated as a side product is not shown). *Right*: Confocal laser scanning microscopy images of A549 cells incubated with the endoperoxide Ir(III) prodrug which is converted into the anthracene Ir(III) complex upon irradiation (λ_{ex}=750 nm) by luminescence lifetime microscopy. Scale bar=10 μm. (Reproduced by permission from Ref. [32]; Copyright 2022 American Chemical Society.)

which provided the necessary photon flux density for this photophysical phenomena. In honor of her contributions to this field, the unit in which a chromophore is measured to absorb two photons simultaneously, also referred to as the two-photon absorption cross-section, is termed as Göppert-Mayer (1 GM = 10^{-50} cm^4 s^{-1} photon^{-1}). Besides the proof of concept of the existence of two-photon processes, this field of research started to receive increasing attention with the development of sub-picosecond pulsed lasers and in particular the Ti-sapphire laser in the 1990s, which enabled the commercialization and easy accessibility of such instruments. A milestone for the use in biomedical applications was the development of the two-photon fluorescence microscope by Webb and coworkers [35]. Within the following section, the concept and the use of metal-based two-photon excited chromophores for their detection in cancer cells will be discussed. Several of these compounds can also be used for phototherapeutic applications which will not be covered here but has been critically reviewed recently [3, 36–39].

4.1 Advantages of Two-Photon Excitation Over One-Photon Excitation

During a typical (one-photon) luminescence process, the chromophore is excited from the ground state at a specific wavelength to an excited singlet state. Through vibrational non-radiative decay, this state is relaxed to an excited singlet state (S_2) for chromophores which interact by fluorescence or an excited triplet state (T_1) for chromophores which interact by phosphorescence (see Figure 7 above). Upon relaxation of this state, the chromophore emits light, which can be detected. Contrary to the one-photon mechanism, in a two-photon process, the initial excitation is performed through the simultaneous absorption of two photons of low energy/long wavelength (Figure 14), presenting several potential advantageous:

1. Selective excitation: As the excitation with a one-photon light source involves a single transition from the ground state to an excited state though a linear relationship between excitation and luminescence intensity, various molecules and chromophores can be excited along the z-axes of the laser beam, generating a focal plane. In contrast, a two-photon excitation shows a quadratic dependency to the luminescence intensity, allowing for an excitation only at the focal point (see photograph of the excitation of a fluorophore in Figure 15).
2. Reduced photodamage: One-photon laser excitations in particular with highly energetic UV-light may generate a number of undesired chemical modifications such as bond cleavage, isomerization, or even molecule decomposition. As two-photon excitations are characterized by the use two photons to reach the excited state, low energetic light sources can be used which results in much reduced photodamage.
3. Deeper light tissue penetration: One-photon light sources within the UV/VIS region have a very limited tissue penetration depth, allowing

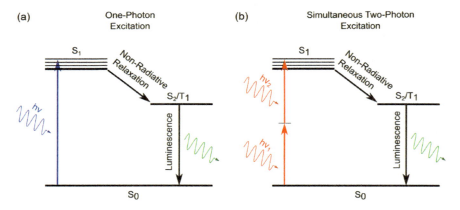

FIGURE 14 Jablonski diagram of (a) one-photon or (b) two-photon excitation. S = Singlet state, T = Triplet state.

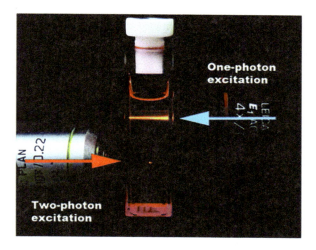

FIGURE 15 Photograph of the luminescence of a diketopyrrolopyrrole dye in a cuvette upon excitation with a one-photon (λ_{ex}=405 nm) or two-photon laser (λ_{ex}=800 nm). (Reproduced by permission from Ref. [40]; Copyright 2017 The Royal Society of Chemistry.)

only for superficial applications. Contrary, less energetic two-photon light has a longer wavelength which allows for significantly deeper tissue penetration (λ_{ex} = 405 vs. 800 nm in Figure 15).

4.2 Advantages of Metal Complexes as Two-Photon Excited Chromophores

Since the discovery of two-photon excitations, much research effort has been invested in the development of efficient two-photon chromophores. Although some structure-activity relationships have been established, there remains a lack of fundamental understanding for the rational design of such compounds. Studies have shown that in particular the extension of the conjugated π-system has an improved effect on the two-photon absorption properties. Further, terminal functionalization, which is able to influence the electron density in the conjugated system, showed a strong effect toward the two-photon absorption. Generally, D-π-D and D-π-A-π-D systems were found with enhanced properties in comparison to A-π-A and A-π-D-π-A systems (D=electron donating moiety, A=electron accepting moiety) [41–43].

Besides organic molecules, some attention has also been devoted to metal complexes. The first reported metal complex with two-photon absorption properties was dipyridinium thallium(III) pentachloride by Srivastava and Gupta in 1974. While their findings established the ability of metal-containing compounds to interact by a two-photon absorption process, the obtained results were of rudimentary and qualitative nature [44]. Investigations into the nature of the transition and the ability of metal complexes to interact in two-photon absorption processes were provided in 1997 by Lakowicz and coworkers, using ruthenium(II) polypyridine complexes of the type $[Ru(2,2'-bipyridine)_3]^{2+}$ as luminescent model compounds. The photophysical properties of the compounds were compared upon one-photon ($\lambda_{ex}=440\,nm$) and two-photon ($\lambda_{ex}=880\,nm$) excitation by steady-state and time-resolved emission spectroscopy. The results clearly indicated that the excited triplet metal-to-ligand charge transfer state (^{3}MLCT) can be populated through one- and two-photon excitation [45]. Following this study, various types of metal complexes have been studied and were found to possess two-photon absorption properties including complexes obtained from ruthenium [46–49], nickel [50], copper [51], silver [51], zinc [51, 52], platinum [25, 53, 54], mercury [55], iridium [56–58], europium [58–60], and terbium [60, 61]. Besides these findings, there remains still much to understand and learn about the structure-activity relationship and what makes a compound a good two-photon absorbing chromophore. The vast majority of studies have focused on incorporating organic moieties with known two-photon absorbing moieties into the ligand scaffold of metal complexes. However, recently a study has demonstrated that two-photon absorption could also be predicted by density functional theory calculations, indicating a path toward the rational design of metal complexes as efficient two-photon absorbing chromophores [62]. In addition to their ability to interact in two-photon absorption processes, metal complexes have been investigated as imaging probes due to a number of potential advantages:

1. Versatile modification of the photophysical properties by extension or functionalization of the ligand scaffold;
2. Large Stokes shift resulting in minimal interference between excitation and emission;
3. Emission properties are susceptible to the environment, allowing for the detection of trace or reactive species;
4. Strong emission and long luminescence lifetime due to promotion of the intersystem crossing process toward the excited triplet state by the heavy atom effect of the metal ion.

4.3 Selected Biomedical Problems Investigated by Two-Photon Excitation Microscopy of Metal Complexes

4.3.1 Metal Complexes as Two-Photon Excited Cell Organelle Dyes

Based on the strong photophysical properties of certain metal complexes, their subcellular localization can be tracked by confocal laser scanning microscopy. To avoid interference with other biologically present compounds, the metal complexes can be excited by a two-photon irradiation and their emission detected. The one- and two-photon excited channels can also be used in parallel. To date, metal complexes that can be excited by a two-photon light source and selectively

Elucidating the Localization of Metal Complexes in Cancer Cells 257

localize in the nucleus [63, 64], cytoplasm [65–67], cytomembrane [68], lysosomes [69–73], mitochondria [74–76], endoplasmic reticulum [77], and Golgi apparatus [78] have been reported. A recent review describes the subcellular localization of metal complexes in cancer cells as well as design strategies toward a specific cell organelle [79]. As an exemplary example, the confocal scanning laser microscopy images of HeLa cancer cells upon incubation with a luminescent Ru(II) polypyridine complex functionalized with a triphenylphosphonium group as a mitochondria-targeting moiety upon one- and two-photon excitation are presented. As expected, the one- and two-photon excited images were found to be congruent; however, a significantly better signal-to-noise ratio was observed upon two-photon excitation (Figure 16) [74].

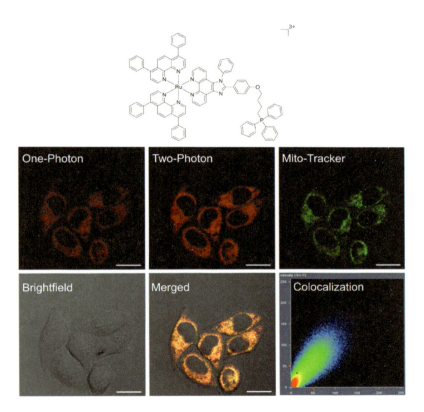

FIGURE 16 *Top*: Structure of a luminescent Ru(II) polypyridine complex functionalized with triphenylphosphine as a mitochondria-targeting moiety. *Bottom*: Confocal laser scanning microscopy images of HeLa cells incubated with a commercial mitochondria selective dye (Mito-Tracker) and a luminescent Ru(II) polypyridine complex functionalized with a triphenylphosphonium group as a mitochondria-targeting moiety. The metal complex was excited using one- (λ_{ex}=458 nm) or two-photon (λ_{ex}=830 nm) light sources and its emission detected (λ_{em}=580–640 nm). Scale bar=20 µm. (Reproduced by permission from Ref. [74]; Copyright 2015 Elsevier.)

4.3.2 Metal Complexes as Two-Photon Excited Sensors for Small Molecules

Various small molecules are involved in cellular processes or in the mechanism of action of therapeutic compounds. In an effort to understand certain cellular pathways, the generation and localization of these small and often reactive species is of high importance. Capitalizing on this, metal complexes that are able to selectively interact with a specific small molecule as well as show a modification of their photophysical properties upon that interaction could be used as two-photon excited sensors. To date, metal complexes have been reported as two-photon excited luminescent sensors for hydrogen peroxide [80], nitric oxide [81, 82], hydrogen sulfide [83], carbon monoxide [84], hypochlorous acid [85], sulfur dioxide [86], and oxygen [87–91]. Herein, the use of a Pd(II) carbazole-coumarin fused metal complex as a sensor for the detection of carbon monoxide is highlighted. While the metal complex itself is non-luminescent, upon interaction with carbon monoxide, the metal ion is released and the carbazole-coumarin construct is able to emit green light, upon one- or two-photon excitation (Figure 17) [84]. In this particular

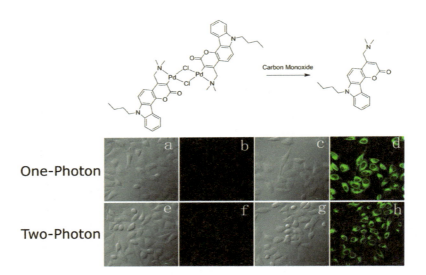

FIGURE 17 *Top*: Interaction of the non-luminescent Pd(II) complex with carbon monoxide to release the strong one- or two-photon luminescent organic chromophore. *Bottom*: Confocal laser scanning microscopy images of HeLa cells incubated with the Pd(II) complex (5 µM) and CORM-2 (200 µM) as a carbon monoxide source. (a/e) Brightfield microscopy image of HeLa cells incubated with CORM-2, (b/f) Fluorescence microscopy image of HeLa cells incubated with CORM-2 upon one- (λ_{ex}=405 nm) or two-photon (λ_{ex}=740 nm) excitation. (c/g) Brightfield microscopy image of HeLa cells incubated with the carbon monoxide-releasing compound $Ru_2Cl_4(CO)_6$ (CORM-2) as a source for carbon monoxide and the Pd(II) complex, (d/h) Fluorescence microscopy image of HeLa cells incubated with CORM-2 and the Pd(II) complex upon one- (λ_{ex}=405 nm) or two-photon (λ_{ex}=740 nm) excitation. (Reproduced by permission from Ref. [84]; Copyright 2014 Royal Society of Chemistry.)

Elucidating the Localization of Metal Complexes in Cancer Cells 259

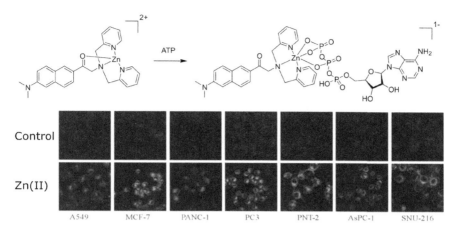

FIGURE 18 *Top*: Interaction of the poorly luminescent Zn(II) complex with adenosine triphosphate (ATP) to form a two-photon excited luminescent adduct. *Bottom*: Confocal laser scanning microscopy images of various types of cells incubated with the Zn(II) complex (Zn(II), 100 µM) upon two-photon (λ_{ex}=740 nm) excitation. (Reproduced by permission from Ref. [92]; Copyright 2012 Royal Society of Chemistry.)

experiment, the carbon monoxide-releasing compound, $Ru_2Cl_4(CO)_6$ (CORM-2), is actually the source of carbon monoxide and the Pd(II) complex serves as a sensor, thus beautifully highlighting the therapeutic as well as analytic/diagnostic properties of metal complexes in biomedical experiments.

4.3.3 Metal Complexes as Two-Photon Excited Luminophores for Biomolecules

Biomolecules play a fundamental role in the function of human cells. To unveil the cellular pathways these are involved in, selective and efficient luminescent probes are needed. To date, metal complexes that act as two-photon excited luminophores for adenosine triphosphate (ATP) [92–93], deoxyribonucleic acid (DNA) [94, 95], and biological thiols [96] have been described. Herein, the use of a Zn(II) complex as a selective cellular probe for the presence of ATP is discussed. The metal complex itself is poorly emissive in aqueous solution but is able to selectively interact with ATP. The generated metal complex-ATP adduct was found to be highly luminescent upon two-photon excitation (Figure 18) [92].

5 CONCLUSIONS

The localization of a metal complex within cancer cells has a strong impact on its biological effect. Within this chapter, some advanced methods for detection of metal complexes in cancerous cells have been highlighted. X-ray fluorescence microscopy allows for the detection of specific metals in cancerous cells. This technique is specifically suited for the identification of the localization of metal complexes based on non-naturally occurring metal ions. Also, it is the most direct method for detecting the co-localization of two (or several) different metal ions. Luminescence lifetime imaging microscopy enables the detection of changes in the chemical structure or specific interactions of luminescent metal complexes in cancerous cells. Luminescence lifetime imaging offers another dimension for detection beyond excitation and emission wavelengths. Luminescent two-photon chromophores could be specifically excited and detected by two-photon excitation microscopy, allowing for the precise determination of the subcellular localization of the metal complex. By exciting the probe with lower energy light, two-photon microscopy is potentially much less harmful to cells than traditional (confocal) microscopy, and also less damaging to the chromophores, allowing longer observation under less damaging conditions. We are confident that these techniques will pave the way into a better understanding of the localization and biochemical mechanism of action of metal complexes in cancer cells, thereby fostering the ability to rationally design novel compounds with tailored biological properties.

ACKNOWLEDGMENTS

J.K. gratefully acknowledges the financial support with a Liebig fellowship from the Chemical Industry Fund of the German Chemical Industry Association. N. M.-N. acknowledges support for the group from the German Science Foundation (DFG) through several grants over the years, most recently as a member of the RTG 2341 "Microbial Substrate Conversion." He is also grateful for the many and diverse coworkers, international visitors, and collaborators that have all contributed to the success of the group over the years.

ABBREVIATIONS

A	electron accepting moiety
ATP	adenosine triphosphate
A2780 cell	human ovarian cancer cell
A549 cell	human alveolar basal epithelial cell
CLD-1 cell	human colon carcinoma cell
CHO cell	Chinese hamster ovary cell
D	electron donating moiety
DNA	deoxyribonucleic acid
HeLa	human cervical carcinoma cell
IGROV1 cell	human ovarian adenocarcinoma cell
IGROV1-DDP cell	cisplatin-resistant human ovarian adenocarcinoma cell
^{3}MLCT	excited triplet metal-to-ligand charge transfer state
MCF-7 cell	human breast cancer cell
S_1/S_2	excited singlet state
T_1	excited triplet state
XRF imaging	X-ray fluorescence imaging

REFERENCES

[1] C. J. Fahrni, *Curr. Op. Chem. Biol.* **2007**, *11*, 121–127.

[2] S. W. Botchway, M. Charnley, J. W. Haycock, A. W. Parker, D. L. Rochester, J. A. Weinstein, J. A. G. Williams, *Proc. Natl. Acad. Sci.* **2008**, *105*, 16071–16076.

[3] Y. Chen, R. Guan, C. Zhang, J. Huang, L. Ji, H. Chao, *Coord. Chem. Rev.* **2016**, *310*, 16–40.

[4] M. J. Pushie, I. J. Pickering, M. Korbas, M. J. Hackett, G. N. George, *Chem. Rev.* **2014**, *114*, 8499–8541.

[5] A. A. Hummer, A. Rompel, *Metallomics* **2013**, *5*, 597–614.

[6] S. A. James, A. V. D. Ent, H. H. Harris, *Encycl. Inorg. Bioinorg. Chem.* **2019**, *1* 1–18.

[7] S. P. Roudeau, A. Carmona, L. Perrin, R. Ortega, *Anal. Bioanal. Chem.* **2014**, *406*, 6979–6991.

[8] S. C. Leary, M. Ralle, *Curr. Op. Chem. Biol.* **2020**, *55*, 19–25.

[9] E. R. Jamieson, S. J. Lippard, *Chem. Rev.* **1999**, *99*, 2467–2498.

[10] R. Ortega, P. Moretto, A. Fajac, J. Benard, Y. Llabador, M. Simonoff, *Cell. Mol. Biol.* **1996**, *42*, 77–88.

[11] P. Ilinski, B. Lai, Z. Cai, W. Yun, D. Legnini, T. Talarico, M. Cholewa, L. K. Webster, G. B. Deacon, S. Rainone, D. R. Phillips, A. P. J. Stampfl, *Cancer Res.* **2003**, *63*, 1776–1779.

[12] M. D. Hall, R. A. Alderden, M. Zhang, P. J. Beale, Z. Cai, B. Lai, A. P. J. Stampfl, T. W. Hambley, *J. Struct. Biol.* **2006**, *155*, 38–44.

[13] V. Fernandez-Moreira, M. C. Gimeno, *Chem. Eur. J.* **2018**, *24*, 3345–3353.

[14] E. L. Crossley, J. B. Aitken, S. Vogt, H. H. Harris, L. M. Rendina, *Angew. Chem. Int. Ed.* **2010**, *49*, 1231–1233.

[15] J. L. Wedding, H. H. Harris, C. A. Bader, S. E. Plush, R. Mak, M. Massi, D. A. Brooks, B. Lai, S. Vogt, M. V. Werrett, P. V. Simpson, B. W. Skelton, S. Stagni, *Metallomics* **2017**, *9*, 382–390.

[16] C. C. Konkankit, J. Lovett, H. H. Harris, J. J. Wilson, *Chem. Commun.* **2020**, *56*, 6515–6518.

[17] Z. Y. Huang, A. P. King, J. Lovett, B. Lai, J. J. Woods, H. H. Harris, J. J. Wilson, *Chem. Commun.* **2021**, *57*, 11189–11192.

[18] R. A. Alderden, H. R. Mellor, S. Modok, M. D. Hall, S. R. Sutton, M. G. Newville, R. Callaghan, T. W. Hambley, *J. Am. Chem. Soc.* **2007**, *129*, 13400–13401.

[19] C. Sanchez-Cano, I. Romero-Canelon, K. Geraki, P. J. Sadler, *J. Inorg. Biochem.* **2018**, *185*, 26–29.

[20] J. Z. Zhang, N. S. Bryce, A. Lanzirotti, C. K. J. Chen, D. Paterson, M. D. de Jonge, D. L. Howard, T. W. Hambley, *Metallomics* **2012**, *4*, 1209–1217.

[21] E. Becquerel, *Ann. Chimie Phys.* **1859**, *3*, 5.

[22] R. W. Wood, *Proc. R. Soc. London, Ser. A* **1921**, *99*, 362.

[23] E. Gaviola, Z. *Phys.* **1926**, *35*, 748.

[24] R. R. de Haas, R. P. M. van Gijlswijk, E. B. van der Tol, H. J. M. A. A. Zijlmans, T. Bakker-Schut, J. Bonnet, N. P. Verwoerd, H. J. Tanke, *J. Histochem. Cytochem.* **1997**, *45*, 1279–1292.

[25] R. R. de Haas, R. P. M. van Gijlswijk, E. B. van der Tol, J. Veuskens, H. E. van Gijssel, R. B. Tijdens, J. Bonnet, N. P. Verwoerd, H. J. Tanke, *J. Histochem. Cytochem.* **1999**, *47*, 183–196.

[26] E. Baggaley, I. V. Sazanovich, J. A. G. Williams, J. W. Haycock, S. W. Botchway, J. A. Weinstein, *RSC Adv.* **2014**, *4*, 35003–35008.

[27] E. Baggaley, S. W. Botchway, J. W. Haycock, H. Morris, I. V. Sazanovich, J. A. G. Williams, J. A. Weinstein, *Chem. Sci.* **2014**, *5*, 879–886.

[28] E. Baggaley, M. R. Gill, N. H. Green, D. Turton, I. V. Sazanovich, S. W. Botchway, C. Smythe, J. W. Haycock, J. A. Weinstein, J. A. Thomas, *Angew. Chem. Int. Ed.* **2014**, *53*, 3367–3371.

[29] J. Lecoq, A. Parpaleix, E. Roussakis, M. Ducros, Y. G. Houssen, S. A. Vinogradov, S. Charpak, *Nat. Med.* **2011**, *17*, 893–898.

[30] O. S. Finikova, A. Y. Lebedev, A. Aprelev, T. Troxler, F. Gao, C. Garnacho, S. Muro, R. M. Hochstrasser, S. A. Vinogradov, *ChemPhysChem* **2008**, *9*, 1673–1679.

[31] R. I. Dmitriev, A. V. Zhdanov, Y. M. Nolan, D. B. Papkovsky, *Biomaterials* **2013**, *34*, 9307–9317.

[32] S. Kuang, F. Wei, J. Karges, L. Ke, K. Xiong, X. Liao, G. Gasser, L. Ji, H. Chao, *J. Am. Chem. Soc.* **2022**, *144*, 4091–4101.

[33] M. Göppert-Mayer, *Ann. Phys.* **1931**, *401*, 273–294.

[34] W. Kaiser, C. G. B. Garrett, *Phys. Rev. Lett.* **1961**, *7*, 229–231.

[35] W. Denk, J. H. Strickler, W. W. Webb, *Science* **1990**, *248*, 73–76.

[36] J. Karges, H. Chao, G. Gasser, *J. Biol. Inorg. Chem.* **2020**, *25*, 1035–1050.

[37] L. K. McKenzie, H. E. Bryant, J. A. Weinstein, *Coord. Chem. Rev.* **2019**, *379*, 2–29.

[38] F. Heinemann, J. Karges, G. Gasser, *Acc. Chem. Res.* **2017**, *50*, 2727–2736.

[39] Z. Sun, L.-P. Zhang, F. Wu, Y. Zhao, *Adv. Funct. Mater.* **2017**, *27*, 1704079.

[40] F. Bolze, S. Jenni, A. Sour, V. Heitz, *Chem. Commun.* **2017**, *53*, 12857–12877.

[41] M. Pawlicki, H. A. Collins, R. G. Denning, H. L. Anderson, *Angew. Chem. Int. Ed.* **2009**, *48*, 3244–3266.

[42] S. Yao, K. D. Belfield, *Eur. J. Org. Chem.* **2012**, *2012*, 3199–3217.

[43] F. Terenziani, C. Katan, E. Badaeva, S. Tretiak, M. Blanchard-Desce, *Adv. Mater.* **2008**, *20*, 4641–4678.

[44] G. P. Srivastava, S. C. Gupta, *Optica Acta* **1974**, *21*, 43–49.

[45] F. N. Castellano, H. Malak, I. Gryczynski, J. R. Lakowicz, *Inorg. Chem.* **1997**, *36*, 5548–5551.

[46] C. Girardot, G. Lemercier, J. C. Mulatier, J. Chauvin, P. L. Baldeck, C. Andraud, *Dalton Trans.* **2007**, 3421–3426.

[47] S. C. Boca, M. Four, A. Bonne, B. van der Sanden, S. Astilean, P. L. Baldeck, G. Lemercier, *Chem. Commun.* **2009**, 4590–4592.

[48] J. Karges, S. Kuang, Y. C. Ong, H. Chao, G. Gasser, *Chem. Eur. J.* **2021**, *27*, 362–370.

[49] C. Girardot, B. Cao, J.-C. Mulatier, P. L. Baldeck, J. Chauvin, D. Riehl, J. A. Delaire, C. Andraud, G. Lemercier, *ChemPhysChem* **2008**, *9*, 1531–1535.

[50] Q. Zheng, G. S. He, P. N. Prasad, *J. Mater. Chem.* **2005**, *15*, 579–587.

[51] H. Akdas-Kilig, J.-P. Malval, F. Morlet-Savary, A. Singh, L. Toupet, I. Ledoux-Rak, J. Zyss, H. Le Bozec, *Dyes Pigments* **2012**, *92*, 681–688.

[52] Y. Gao, J. Wu, Y. Li, P. Sun, H. Zhou, J. Yang, S. Zhang, B. Jin, Y. Tian, *J. Am. Chem. Soc.* **2009**, *131*, 5208–5213.

[53] C.-K. Koo, K.-L. Wong, C. W.-Y. Man, Y.-W. Lam, L. K.-Y. So, H.-L. Tam, S.-W. Tsao, K.-W. Cheah, K.-C. Lau, Y.-Y. Yang, J.-C. Chen, M. H.-W. Lam, *Inorg. Chem.* **2009**, *48*, 872–878.

[54] T. Goudreault, Z. He, Y. Guo, C.-L. Ho, H. Zhan, Q. Wang, K. Y.-F. Ho, K.-L. Wong, D. Fortin, B. Yao, Z. Xie, L. Wang, W.-M. Kwok, P. D. Harvey, W.-Y. Wong, *Macromolecules* **2010**, *43*, 7936–7949.

[55] H. Zhou, F. Zhou, P. Wu, Z. Zheng, Z. Yu, Y. Chen, Y. Tu, L. Kong, J. Wu, Y. Tian, *Dyes Pigments* **2011**, *91*, 237–247.

[56] J. Liu, C. Jin, B. Yuan, X. Liu, Y. Chen, L. Ji, H. Chao, *Chem. Commun.* **2017**, *53*, 2052–2055.

Elucidating the Localization of Metal Complexes in Cancer Cells 263

[57] X. Liao, J. Shen, W. Wu, S. Kuang, M. Lin, J. Karges, Z. Tang, H. Chao, *Inorg. Chem. Front.* **2021**, *8*, 5045–5053.

[58] E. Baggaley, D.-K. Cao, D. Sykes, S. W. Botchway, J. A. Weinstein, M. D. Ward, *Chem. Eur. J.* **2014**, *20*, 8898–8903.

[59] A. Picot, A. D'Aléo, P. L. Baldeck, A. Grichine, A. Duperray, C. Andraud, O. Maury, *J. Am. Chem. Soc.* **2008**, *130*, 1532–1533.

[60] A. D'Aléo, G. Pompidor, B. Elena, J. Vicat, P. L. Baldeck, L. Toupet, R. Kahn, C. Andraud, O. Maury, *ChemPhysChem* **2007**, *8*, 2125–2132.

[61] D. Li, N. Shao, X. Sun, G. Zhang, S. Li, H. Zhou, J. Wu, Y. Tian, *Spectrochim. Acta A* **2014**, *133*, 134–140.

[62] J. Karges, S. Kuang, F. Maschietto, O. Blacque, I. Ciofini, H. Chao, G. Gasser, *Nat. Commun.* **2020**, *11*, 3262.

[63] C.-K. Koo, L. K.-Y. So, K.-L. Wong, Y.-M. Ho, Y.-W. Lam, M. H.-W. Lam, K.-W. Cheah, C. C.-W. Cheng, W.-M. Kwok, *Chem. Eur. J.* **2010**, *16*, 3942–3950.

[64] A. D'Aléo, A. Bourdolle, S. Brustlein, T. Fauquier, A. Grichine, A. Duperray, P. L. Baldeck, C. Andraud, S. Brasselet, O. Maury, *Angew. Chem. Int. Ed.* **2012**, *51*, 6622–6625.

[65] S.-S. Zhou, X. Xue, J.-F. Wang, Y. Dong, B. Jiang, D. Wei, M.-L. Wan, Y. Jia, *J. Mater. Chem.* **2012**, *22*, 22774–22780.

[66] C. Nie, Q. Zhang, H. Ding, B. Huang, X. Wang, X. Zhao, S. Li, H. Zhou, J. Wu, Y. Tian, *Dalton Trans.* **2014**, *43*, 599–608.

[67] W. Xu, J. Zuo, L. Wang, L. Ji, H. Chao, *Chem. Commun.* **2014**, *50*, 2123–2125.

[68] K. Qiu, J. Wang, C. Song, L. Wang, H. Zhu, H. Huang, J. Huang, H. Wang, L. Ji, H. Chao, *ACS Appl. Mater. Interfaces* **2017**, *9*, 18482–18492.

[69] Y.-M. Ho, N.-P. B. Au, K.-L. Wong, C. T.-L. Chan, W.-M. Kwok, G.-L. Law, K.-K. Tang, W.-Y. Wong, C.-H. E. Ma, M. H.-W. Lam, *Chem. Commun.* **2014**, *50*, 4161–4163.

[70] L. He, C.-P. Tan, R.-R. Ye, Y.-Z. Zhao, Y.-H. Liu, Q. Zhao, L.-N. Ji, Z.-W. Mao, *Angew. Chem. Int. Ed.* **2014**, *53*, 12137–12141.

[71] J. Jing, J.-J. Chen, Y. Hai, J. Zhan, P. Xu, J.-L. Zhang, *Chem. Sci.* **2012**, *3*, 3315–3320.

[72] C. A. Bader, R. D. Brooks, Y. S. Ng, A. Sorvina, M. V. Werrett, P. J. Wright, A. G. Anwer, D. A. Brooks, S. Stagni, S. Muzzioli, M. Silberstein, B. W. Skelton, E. M. Goldys, S. E. Plush, T. Shandala, M. Massi, *RSC Adv.* **2014**, *4*, 16345–16351.

[73] J. Karges, J. Li, L. Zeng, H. Chao, G. Gasser, *ACS Appl. Mater. Interfaces* **2020**, *12*, 54433–54444.

[74] J. Liu, Y. Chen, G. Li, P. Zhang, C. Jin, L. Zeng, L. Ji, H. Chao, *Biomaterials* **2015**, *56*, 140–153.

[75] J. Shen, J. Karges, K. Xiong, Y. Chen, L. Ji, H. Chao, *Biomaterials* **2021**, *275*, 120979.

[76] H. Huang, L. Yang, P. Zhang, K. Qiu, J. Huang, Y. Chen, J. Diao, J. Liu, L. Ji, J. Long, H. Chao, *Biomaterials* **2016**, *83*, 321–331.

[77] J. S. Nam, M.-G. Kang, J. Kang, S.-Y. Park, S. J. C. Lee, H.-T. Kim, J. K. Seo, O.-H. Kwon, M. H. Lim, H.-W. Rhee, T.-H. Kwon, *J. Am. Chem. Soc.* **2016**, *138*, 10968–10977.

[78] C. L. Ho, K. L. Wong, H. K. Kong, Y. M. Ho, C. T. L. Chan, W. M. Kwok, K. S. Y. Leung, H. L. Tam, M. H. W. Lam, X. F. Ren, A. M. Ren, J. K. Feng, W. Y. Wong, *Chem. Commun.* **2012**, *48*, 2525–2527.

[79] K. Qiu, Y. Chen, T. W. Rees, L. Ji, H. Chao, *Coord. Chem. Rev.* **2019**, *378*, 66–86.

[80] J. Jing, J.-L. Zhang, *Chem. Sci.* **2013**, *4*, 2947–2952.

[81] M. Ghosh, N. M. S. van den Akker, K. A. P. Wijnands, M. Poeze, C. Weber, L. E. McQuade, M. D. Pluth, S. J. Lippard, M. J. Post, D. G. M. Molin, M. A. M. J. van Zandvoort, *PLOS One* **2013**, *8*, e75331.

[82] X. Chen, L. Sun, Y. Chen, X. Cheng, W. Wu, L. Ji, H. Chao, *Biomaterials* **2015**, *58*, 72–81.

[83] A. Zhu, Z. Luo, C. Ding, B. Li, S. Zhou, R. Wang, Y. Tian, *Analyst* **2014**, *139*, 1945–1952.

[84] K. Zheng, W. Lin, L. Tan, H. Chen, H. Cui, *Chem. Sci.* **2014**, *5*, 3439–3448.

[85] G. Li, Q. Lin, L. Sun, C. Feng, P. Zhang, B. Yu, Y. Chen, Y. Wen, H. Wang, L. Ji, H. Chao, *Biomaterials* **2015**, *53*, 285–295.

[86] G. Li, Y. Chen, J. Wang, J. Wu, G. Gasser, L. Ji, H. Chao, *Biomaterials* **2015**, *63*, 128–136.

[87] X.-D. Wang, D. E. Achatz, C. Hupf, M. Sperber, J. Wegener, S. Bange, J. M. Lupton, O. S. Wolfbeis, *Sens. Actuators B Chem.* **2013**, *188*, 257–262.

[88] A. V. Kondrashina, R. I. Dmitriev, S. M. Borisov, I. Klimant, I. O'Brien, Y. M. Nolan, A. V. Zhdanov, D. B. Papkovsky, *Adv. Funct. Mater.* **2012**, *22*, 4931–4939.

[89] O. S. Finikova, T. Troxler, A. Senes, W. F. DeGrado, R. M. Hochstrasser, S. A. Vinogradov, *J. Phys. Chem. A* **2007**, *111*, 6977–6990.

[90] P. Zhang, H. Huang, Y. Chen, J. Wang, L. Ji, H. Chao, *Biomaterials* **2015**, *53*, 522–531.

[91] E. Roussakis, J. A. Spencer, C. P. Lin, S. A. Vinogradov, *Anal. Chem.* **2014**, *86*, 5937–5945.

[92] A. Sreenivasa Rao, D. Kim, H. Nam, H. Jo, K. H. Kim, C. Ban, K. H. Ahn, *Chem. Commun.* **2012**, *48*, 3206–3208.

[93] S. J. Lee, A. S. Rao, Y. H. Shin, H.-J. Chung, Y. Huh, K. H. Ahn, J. Jung, *J. Mol. Hist.* **2013**, *44*, 241–247.

[94] P. Hanczyc, B. Norden, M. Samoc, *Dalton Trans.* **2012**, *41*, 3123–3125.

[95] X. Wang, X. Tian, Q. Zhang, P. Sun, J. Wu, H. Zhou, B. Jin, J. Yang, S. Zhang, C. Wang, X. Tao, M. Jiang, Y. Tian, *Chem. Mater.* **2012**, *24*, 954–961.

[96] P. Zhang, J. Wang, H. Huang, H. Chen, R. Guan, Y. Chen, L. Ji, H. Chao, *Biomaterials* **2014**, *35*, 9003–9011.

10 Metalloproteomics: *A Powerful Technique for Metals in Medicine*

Tiffany Ka-Yan Ip, Ying Zhou,
Hongyan Li*, and Hongzhe Sun*
Department of Chemistry and CAS-HKU Joint
Laboratory of Metallomics on Health and Environment
The University of Hong Kong, Pokfulam Road,
Hong Kong SAR, China
hylichem@hku.hk, hsun@hku.hk

CONTENTS

1 Introduction 266
2 Methodology of Metallomics and Metalloproteomics 267
    2.1 Mass Spectrometry: Inductively Coupled Plasma-Mass
        Spectrometry (ICP-MS) and Mass Cytometry 267
    2.2 Photoaffinity Chemical Probes for Mining Metalloproteins 270
    2.3 Nuclear-Based Techniques 272
    2.4 Immobilized Metal Affinity Chromatography (IMAC) 272
    2.5 Integration of Metalloproteomics with Other-Omics and Deep
        Learning 272
3 Implementation on Biomedical Studies 273
    3.1 Anticancer Drugs 274
    3.2 Antimicrobial Drugs... 278
4 Conclusion and Outlook 282
Acknowledgments.. 283
Abbreviations 283
References... 284

ABSTRACT

Metal ions are essential for the living process of organisms physiologically and
pathologically, interacting with numerous proteins in biological systems. Metal
ions have also been incorporated into pharmaceuticals for diagnostic and therapeutic purposes. However, their mechanisms of action remain uncharted due to
the difficulty in mapping their interactive proteomes in the complex biological

---

* Corresponding authors

DOI: 10.1201/9781003272250-10

265

system. Recently, the introduction and development of metalloproteomics facilitates the metal-associated proteomes to be tracked, which provides a fundamental basis for further unveiling the modes of action of metallo-drugs. In this chapter, we introduce the development of metalloproteomics, including the methodology, its implementation in biomedical studies such as anticancer and antimicrobial mechanistic studies of metallo-drugs, and pinpoint the potential application of metalloproteomics in other research areas in the future.

KEYWORDS

Metalloproteomics; Metallo-drugs; Mechanism of Action; Bioinorganic Chemistry; Proteomics; Anticancer Drug; Antibacterial Drug

1 INTRODUCTION

Metal ions play a vital role in living organisms. Within bacteria, metal homeostasis is maintained to assure appropriate functioning of enzymes that utilize essential metal ions such as zinc, iron, and manganese as cofactors, and to prevent metal overload, which may cause bacterial death [1, 2]. Metal ions are also necessary for human physiology and pathology. Copper and iron are responsible for the function of critical enzymes and proteins in mammalian cells for sustaining human health [3, 4]. In contrast, the introduction of heavy metals into the human body, such as platinum, arsenic, and gold, may induce malignant cell death, boosting the development of numerous anticancer metallo-drugs [5]. By virtue of the extensive proteins in living organisms and the multi-targeted mode of action of metal ions, understanding the complex relationship between metals and proteins are extremely challenging, and there are only limited studies at a systemic level to unveil the mechanism of action of these metallo-drugs.

The concept of "metallome" was first introduced by Robert J. P. Williams in 2003. In parallel to the term "proteome," metallome represents a pool of soluble elements (mostly metal ions) which distributes within cells; whereas proteome represents a pool of proteins in biological systems [6]. Later, Hiroki Haraguchi further proposed metallomics as a new research field, and stated its importance corresponding to genomics, proteomics, and metabolomics [7]. This offers a more comprehensive way to analyze the distribution of metals within cellular compartments. In his definition, any metal-containing biomolecules are considered as metallomes, which include metalloproteins and metalloenzymes. These metalloproteins are crucial, and they not only cover one quarter of the protein bank, but also work as catalysts in metabolism, DNA and RNA synthesis, antioxidation, and so on. Due to the importance of metalloproteins, the term "metalloproteome" was proposed, some also suggested that this category should not only be limited to metalloproteins, but also any proteins that possess metal-binding capability or having metal-binding sites [8]. The related studies have further evolved as "metalloproteomics," serving as a sub-discipline of metallomics and proteomics, which helps elucidate cellular disposition and function of metals in metabolism.

In terms of pathological studies, metalloproteomics helps to unveil the disease mechanisms related to metals or complicated by abnormal disposition of metals.

2 METHODOLOGY OF METALLOMICS AND METALLOPROTEOMICS

For metalloproteomics studies, four steps are normally involved (Figure 1). Metallo-drugs or metal-containing photoaffinity chemical probes are applied to the cells or tissues, metal-associated proteins are then differentiated from the pool of proteins by separation techniques. After that, metalloproteins are detected and identified using analytical tools. The binding of metals to the proteins is further validated by different techniques including ultraviolet (UV)-vis spectroscopy [9], isothermal titration calorimetry (ITC) [10], mass spectrometry [11], and circular dichroism (CD) [12] and *in cellulo* binding can be confirmed by cellular thermal shift assay (CETSA) [13]. The structure of metalloproteins can also be determined by protein crystallography [14], nuclear magnetic resonance (NMR) spectroscopy [15], or cryogenic electron microscopy (CryoEM) [16]. It will be useful if these metalloproteomics data are integrated with other -omics data to map a more comprehensive picture of the molecular mechanisms. Recently, artificial intelligence (AI) has been developed to facilitate metalloprotein investigation efficiently in a computational way. In the following section, we introduce the analytical techniques commonly used in metalloproteomics research.

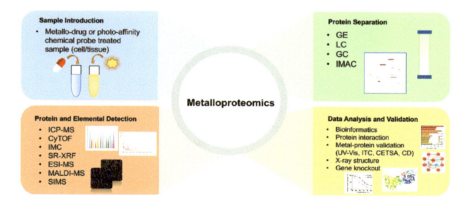

FIGURE 1 Workflow of a metalloproteomics study.

2.1 Mass Spectrometry: Inductively Coupled Plasma-Mass Spectrometry (ICP-MS) and Mass Cytometry

Biological samples treated with metallo-drugs may contain a collection of proteins and metalloproteins. Prior to mass spectrometry, partition of these proteins required the use of several separation techniques, such as liquid chromatography (LC), capillary electrophoresis (CE), and gel electrophoresis (GE). While LC provides a milder separation condition by separating proteins according to their affinities for the mobile phase and the porous solid, the resolution is quite low and usually requires multidimensional separations [17]. In contrast, CE uses applied voltage to separate proteins and peptides based on isoelectric points; however, protein separation is difficult to optimize [18]. CE is also hard to integrate with ICP-MS due to the insufficient detection limit [19], therefore it is not commonly used now in protein separation. On the other hand, GE provides a completely different approach to separate proteins running through polyacrylamide gel by applying an electric field and it is now the most often used technique in proteomics. For 1-dimensional (1D) electrophoresis, separation is facilitated according to protein size, in which smaller proteins move faster and larger proteins migrate slower [20]. For 2D-electrophoresis, proteins can be further separated perpendicularly right after the first dimension. It allows separation of proteins according to their isoelectric point and protein mass [21].

In favor of characterizing metalloproteins, detection of metal ions is necessary. This can be achieved by mass spectrometry (MS), which is an analytical technique to measure the mass-to-charge (m/z) ratio of ions in a sample. This technique goes through three major processes: creating ions from the sample, separating these ions, and then detecting these ions for analysis [22]. The ionization source, mass analyzer, and detector vary on different mass spectrometers according to their applications. One of the commonly used MS techniques for detecting metals is inductively coupled plasma-mass spectrometry (ICP-MS). The sample is nebulized on being introduced to the ICP, and then reaches the plasma, where the sample is atomized and ionized under high temperature. The ions are guided to the mass analyzer, which separates the ions according to their m/z ratio, and finally, the analyte strikes the detector and generates a signal [23]. To ease the workflow of metalloproteomics studies, separation and detection techniques are often hyphenated. LC-ICP-MS is a rather straightforward connection of column outlet of LC with the nebulizer of ICP-MS [24]; however, the separation resolution of LC is poor, and thus multidimensional separation is required. On the other hand, GE-ICP-MS was developed using column-type gel instead of slab gel in the GE system to achieve continuous flow, and the separated elutes are then subjected to two parts: ICP-MS for metal measurement and biological mass spectrometry for protein identification [25]. The major drawback for GE-ICP-MS is its poor separation resolution due to the use of 1D-GE in the system. Recently, LC-GE-ICP-MS was built to address this problem (Figure 2). In this approach, LC is used to separate proteins according to isoelectric points while GE differentiates proteins based on molecular weights, achieving multidimensional separation in continuous flow [26].

Single cell analysis is currently a prominent field in cellular biology. Since cells may differ in terms of cell type and diseases, traditional analysis from bulk samples may not acquire information reflecting on cell heterogeneity [27]. In fact, single cell analysis provides useful information in the study of genomics, proteomics, and cell-cell interactions [28]. Given the unique advantages of ICP-MS for metal quantification, ICP-MS, in its time-resolved analysis mode (TR-ICP-MS), has been expanded for single cell studies. Monitoring metallo-drug-treated single bacterial cells by TR-ICP-MS demonstrates individual

Metalloproteomics

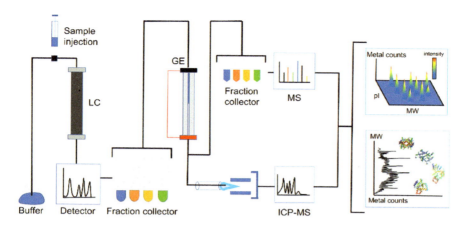

FIGURE 2 Workflow of LC-GE-ICP-MS.

growing stages of a cell and its respective metal uptake, which offers insight into metal-related bioprocesses [29]. Exploring the mechanism of action of the anticancer metallo-drug arsenic trioxide, based on TR-ICP-MS, reveals the apoptosis-inducing effects of arsenic trioxide as its major pathway for killing leukemia cells [30]. Additionally, the cell cycle-dependent uptake and cytotoxicity of arsenic-based drugs uncovered by TR-ICP-MS provide an additional basis for anticancer drug design [31]. Mass cytometry (CyTOF) may also offer detailed information at the single cell level. Prior to CyTOF, cellular proteins in samples were labeled with lanthanide tag-conjugated antibodies. The labeled samples will be injected to CyTOF, nebulized and ignited in argon plasma, and then the ion clouds generated were quantified by ICP-MS detector. This technology has overcome the limitation of flow cytometry and doesn't require any fluorescent tag that may cause emission overlap [32], providing the most highly multiplexed capability for single cell proteome quantification. With the help of CyTOF, cisplatin accumulation in cisplatin-sensitive and -resistant cells can be accurately determined, aiding in screening inhibitors of the cisplatin efflux ABCC2 pump [33]. Additionally, through simultaneous monitoring of intracellular cisplatin, the cell cycle and cell proliferation status, the dose, and the time-dependent cell cycle arrest of tumor cells (BxPC-3 and ME-180) induced by cisplatin were noted [34]. In addition to the application of mass cytometry for uncovering the mechanism of action of metallo-drugs, it has also been used to study the accumulation and interaction of nanoparticles with different types of immune cells, providing an additional basis for the nanomedicine design [35, 36].

In addition, the two types of mass cytometry imaging (MCI), imaging mass cytometry (IMC) and multiplexed ion beam imaging (MIBI), endow visualization of the tissue microenvironment by ablating stained tissue and directing ions to the CyTOF. The two work similarly except for the ablation methods and resolution where IMC ablates by a laser with a fixed resolution, while MIBI uses a tunable ion beam with varying image resolution [37]. The MCI technique provides highly multiplexed imaging for comprehensive analysis of tissue heterogeneity and thus benefits diagnoses and therapies [38]. With MCI, visualization of Pt localization and phenotypes associated with cellular responses in tissues (malignant and normal) of cisplatin-treated mice has been achieved, uncovering the extensive binding of Pt to collagen fibers and the slow release of stroma-bound Pt [39].

2.2 PHOTOAFFINITY CHEMICAL PROBES FOR MINING METALLOPROTEINS

The ease of metalloprotein detection is highly related to the metal-binding affinity of proteins. In response to proteins with weak and transient metal binding, ICP-MS is not a favorable technique as metals might be dissociated during protein separation. Alternatively, small molecule fluorescent probes are more useful for identifying these metalloproteins, which are designed to be highly specific and have less perturbation on the proteins; besides, it offers chances to mapping of metalloproteins and real-time visualization [40]. Being the most representative chemical probe, fluorescein arsenical hairpin binder-ethanedithiol (FlAsH-EDT_2) (Figure 3e) achieves site-specific labeling by the interaction of arsenic and the tetracysteine motif in a protein, and fluorescence is turned on upon the binding [41]. The debut of FlAsH-EDT_2 stimulates the development of heterogeneous fluorescent chemical probes.

Nitrilotriacetic acid (NTA) works akin to ethylenediaminetetraacetic acid (EDTA), its metal chelating properties make it a powerful tool for both protein purification and recognition. Since the first report on using Ni^{2+}-NTA beads (Figure 3a) to purify polyhistidine-tagged proteins [42], further modifications have been made such as adding fluorochrome on a His_6-Ni^{2+}-NTA system, to achieve site-specific fluorescent labeling [43]. Later, diverse NTA-based fluorescent probes have been developed via conjugation of mono-, di-, tri-, or tetra-NTA derivatives (Figure 3b) to resemble the concept of FlAsH [44–47]; however, low cell permeability remains a major problem of these probes, restraining their application on intracellular proteins [45]. To address this issue, Ni-NTA-AC (Figure 3c) was designed, which consists of a membrane-permeable fluorophore, a mono-NTA moiety, and an arylazide moiety [48]. Following the introduction of Ni-NTA-AC, other NTA-based probes (Figure 3d) have been developed with diverse fluorophores to expand the spectrum of applications [49, 50]. The concept of an NTA probe has been further extended by replacing Ni^{2+} with other metal ions, such as $Bi^{3+,}$ $Fe^{2+,}$ and Ga^{3+}, constructing an array of metal-tunable and membrane-permeable fluorescent probes (M^{n+}-TRACER) [51–53]. This facilitates the separation of proteins for further downstream analysis on metalloproteomics. By replacing the metal tagging group, the Ni-NTA moiety, with an arsenic targeting group, new organic arsenic EDT-containing probe NPE and As-AC (Figure 3g) were obtained [54, 55]. The probe As-AC selectively targets arsenic-binding proteins and arylazide is critical for significant fluorescence turn-on upon UV activation, and over 30 arsenic-binding proteins were tracked by applying this probe to NB4 cells. Apart from the EDT-containing probe, arsenical probes with two hydroxyl groups were also designed to target arsenic-binding proteins (Figure 3f), and was further proved by assay using thioredoxin as an arsenic-binding protein model [56].

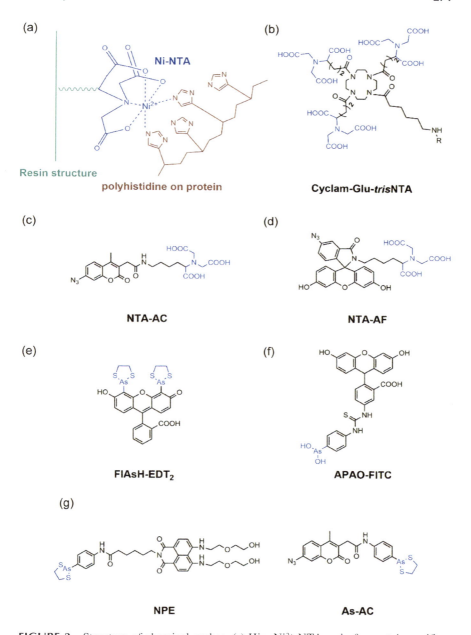

FIGURE 3 Structure of chemical probes. (a) His$_6$-Ni^{2+}-NTA resin for protein purification; (b) di- and tri-NTA probes; (c) cell permeable NTA-AC probe (AC=azide-coumarin); (d) other cell permeable NTA probe: NTA-AB (AB=azide-BODIPY) and NTA-AF (AF=azide-fluorescein); (e) membrane-permeable and non-fluorescent FlAsH-EDT$_2$ (EDT=ethanedithiol); (f) hydroxyl-containing arsenical probe APAO-FITC; (g) fluorescent EDT-containing arsenical probe: As-AC and NPE.

2.3 Nuclear-Based Techniques

For elemental analysis of metalloproteins, a highly precise and non-invasive technique, X-ray absorption spectrometry (XAS), is introduced. Once the X-ray beam strikes the sample, absorption edge energy of each element can be observed. With the help of XAS, active site geometries and accurate bond lengths can be resolved, which is notably helpful for metalloproteomics research [57]. Furthermore, XAS successfully revealed 10.2% first-row transition metal-containing proteins from a pool of 654 proteins, which is consistent with the structures deposited in the protein data bank (PDB) [58]. Synchrotron radiation X-ray fluorescence (SR-XRF) is another useful tool for elemental analysis, and X-ray irradiation on an atom of the sample generates fluorescent X-ray because of the energy differences of outer- and inner-shell electrons. Fluorescent X-rays vary between elements, and thus they can be used for elemental analysis [59]. With synchrotron radiation, which is generated from accelerating electrons in magnetic fields of the particle accelerator, high intensity and penetrating power to the analyte can be achieved. This technique has effectively enhanced sensitivity and reduced scattered background compared to traditional XRF [60]. It has currently been applied in disease investigation, such as confirming the colocalization of trace metals within human plaque correlated with Alzheimer's disease (AD) [61]. Recently, 3D X-ray imaging can be carried out by Cryo-XRF, providing 3D elemental localization and cell structural information. In addition, the adoption of cryogenic samples avoids metal intercellular flux that may affect imaging resolution [61].

2.4 Immobilized Metal Affinity Chromatography (IMAC)

Apart from GE and LC, there is a more direct way to achieve metalloprotein separation. Introduced in 1975, immobilized metal affinity chromatography (IMAC) separates proteins according to their affinity to specific metal ions [42]. Metal ions are immobilized on a matrix and packed in a column, proteins with the specific metal-binding ability will attach to the column and finally be eluted out by adding EDTA, reducing pH or increasing the mobile phase ion strength [62]. Various metal ions are applicable for this technique, for instance, Co(II), Zn(II), Cu(II), Bi(III), and Ga(III), widening the scope of metalloprotein analysis [63–66]. The only disadvantage is that proteins with metal-binding sites which are buried or occupied will be hardly recognized by this technique, and therefore it is often used in combination with 2D-GE or LC with matrix-assisted laser desorption/ionization (MALDI), to facilitate a more comprehensive exploration of metal-binding proteins and biocoordination of metals within cells [67, 68].

2.5 Integration of Metalloproteomics with Other-Omics and Deep Learning

The analysis of metalloproteome can be extremely complicated, as such, it is necessary to not only focus on the targeted protein, but also other proteins within

Metalloproteomics 273

the intracellular environment as proteins are intercorrelated. To search for new metallo-drug targets, an integration of metalloproteomics with proteomics and genomics is necessary to give a comprehensive picture of the entire system in response to drug treatment. Quantitative proteomics is sometimes necessary to determine the expression level of critical proteins, especially for comparative analysis of drug treated and untreated samples. Isobaric labeling strategies such as isobaric tags for relative and absolute quantitation (iTRAQ) [69] and tandem mass tag (TMT) [70] are applied; these tags have identical masses but with different heavy isotopes to differentiate proteins of different samples. These mass tags will be eventually cleaved by MS/MS.

On the other hand, genomic and proteomic data can be interpreted computationally; this can be done with the help of bioinformatics, which eases the interpretation of massive omics data by software tools. Gene ontology (GO) is a universal system that integrates several model organism databases to describe the roles of genes and gene products in organisms. Three independent ontologies were constructed for the ease of classification: biological process, molecular function, and cellular component which are the basic attributes of genes [71]. Using database for annotation, visualization, and integrated discovery (DAVID) [72], GO terms are identified and taken for enrichment analysis to summarize biological pathways the proteins are involved in. In terms of proteomics, STRING database enables the integration of known and predicted association between proteins, generating protein-protein interaction networks by Cytoscape [73].

With extensive biological data processed in computational systems, advanced algorithms are developed to manage these data and thus deep learning on bioinformation is gradually realized. For example, a deep learning approach was developed to allow prediction of disease-associated mutations at metal-binding sites. Sequential and spatial features of metal-binding sites are collected from different databases and implemented into a multichannel convolutional neural network (MCCNN), the model was successfully trained and deployed to predict mutations of zinc-binding sites in metalloproteins [74]. Recently, a machine learning model was built to distinguish enzymatic and non-enzymatic metals in proteins, which can correctly recognize active sites that are accountable for enzymatic activity [75]. The increasing acquirement of metalloproteomics data will be beneficial to the training and designing of the machine learning models, improving the prediction accuracy.

3 IMPLEMENTATION ON BIOMEDICAL STUDIES

With the aid of the abovementioned techniques used in metalloproteomics studies, mechanisms of action of metallo-drugs that target metalloproteins are revealed. In the following section, certain metal ions, which possess anticancer or antimicrobial activities, and their interactions with metalloproteins, are introduced.

3.1 ANTICANCER DRUGS

Cisplatin is the most well-known metallo-drug in chemotherapy, it also paved the way for the development of metallo-drugs. This platinum complex bearing two chloride and two ammine ligands shows cell division inhibitory activity, first discovered by Rosenburg in 1965, and then later proposed as an anticancer drug. It was finally approved by the Food and Drug Administration (FDA) in 1978 [76]. The widely accepted mechanism of action of cisplatin is its binding with DNA which induces cytotoxicity [77], but in fact, the platinum ion also interacts with several proteins and enzymes which eventually leads to cell death [78]. At the same time, drug resistance is a worrying issue, thus a deeper understanding of the underlying mechanism is needed. As a result, a comprehensive platinum-proteomic study is necessary for developing new analogues to combat resistance.

A cisplatin derivative has been modified as a fluorescent carboxyfluorescein-diacetate-labeled analog (CFDA-cisplatin) probe, this probe was subjected to A2780 tumor cells, together with the use of 2D-GE and ESI-MS/MS, a set of cisplatin binding proteins were successfully identified, such as protein disulfide isomerase (PDI) and glucose-regulated protein GRP78 [79]. These proteins are unfolded protein response regulators that are activated when there are stress signals, taking part in cisplatin resistance in certain cancers [80]. Another platinum-based fluorescent probe is azidoplatin (AzPt), incorporating an azide which enables a click reaction with a fluorophore for gel visualization or a biotin streptavidin bead for LC-MS/MS protein identification. A total of 152 proteins were identified in Pt(II)-treated *Saccharomyces cerevisiae*, and proteins related to endoplasmic reticulum (ER) stress response were monitored, which proves cisplatin's cytotoxicity. This study also identified PDI protein as a Pt binding protein, suggesting its significance on platinum cytotoxicity in multiple cell types [81]. Rat serum and renal proximal tubule epithelial cells (RPTECs) were treated with cisplatin and subjected to GE and LA-ICP-MS, and further identified by nano liquid chromatography coupled to electrospray linear ion trap tandem mass spectrometry (nHPLC-ESI-LTQ-FT-MS/MS). A number of proteins were discovered in rat serum, such as transferrin, albumin, alpha-2-macroglobulin, and hemoglobin, while core histones, 40S and 60S ribosomal proteins, malate dehydrogenase, elongation factor Tu, and vimentin were found in RPTECs treated with cisplatin, which contribute to the enzymatic changes in cancer cell upon cisplatin treatment [82]. Platinum(II) N-heterocyclic carbene complexes are considered as promising anticancer agents, binding to the same cellular target as their gold(III) and palladium(II) analogues. These targets were determined by incubating a gold-NHC probe in various cancer cells followed by UV irradiation and a click reaction with biotin azide for imaging (Figure 4a). Cellular proteins such as hsp60, vimentin, nucleophosmin, nucleoside diphosphate kinase A, and peroxiredoxin 1 were detected by MALDI-TOF-MS as anticancer molecular targets [83].

Ruthenium compounds are found to have some anticancer effects with lower systemic toxicity. Some ruthenium complexes have already entered clinical trials, particularly KP109/KNP1339 and NAMI-A [84]. They are treated as anticancer

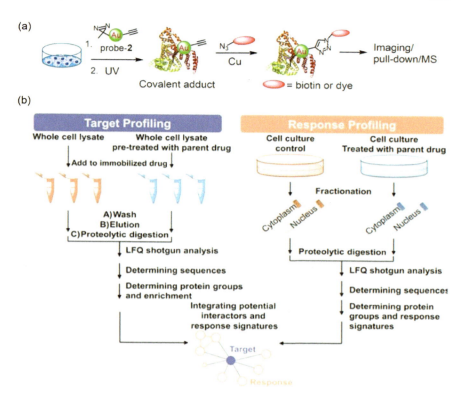

FIGURE 4 (a) The procedure of identifying cellular protein targets with gold-NHC probe; (b) the workflow of integrated target-response profiling of plecstatin. (Reproduced by permission from Refs. [83, 89]; copyright 2017, Wiley-VCH.)

agents either by reducing tumor volume or preventing metastasis [85], but their underlying mechanisms are still yet to be confirmed.

Ruthenium-arene compounds exhibit anti-proliferative activity and can be linked to several Ru-immobilized beads for metallo-drug pull-down studies. The ruthenium-based RAPTA complexes ([Ru(arene)(PTA)X$_2$], PTA = 1,3,5-triaza-7-phosphaadamantane, X = halogenide) are a family of ruthenium compounds with arene and PTA ligands, which retain antimetastatic activity with selective cytotoxicity toward malignant cells over normal cells [86]. Among the RAPTA derivatives, RAPTA-T and RAPTA-EA were introduced to invasive breast cancer cells MDA-MB-231 and non-invasive MCF-7 cells for exploring their metallo-drug targets. After separation and identification by LC-MS/MS, the data was analyzed by functional identification of target by expression proteomics (FITExP) and referenced against positive controls with known biological targets. This enabled the prediction of potential protein targets of RAPTA-T and RAPTA-EA. Under FITExP analysis, 2-adenosylmethionine synthase isoform type-2, metallotheinein-2, heat shock 70 kDa protein 1A/1B, and heme oxygenase

1 were found to be significantly regulated following RAPTA-T and RAPTA-EA treatment [87]. These proteins are involved in cancer cell growth, gene regulation, protein folding and trafficking, and oxidative stress. Both RAPTA derivatives can also be modified as streptavidin beads by attaching biotin *via* a linker to arene for affinity chromatography, pulling down proteins that are related to angiogenesis, cell proliferation, DNA binding, transcription processes, and protein biosynthesis [88]. A series of ruthenium-arene compounds named plecstatin (ruthenium(arene) pyridinecarbothioamide) were reported and applied on an integrated proteomics-based target-response profiling approach to search for cellular target of metallo-drugs (Figure 4b), with the aid of label-free quantitative mass-spectrometric shotgun analysis. It was found that scaffold protein and cytolinker plectin is a main target of plecstatin, the targeting reorganizes the non-mitotic MT network that may lead to G0/G1 arrest. The anticancer activity of plecstatin was further confirmed by treating it on tumor models [89].

Arsenic is well known as a dangerous compound with high toxicity, right until a group of Chinese scientists developed "Ailing-1," a mixture of arsenic trioxide (ATO) with trace amounts of mercury and found it to be effective for the treatment of cancer patients, particularly acute promyelocytic leukemia (APL) [90]. Later, a single dose of ATO also provided encouraging results on its anticancer ability to cure APL patients [91]. The repurposing of arsenic drugs boosts the development of other organoarsenic compounds such as darinasparsin (ZIO-101), 4-(N-(S-glutathionylacetyl)amino) phenylarsonous acid (GSAO), and 4-(N-(S-penicillaminylacetyl)amino) phenylarsonous acid (PENAO), as anticancer drugs [92–94]. However, the cytotoxicity of these drugs is still a concern and their use as drugs are regulated in most of the countries. Therefore, a full understanding of their mechanisms of action is needed to improve drug design and alleviate the side effects caused.

A systematic identification of arsenic-binding proteins was achieved by incubating biotinylated *p*-aminophenylarsenoxide (Biotin-As) with a human proteome microarray, arsenic-binding proteins were then identified with fluorescent Cy3-streptavidin. Three hundred and sixty arsenic-binding proteins were discovered by this approach and were examined for enrichment using several databases to reveal their biological interaction network. Proteins that participate in the glycolysis pathway were found to form the densest cluster, such as hexokinase-1 (HK1), triosephosphate isomerase (TPI1), and transketolase (TKT). After the investigation on HK1, its highly homologous form HK2 was also studied and showed arsenic-binding affinity. As a glycolysis facilitator and apoptosis repressor, HK2 is considered as a drug target in which arsenic can inhibit HK2 and glycolysis [95]. Besides, arsenic-binding proteins in MCF-7 breast cancer cells were explored by treating MCF-7 cells with arsenic-biotin conjugate, loaded on gel for separation, and subjected to MALDI-MS analysis [96]. Around 50 proteins were isolated, they are mainly proteins that are involved in metabolism, cell structure, and stress response. Although arsenic-biotin conjugates are commonly used to explore arsenic-binding proteins, the size of the conjugate may interfere with endogenous biotin in metabolic pathways [97]. Another arsenical probe,

Metalloproteomics 277

p-azidophenylarsenoxide (PAzPAO), was designed and introduced inside living cells, the azide group on the probe was able to click with biotin-dibenzylcyclooctyne (DIBO), capturing arsenic-binding proteins through non-enzymatic click chemistry. This probe was tested on A549 human lung carcinoma cells and eventually 48 arsenic-binding proteins were identified. Among them, two antioxidant proteins, namely, thioredoxin and peroxiredoxin-1, were found to be most abundant proteins, and binding of arsenic may elevate oxidative stress and induce cell damage [98]. Recently, a new arsenic-based fluorescent probe As^{III}-AC, which consists of a fluorophore coumarin and arylazide, was designed (Figure 5a). This probe was applied to NB4 APL cells, and it successfully tracked 37 putative

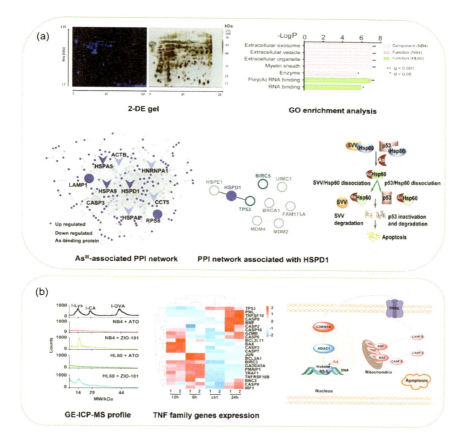

FIGURE 5 Integrative approaches on arsenic-binding proteins studies. (a) Fluorescent probe As^{III}-AC helps identifying arsenic-binding protein Hsp60 as a protein target eventually leading to apoptosis; (b) arsenic-based drug ZIO-101 shows a unique protein target histone H3.3 which induces downregulation of HDAC1, results in TRAIL-induced apoptosis. (Reproduced by permission from Refs. [54, 99]; copyright 2019 and 2021, Royal Society of Chemistry.)

arsenic-binding proteins. A TMT quantitative experiment was further performed to investigate protein expression by LC-MS/MS. About 141 upregulated and 109 downregulated proteins were identified to be significant differential proteins and some of them are the arsenic-binding proteins, together with the 37 arsenic-binding proteins, a protein-protein interaction network was generated. Among them, HSPD1 (Hsp60) is the most upregulated arsenic-binding protein, which is highly associated with two apoptosis proteins, survivin (BIRC5), and tumor protein P53 [54]. By using GE-ICP-MS and MALIDI-TOF-MS (Figure 5b), an arsenic-associated protein, histone H3.3, was found to be the targeted protein of ZIO-101. The binding of ZIO-101 hampers the formation of the histone H3.3 dimer and destabilizes nucleosomes. Through real-time polymerase chain reaction (RT-PCR), the histone H3.3-related genes involved in transcriptional misregulation were monitored, and the up- and downregulation of cyclin-dependent kinase inhibitor 1A (CDKN1A) and histone deacetylase 1 (HDAC1 were observed, inducing the expression of tumor necrosis factor TNF family genes and eventually leads to TRAIL-induced apoptosis) [99]. Furthermore, a genome-wide transcriptional and GO analysis was carried out on ZIO-101 treated NB4 cells and it was found that ferroptosis was most notably activated among the other enriched pathways at the early stage. This was further evidenced by observing the upregulated expression of cellular iron homeostasis genes HMOX1, inducing abnormal intracellular iron accumulation and lipid peroxidation. The discovery of a new apoptotic pathway by ZIO-101 stimulated the application of kinase inhibitors Dasatinib or Dactolisib for combination therapy on drug-resistant leukemia [100].

3.2 Antimicrobial Drugs

Bismuth compounds are commonly used in the treatment of gastrointestinal disorders, with very low toxicity as a heavy metal. Numerous commercially available bismuth drugs are still on the market since their discoveries in 1970s. Bismuth subsalicylate, well known as pink bismuth and Pepto-Bismol, is used to treat diarrhea and dyspepsia. Peptic ulcer drug colloidal bismuth subcitrate (CBS) and stomach ulcer drug ranitidine bismuth citrate (RBC) are found to have antibacterial effects against *H. pylori* [101]. Recently, CBS and other bismuth compounds have been shown to inhibit New Delhi metallo-β-lactamases NDM-1, thus serving as β-lactam adjuvants to treat infections by drug-resistant superbugs [102]. In addition, bismuth compounds also exhibit potent anti-SARS-CoV and anti-SARS-CoV-2 activity both *in vitro* and *in vivo* [103–105].

The mechanism of action of bismuth drugs for the treatment of *H. pylori* infection was revealed by proteomic analysis of *H. pylori* cells before and after treatment of CBS. Bismuth-loaded IMAC was used to screen proteins with bismuth-binding affinity and these proteins were eluted to carry out 2D-GE, the two gels from untreated and CBS-treated *H. pylori* cells were compared [106]. Differentially expressed proteins were selected and subjected to MALDI-MS analysis. Heat shock proteins HspA and HspB, neutrophil-activating protein (NapA), and putative alkyl hydroperoxide reductase (TsaA) are highly influenced

Metalloproteomics

279

by bismuth treatment, which induces oxidative stress and inhibits the functions of enzymes. Later, a more comprehensive study on bismuth-binding *H. pylori* proteins was carried out through Bi-IMAC and LC-MS [64]. In this study, 166 proteins were subjected to the system and over 300 peptides were found to be bismuth binding. It shows that bismuth has a preferable biocoordination with peptides containing thiolate sulfur cysteine and imidazolium nitrogen histidine, building a valuable Bi-binding motif data bank. Bismuth's favorable binding toward cysteine and histidine was later proved, by the fact that bismuth failed to bind the mutated C-terminal histidine and cysteine-rich domain in HpSlyD [25]. These bismuth-binding proteins were then categorized into translation, oxidation-reduction process, transcription, protein folding, and transition metal ion binding, which most of the proteins lies on the category of translation. Apart from IMAC, bismuth-associated proteins were also detected by column-type gel electrophoresis with ICP-MS, such as UreA and UreB, which neutralizes the acid environment for bacterial colonization, Ef-Tu for protein biosynthesis and CeuE, an iron-binding protein [25]. Recently, a fluorescent probe Bi^{3+}-TRACER was introduced to *H. pylori*, following with GE-ICP-MS analysis; around 26 bismuth-binding proteins were identified (Figure 6a) [107], and some of the pH-buffering enzymes had been detected previously [25, 106]. With the help of quantitative iTRAQ experiment and LC-MS/MS, 34 upregulated and 85 downregulated proteins were identified (Figure 6b). Bismuth shows disruption of multiple biological pathways in *H. pylori*, reducing bacterium-host cell adhesion, damaging oxidative defense systems of bacteria and prohibiting pH-buffering by binding key enzymes (Figure 6d). Through construction of bismuth protein-protein interaction networks (Figure 6c), three central nodes are newly uncovered to be targets of bismuth drugs, namely, DnaK, RpoA, and NusG. More investigation is needed to examine these central nodes, which are potential drug targets with less likelihood to develop drug resistance. Together with RNA sequencing and metabolic profiling, it was discovered that the bismuth toxicity toward *H. pylori* is due to the intrusion of iron and nickel homeostasis, disruption of central carbon metabolism, reduction of amino acid abundance, and impairment of oxidative defense systems [108]. Other proteomic and metabolomic studies on clinically isolated *H. pylori* strains show inhibition of virulence proteins vacuolating cytoxin A (VacA) and cytotoxin-associated gene A (CagA), disruption of bacterial colonization, and hindrance of several antioxidant enzymes prior to bismuth treatment [109].

Gallium ions share similar chemical properties with iron ions, such as octahedral and tetrahedral ionic radii, ionization potential and electron affinity; it thus serves as a perfect mimetic of iron in biological systems [110]. Iron plays an important role in sustaining microbial pathogens, bacteria have even developed several methods to obtain iron either by developing receptors such as transferrin or using siderophores to acquire iron from host proteins [111]. By substituting iron with gallium, protein function and metabolism are disrupted, leading to microbial suppression [112], therefore several gallium compounds have been developed as antimicrobial agents. Gallium-protoporphyrin IX (GaPPIX) shows inhibition on strains containing hemT and hemO gene clusters such as *S. aureus*

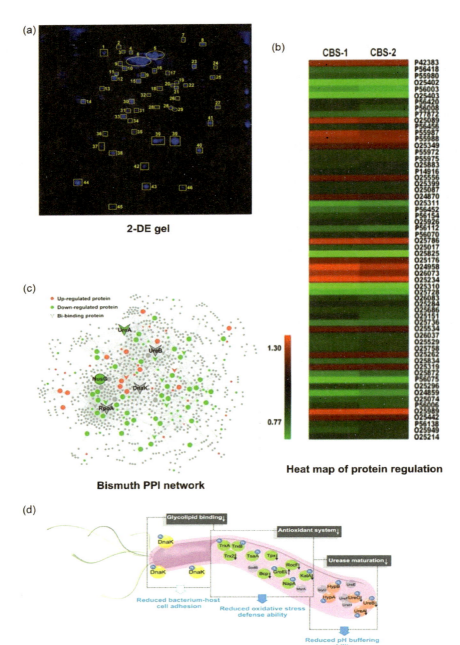

FIGURE 6 Integrative approach for the analysis of bismuth-binding proteins in *H. pylori*. (a) 2-DE gel of *H. pylori* 26695 cell lysates pre-incubated with Bi^{3+}-TRACER; (b) heat map of the bismuth-regulated proteins; (c) bismuth-influenced protein-protein interaction network; (d) model for the multi-targeted mode of action of colloidal bismuth subcitrate. (Reproduced by permission from Ref. [107]; copyright 2017, Royal Society of Chemistry.)

Metalloproteomics

281

and *A. baumannii* [113]. Desferrioxamine-gallium (DFO-Ga) is a metal complex, in which the siderophore is designed to complex with gallium(III), this trojan horse delivery system shows promising results in treating *P. aeruginosa* infections [114]. Gallium-loaded carboxymethyl cellulose (Ga-CMC) shows inhibitory activity on the growth of *P. aeruginosa*, *E. coli*, and *S. aureus* compared to iron-loaded polysaccharide [115].

Recently, the mechanism of action of gallium(III)-based drugs was finally revealed by metalloproteomics approach. Live *P. aeruginosa* were incubated with a Ga-coordinated fluorescent probe Ga(III)-TRACER, and Ga-IMAC was also employed to identify gallium-binding proteins [53]. Through intense fluorescent bands on SDS PAGE (sodium dodecyl sulfate–polyacrylamide gel electrophoresis) and the eluted proteins from Ga-IMAC, PaRpoB, and PaRpoC were identified as gallium-binding proteins with high enrichment factors. These are the two subunits of RNA polymerase that regulate transcription and gene expression. By targeting these proteins, gallium shows bacteriostatic activity against *P. aeruginosa*. Moreover, a GC-MS metabolomic study was conducted to analyze changes in metabolites upon gallium treatment. Among 62 metabolites detected, several metabolites were observed to have a significant increase in abundance after 4 h treatment, it is noticed that addition of metabolites may induce stimuli, either bacterial growth or inhibition. Through transcriptomics and metabolomics studies, it was suggested that the co-treatment of gallium with carbon source metabolites such as acetate enhanced bacteriostatic activity of gallium through certain pathways.

Silver in medical use has an exceedingly long history dating back to the 16th century, where physicians used silver nitrate to treat wounds. During war times in the 20th century, silver was applied for wound dressings and silver sutures were used in surgical tools [116]. Till now, it is still widely applied in the clinic, such as in the form of an antibacterial cream containing silver sulfadiazine or silver nanomaterials to prevent infection on burns [117] and silver coatings on endotracheal tubes and catheters [118]. Silver has also been shown to boost antibiotic activity by 1,000 times and could resensitize superbugs to conventional antibiotics [119]. Moreover, silver was shown to resensitize mcr-1 carrying bacteria to colistin owing to its ability to inhibit the MCR-1 enzyme through displacement of zinc cofactors [120]. Though silver has limited toxicity, excess silver accumulation in the body may cause skin to turn blue or gray which is a symptom of argyria [116]. Therefore, it is necessary to investigate the mechanism of silver in the body, designing effective silver-based compounds which prevent excess silver intake.

Recently, metalloproteomics together with metabolomic studies were made to depict a complete cellular response to silver drugs. Silver nitrate-treated *E. coli* were subjected to LC-GE-ICP-MS, where silver-binding proteins were separated, identified, and validated [26]. Apart from glutaredoxin 2 (GrxB) and tryptophanase (TnaA) that were previously identified [121], 32 proteins were recognized as silver-binding targets for the first time. These proteins were then subjected to GO and DAVID analysis, showing their involvement in the TCA cycle (citric acid cycle), glycolysis, translation, intercellular pH regulation, and oxidative stress response. The changes of metabolites entailed in these pathways were also shown upon drug treatment, demonstrating metabolism disruption by silver-based drugs. It was also found that metabolites involved in the TCA cycle, such as citrate and acetate, potentiate bactericidal efficacy against bacteria, and this was further proved by the significantly reduced bacterial load in a mouse urinary tract infection (UTI) model, upon combination treatment of silver and sodium citrate. Lately, an LC-GE-ICP-MS approach has also been applied on silver-binding proteins in *S. aureus*, resulting in 38 silver-associated proteins being identified [122]. Several enzymes from glycolysis and the oxidative pentose phosphate pathway (OxPPP) were newly discovered as protein targets of silver. Among them, the binding of silver to 6-phosphogluconate dehydrogenase (6PGDH) inhibits its activity, leading to 6-phosphogluconate (6PG) accumulation and nicotinamide adenine dinucleotide phosphate (NADPH) deficiency, which is toxic to cells. This may explain the bactericidal activity of silver against *S. aureus*.

4 CONCLUSION AND OUTLOOK

By taking advantage of metalloproteomics, scientists are now able to investigate the interaction between metals and proteins at a systemic level, exploring how metals play their role in physiological and pathological processes in a whole cell scale. In this chapter, we have introduced the commonly used techniques for protein separation, metalloprotein identification, and bioinformatics analysis. With the help of these approaches, the previously unsolvable and complicated myths on the role of metals in biology and medicine are likely to be resolved. Development of metalloproteomics is still ongoing, techniques like single cell RNA sequencing [123, 124] are useful for characterizing transcriptomes of individual cells, yielding comprehensive profiling of tissue composition and cell plasticity in dynamic systems, which provides valuable genome-wide data for metalloproteomics-related research. In the future, protein research will benefit from the evolution of AI, e.g., protein structures can be predicted by end-to-end deep neural network, which performs residue co-evolution analysis on the multiple sequence alignment for a target protein [125].

In this chapter, we have also introduced metalloproteomics studies on anticancer and antimicrobial metallo-drugs, and more metalloproteins are dug out and investigated to draw a comprehensive picture on their modes of action. Henceforward, a metalloproteomics approach might well be applied to other research areas such as neurological disorders (e.g., Alzheimer's and Parkinson's diseases) given that these diseases are highly correlated with zinc, copper, and iron, which play important roles in the proteins related to the neural system [126]. Comprehensive studies of neurological diseases at a systemic level may enable the development of diagnostic tools and design of therapeutic drugs. Other research areas that metalloproteomics can be well applied may include the nutritional aspect of metals, microbial metalloproteomes, which is largely uncharacterized [127], as well as understanding the role of metals in (patho)physiology. We hope this chapter may stimulate interest of researchers to apply the metalloproteomics approach to investigate the roles of metal ions in medicine and biological processes at a systemic level.

Metalloproteomics

ACKNOWLEDGMENTS

We thank the Research Grants Council (RGC) of Hong Kong (17307017, R7070-18, C7034-20E, ITS/278/20, 17308921, 2122–7S04, T11–709/21N), Innovation Technology Commission (ITS/124/17, ITS/278/20), and the University of Hong Kong (Norman & Cecilia Yip Foundation and URC (202107185074)) for support.

ABBREVIATIONS

AI	artificial intelligence
APL	acute promyelocytic leukemia
ATO	arsenic trioxide
CBS	colloidal bismuth subcitrate
CE	capillary electrophoresis
CETSA	cellular thermal shift assay
CD	circular dichroism
CryoEM	cryo-electron microscopy
CyTOF	mass cytometry
DAVID	database for annotation, visualization and integrated discovery
EDTA	ethylenediamine tetraacetic acid
ESI-MS/MS	electrospray ionization tandem mass spectrometry
FlAsH-EDT$_2$	fluorescein arsenical hairpin binder-ethanedithiol
FITExP	functional identification of target by expression proteomics
FT	Fourier transform
GE	gel electrophoresis
GO	gene ontology
ICP-MS	inductively coupled plasma-mass spectrometry
IMAC	immobilized metal affinity chromatography
IMC	imaging mass cytometry
ITC	isothermal titration calorimetry
iTRAQ	isobaric tags for relative and absolute quantitation
LA	laser ablation
LC	liquid chromatography
LTQ	linear ion trap
MALDI	matrix-assisted laser desorption/ionization
MCCNN	multichannel convolutional neural network
MCI	mass cytometry imaging
MIBI	multiplexed ion beam imaging
MS	mass spectrometry
NHC	nitrogen functionalized N-heterocyclic carbene
NTA	nitrilotriacetic acid
PDB	protein data bank
PDI	protein disulfide isomerase
RBC	ranitidine bismuth citrate
RPTEC	renal proximal tubule epithelial cell

RT-PCR	real-time polymerase chain reaction
SR-XRF	synchrotron radiation X-ray fluorescence
TMT	tandem mass tag
TR-ICP-MS	time resolved analysis
TRACER	"metal-tunable" fluorescent probe
TRAIL	TNF-related-apoptosis-inducing ligand
UV	ultraviolet
XAS	X-ray absorption spectrometry
ZIO-101	darinaparsin

REFERENCES

[1] P. Chandrangsu, C. Rensing, J. D. Helmann, *Nat. Rev. Microbiol.* **2017**, *15*, 338–350.

[2] L. D. Palmer, E. P. Skaar, *Annu. Rev. Genet.* **2016**, *50*, 67–91.

[3] H. Tapiero, D. M. Townsend, K. D. Tew, *Biomed. Pharmacother.* **2003**, *57*, 386–398.

[4] N. Abbaspour, R. Hurrell, R. Kelishadi, *J. Res. Med. Sci.* **2014**, *19*, 164–174.

[5] B. Desoize, *Anticancer Res.* **2004**, *24*, 1529–1544.

[6] R. J. P. Williams, *Coord. Chem. Rev.* **2001**, *216–217*, 583–595.

[7] H. Haraguchi, *J. Anal. At. Spectrom.* **2004**, *19*, 5–14.

[8] E. A. Roberts, B. Sarkar, *Curr. Opin. Clin. Nutr. Metab. Care* **2014**, *17*, 425–430.

[9] W. Xia, H. Li, H. Sun, *Chem. Commun.* **2014**, *50*, 1611–1614.

[10] F. Bou-Abdallah, T. R. Giffune, *Biochim. Biophys. Acta* **2016**, *1860*, 879–891.

[11] X. Wang, X. Du, H. Li, D. S. Chan, H. Sun, *Angew. Chem. Int. Ed. Engl.* **2011**, *50*, 2706–2711.

[12] L. Quintanar, L. Rivillas-Acevedo, *Methods Mol. Biol.* **2013**, *1008*, 267–297.

[13] D. Martinez Molina, R. Jafari, M. Ignatushchenko, T. Seki, E. A. Larsson, C. Dan, L. Sreekumar, Y. Cao, P. Nordlund, *Science* **2013**, *341*, 84–87.

[14] S. E. Bowman, J. Bridwell-Rabb, C. L. Drennan, *Acc. Chem. Res.* **2016**, *49*, 695–702.

[15] K. Wüthrich, *J. Biol. Chem.* **1990**, *265*, 22059–22062.

[16] K. M. Yip, N. Fischer, E. Paknia, A. Chari, H. Stark, *Nature* **2020**, *587*, 157–161.

[17] A. Hagège, T. N. S. Huynh, M. Hébrant, *Trends Analyt. Chem.* **2015**, *64*, 64–74.

[18] D. Burgi, A. J. Smith, *Curr. Protoc. Protein Sci.* **2001**, *2*, 10.9.1–10.9.13.

[19] X.-B. Yin, Y. Li, X.-P. Yan, *Trends Anal. Chem.* **2008**, *27*, 554–565.

[20] J. L. Brunelle, R. Green, *Methods Enzymol.* **2014**, *541*, 151–159.

[21] S. Magdeldin, S. Enany, Y. Yoshida, B. Xu, Y. Zhang, Z. Zureena, I. Lokamani, E. Yaoita, T. Yamamoto, *Clin. Proteomics* **2014**, *11*, 16.

[22] G. L. Glish, R. W. Vachet, *Nat. Rev. Drug Discov.* **2003**, *2*, 140–150.

[23] S. C. Wilschefski, M. R. Baxter, *Clin. Biochem. Rev.* **2019**, *40*, 115–133.

[24] K. Coufalíková, I. Benešová, T. Vaculovič, V. Kanický, J. Preisler, *Anal. Chim. Acta* **2017**, *968*, 58–65.

[25] L. Hu, T. Cheng, B. He, L. Li, Y. Wang, Y. T. Lai, G. Jiang, H. Sun, *Angew. Chem. Int. Ed. Engl.* **2013**, *52*, 4916–4920.

[26] H. Wang, A. Yan, Z. Liu, X. Yang, Z. Xu, Y. Wang, R. Wang, M. Koohi-Moghadam, L. Hu, W. Xia, H. Tang, Y. Wang, H. Li, H. Sun, *PLoS Biol.* **2019**, *17*, e3000292.

[27] S. J. Altschuler, L. F. Wu, *Cell* **2010**, *141*, 559–563.

[28] D. Wang, S. Bodovitz, *Trends Biotechnol.* **2010**, *28*, 281–290.

[29] C. N. Tsang, K. S. Ho, H. Sun, W. T. Chan, *J. Am. Chem. Soc.* **2011**, *133*, 7355–7357.

[30] Y. Zhou, H. Li, H. Sun, *Chem. Commun.* **2017**, *53*, 2970–2973.

Metalloproteomics

[31] Y. Zhou, H. Wang, E. Tse, H. Li, H. Sun, *Anal. Chem.* **2018**, *90*, 10465–10471.

[32] D. R. Bandura, V. I. Baranov, O. I. Ornatsky, A. Antonov, R. Kinach, X. Lou, S. Pavlov, S. Vorobiev, J. E. Dick, S. D. Tanner, *Anal. Chem.* **2009**, *81*, 6813–6822.

[33] E. Comsa, K. A. Nguyen, F. Loghin, A. Boumendjel, M. Peuchmaur, T. Andrieu, P. Falson, *Future Med. Chem.* **2018**, *10*, 1349–1360.

[34] Q. Chang, O. I. Ornatsky, C. J. Koch, N. Chaudary, D. T. Marie-Egyptienne, R. P. Hill, S. D. Tanner, D. W. Hedley, *Int. J. Cancer* **2015**, *136*, 1202–1209.

[35] A. Lopez-Serrano Oliver, A. Haase, A. Peddinghaus, D. Wittke, N. Jakubowski, A. Luch, A. Grutzkau, S. Baumgart, *Anal. Chem.* **2019**, *91*, 11514–11519.

[36] M. K. Ha, S. J. Kwon, J. S. Choi, N. T. Nguyen, J. Song, Y. Lee, Y. E. Kim, I. Shin, J. W. Nam, T. H. Yoon, *Small* **2020**, *16*, e1907674.

[37] H. Baharlou, N. P. Canete, A. L. Cunningham, A. N. Harman, E. Patrick, *Front. Immunol.* **2019**, *10*, 2657.

[38] C. Giesen, H. A. Wang, D. Schapiro, N. Zivanovic, A. Jacobs, B. Hattendorf, P. J. Schuffler, D. Grolimund, J. M. Buhmann, S. Brandt, Z. Varga, P. J. Wild, D. Gunther, B. Bodenmiller, *Nat. Methods* **2014**, *11*, 417–422.

[39] Q. Chang, O. I. Ornatsky, I. Siddiqui, R. Straus, V. I. Baranov, D. W. Hedley, *Sci. Rep.* **2016**, *6*, 36641.

[40] N. Jiang, H. Li, H. Sun, *Front. Chem.* **2019**, *7*, 560.

[41] S. R. Adams, R. Y. Tsien, *Nat. Protoc.* **2008**, *3*, 1527–1534.

[42] J. Porath, J. Carlsson, I. Olsson, G. Belfrage, *Nature* **1975**, *258*, 598–599.

[43] A. N. Kapanidis, Y. W. Ebright, R. H. Ebright, *J. Am. Chem. Soc.* **2001**, *123*, 12123–12125.

[44] E. G. Guignet, R. Hovius, H. Vogel, *Nat. Biotechnol.* **2004**, *22*, 440–444.

[45] C. R. Goldsmith, J. Jaworski, M. Sheng, S. J. Lippard, *J. Am. Chem. Soc.* **2006**, *128*, 418–419.

[46] K. Gatterdam, E. F. Joest, V. Gatterdam, R. Tampe, *Angew. Chem. Int. Ed. Engl.* **2018**, *57*, 12395–12399.

[47] C. Jing, V. W. Cornish, *Acc. Chem. Res.* **2011**, *44*, 784–792.

[48] Y. T. Lai, Y. Y. Chang, L. Hu, Y. Yang, A. Chao, Z. Y. Du, J. A. Tanner, M. L. Chye, C. Qian, K. M. Ng, H. Li, H. Sun, *Proc. Natl. Acad. Sci. U.S.A.* **2015**, *112*, 2948–2953.

[49] A. Chao, N. Jiang, Y. Yang, H. Li, H. Sun, *J. Mater. Chem. B* **2017**, *5*, 1166–1173.

[50] Y. Yang, N. Jiang, Y. T. Lai, Y. Y. Chang, X. Yang, H. Sun, H. Li, *ACS Sens.* **2019**, *4*, 1190–1196.

[51] X. Yang, M. Koohi-Moghadam, R. Wang, Y. Y. Chang, P. C. Y. Woo, J. Wang, H. Li, H. Sun, *PLoS Biol.* **2018**, *16*, e2003887.

[52] N. Jiang, T. Cheng, M. Wang, G. C. Chan, L. Jin, H. Li, H. Sun, *Metallomics* **2018**, *10*, 77–82.

[53] Y. Wang, B. Han, Y. Xie, H. Wang, R. Wang, W. Xia, H. Li, H. Sun, *Chem. Sci.* **2019**, *10*, 6099–6106.

[54] X. Hu, H. Li, T. K.-Y. Ip, Y. F. Cheung, M. Koohi-Moghadam, H. Wang, X. Yang, D. N. Tritton, Y. Wang, Y. Wang, R. Wang, K. M. Ng, H. Naranmandura, E. W. Tse, H. Sun, *Chem. Sci.* **2021**, *12*, 10893–10900.

[55] C. Huang, Q. Yin, W. Zhu, Y. Yang, X. Wang, X. Qian, Y. Xu, *Angew. Chem. Int. Ed. Engl.* **2011**, *50*, 7551–7556.

[56] A. L. Femia, C. F. Temprana, J. Santos, M. L. Carbajal, M. S. Amor, M. Grasselli, V. Alonso Sdel, *Protein J.* **2012**, *31*, 656–666.

[57] R. Ortega, A. Carmona, I. Llorens, P. L. Solari, *J. Anal. At. Spectrom.* **2012**, *27*, 2054–2065.

[58] W. Shi, C. Zhan, A. Ignatov, B. A. Manjasetty, N. Marinkovic, M. Sullivan, R. Huang, M. R. Chance, *Structure* **2005**, *13*, 1473–1486.

[59] A. Iida, in *Encyclopedia of Analytical Chemistry*, Eds R. A. Meyers, John Wiley & Sons, New York, 2013, pp. 1–23.

[60] M. J. Pushie, I. J. Pickering, M. Korbas, M. J. Hackett, G. N. George, *Chem. Rev.* **2014**, *114*, 8499–8541.

[61] J. J. Conesa, A. C. Carrasco, V. Rodriguez-Fanjul, Y. Yang, J. L. Carrascosa, P. Cloetens, E. Pereiro, A. M. Pizarro, *Angew. Chem. Int. Ed. Engl.* **2020**, *59*, 1270–1278.

[62] H. Block, B. Maertens, A. Spriestersbach, N. Brinker, J. Kubicek, R. Fabis, J. Labahn, F. Schafer, *Methods Enzymol.* **2009**, *463*, 439–473.

[63] E. Zatloukalova, Z. Kucerova, *J. Chromatogr. B Analyt. Technol. Biomed. Life Sci.* **2004**, *808*, 99–103.

[64] Y. Wang, C. N. Tsang, F. Xu, P. W. Kong, L. Hu, J. Wang, I. K. Chu, H. Li, H. Sun, *Chem. Commun.* **2015**, *51*, 16479–16482.

[65] M. C. Posewitz, P. Tempst, *Anal. Chem.* **1999**, *71*, 2883–2892.

[66] Y. M. She, S. Narindrasorasak, S. Yang, N. Spitale, E. A. Roberts, B. Sarkar, *Mol. Cell Proteomics* **2003**, *2*, 1306–1318.

[67] P. Jungblut, H. Baumeister, J. Klose, *Electrophoresis* **1993**, *14*, 638–643.

[68] J. G. Abelin, P. D. Trantham, S. A. Penny, A. M. Patterson, S. T. Ward, W. H. Hildebrand, M. Cobbold, D. L. Bai, J. Shabanowitz, D. F. Hunt, *Nat. Protoc.* **2015**, *10*, 1308–1318.

[69] S. Wiese, K. A. Reidegeld, H. E. Meyer, B. Warscheid, *Proteomics* **2007**, *7*, 340–350.

[70] A. Thompson, J. Schafer, K. Kuhn, S. Kienle, J. Schwarz, G. Schmidt, T. Neumann, R. Johnstone, A. K. Mohammed, C. Hamon, *Anal. Chem.* **2003**, *75*, 1895–1904.

[71] M. Ashburner, C. A. Ball, J. A. Blake, D. Botstein, H. Butler, J. M. Cherry, A. P. Davis, K. Dolinski, S. S. Dwight, J. T. Eppig, M. A. Harris, D. P. Hill, L. Issel-Tarver, A. Kasarskis, S. Lewis, J. C. Matese, J. E. Richardson, M. Ringwald, G. M. Rubin, G. Sherlock, *Nat. Genet.* **2000**, *25*, 25–29.

[72] G. Dennis, B. T. Sherman, D. A. Hosack, J. Yang, W. Gao, H. C. Lane, R. A. Lempicki, *Genome Biol.* **2003**, *4*, R60.

[73] N. T. Doncheva, J. H. Morris, J. Gorodkin, L. J. Jensen, *J. Proteome Res.* **2019**, *18*, 623–632.

[74] M. Koohi-Moghadam, H. Wang, Y. Wang, X. Yang, H. Li, J. Wang, H. Sun, *Nat. Mac. Intell.* **2019**, *1*, 561–567.

[75] R. Feehan, M. W. Franklin, J. S. G. Slusky, *Nat. Commun.* **2021**, *12*, 3712.

[76] S. Trzaska, *Chem. Eng. News* **2005**, *83*, 52.

[77] S. Dasari, P. B. Tchounwou, *Eur. J. Pharmacol.* **2014**, *740*, 364–378.

[78] P. M. Bruno, Y. Liu, G. Y. Park, J. Murai, C. E. Koch, T. J. Eisen, J. R. Pritchard, Y. Pommier, S. J. Lippard, M. T. Hemann, *Nat. Med.* **2017**, *23*, 461–471.

[79] S. Kotz, M. Kullmann, B. Crone, G. V. Kalayda, U. Jaehde, S. Metzger, *Electrophoresis* **2015**, *36*, 2811–2819.

[80] S. Xu, A. N. Butkevich, R. Yamada, Y. Zhou, B. Debnath, R. Duncan, E. Zandi, N. A. Petasis, N. Neamati, *Proc. Natl. Acad. Sci. U. S. A.* **2012**, *109*, 16348–16353.

[81] R. M. Cunningham, V. J. DeRose, *ACS Chem. Biol.* **2017**, *12*, 2737–2745.

[82] E. Moreno-Gordaliza, D. Esteban-Fernández, C. Giesen, K. Lehmann, A. Lázaro, A. Tejedor, C. Scheler, B. Cañas, N. Jakubowski, M. W. Linscheid, M. M. Gómez-Gómez, *J. Anal. Atom. Spec.* **2012**, *27*, 1474–1483.

[83] S. K. Fung, T. Zou, B. Cao, P. Y. Lee, Y. M. Fung, D. Hu, C. N. Lok, C. M. Che, *Angew. Chem. Int. Ed. Engl.* **2017**, *56*, 3892–3896.

Metalloproteomics 287

[84] A. Valente, T. S. Morais, R. G. Teixeira, C. P. Matos, A. I. Tomaz, M. H. Garcia, in *Synthetic Inorganic Chemistry*, Eds E. J. M. Hamilton, Elsevier, Amsterdam, 2021, pp. 223–276.

[85] E. Alessio, L. Messori, *Molecules* **2019**, *24*(10),1995.

[86] B. S. Murray, M. V. Babak, C. G. Hartinger, P. J. Dyson, *Coord. Chem. Rev.* **2016**, *306*, 86–114.

[87] R. F. S. Lee, A. Chernobrovkin, D. Rutishauser, C. S. Allardyce, D. Hacker, K. Johnsson, R. A. Zubarev, P. J. Dyson, *Sci. Rep.* **2017**, *7*, 1590.

[88] M. V. Babak, S. M. Meier, K. V. M. Huber, J. Reynisson, A. A. Legin, M. A. Jakupec, A. Roller, A. Stukalov, M. Gridling, K. L. Bennett, J. Colinge, W. Berger, P. J. Dyson, G. Superti-Furga, B. K. Keppler, C. G. Hartinger, *Chem. Sci.* **2015**, *6*, 2449–2456.

[89] S. M. Meier, D. Kreutz, L. Winter, M. H. M. Klose, K. Cseh, T. Weiss, A. Bileck, B. Alte, J. C. Mader, S. Jana, A. Chatterjee, A. Bhattacharyya, M. Hejl, M. A. Jakupec, P. Heffeter, W. Berger, C. G. Hartinger, B. K. Keppler, G. Wiche, C. Gerner, *Angew. Chem. Int. Ed. Engl.* **2017**, *56*, 8267–8271.

[90] H. D. Sun, Y. S. Li, L. Ma, X. C. Hu, T. D. Zhang, *Chin. J. Integrat. Chin. Trad. Med. West. Med.* **1992**, *12*, 170–171.

[91] P. Zhang, S. Y. Wang, L. H. Hu, *J. Harbin Med. Univ.* **1995**, *29*, 243.

[92] K. K. Mann, B. Wallner, I. S. Lossos, W. H. Miller, Jr., *Expert Opin. Investig. Drugs* **2009**, *18*, 1727–1734.

[93] P. J. Dilda, S. Decollogne, L. Weerakoon, M. D. Norris, M. Haber, J. D. Allen, P. J. Hogg, *J. Med. Chem.* **2009**, *52*, 6209–6216.

[94] A. S. Don, O. Kisker, P. Dilda, N. Donoghue, X. Zhao, S. Decollogne, B. Creighton, E. Flynn, J. Folkman, P. J. Hogg, *Cancer Cell* **2003**, *3*, 497–509.

[95] H. N. Zhang, L. Yang, J. Y. Ling, D. M. Czajkowsky, J. F. Wang, X. W. Zhang, Y. M. Zhou, F. Ge, M. K. Yang, Q. Xiong, S. J. Guo, H. Y. Le, S. F. Wu, W. Yan, B. Liu, H. Zhu, Z. Chen, S. C. Tao, *Proc. Natl. Acad. Sci. U. S. A.* **2015**, *112*, 15084–15089.

[96] X. Zhang, F. Yang, J. Y. Shim, K. L. Kirk, D. E. Anderson, X. Chen, *Cancer Lett.* **2007**, *255*, 95–106.

[97] D. Pacheco-Alvarez, R. S. Solorzano-Vargas, A. L. Del Rio, *Arch. Med. Res.* **2002**, *33*, 439–447.

[98] X. Yan, J. Li, Q. Liu, H. Peng, A. Popowich, Z. Wang, X. F. Li, X. C. Le, *Angew. Chem. Int. Ed. Engl.* **2016**, *55*, 14051–14056.

[99] X. Xu, H. Wang, H. Li, X. Hu, Y. Zhang, X. Guan, P. H. Toy, H. Sun, *Chem. Commun.* **2019**, *55*, 13120–13123.

[100] X. Xu, H. Wang, H. Li, H. Sun, *CCS Chem.* **2022**, *4*, 963–974.

[101] P. J. Sadler, H. Li, H. Sun, *Coord. Chem. Rev.* **1999**, *185–186*, 689–709.

[102] R. Wang, T. P. Lai, P. Gao, H. Zhang, P. L. Ho, P. C. Woo, G. Ma, R. Y. Kao, H. Li, H. Sun, *Nat. Commun.* **2018**, *9*, 439.

[103] N. Yang, J. A. Tanner, B. J. Zheng, R. M. Watt, M. L. He, L. Y. Lu, J. Q. Jiang, K. T. Shum, Y. P. Lin, K. L. Wong, M. C. Lin, H. F. Kung, H. Sun, J. D. Huang, *Angew. Chem. Int. Ed. Engl.* **2007**, *46*, 6464–6468.

[104] S. Yuan, R. Wang, J. F. Chan, A. J. Zhang, T. Cheng, K. K. Chik, Z. W. Ye, S. Wang, A. C. Lee, L. Jin, H. Li, D. Y. Jin, K. Y. Yuen, H. Sun, *Nat. Microbiol.* **2020**, *5*, 1439–1448.

[105] R. Wang, J. F. Chan, S. Wang, H. Li, J. Zhao, T. K. Y. Ip, Z. Zuo, K. Y. Yuen, S. Yuan, H. Sun, *Chem. Sci.* **2022**, *13*, 2238–2248.

[106] R. Ge, X. Sun, Q. Gu, R. M. Watt, J. A. Tanner, B. C. Wong, H. H. Xia, J. D. Huang, Q. Y. He, H. Sun, *J. Biol. Inorg. Chem.* **2007**, *12*, 831–842.

[107] Y. Wang, L. Hu, F. Xu, Q. Quan, Y. T. Lai, W. Xia, Y. Yang, Y. Y. Chang, X. Yang, Z. Chai, J. Wang, I. K. Chu, H. Li, H. Sun, *Chem. Sci.* **2017**, *8*, 4626–4633.

[108] B. Han, Z. Zhang, Y. Xie, X. Hu, H. Wang, W. Xia, Y. Wang, H. Li, Y. Wang, H. Sun, *Chem. Sci.* **2018**, *9*, 7488–7497.

[109] X. Yao, S. Xiao, L. Zhou, *Helicobacter* **2021**, *26*, e12846.

[110] C. R. Chitambar, *Biochim. Biophys. Acta* **2016**, *1863*, 2044–2053.

[111] E. D. Weinberg, *Biochim. Biophys. Acta* **2009**, *1790*, 600–605.

[112] C. H. Goss, Y. Kaneko, L. Khuu, G. D. Anderson, S. Ravishankar, M. L. Aitken, N. Lechtzin, G. Zhou, D. M. Czyz, K. McLean, O. Olakanmi, H. A. Shuman, M. Teresi, E. Wilhelm, E. Caldwell, S. J. Salipante, D. B. Hornick, R. J. Siehnel, L. Becker, B. E. Britigan, P. K. Singh, *Sci. Transl. Med.* **2018**, *10*(460), eaat7520.

[113] S. Hijazi, D. Visaggio, M. Pirolo, E. Frangipani, L. Bernstein, P. Visca, *Front. Cell. Infect. Microbiol.* **2018**, *8*, 316.

[114] E. Banin, A. Lozinski, K. M. Brady, E. Berenshtein, P. W. Butterfield, M. Moshe, M. Chevion, E. P. Greenberg, E. Banin, *Proc. Natl. Acad. Sci. U. S. A.* **2008**, *105*, 16761–16766.

[115] M. G. Best, C. Cunha-Reis, A. Y. Ganin, A. Sousa, J. Johnston, A. L. Oliveira, D. G. E. Smith, H. H. P. Yiu, I. R. Cooper, *ACS Appl. Bio. Mater.* **2020**, *3*, 7589–7597.

[116] J. W. Alexander, *Surg. Infect. (Larchmt)* **2009**, *10*, 289–292.

[117] A. Adhya, J. Bain, O. Ray, A. Hazra, S. Adhikari, G. Dutta, S. Ray, B. K. Majumdar, *J. Basic Clin. Pharm.* **2014**, *6*, 29–34.

[118] A. D. Politano, K. T. Campbell, L. H. Rosenberger, R. G. Sawyer, *Surg. Infect. (Larchmt)* **2013**, *14*, 8–20.

[119] J. R. Morones-Ramirez, J. A. Winkler, C. S. Spina, J. J. Collins, *Sci. Transl. Med.* **2013**, *5*, 190ra181.

[120] Q. Zhang, R. Wang, M. Wang, C. Liu, M. Koohi-Moghadam, H. Wang, P. L. Ho, H. Li, H. Sun, *Proc. Natl. Acad. Sci. U. S. A.* **2022**, *119*, e2119417119.

[121] N. S. Wigginton, A. de Titta, F. Piccapietra, J. Dobias, V. J. Nesatyy, M. J. Suter, R. Bernier-Latmani, *Environ. Sci. Technol.* **2010**, *44*, 2163–2168.

[122] H. Wang, M. Wang, X. Xu, P. Gao, Z. Xu, Q. Zhang, H. Li, A. Yan, R. Y.-T. Kao, H. Sun, *Nat. Commun.* **2021**, *12*, 3331.

[123] E. Mereu, A. Lafzi, C. Moutinho, C. Ziegenhain, D. J. McCarthy, A. Alvarez-Varela, E. Batlle, Sagar, D. Grun, J. K. Lau, S. C. Boutet, C. Sanada, A. Ooi, R. C. Jones, K. Kaihara, C. Brampton, Y. Talaga, Y. Sasagawa, K. Tanaka, T. Hayashi, C. Braeuning, C. Fischer, S. Sauer, T. Trefzer, C. Conrad, X. Adiconis, L. T. Nguyen, A. Regev, J. Z. Levin, S. Parekh, A. Janjic, L. E. Wange, J. W. Bagnoli, W. Enard, M. Gut, R. Sandberg, I. Nikaido, I. Gut, O. Stegle, H. Heyn, *Nat. Biotechnol.* **2020**, *38*, 747–755.

[124] B. J. Auerbach, J. Hu, M. P. Reilly, M. Li, *Genome Res.* **2021**, *31*, 1728–1741.

[125] F. Ju, J. Zhu, B. Shao, L. Kong, T. Y. Liu, W. M. Zheng, D. Bu, *Nat. Commun.* **2021**, *12*, 2535.

[126] C. J. Frederickson, J. Y. Koh, A. I. Bush, *Nat. Rev. Neurosci.* **2005**, *6*, 449–462.

[127] A. Cvetkovic, A. L. Menon, M. P. Thorgersen, J. W. Scott, F. L. Poole, 2nd, F. E. Jenney, Jr., W. A. Lancaster, J. L. Praissman, S. Shanmukh, B. J. Vaccaro, S. A. Trauger, E. Kalisiak, J. V. Apon, G. Siuzdak, S. M. Yannone, J. A. Tainer, M. W. Adams, *Nature* **2010**, *466*, 779–782.

11 Metal-Based Nanoclusters for Biomedical Applications

Edit Csapó

MTA-SZTE Lendület "Momentum" Noble
Metal Nanostructures Research Group

Interdisciplinary Excellence Center, Department of
Physical Chemistry and Materials Science, University of
Szeged, Rerrich B. square 1, H-6720 Szeged, Hungary
juhaszne@chem.u-szeged.hu

CONTENTS

1   Introduction 290
2   Characterization of Nanoclusters 291
    2.1   Metal Nanoclusters: Basic Concepts and Preparation Possibilities ... 291
    2.2   Structural Characteristics 294
    2.3   Optical Characteristics 295
3   Biomedical Applications of Noble Metal Nanoclusters 297
    3.1   Detection and Other Sensor Possibilities 297
        3.1.1   Detection of Metal Ions and Inorganic Anions 298
        3.1.2   Detection of Small Molecules 301
        3.1.3   Detection of Proteins and Nucleic Acids 303
    3.2   Bioimaging and Biolabeling 304
    3.3   Drug Delivery 307
    3.4   Diagnostics and Therapy 309
4   General Conclusions 312
Acknowledgments 312
Abbreviations and Definitions 312
References 314

ABSTRACT

Within the large group of nanostructured materials, metal-based nano-objects have prominent optical and structural features; their applications are attracting increasing attention in many research fields. Within metals, the noble metals like gold (Au), silver (Ag), copper (Cu), platinum (Pt), palladium (Pd), rhodium (Rh), and ruthenium (Ru) have the most versatile function. Classical nanoparticles (NPs) can be produced from almost all these mentioned noble metals via different synthesis

DOI: 10.1201/9781003272250-11

protocols, but there are significantly fewer publications on sub-nanometer-sized noble metal nanoclusters (MeNCs), especially for the last three metals. Metal nanoclusters (MeNCs) typically have a smaller size than ~2 nm and thus provide a bridge between metal atoms and NPs. Because of the unique physico-chemical and structural properties like ultra-small size, easy functionalization, good biocompatibility, excellent photostability, and structure-dependent unique photoluminescence (PL) features, they are extremely important nano-objects for diverse research fields. Among the noble metals, this chapter summarizes the preparation possibilities of mainly Au-, Ag-, and Cu-containing NCs, the interpretation of their structural and optical properties and their potential applications in several biomedical fields are also summarized. This chapter particularly focuses on the presentation of MeNCs as potential sensors for detection of several analytes (metal ions, anions, small (bio)molecules, peptides, proteins, and nucleic acids). Moreover, the possible use of MeNCs for bioimaging/biolabeling, drug delivery, diagnostics, and therapy is also demonstrated.

KEYWORDS

Metallic Nanostructures; Metal Nanoclusters; Noble Metals; (Bio)Sensors; Drug Delivery by Noble Metal Nanoclusters; Diagnostics and Therapy

1 INTRODUCTION

Nanostructured materials, which have unique properties such as high surface area to volume ratio, stability, inertness, easy functionalization, as well as novel optical, electrical, catalytic, and magnetic behaviors, are playing an increasingly important role in a diverse range of fields including but not limited to chemistry, physics, biology, catalytic processes, food processing industries, electronics, energy sectors, optoelectronics, sensing as well as medicine. These nanostructures can be classified according to several aspects (e.g., material quality, size, morphology, composition, structure), but perhaps the most commonly used is the material quality. Based on these, we distinguish between organic- and inorganic-based nanostructures. Namely, the polymeric nanospheres/nanocapsules, polymeric micelles, liposomes, dendrimers, and protein-based nanostructures are the main representatives of organic-based systems, while the mesoporous silica, carbon nanotubes, quantum dots, and, decisively, the transition metal-based nanostructures form a group of the inorganic-based nano-objects. While the former systems play a more dominant role in pharmaceutical applications as potential drug delivery and controlled release nano-sized systems, the latter group is becoming increasingly important in both material and life science research as well. Several groups can be also distinguished according to the size of the nanostructures: nanoclusters ($d < 2$ nm or sub-nano-sized), nanoparticles ($d < 100$ nm), colloidal particles ($d < 500$ nm), and sub-micro-sized particles ($d < 1,000$ nm).

This chapter exclusively focuses on the interpretation of the preparation possibilities and the structure-dependent optical features of the sub-nanometer-sized transition metal-based nanoclusters (mainly noble metals). Moreover, a comprehensive presentation of their possible applications in biomedical fields like selective and sensitive detection of various analytes, and novel possibilities in bioimaging/biolabeling, drug delivery, diagnostics, and therapy are an integral part of this chapter.

2 CHARACTERIZATION OF NANOCLUSTERS

2.1 METAL NANOCLUSTERS: BASIC CONCEPTS AND PREPARATION POSSIBILITIES

Metal nanoclusters (MeNCs) typically have a smaller size than ~2 nm and thus provide a bridge between metal atoms and nanoparticles (NPs) [1]. Figure 1 clearly represents the determining size range of MeNCs on nanoscale.

In some cases, the "cluster" definition is used for the designation of larger nano-objects containing nanoparticle assemblies, but in this chapter the firstly mentioned definition, which is the first sentence of this chapter, is used. In addition to size, another important feature is that the metals in the clusters are predominantly in non-ionic form. This property/structure essentially distinguishes between the classical metal complexes and MeNCs. Depending on the nanostructure, in several cases the "hybrid" distribution of the metal atoms and ions (e.g., atoms with zero oxidation number locate in metal "core," while the ions having positive charge in the "shell") often occurs which gives the clusters advantageous optical and electrical properties [2].

According to material quality, several types of metal-based clusters can be distinguished, of which the dominant group belongs to the transitional metal-based nanostructures. As a result of their unique optical and catalytic features, noble metals such as gold (Au) [3], silver (Ag) [4], copper (Cu) [5], platinum (Pt) [6], palladium (Pd) [7], rhodium (Rh) [8], and ruthenium (Ru) [9] play a key role, but the metal clusters having outstanding magnetic features (e.g., Fe_xO_y) are also of particular interest [10]. Moreover, in the literature we can find articles for other metal-based clusters, like cobalt (Co) [11], cadmium (Cd), or nickel (Ni) [11], but there are also promising experimental results for "hybrid" assemblies (e.g.,

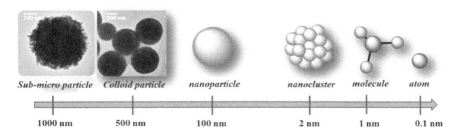

FIGURE 1 Representative size ranges from simple metal atoms to complex metal nanostructures in the range of 0.1–1,000 nm (arbitrarily scaled).

Zn-lantanoides [12], Gd-doped metallic structures) both in materials and life science applications.

Several fabrication routes for sub-nanometer-sized MeNCs have been established in the last two decades, including both "top-down" and "bottom-up" approaches [1], as Figure 2 summarizes, especially for Au nanoclusters (Au NCs). The *"direct synthesis methods"* provide simple and universal preparation routes for dominantly thiol-protected NCs. Taking Au NCs as an example, Au(III) ions are converted to -Au(I)-SR$_n$- complexes, in the presence of thiol ligand precursors, and then directly reduced to fluorescent Au NCs by a reducing agent (e.g., NaBH$_4$, hydrazine, or bioligands (mainly amine derivatives)) [13].

In the case of *"bottom-up methods,"* the clusters are formed via a reduction of the precursor ions by assembling individual atoms one-by-one. Among them, the ultra-facile, one-step synthetic processes are of particular interest, according to strict criteria for biomedical applications of these metal NCs, where the execution of the reactions is very convenient, rapid, and mild, exempted from the application of harsh reducing agents, special ambience and media, and high pressure. Numerous articles have been published, reporting the preparation of biocompatible Au NCs, synthesized by template-assisted preparation protocols using proteins and peptides, polymers, DNA, dendrimers [1], etc., but only a few publications present the possible applicability of simple amino acids, amino acid derivatives, vitamins, or nucleotides as reducing and stabilizing agents [13]. For these template-assisted routes, it is well known that the main experimental

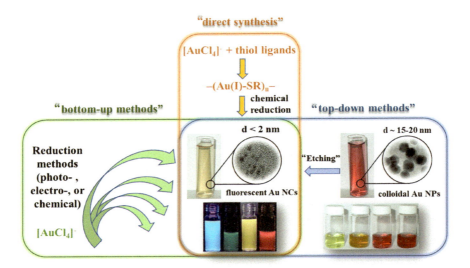

FIGURE 2 Generally applied preparation protocols of gold nanoclusters (Au NCs).

Metal-Based Nanoclusters for Biomedical Applications

conditions (ratio of the metal to reducing/stabilizing agents, pH, ionic strength, temperature, synthesis time, etc.) have dominant effects on both the optical and structural properties of these materials, which will be discussed in detail in Sections 2.2 and 2.3.

For "top-down methods," the larger colloidal particles undergo so-called "etching" to produce smaller metal clusters. In addition to noble metals, the magnetic nanoparticles (MNPs) are also becoming increasingly important within the group of metallic nanoparticles/nanoclusters [10]. In the last 10–15 years, many publications about MNPs have described efficient synthetic routes to provide shape-controlled, highly stable MNPs having narrow size distribution. Namely, the co-precipitation, microemulsion, thermal decomposition, solvothermal, sono-chemical, microwave assisted, chemical vapor deposition, combustion synthesis, carbon arc, and laser pyrolysis methods have been reported for the synthesis of MNPs. In terms of size, these magnetic nanostructures belong to the size range of classical nanoparticles ($d \sim$ 10–100 nm), so we will not discuss their detailed characterization in this chapter. With respect to several synthesis techniques described above, the application fields of the metal nanostructures may limit the use of the preparation processes. Because of the sub-nanometer size, as well as the excellent catalytic activity of metallic NCs, one of the major application areas of metallic NCs (mainly for Au, Pt, Pd) is heterogeneous catalysis. Several articles can be found in the literature for the possible utilization of metallic NCs for catalytic oxidation or hydrogeneration processes, for C-C coupling reactions, or in electron-transfer catalysis. Moreover, they are potent candidates as effective photo- or electrocatalysts [14]. In the latter case, one of the most intensively researched areas focuses on the design of effective electrocatalysts for controlled decomposition of carbon dioxide [15]. Among them, our research group successfully produced various Au-containing bimetallic particles as potential electrocatalysts for the decomposition of CO_2 in the last 4 years [16–18]. We successfully synthesized many types of bimetallic systems with different compositions (Au-Ag, Au-Sn, Au-Pb) and morphology (core-shell, alloy), and we studied the effects of the structure and composition on catalytic activity and product quality. Using the Au-Pb BNPs, we could reach the formation of the CH_4 reduction product from the CO_2 conversion processes, which has only been observed on very few Cu-free electrodes [16]. Besides the catalytic function, the application of MeNCs has been extended to nanoelectronics and photonics due to their excellent optical features. The self-assembled NCs have been used to construct multicolor light-emitting diodes (LEDs), in which NC assembly act as a color conversion layer [19]. This chapter mainly focuses on the biomedical utilizations, so the above-mentioned fields are listed only referred to briefly. The biomedical applications (cancer therapy, diagnostics, and bioimaging, etc.) of nano-sized functionalized metallic particles/clusters require biocompatible (so-called "green") preparation routes with mild reaction conditions [1, 20, 21]. During these one-step "green" synthetic approaches, mainly the template-assisted preparation approaches, are used, where predominantly amines, like simple amino acids, peptides or proteins, dendrimers, and nucleotides are applied, which have simultaneously a dual role as reducing and stabilizing ligands. The main advantages of this relatively simple template-directed reduction technique are that no additional reducing agent is required and based on the well-defined structure of polypeptides and proteins, uniform nanostructures with tunable optical features can be synthesized. Besides the type of the reducing ligands, the ratio of the metal ion to organic molecule as well as the pH and the type of the solvent have also dominant effect on the structure and the optical features of the metallic nanostructures. Section 2.2 clearly summarizes the main structural properties of metallic NCs, while Section 2.3 focuses on the presentation of the unique structure-dependent optical features.

2.2 STRUCTURAL CHARACTERISTICS

The MeNCs, consisting of several to a few tens metal atoms with a diameter of <2 nm, have attracted significant attention due to their unique molecule-like features, such as their well-defined molecular structures, explicit HOMO–LUMO transitions, quantized charge, and strong photoluminescence (PL) [2, 3, 13, 22]. The threshold of 2 nm was calculated by free-electron theory. Among metals, the noble metals, especially Au, have perhaps the largest literature relating to the presentation and confirmation of possible structures. Structures building on an increasing number of Au atoms can have increasingly complicated geometries, the basic kernel structures are summarized in Figure 3, as examples of few-atom clusters (Au < 13) [3]. By linking individual basic structures presented in Figure 3, larger, more complex nanostructures can be formed, e.g., Au_{25}, Au_{36}, Au_{38}, or Au_{102}.

For Au-based NCs, depending on the surface-bounded ligands (thiols, amines, phosphenes, etc.), a nano-object containing about ~150-200 Au atoms can be called a "nanocluster," but systems with a larger number of atoms are more in the size range of "nanoparticles." The Au NPs, containing more than ~150-200 atoms, exhibit a single localized surface plasmon resonance (LSPR) band based on the collective oscillation of the conduction electrons [23]. This LSPR phenomenon

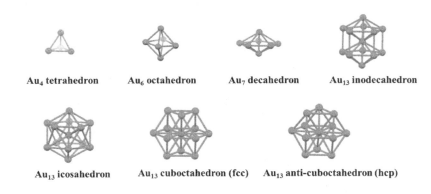

FIGURE 3 The basic kernel structures of Au NCs. (Copyright (2016) ACS Publications. Used with permission from Ref. [3].)

Metal-Based Nanoclusters for Biomedical Applications

will be mentioned in detail in Section 2.3 (Optical Characteristics). However, various Au NCs have already been structurally determined by X-ray diffraction techniques, but the number of structurally determined Ag NCs has been limited due to their weaker stability, atmospheric oxidation, and lower purity. Most of the representative structures of Ag NCs could be considered as being built from similar basic kernel units such as Ag_4, Ag_6, Ag_7, and Ag_{13} polyhedrons and peripheral ligands including thiols, phosphines, alkynyls, or their combination are used to protect Ag NCs [3, 4]. For the synthesis of atomically precise Cu NCs, similar strategies can be employed as for Au clusters [5]. Considering the high susceptibility of Cu toward oxidation, reactions require an inert atmosphere generally. Moreover, the choice of the protecting ligand as well as its chemical structure and the chalcogen precursor play a crucial role in the formation of certain cluster sizes. Although most of the reported structures have Cu atoms in the +1 oxidation state or even in a mixed-valence state due to the presence of non-stoichiometric phases and electron deficiency, recently, a few "metallic" Cu NCs have also been reported. In case of Cu NCs references describing Cu NCs containing a few atoms (e.g., Cu_6 stabilized by C_7H_5NOS ligand) to a cluster of 136 atoms can be found in the literature [5]. In conclusion, similar structures can be obtained for all noble metal-based NCs as presented for Au NCs, but primary differences can be found in their optical features, which is the main topic of the next section.

2.3 OPTICAL CHARACTERISTICS

One of the most outstanding properties of MeNCs—particularly preferred for biomedical applications—is the PL originated from the above-mentioned molecular structure [24], which can be easily and controllably tuned by the number of atoms forming the clusters and the quality of the surface stabilizing ligands [1–3, 25]. This PL is predominantly presented for pure Au, Ag, and Cu NCs and their alloys, but there are a few publications in the literature for the synthesis of blue-green emitting Pd NCs stabilized by thiols and polyelectrolytes or poly(amido) amine (PAMAM) dendrimer-stabilized Pt NCs having red PL [26]. As presented in Section 2.1, proteins are commonly used macromolecules for the synthesis of fluorescent MeNCs via template-assisted synthesis protocols. Bovine serum albumin (BSA) has been successfully used to prepare Au- [27, 28], Ag- [29], Cu- [30], Pt- [31], and Ni-based NCs [32], but these structures show different PL based on the quality of the metals. While for BSA-stabilized Au and Ag NCs the characteristic emission band is detected at 650 and 635 nm (red-emitting NCs), the BSA-directed Cu NCs possess intense blue emission (405 nm) with quantum yield (QY(%)) of *ca.* 7.5%. The characteristic PL band is observed at 403 nm for BSA-Ni NCs (QY(%) ~ 8%), which totally disappears, if the Ni is replaced by Pt.

Two major theories on the origin of PL of MeNCs have become generally accepted by scientists [24]. On the one hand, the simple metal quantum confinement effect is interpreted, whereby if the cluster size reaches the Fermi wavelength of metals (usually <1 nm), the continuous band of energy level becomes discrete resulting in the emerging of molecular-like features. On the other hand, the charge transfer on the shell of metal clusters is explained due to the interaction between the surface-bounded (bio)molecules (e.g., thiols, peptides, or small ligands) and the metal "core." For the latter case "two options" could be considered such as ligand-to-metal charge transfer (LMCT) and the ligand-to-metal-metal charge transfer (LMMCT) [24]. Because of the huge number of publications, as well as the length limitation of this chapter, the detailed interpretation of the metal-centered and ligand-centered emissions is not mentioned here.

As was mentioned previously, one of the main factors in determining the characteristic of the PL is the size of the clusters, specifically the number of atoms that build them. For example, for Au NCs, it is well known that, if the Au NCs consist of only a few atoms, blue emission can be detected; the appearance of the emission band mostly depends only on the number of metal atoms in the clusters [13]. Their PL lifetimes are usually of the order of nanoseconds although the surface ligands could have some influence on the fluorescence features. As the number of atoms increases, green, yellow, orange, and red emission can be detected gradually. If the NC size reaches ~1.5–2.0 nm (red-emitting NCs), both the oxidation state of the surface metal atoms and the surface ligand effect influence the wavelength of the emission maximum. These NCs possess a characteristic PL in the orange/red (Vis) or in the near-infrared (NIR) region and they have a PL lifetime as well in the microsecond range. Upon further increase in size, the few nanometers Au NPs ($d > 2$ nm) show plasmonic feature, because the collective oscillation of the free electron occurs. However, the smaller ($d < 20$–30 nm) plasmonic Au NPs may also exhibit characteristic short-time fluorescence, which depends on the surface roughness or the grain size effect [13].

Figure 4 shows representative absorbance (Figure 4a) and emission (Figure 4b) spectra for Au- and Ag-based NPs and NCs [33]. If size were the sole determinant (based only on the size-dependent quantum confinement effect (QCE)), metals from the same family, with nearly identical size, should show similar fluorescence. Several experimental examples can be found in the literature to

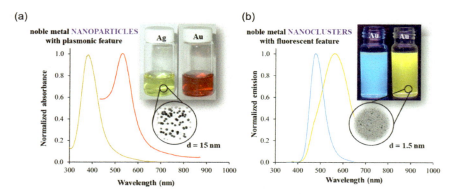

FIGURE 4 Representative LSPR bands and emission spectra of (a) Au- and Ag-based NPs and (b) NCs with the photos of the dispersions in daylight (a) and under UV lamp (b). (Copyright (2022) Elsevier. Used with permission from Ref. [33].)

Metal-Based Nanoclusters for Biomedical Applications 297

the contrary. Differences between the experimental and theoretical data indicate the invalidity of metal-centered QCE. An interesting example for mercaptosuccinic acid-stabilized Ag NCs having the same size (Ag_7 and Ag_8) clearly confirms the above-mentioned hypothesis. Namely, the characteristic PL band was detected at 440 nm (blue PL) for Ag_7 NCs, while the Ag_8 NCs exhibit red PL (650 nm). The main conclusion is that the chemical nature and the surface coverage of the stabilizing ligand(s) have a more dominant effect on the PL of MeNCs [3]. To give an example, Luo et al. synthesized glutathione-directed Au NCs having M_xL_y structure, where x is the number of Au atoms, while y is the number of the glutathione molecules (L) in the NCs. Their results clearly showed that a series of NCs (from $Au_{29}L_{27}$, $Au_{30}L_{28}$ ... to $Au_{43}L_{37}$) with the same characteristic PL (610 nm) can be prepared, but the systematic change of the surface coverage results in the tune of the PL from 610 to 800 nm. Fine-tuning was achieved by changing the metal/ligand ratio during the synthesis [34]. However, the sizes of the NC cores are larger than 2 nm, but the absorbance spectra confirm the absence of the LSPR band, thus the formation of plasmonic Au NPs is excluded.

One interesting optical phenomenon worthy of mention in this chapter is the aggregation-induced emission (AIE) known since 2001 [35]. Many MeNCs only possess PL property with low intensity, or the characteristic PL feature is observed under low temperature or in special solvent, etc., which limits their applications. The previously mentioned AIE phenomenon is an excellent possibility to enhance the PL property of these MeNCs, but in some cases quenching can also occur due to the aggregation of these nano-assemblies [35]. This phenomenon can be caused by a change in pH, temperature, or solvent, or by the addition of a reagent (a small biomolecule, an ion, or large colloidal particle on whose surface they can aggregate) which is generally observed for biosensor applications [36]. Several examples for AIE will be presented in Section 3.1.

3 BIOMEDICAL APPLICATIONS OF NOBLE METAL NANOCLUSTERS

3.1 DETECTION AND OTHER SENSOR POSSIBILITIES

Because of their unique physico-chemical and structural properties like ultrasmall size, easy functionalization, good biocompatibility, excellent photostability, the MeNCs are playing an increasingly important role in sensing utilizations [21, 25]. For a MeNC to perform excellently as an optical sensor, it must meet at least three important criteria: high sensitivity, selectivity, and fast response. On the one hand, the selectivity is ensured by the targeted surface modification(s) of the metal core by different ligands. On the other hand, the change of the optical signal is simple: the applicability of MeNCs is crucially based on the fact that their characteristic fluorescence is quenched, enhanced, or even systematically shifted, as Figure 5 represents, because of the direct or indirect interaction with an analyte to be detected [25].

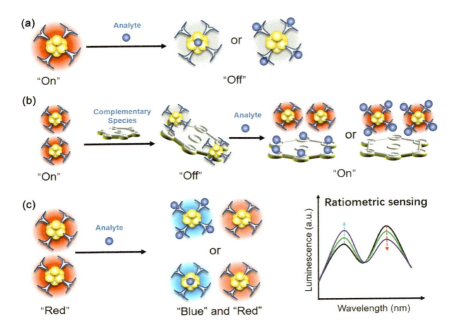

FIGURE 5 Schematic representation of the different sensing modes of fluorescent MeNCs. (Copyright (2022) Elsevier. Used with permission from Ref. [25].)

Among the wide range of sensing possibilities, research on the selective detection of heavy metal ions, inorganic anions, small (e.g., glucose, trypsin, amino acids, H_2O_2, dopamine, serotonin) and large (e.g., proteins) biomolecules or nucleic acids is outstanding mainly for noble metal-based NCs (Au, Ag, Cu, and their alloys) [1]. The following subsections present the main advantages and disadvantages and the proposed mechanisms of the utilizations of MeNCs as potent sensors and are categorized according to the type of the analytes being detected.

3.1.1 Detection of Metal Ions and Inorganic Anions

Over the past 15 years, hundreds of scientific papers have been published to demonstrate specifically the metal ion sensing possibilities of fluorescent noble metal NCs. The first article was presented in 2005, in which cadmium-selenide (CdSe) NCs, with 5–10 nm average diameter, have been prepared for selective detection of **Hg(II) ions**, but in terms of size, these systems do not strictly belong to the class termed "clusters" [37]. In the period of 2007–2010, a few articles (*ca.* 4) presented sensor studies for identification of this highly pollutant Hg(II) ion in liquid medium by using 11-mercaptoundecanoic acid- [38] and BSA- [39] stabilized Au NCs, but oligonucleotide- [40] and dihydrolipoic acid- [41] functionalized Ag NCs have also been reported for selective Hg(II) detection. To the best of our knowledge, Hg was the first metal ion for which the applicability of noble MeNCs as sensors was studied. In all but one of these papers, the detection was

Metal-Based Nanoclusters for Biomedical Applications

based on fluorescence quenching; the appropriate limit of detection (LOD) values varied in the range of 0.1–5.0 nM. In the last 10 years (2011–2021), nearly 25 additional publications have been published on the Hg(II) sensing applications of Au-, Ag-, and Cu-based fluorescent NCs modified with different molecules (e.g., cysteine, polyvinylpyrrolidone (PVP), DNA, poly(acrylic) acid (PAA)). A comprehensive review article, published in 2022 [42], summarizes all the articles from 2007 to date. It is also worth pointing out that in most of the articles the quenching effect was observed because of the interaction of the different fluorescent NCs with the Hg ion analyte, but for DNA-stabilized Ag and Cu NCs the turn-on fluorescence was detected. Given this, the direction of the change of the optical signal can be designed by means of targeted surface modification (turn-off or turn-on). In the early years, the **Cu(II) ion** was another one that was intensively studied. Shang and Dong reported the first application of water-soluble fluorescent poly(methacrylic acid) (PMAA)-templated Ag NCs for selective detection of Cu(II) ions based on PL quenching effect [43]. To date, the selective and sensitive identification of some other heavy metal ions like Fe(II) [44], Fe(III) [45], Pb(II) [46], or Cr(III)/Cr(VI) [47] have been carried out by noble metal NCs. Some interesting publications have also been reported. Among them, we were the first to successfully developed a one-step synthesis method for the preparation of both adenosine monophosphate (AMP)-stabilized colloidal Au nanoparticles (AMP-Au NPs) and fluorescent Au nanoclusters (AMP-Au NCs) by varying the $AMP:AuCl_4^-$ molar ratios within the synthesis protocol [45]. The study confirmed that the AMP-Au NPs do not function well as optical sensors, rather the blue-emitting AMP-Au NCs are excellent for detecting Fe(III) ions. The preparation protocols, as well as the results of the sensor tests, are seen on Figure 6.

Among Au- and Ag-based NCs, the investigation of the applicability of Cu NCs-based fluorescent sensors has only become dominant in the last 10 years. The first Cu NCs sensor was developed for Pb(II) detection in dispersion [5]. Another interesting article was published in 2019, similarly based on Pb(II) identification. Dehghani and coworkers synthesized Au/Pt nanoclusters at room temperature using chitosan as a stabilizing macromolecule [48]. Chitosan-protected Au/Pt nanoclusters exhibit strong peroxidase-like activity, and could catalyze the oxidation of 3,3,5,5-tetramethylbenzidine (TMB) in the vicinity of hydrogen peroxide (H_2O_2) and create a visual blue color. The detection mechanism with the LOD of 16 nM is based on the Pb^{2+} ions-induced aggregation of chitosan–Au/Pt NCs that cause changes in size and impair the enzymatic performance of Au/Pt NCs. Their studies indicated that a step-by-step increase in concentration of Pb^{2+} ions gradually decreased peroxidase activity and this reduction was linear.

The number of publications for detection of **inorganic anions** is somewhat less. The most studied inorganic anion is cyanide because of its highly toxic character. The first report, for the identification of cyanide ions in aqueous medium by fluorescent MeNCs, was published in 2010 [49]. The successful applicability of BSA-stabilized red-emitting Au NCs was confirmed with the obtained LOD of

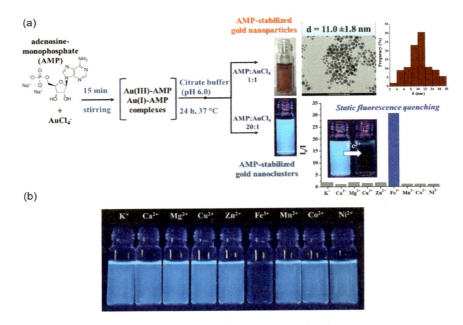

FIGURE 6 Preparation protocol of AMP-stabilized Au NPs and NCs (a) with the photo of the NCs dispersions in presence of metal ions (b). (Copyright (2017) Elsevier. Used with permission from Ref. [45].)

200 nM. To the best of our knowledge, Table 1 summarizes all the publications which reported MeNCs-based fluorescent sensors for cyanide detection [49–56].

As can be seen in Table 1, MeNCs-based fluorescent sensors are almost exclusively Au NCs-based sensors. Another interesting fact is that the metal cores are predominantly functionalized with macromolecules (e.g., proteins or polyelectrolytes) and the characteristic emissions of these NCs are observed in the orange-red range (~590–650 nm). The sensing mechanism is also based on a crucially similar phenomenon and structural change. Namely, the CN^- ions can transform the Au atoms to $[Au(CN)_2^-]$ complex ions in the presence of oxygen, the latter causing the quenching of the characteristic orange or red PL of the MeNCs. In parallel, a new emission band is observed in the blue region (at ca. 410–420 nm) which can be assigned to the cyanide-based complex ions [51]. The function of some sensors is based on a more complex ratiometric detection of cyanide ions [50]. In one case, e.g., a fluorescent copper(II) phthalocyanine (Cu(PcTs)) complex is used as well besides the glutathione-directed Au NCs [50]. In the presence of CN^- anion, the Au NCs and Cu(PcTs) interaction is perturbed, so that the fluorescence of Cu(PcTs), already quenched by Au NCs, is found to be efficiently recovered, while the fluorescence intensity of AuNCs is quenched via the formation of a stable $[Au(CN)_2]^-$ species. The ratiometric variation of Au NCs (λ_{em} = 580 nm) and Cu(PcTs) fluorescence (λ_{em} = 420 nm) intensities leads to designing a highly sensitive probe for cyanide detection.

Metal-Based Nanoclusters for Biomedical Applications

TABLE 1
Different Metal-Only Nanocluster-Based Fluorescent Sensors for Detection of Cyanide Ions in the Period of 2010–2020

Type of MeNCs	Stabilizing Ligand	Emission (nm)	Mechanism of Sensing	LOD (nM)	Year	Reference
Au NCs	BSA	640	From red to blue shift ("etching")	200	2010	[49]
Au(I) NCs	3-mercapto-1,2,4-triazole	640	Turn-off	80	2014	[55]
Au NCs	Lys[a]	650	From red to blue shift ("etching")	190	2014	[51]
Au NCs	LAAOx[b]	630	From red to blue shift ("etching")	180	2015	[56]
Ce/Au NCs	BSA 658	410	Turn-off	50	2016	[53]
Au NCs	OVA[c]	650	Turn-off	68	2018	[52]
Au NCs	hPEI[d]	590	From red to blue shift ("etching")	10	2020	[54]

[a] Lys: lysozyme protein (14.6 kDa),
[b] L-amino acid oxidase.
[c] OVA = ovalbumin.
[d] Hyperbranched polyethyleneimine.

Some articles for detection of other ions like I^-, S^{2-}, and NO_2^- can also be found; detailed results are presented in the following Refs. [1, 5, 21].

3.1.2   Detection of Small Molecules

Small molecules, such as hydrogen peroxide (H_2O_2), glucose, amino acids, small peptides, antioxidants, or neuroactive compounds, play a crucial role in the human body, therefore the continuous monitoring of their levels *in vivo* is extremely important for the diagnosis of various diseases. Similar to metal ions, the first earliest reports were published between 2008 and 2010 [1]. It is well known that H_2O_2 is a key compound in biological processes and an important chemical reagent in industrial applications as well. To the best of our knowledge, *ca.* 100–120 articles have already been published till 2021 relating to the development of different sensors for the identification of H_2O_2 [57]. We can find articles that present the potential role of simple molecules [58], metal hexacyanoferrates [59], metallic [60, 61], or metal oxide [62] nanostructures as H_2O_2 sensors. Among the sensors developed to identify this molecule, MeNCs are not a dominant group; only a few publications are available in the literature [60, 63]. Wen et al. successfully prepared horseradish peroxidase (HRP)-stabilized red-emitting (λ_{em} = 650 nm) HRP–Au NC conjugates having an average cluster size of 2.7 ± 0.6 nm [63]. They found that the fluorescence of HRP–Au NCs can be quenched quantitatively by adding H_2O_2. Upon the addition of H_2O_2 under optimal conditions, the fluorescence intensity quenched linearly over the range of 100 nM to 100 μM with high sensitivity (LOD = 30 nM, S/N = 3). Molaabasi et al. reported a label-free fluorescent detection system based on blue-emitting hemoglobin-stabilized Au NCs [60] which was designed as a fluorescence enhancing-quenching (on-off) sensor for the direct detection of glucose in serum samples. In the presence of glucose as a substrate and glucose oxidase (GOx) as catalyst, H_2O_2 is produced that can intensively enhance the PL intensity of hemoglobin-Au NPs. In the presence of H_2O_2, an intramolecular electron transfer to hemoglobin-Au NCs takes place under the heme degradation and/or Fe release from hemoglobin which is accompanied with the PL enhancement of the Au NCs.

In contrast to H_2O_2, the number of MeNCs as folic acid (FA) sensors is much more significant. Table 2 summarizes nearly all the publications which reported MeNCs-based fluorescent sensors for FA detection [64–72].

As can be clearly seen, Au- [66–68, 72], Ag- [64, 65], and Cu-based [70, 71] NCs have also been prepared and stabilized by different ligands for the identification of FA, and the LOD is also varied within a wide range depending on the mechanism. In most articles, red- and blue-emitting NCs were fabricated, and the identification of FA is based on the quenching of NCs' fluorescence (turn-off), but in one case, however, PL enhancement occurs, when the DPA-FA complex interacts with Cu NCs (linear range 0.1–10 μM) [71]. Meng and coworkers developed a ratiometric fluorescence strategy where they found that the characteristic red PL ($\lambda_{em} = 612$ nm) of the 11-MUA-Au NCs decreases while the emission of

TABLE 2
Various Metal-Only Nanocluster-Based Fluorescent Sensors for Detection of Folic Acid in the Period of 2014–2022

Type of MeNCs	Stabilizing Ligand	Emission (nm)	Mechanism of Sensing	LOD	Year	Reference
Au NCs	BSA	629	Turn-off	41.5 nM	2014	[67]
Ag NCs	PEI	452	Turn-off	0.032 nM	2014	[64]
Au NCs	BSA	640	Turn-off	68 nM	2016	[68]
Au NCs	11-MUA[a]	612	Ratiometric	26 nM	2018	[66]
Cu NCs	DPA[b]	465	Turn-on	69 nM	2019	[71]
Cu NCs	OVA	625	Turn-off	0.18 μM	2019	[70]
Au/Ag NCs	AMP[c]	560	Ratiometric	0.109 μM	2021	[69]
Au NCs	D-Trp[d]	460	Turn-off	5.8 μM	2021	[72]
Ag NCs	PEI[e]	631	Turn-off	12 nM	2022	[65]

[a] 11-mercaptoundecanoic acid.
[b] Diperiodatoargentate(III).
[c] Adenosine monophosphate.
[d] D-tryptophan.
[e] Polyethylenimine.

Metal-Based Nanoclusters for Biomedical Applications

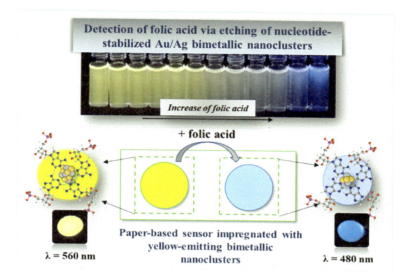

FIGURE 7 Schematic representation of the function of yellow-emitting AMP-directed Au/Ag NCs for detection of folic acid (FA). (Copyright (2021) Elsevier. Used with permission from Ref. [69].)

FA detected at λ_{em} = 446 nm (blue region) increases with titration of FA [66]. D. Ungor et al. synthesized bimetallic Au/Ag NCs stabilized by AMP nucleotide [69]. They found that the characteristic yellow PL of the NCs turns to blue emission after interaction with FA (Figure 7). They confirmed that the FA molecules can cleave the metal atoms from the cluster cores, which explains well the dramatic decrease and blue shifting of the yellow emission. In addition to the standard liquid phase studies, a "paper-based" quick test was also developed to recommend the future usability of their sensor.

Detection of glucose [73], neurotransmitter molecules like dopamine [74, 75] or serotonin, neurotoxic compounds (e.g., kynurenine) [76], bilirubin [77], penicillamine [78], and pramipexole [79] have been carried out by MeNCs. Due to space limitations, it is not possible to present all the publications within the scope of chapter, but detailed results are given in the references. In most of the clusters mentioned above, the material quality of the metal is Au and both turn-off and turn-on sensors can be found depending on the stabilizing ligands (e.g., BSA, HSA, methionine (Met), histidine (His), or papain).

3.1.3 Detection of Proteins and Nucleic Acids

Similar to small molecules, the monitoring of proteins and nucleic acids in the human body is an essential diagnostic tool to identify certain diseases at an early stage. Several protocols can be found in the literature for protein or nucleic acid detection; the first article was published in 2006 [80] for human immunoglobulin G (IgG) using PAMAM dendrimer-stabilized Au NCs (λ_{em} = 450 nm), where the sensing mechanism is based on PL quenching (turn-off sensor) of the NCs after interaction with human IgG. To date, fluorescence-based sensors using noble metal NCs, mainly Au, have been developed for identification of a variety of proteins. Without being exhaustive, we refer the reader to publications on the detection of glutathione-S-transferase [81], breast cancer marker protein [82], concanavalin A [83], protein kinase [84], trypsin [85], heparin [86], matrix metalloproteinase-9 [87], or other specific proteins [88] in the human body or in artificial media modeling it. Relating to nucleic acids, somewhat less articles can be found, but in 2022 a comprehensive review has been published for the presentation of MeNCs in nucleic acid detection [89]. Wang et al. designed a novel Ag NCs-based fluorescent assay to detect single nucleotide modifications in DNA [90]. This was the first article in *ca.* 12 years ago covering this topic. They demonstrated the capability of this method to identify the sickle cell anemia mutation in the hemoglobin beta chain (HBB) gene. It is well known that Ag NCs have longer PL lifetime and better stability compared to Cu-based nanostructures, and higher PL intensity than Au NCs. The Ag(I) ions have stronger capability to bind DNA than other metal ions and it is easier to bind to a single-stranded DNA (ssDNA). In 2022, Lin et al. published an interesting article that clearly summarizes nearly all the articles for nucleic acid detection by MeNCs [89]. PL enhancement and red shift can occur when the G-rich sequence comes close to Ag NCs or the complementary DNA strand hybridizes with Ag NCs tail strand, which can be used for detection. Ag NCs with the abasic site in DNA duplex can distinguish mutant genes. Ag NCs with auxiliary DNA can be used to identify microRNA like miR-21, miR-16-5p, miR-19b-3p, and miR-141. The Cu NCs/Cu NPs can recognize miRNA-155, miR-21, and miR-let-7d without auxiliary DNA. The Au NCs can identify H1N1 gene fragments by PL quenching caused by proximity to the G-rich sequence. Moreover, Au NCs can recognize miRNA-21 and let-7a [89].

3.2 BIOIMAGING AND BIOLABELING

Based on several attractive properties including but not limited to ultra-small size, good biocompatibility, brightness, and excellent photostability, the MeNCs are promising fluorescence probes for biological imaging and labeling (Figure 8). This research area has a history of almost 15 years. In this period *ca.* a few hundred articles have been published showcasing the advantages and possibilities of the use of only MeNCs having controllable PL features for bioimaging and biolabeling applications. Conventional fluorophores, like organic dye molecules or fluorescent proteins, can be generally used for imaging/labeling agents but they have limited photostability, which is one of the main disadvantages for long-term applications. For these reasons, there is a growing demand for the development of new, cost-effective, and efficient fluorescent labeling materials. The semiconductor quantum dots (QDs) have been considered as a promising alternative owing to their excellent photophysical properties such as good photostability and high PL brightness; therefore, they have been under intense investigation for *in vitro* and *in vivo* imaging. However, these QDs have prompted potential safety concerns for *in vivo* use. In addition, their larger dimensions, typically comparable to or larger than the size of proteins, could possibly affect the function of attached (bio)molecules. Besides QDs, the carbon dots (CDs) or the silicon nanoparticles (Si NPs) are also potent candidates. While the CDs are zero-dimensional fluorescent carbonaceous nanomaterials with a typical size of <10 nm, the Si NPs are metal-free and PL nanomaterials containing Si, which is a nontoxic and naturally abundant element. In contrast to all these, fluorescent MeNCs have smaller sizes and possess bright emission and good biocompatibility, whereby they can be applied as excellent fluorescent probes for bioimaging and labeling applications [91].

Among noble metals, the Au, Ag, and Cu NCs are the most reported for such applications. As mentioned previously in Section 2.3, the PL feature of the noble MeNCs can be tuned by changing the cluster size as well as the type of the surface functionalizing ligand, thus MeNCs can be prepared having PL emission in the broad wavelength range (Vis (400–800 nm) or partly NIR (750–2500 nm) range). Within the NIR region, the 650–900 nm is a determinative range, because this is

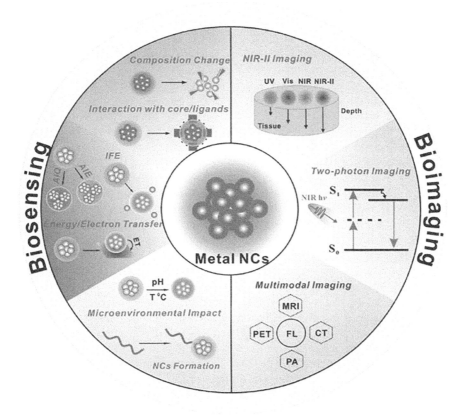

FIGURE 8 Schematic illustration of biosensing and bioimaging strategies based on luminescent MeNCs. (Copyright (2021) Wiley. Used with permission from Ref. [91].)

the first "biological window," which provides enhanced transparency to biological molecules and water. Baskakov and coworkers [92] presented the first imaging application of Ag NCs in combination with a fluorophore, thioflavin T (ThT) in 2005. Fluorescent NCs were generated *in situ* by sensitized photoreduction of Ag^+ ions in the presence of ThT. The prepared Ag NCs showed ultrabright PL in aqueous solution and the applicability of this non-object was confirmed by staining amyloid fibrils. After incubating the protein fibrils with ThT-Ag NCs for 5 min, the amyloid fibrils were observed to be covered by fluorescent NCs. In contrast, amyloid fibrils stained with ThT-Ag NCs displayed a time-dependent increase of fluorescence with no appreciable photobleaching even after 24 h of illumination at 475 nm ($\sim$500 W cm^{-2}), those stained only with ThT showed a rapid decay of the fluorescence and were barely detectable even after 1 min of illumination. Within the scope of this chapter, it is not possible to present all contributions, but some main results and conclusions can be summarized regarding the potential use of MeNCs in bioimaging and biolabeling applications as follows [92]:

i. Regarding *the quality of metals*—based on published articles in the last 15 years—it can be concluded that the most studied noble metal is Au ($\sim$50% of the articles). Moreover, about 25% of the published articles report on the advantages and possibilities of Ag-based clusters, compared to about 10–12% for Cu-based clusters. Beyond this, research on, e.g., Pt-based clusters is scarce [93, 94]. As a point of interest, Tanaka et al. successfully prepared mercaptoacetic acid (MAA)-functionalized Pt_5 NCs [93] by reducing firstly the H_2PtCl_6 with $NaBH_4$ in the presence of PAMAM (G4-OH) and the PAMAM ligand was exchanged with MAA as a second step. The synthesized $Pt_5(MAA)_8$ NCs showed blue fluorescence at 470 nm with the PL lifetime of 8.8 ns. Next, the $Pt_5(MAA)_8$ NCs were conjugated with Protein A using a 1-[(3-dimethylamino)-propyl]-3-ethylcarbodiimide hydrochloride (EDC)/ *N*-hydroxysulfosuccinimide (Sulfo-NHS) coupling reaction. As a final step, the $Pt_5(MAA)_8$-(Protein A) was bound to an anti-chemokine receptor antibody (anti-CXCR4-Ab) through the Fc moiety of the antibody. The applicability of the prepared Pt-based nano-object as a bioimaging agent was tested for human cervical cancer (HeLa) cells. Huang et al. also studied Pt-based NCs [94] as potential HeLa cell imaging, but the MAA was changed to PEI polyelectrolyte. These Pt NCs@PEI-(anti-CXCR4-Ab) conjugates showed yellow PL ($\lambda_{em} = 560$ nm). No significant differences were observed, even considering the different size of the clusters and their different characteristic fluorescence. In addition to monometallic clusters, a few articles are available on the study of bimetallic (Au/Ag) NCs, mainly to demonstrate the labeling possibilities of HeLa cells [95].

ii. Concerning *the type of the surface functionalized ligands*—based on the published articles in the last 15 years [96], it can be stated that serum proteins like BSA and HSA are applied generally (30–35% of the

Metal-Based Nanoclusters for Biomedical Applications

articles); the serum protein stabilized Au NCs possess intense red emission ($\lambda_{em} \sim 640$–660 nm). Besides proteins, peptides (mostly GSH) and small molecules (e.g., DHLA, LA or alkylthiols) are often used as surface-modifying ligands for MeNCs. In addition to the aforementioned molecules, DNA-, polyelectrolyte-, or other macromolecule- (e.g., chitosan, PMAA) stabilized MeNCs have also been tested in bioimaging and biolabeling utilizations [96].

iii. Regarding *the emission feature of the MeNCs*, no profound conclusion can be drawn; MeNCs having blue emission are also tested in the same way as the red-emitting MeNCs [96]. It can be stated that a suitable fluorescent reporter must meet several requirements, such as suitable brightness and solubility, good photo- and chemical stability, low toxicity as well as the absorption and emission are suggested to be in the red and NIR region (~600–900 nm) where biological objects have a negligible auto-absorption and auto-fluorescence. For this reason, systems emitting in the longer wavelength range ($\lambda > 600$ nm) may be more optimal.

iv. Concerning *the type of the labeled biosystems,* it can be concluded that many articles focus on tumor cell imaging [96]. Namely, *ca.* 50% of published papers highlight the imaging possibilities of HeLa cells. Some limitations are worthy of mention for detailed evaluation of the role of MeNCs as excellent labeling/imaging agents. On the one hand, the MeNCs have a unique size-, shape-, and composition-dependent optical feature which is strongly dependent upon methods to synthesize and to purify them. Small changes in size, composition, and type of surface-bound ligands can significantly affect this optical feature. Precision and reproducible syntheses are therefore necessary to produce MeNCs with controllable size, distribution, structure, and high QY(%). On the other hand, from a cost perspective, Au is still an expensive raw material, so there is a continuous demand to use cheaper metals or to develop protocols to produce bimetallic NCs. In many cases, the alloying process is expected to enhance certain optical properties. Furthermore, the number of studies relating to the detailed understanding of the cytotoxicity effect of MeNCs [27, 28] and their behavior in biological environments are relatively less compared to classical noble metal NPs. The safe and efficient utilization of MeNCs in biological applications is extremely important, and therefore there is a high demand to design new MeNCs with tunable optical properties and controlled structures.

3.3 Drug Delivery

Due to the ultra-small size, uniform morphology, stable fluorescence emission, and high biocompatibility, MeNCs have been intensively studied as potential drug delivery nano-objects. To design an effective nano-sized drug delivery system the size and the surface-bounded ligand(s) of the particles/clusters have important roles in targeted delivery and controlled release. There are thousands of publications demonstrating the applicability of classical colloidal NPs, including metal-based particles, as potent drug delivery systems. In contrast to particles, the MeNCs have sub-nanometer sizes which are below the kidney filtration threshold (KFT, *ca.* 5.5 nm), and thus they can be cleared rapidly via the kidney. This size is a defining requirement to design effective drug delivery nano-objects with high stability. The study of the applicability of MeNCs (not particles) as drug delivery systems dates back only 6–7 years. The first articles were presented in 2015 for doxorubicin (DOX) encapsulation [97–100]. Doxorubicin is one of the most common anticancer drugs, thus it is generally used as a model compound. Khandelia et al. published the preparation of nanotheranostic BSA NPs with Au NCs as the luminescent probe, and their application for *in vitro* delivery of DOX to cancer cells [98]. They found that the fabricated nano-objects showed biocompatible, noncytotoxic, and highly photostable features and they possessed suitable quantum yield and large Stokes shifted emission [98]. Other multifunctional luminescent MeNCs with the characteristics of being ultrastable [97] and temperature- [99] and pH-sensitive were also designed and tested for encapsulation of DOX for chemotherapy of lung and liver cancers. Namely, in the case of the ultrastable system, the thiol-terminated (-SH), alkyl-chain-containing (-C$_{11}$-) with short-chain PEGs (-EG$_6$-) (HS–C$_{11}$–EG$_6$–X; X = X = OH, COOH, NH$_2$, GRGD)-capped Au NCs were fabricated which exhibited high stability under different experimental conditions (e.g., extreme pH, high salt concentration, PBS and cell medium) for at least 6 months, even after conjugation with anticancer DOX. Zhao et al. synthesized DNA-stabilized Ag NCs with a fluorescence emission at 610 nm using a special hairpin DNA sequence [99]. They found that the clusters had a good fluorescence reversible sense for temperatures in the range of 25–66°C. Moreover, the fluorescence analytical results demonstrated that the Dox in Dox-loaded DNA-AgNCs system can be selectively released by the sense of the HepG-2 cells [99]. In addition, pH-sensitive drug delivery vehicles were also fabricated for DOX encapsulation [100]. Zhang and coworkers synthesized novel multifunctional spherical Au NCs assemblies encapsulated by a polyacrylic acid (PAA)/calcium phosphate (CaP) shell with aggregation-enhanced fluorescence property (designated as AuNCs-A@PAA/CaP). The prepared AuNCs-A@PAA/CaP NPs possess a high payload of DOX as a synergetic pH-sensitive drug delivery system to employ for dual-modal computed tomography (CT) and fluorescence imaging-guided liver cancer chemotherapy *in vivo* [100]. Besides DOX, cisplatin is the other commonly studied anticancer agent and we can find articles relating to the design of cisplatin-loaded MeNCs-based drug delivery systems as well [101, 102]. Zhou et al. published the preparation protocol of a cisplatin prodrug and folic acid-loaded fluorescent Au NCs (FA-GNC-Pt NPs) for fluorescence imaging and targeted chemotherapy of breast cancer. They found that FA modification significantly accelerated the cellular uptake and increased the cytotoxicity in murine 4T1 breast cancer cells. They also confirmed that FA-GNC-Pt NPs can predominantly inhibit the growth and lung metastasis of the orthotopically implanted 4T1 breast tumors [102]. In 2018, Chatterjee and coworkers successfully prepared PEG-coated deoxyguanosine 5′-triphosphate (dGTP)-templated fluorescent Au NCs having a spherical shape and size of 2.05 ± 0.43 nm in the presence of cisplatin. They confirmed that the composite NPs delivered the cisplatin efficiently into HeLa cells to induce apoptosis-mediated cell death, and simultaneously bio-imaged the cellular uptake [101]. In the last few years, the utilization of MeNCs has been extended to more classes of model compounds, such as tumor-targeting aptamer [103] or paclitaxel [104].

Chen and coworkers prepared a multifunctional oligonucleotide nanocarrier complex composed of a tumor-targeting aptamer sequence specific to mucin 1 (MUC1), poly-cytosine region for AgNCs synthesis, and complimentary sequence for microRNA miR-34a loading. They proved that this complex nano-object was able to enter MCF-7 breast cancer cells. This novel multifunctional AgNC-based nanocarrier can aid in improving the efficacy of breast cancer theranostics [103]. The role of MeNCs is more and more dominant in colorimetric clinical applications as well [105, 106].

3.4 Diagnostics and Therapy

In addition to the areas of application mentioned in the previous subsections, there is one major area worth mentioning, namely, the usability of NCs to act as diagnostics and therapeutic agents. Concerning therapeutic uses, different articles can be read on the area of gene, immuno-, photodynamic, and the

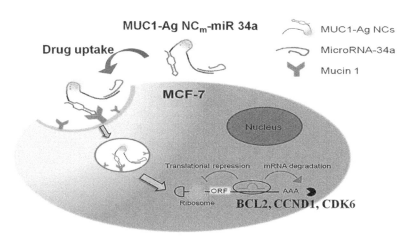

FIGURE 9 Schematic representation of the delivery of tumor-targeting aptamer into MCF-7 cells by functionalized Ag NCs. (Copyright (2017) Elsevier. Used with permission from Ref. [103].)

optical imaging-guided cancer therapies [107]. The following are two to three examples for each area. The *optical imaging-guided cancer therapy* also includes simultaneous tumor cell(s) imaging as well as the targeted therapy. Irudayaraj and colleagues were among the first to publish work in 2011 on the enhancement of the therapeutic efficacy of herceptin (chemical name: trastuzumab) by immobilizing this antineoplastic agent ($M_w \sim 145$ kDa) on BSA-covered Au NCs [108]. They confirmed that this Au NC-herceptin conjugate can penetrate cancer cells. The above-mentioned BSA-Au NCs have also been successfully applied for other tumor diagnosis and therapy. Namely, the protein-directed AuNCs were functionalized with Met amino acid and labeled with a fluorescent dye molecule (indocyanine-green derivative (MPA)). These functionalized NCs were able to transport the anticancer drug DOX to tumor cells. The preparation steps of the final nano-object are presented in Figure 10. By using MeNCs, the anti-tumor activity of DOX was enhanced [109].

Photodynamic therapy (PDT) is suitable for destroying cancer cells upon selective light irradiation without significant damage to healthy cells. For example, Jayasree and Ajayaghosh developed a fluorescence imaging-assisted PDT by using photosensitizer-linked Au NCs. The NIR-emitting lipoic acid-functionalized Au NCs, incorporating a tumor-targeting agent (folic acid) and a photosensitizer (protoporphyrin IX), showed excellent tumor reduction properties. Moreover, the NIR emission of Au NCs facilitated real-time tracking of the progress in PDT [110]. Chen et al. successfully developed a phototherapy agent

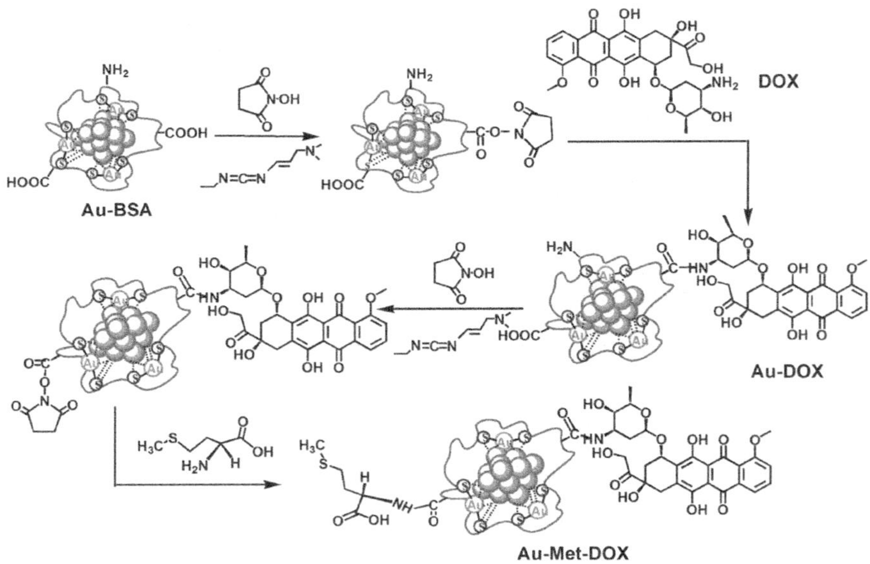

FIGURE 10 Synthesis routine and structures of Au-Met-DOX and Au-DOX. (Copyright (2017) Elsevier. Used with permission from Ref. [109].)

Metal-Based Nanoclusters for Biomedical Applications

based on chlorin e6 (Ce6) photosensitizer-conjugated Au NCs coated by silica (AuNC@SiO$_2$–Ce6). The AuNC@SiO$_2$–Ce6 objects possess excellent properties, such as high Ce6 photosensitizer loading, no nonspecific release of Ce6 during its circulation and significantly enhanced cellular uptake efficiency of Ce6, offering a remarkably improved PDT efficacy compared to free Ce6 [111]. The selectively functionalized MeNCs are also promising platforms for *gene therapy*. The polyelectrolytes like PEI or PSS have a dominant role in NCs stabilization. Chen's group studied the red-emitting PEI-modified Au NCs as a novel gene carrier by using PEI with relatively low molecular weight (1.8K). The PEI–AuNCs exhibited two to three times higher transfection efficiency in cells than that of PEI having a molecular weight of 25K [112]. Similar results have been obtained by other groups [113]. Some examples can also be found in the literature for *immunotherapy* application. X. Qu et al. reported ovalbumin (OVA)-stabilized oligodeoxynucleotides (ODNs), which were capable of being used as a template to produce fluorescent Au NCs (OVA–AuNC–CpG conjugates, OACs) [113]. Through dual-delivery of protein antigens and CpG ODNs on AuNCs, the as-prepared OACs could act as smart self-vaccines to assist in the generation of high immunostimulatory activity while simultaneously acting as an imaging agent. Both *in vitro* and *in vivo* experiments demonstrated that these engineered vaccines possessed high immunogenicity. All these findings suggested that the OACs might be utilized as safe and efficient immunostimulatory agents that were capable of preventing and/or treating a variety of ailments [114]. Besides Au, it is worth mentioning the role of other metal NCs (like Gd or Pt) in photothermal therapy (PTT). Namely, Lu et al. prepared BSA and PEG macromolecules to cover RuS NCs. RuS-based NCs have shown enhanced PTT activity using 808-nm laser irradiation [115]. These NCs accumulated in tumor cells to unprecedented levels, presumably due to their long circulation times. While all the control treatments showed no change in tumor growth, mice treated with BSA/PEG-(RuS)NCs had tumors that were eradicated within 4 days after treatment. These novel BSA/PEG-(RuS)NCs represent a potent agent for cancer PTT. Moreover, Wang and coworkers prepared BSA-stabilized gadolinium oxide nanostructures (Gd$_2$O$_3$) functionalized with cypate, which is a NIR dye with potential as a clinical theranostic agent. These nanocrystals were suitable for trimodal imaging, magnetic resonance, photoacoustic, and NIR fluorescence, plus mediating PTT as a therapy [116]. The fabricated BSA-Gd-oxide NCs showed good tumor ablation under NIR irradiation and increased tumor accumulation and cellular internalization as well. The advantage of this nano-object was the pH-responsive PT effect. Moreover, Yang et al. successfully synthesized BSA-coated Gd:CuS hybrid nano-objects for PTT as well as dual imaging, magnetic resonance, and photoacoustic effects [117]. These protein-coated MeNCs showed a strong NIR photothermal conversion, and potent tumor ablation capacity when irradiated with a laser having 980 nm wavelength. Tumor-bearing mice treated with BSA-(Gd:CuS)NCs showed a remarkable regression in tumor growth, some of which were eliminated after 6 days treatment.

4 GENERAL CONCLUSIONS

Metal nanostructures are gaining ground not only in materials science but also in biomedical applications. Among nanostructures, this chapter focuses specifically on nanoclusters, which are the transition between molecules and colloidal particles. Within metals, the noble metal-based nanostructures play an important role in nanomedicine since *ca.* 2005. The fabrication possibilities of noble metal-based nanostructures, as well as their structural and main optical properties, have been summarized in the first section. These nanoclusters exhibit molecule-like characteristics as their size approaches the Fermi wavelength of electrons. Due to the discrete energy levels, metal nanoclusters possess different electric, optical, and chemical properties from those of larger metal nanoparticles. Their characteristic feature is their strong photoluminescence. Due to their facile synthesis, good quantum yields, tunable fluorescence emission, large Stokes shift, and high photostability, they are excellent nano-objects in biomedical applications as well. Their main biomedical applications include detection of several type of analytes, drug delivery, imaging and diagnostics, and therapy and these have been highlighted in this chapter through several examples. This chapter has been compiled to the best of my knowledge, not only based on my own scientific results in the field over the past 12 years, but also includes the main results from publications in the most highly cited international journals (Nature, Small, ACS Nano, Chem. Rev., Nanoscale, etc.) in this exciting field.

ACKNOWLEDGMENTS

Project no. TKP2021-EGA-32 has been implemented with the support provided by the Ministry of Innovation and Technology of Hungary from the National Research, Development, and Innovation Fund, financed under the TKP2021-EGA funding scheme. This research was also supported by the National Research, Development, and Innovation Office through FK131446 project.

ABBREVIATIONS AND DEFINITIONS

AIE	aggregation-induced emission
AMP	adenosine monophosphate
anti-CXCR4-Ab	anti-chemokine receptor antibody
BSA	bovine serum albumin
CaP	calcium phosphate
CDs	carbon dots
CdSe	cadmium-selenide
Cu(PcTs)	copper(II) phthalocyanine
CT	computed tomography
Cys	cysteine
dGTP	deoxyguanosine 5′-triphosphate
DOX	doxorubicin

DPA	diperiodatoargentate(III)
D-**Trp**	*D*-tryptophan
EDC	3-ethylcarbodiimide hydrochloride
FA	folic acid
GOx	glucose oxidase
HBB	hemoglobin beta chain
HeLa	human cervical cancer cell
His	histidine
hPEI	hyperbranched polyethyleneimine
HRP	horseradish peroxidase
HSA	human serum albumin
IgG	immunoglobulin G
LAAOx	*L*-amino acid oxidase
LEDs	light-emitting diodes
LMCT	ligand-to-metal charge transfer
LMMCT	ligand-to-metal-metal charge transfer
LOD	limit of detection
LSPR	localized surface plasmon resonance
Lys	lysozyme
MAA	mercaptoacetic acid
MeNCs	metal nanoclusters
Met	methionine
MNPs	magnetic nanoparticles
11-MUA	11-mercaptoundecanoic acid
MUC1	mucin 1
NIR	near infrared
NPs	nanoparticles
NCs	nanoclusters
ODNs	oligodeoxynucleotides
OVA	ovalbumin
PAA	poly(acrylic) acid
PEI	polyethyleneimine
PL	photoluminescence
PDT	photodynamic therapy
PTT	photothermal therapy
PVP	polyvinylpyrrolidone
QCE	quantum confinement effect
QDs	quantum dots
QY(%)	quantum yield
Si NPs	silicon nanoparticles
ssDNA	single-stranded DNS
Sulfo-NHS	*N*-hydroxysulfosuccinimide
ThT	thioflavin T
TMB	3,3,5,5-tetramethylbenzidine

REFERENCES

[1] L. Shang, S. Dong, G. U. Nienhaus, *Nano Today* **2011**, *6*, 401–418.

[2] I. Chakraborty, T. Pradeep, *Chem. Rev.* **2017**, *117*, 8208–8271.

[3] R. Jin, C. Zeng, M. Zhou, Y. Chen, *Chem. Rev.* **2016**, *116*, 10346–10413.

[4] Y. P. Xie, Y. L. Shen, G. X. Duan, J. Han, L. P. Zhang, X. Lu, *Mater. Chem. Front.* **2020**, *4*, 2205–2222.

[5] A. Baghdasaryan, T. Bürgi, *Nanoscale.* **2021**, *13*, 6283–6340.

[6] Z. Guo, C. Xiao, R. V. Maligal-Ganesh, L. Zhou, T. W. Goh, X. Li, D. Tesfagaber, A. Thiel, W. Huang, *ACS Catal.* **2014**, *4*, 1340–1348.

[7] C. Xu, J. Lin, D. Yan, Z. Guo, D. J. Austin, H. Zhan, A. Kent, Y. Yue, *ACS Appl. Nano Mater.* **2020**, *3*, 6416–6422.

[8] H. Zhang, M. Huang, J. Wen, Y. Li, A. Li, L. Zhang, A. M. Ali, Y. Li, *Chem. Commun.* **2019**, *55*, 4699–4702.

[9] Q. Song, W. D. Wang, X. Hu, Z. Dong, *Nanoscale.* **2019**, *11*, 21513–21521.

[10] H. Gavilán, S. K. Avugadda, T. Fernández-Cabada, N. Soni, M. Cassani, B. T. Mai, R. Chantrell, T. Pellegrino, *Chem. Soc. Rev.* **2021** *50*, 11614–11667.

[11] S. Gutiérrez-Tarriño, S. Rojas-Buzo, C.W. Lopes, G. Agostini, J. J. Calvino, A. Corma, P. Oña-Burgos, *Green Chem.* **2021**, *23*, 4490–4501.

[12] H. Chen, X. Yang, L. Bo, S. Wang, D. Jiang, D. Shi, D. Schipper, R. A. Jones, *J. Lumin.* **2019**, *213*, 440–445.

[13] D. Ungor, I. Dékány, E. Csapó, *Nanomaterials* **2019**, *9*, 1229.

[14] X. Du, R. Jin, *ACS Nano.* **2019**, *13*, 7383–7387.

[15] B. Liu, H. Yao, W. Song, L. Jin, I. M. Mosa, J. F. Rusling, S. L. Suib, J. He, *J. Am. Chem. Soc.* **2016**, *138*, 4718–4721.

[16] A. M. Ismail, G. F. Samu, H. C. Nguyën, E. Csapó, N. López, C. Janáky, *ACS Catal.* **2020**, *10*, 5681–5690.

[17] A. M. Ismail, G. F. Samu, Á. Balog, E. Csapó, C. Janáky, *ACS Energy Lett.* **2019**, *4*, 48–53.

[18] A. M. Ismail, E. Csapó, C. Janáky, *Electrochim. Acta* **2019**, *313*, 171–178.

[19] J. V. Rival, P. Mymoona, K. M. Lakshmi, Nonappa, T. Pradeep, E. S. Shibu, *Small* **2021**, *17*, 2005718.

[20] Y. Tao, M. Li, J. Ren, X. Qu, *Chem. Soc. Rev.* **2015**, *44*, 8636–8663.

[21] Y. Xiao, Z. Wu, Q. Yao, J. Xie, *Aggregate.* **2021**, *2*, 114–132.

[22] Y. Du, H. Sheng, D. Astruc, M. Zhu, *Chem. Rev.* **2020**, *120*, 526–622.

[23] J. Pérez-Juste, I. Pastoriza-Santos, L. M. Liz-Marzán, P. Mulvaney, *Coord. Chem. Rev.* **2005**, *249*, 1870–1901.

[24] T. Q. Yang, B. Peng, B. Q. Shan, Y. X. Zong, J. G. Jiang, P. Wu, K. Zhang, *Nanomaterials* **2020**, *10*, 261.

[25] S. Qian, Z. Wang, Z. Zuo, X. Wang, Q. Wang, X. Yuan, *Coord. Chem. Rev.* **2022**, *451*, 214268.

[26] C. Deraedt, G. Melaet, W.T. Ralston, R. Ye, G. A. Somorjai, *Nano Lett.* **2017**, *17*, 1853–1862.

[27] D. Ungor, A. Barbasz, A. Czyżowska, E. Csapó, M. Oćwieja, *Coll. Surf. B.* **2021**, *200*, 111593.

[28] A. Czyżowska, A. Barbasz, L. Szyk-Warszyńska, M. Oćwieja, E. Csapó, D. Ungor, *Coll. Surf. A.* **2021**, *620*, 126569.

[29] Y. Chen, T. Feng, L. Chen, Y. Gao, J. Di, *Opt. Mater.* **2021**, *114*, 111012.

[30] R. Singh, S. Majhi, K. Sharma, M. Ali, S. Sharma, D. Choudhary, C. S. P. Tripathi, D. Guin, *Chem. Phys. Lett.* **2022**, *787*, 139226.

Metal-Based Nanoclusters for Biomedical Applications

[31] W. Li, B. Chen, H. Zhang, Y. Sun, J. Wang, J. Zhang, Y. Fu, *Biosens. Bioelectron.* **2015**, *66*, 251–258.

[32] Y. Wang, Y. Mu, J. Hu, Q. Zhuang, Y. Ni, *Spectrochim. Acta - Part A Mol. Biomol. Spectrosc.* **2019**, *214*, 445–450.

[33] D. Ungor, Á. Juhász, N. Varga, E. Csapó, *Adv. Colloid Interface Sci.* **2022**, *301*, 102616.

[34] J. Liu, P. N. Duchesne, M. Yu, X. Jiang, X. Ning, R. D. Vinluan, P. Zhang, J. Zheng, *Angew. Chemie* **2016**, *55*, 8894–8898.

[35] J. Mei, N. L. C. Leung, R. T. K. Kwok, J. W. Y. Lam, B. Z. Tang, *Chem. Rev.* **2015**, *115*, 11718–11940.

[36] F. Xue, F. Qu, W. Han, L. Xia, J. You, *Anal. Chim. Acta* **2019**, *1046*, 170–178.

[37] J. Chen, Y. C. Gao, Z. B. Xu, G. H. Wu, Y. C. Chen, C. Q. Zhu, *Anal. Chim. Acta.* **2006**, *577*, 77–84.

[38] C.C. Huang, Z. Yang, K.H. Lee, H.T. Chang, *Angew. Chemie* **2007**, *46*, 6824–6828.

[39] J. Xie, Y. Zheng, J.Y. Ying, *Chem. Commun.* **2010**, *46*, 961–963.

[40] W. Guo, J. Yuan, E. Wang, *Chem. Commun.* **2009**, 3395–3397.

[41] B. Adhikari, A. Banerjee, *Chem. Mater.* **2010**, *22*, 4364–4371.

[42] G. Panthi, M. Park, *J. Hazard. Mater.* **2022**, *424*, 127565.

[43] Q. Hong, C. Rogero, J. H. Lakey, B. A. Connolly, A. Houlton, B. R. Horrocks, F. Mckenzie, A. Ingram, R. Stokes, D. Graham, Z. Wang, Y. Lu, F. Rowell, K. Hudson, J. Seviour, S.-K. Kim, S. B. Lee, H. Lord, S. O. Kelley, J. Jeon, D.-K. Lim, J.-M. Nam, M. R. Guerra, I. Chianella, E. V. Piletska, K. Karim, A. P. F. Turner, S. A. Piletsky, L. Shang, S. Dong, *J. Mater. Chem.* **2008**, *18*, 4636–4640.

[44] Z.S. Kardar, F. Shemirani, R. Zadmard, *Microchim. Acta.* **2020**, *187*, 1–9.

[45] D. Ungor, E. Csapó, B. Kismárton, A. Juhász, I. Dékány, *Coll. Surf. B.* **2017**, *155*, 135–141.

[46] P. Nath, M. Chatterjee, N. Chanda, *ACS Appl. Nano Mater.* **2018**, *1*, 5108–5118.

[47] H. Zhang, Q. Liu, T. Wang, Z. Yun, G. Li, J. Liu, G. Jiang, *Anal. Chim. Acta* **2013**, *770*, 140–146.

[48] Z. Dehghani, M. Hosseini, J. Mohammadnejad, M. R. Ganjali, *Anal. Methods.* **2019**, *11*, 684–690.

[49] Y. Liu, K. Ai, X. Cheng, L. Huo, L. Lu, *Adv. Funct. Mater.* **2010**, *20*, 951–956.

[50] Z. Shojaeifard, B. Hemmateenejad, M. Shamsipur, *ACS Appl. Mater. Interfaces.* **2016**, *8*, 15177–15186.

[51] D. Lu, L. Liu, F. Li, S. Shuang, Y. Li, M. M. F. Choi, C. Dong, *Spectrochim. Acta - Part A Mol. Biomol. Spectrosc.* **2014**, *121*, 77–80.

[52] R. Rajamanikandan, M. Ilanchelian, *ACS Omega* **2018**, *3*, 14111–14118.

[53] C. W. Wang, Y. N. Chen, B. Y. Wu, C. K. Lee, Y. C. Chen, Y. H. Huang, H. T. Chang, *Anal. Bioanal. Chem.* **2016**, *408*, 287–294.

[54] H. Yang, Y. Yang, S. Liu, X. Zhan, H. Zhou, X. Li, Z. Yuan, *Anal. Bioanal. Chem.* **2020**, *412*, 5819–5826.

[55] C. Zong, L. R. Zheng, W. He, X. Ren, C. Jiang, L. Lu, *Anal. Chem.* **2014**, *86*, 1687–1692.

[56] G. Zhang, Y. Qiao, T. Xu, C. Zhang, Y. Zhang, L. Shi, S. Shuang, C. Dong, *Nanoscale* **2015**, *7*, 12666–12672.

[57] R. M. Trujillo, D. E. Barraza, M. L. Zamora, A. Cattani-Scholz, R. E. Madrid, *Sensors*, **2021**, *21*, 2204.

[58] M. Atar, Ö. Taspinar, S. Hanft, B. Goldfuss, H. G. Schmalz, A. G. Griesbeck, *J. Org. Chem.* **2019**, *84*, 15972–15977.

[59] N. A. Sitnikova, M. A. Komkova, I. V. Khomyakova, E. E. Karyakina, A. A. Karyakin, *Anal. Chem.* **2014**, *86*, 4131–4134.

[60] F. Molaabasi, S. Hosseinkhani, A. A. Moosavi-Movahedi, M. Shamsipur, *RSC Adv.* **2015**, *5*, 33123–33135.

[61] T. Marimuthu, M. R. Mahmoudian, S. Mohamad, Y. Alias, *Sensors Act. B.* **2014**, *202*, 1037–1043.

[62] A. Salimi, R. Hallaj, S. Soltanian, H. Mamkhezri, *Anal. Chim. Acta* **2007**, *594*, 24–31.

[63] F. Wen, Y. Dong, L. Feng, S. Wang, S. Zhang, X. Zhang, *Anal. Chem.* **2011**, *83*, 1193–1196.

[64] J. R. Zhang, Z. L. Wang, F. Qu, H. Q. Luo, N. B. Li, *J. Agric. Food Chem.* **2014**, *62*, 6592–6599.

[65] Z. Li, T. Zhang, M. Zhang, W. Hu, *Dye. Pigment* **2022**, *198*, 109984.

[66] L. Meng, J.H. Yin, Y. Yuan, N. Xu, *RSC Adv.* **2018**, *8*, 9327–9333.

[67] B. Hemmateenejad, F. Shakerizadeh-Shirazi, F. Samari, *Sensors Act. B.* **2014**, *19*, 942–46.

[68] H. Li, Y. Cheng, Y. Liu, B. Chen, *Talanta* **2016**, *158*, 118–124.

[69] D. Ungor, I. Szilágyi, E. Csapó, *J. Mol. Liq.* **2021**, *338*, 116695.

[70] X. Li, X. Wu, F. Zhang, B. Zhao, Y. Li, *Talanta* **2019**, *195*, 372–380.

[71] S. Han, X. Chen, *Spectrochim. Acta - Part A* **2019**, *210*, 315–320.

[72] X. Li, J. Qiao, Y. Sun, Z. Li, L. Qi, *J. Anal. Sci. Technol.* **2021**, *12*, 1–8.

[73] X. Gao, X. Du, D. Liu, H. Gao, P. Wang, J. Yang, *Sci. Reports* **2020**, *10*, 1–10.

[74] H. Peng, H. Deng, M. Jian, A. Liu, F. Bai, X. Lin, W. Chen, *Microchim. Acta* **2017**, *184*, 735–743.

[75] S. Govindaraju, S. R. Ankireddy, B. Viswanath, J. Kim, K. Yun, *Sci. Reports* **2017**, *71*, 1–12.

[76] D. Ungor, K. Horváth, I. Dékány, E. Csapó, *Sensors Act. B.* **2019**, *288*, 728–733.

[77] M. Santhosh, S. R. Chinnadayyala, A. Kakoti, P. Goswami, *Biosens. Bioelectron.* **2014**, *59*, 370–376.

[78] Y. Chen, J. Qiao, Q. Liu, M. Zhang, L. Qi, *Anal. Chim. Acta* **2018**, *1026*, 133–139.

[79] N. T. Si, N. T. A. Nhung, T. Q. Bui, M. T. Nguyen, P. V. Nhat, *RSC Adv.* **2021**, *11*, 16619–16632.

[80] R. C. Triulzi, M. Micic, S. Giordani, M. Serry, W. A. Chiou, R. M. Leblanc, *Chem. Commun.* **2006**, 5068–5070.

[81] C. T. Chen, W. J. Chen, C. Z. Liu, L. Y. Chang, Y. C. Chen, *Chem. Commun.* **2009**, 7515–7517.

[82] C. C. Huang, C. K. Chiang, Z. H. Lin, K. H. Lee, H. T. Chang, *Anal. Chem.* **2008**, *80*, 1497–1504.

[83] C. C. Huang, C. T. Chen, Y. C. Shiang, Z. H. Lin, H. T. Chang, *Anal. Chem.* **2009**, *81*, 875–882.

[84] Q. Liu, N. Li, M. Wang, L. Wang, X. Su, *Anal. Chim. Acta* **2018**, *1013*, 71–78.

[85] L. Hu, S. Han, S. Parveen, Y. Yuan, L. Zhang, G. Xu, *Biosens. Bioelectron.* **2012**, *32*, 297–299.

[86] Z. Zhang, S. Li, P. Huang, J. Feng, F. Y. Wu, *Microchim. Acta* **2019**, *186*, 1–8.

[87] P. D. Nguyen, V. T. Cong, C. Baek, J. Min, *Biosens. Bioelectron.* **2017**, *89*, 666–672.

[88] J. Sharma, H. C. Yeh, H. Yoo, J. H. Werner, J. S. Martinez, *Chem. Commun.* **2011**, *47*, 2294–2296.

[89] X. Lin, L. Zou, W. Lan, C. Liang, Y. Yin, J. Liang, Y. Zhou, J. Wang, *Dalt. Trans.* **2021**, *51*, 27–39.

[90] W. Guo, J. Yuan, Q. Dong, E. Wang, *J. Am. Chem. Soc.* **2010**, *132*, 932–934.

[91] Y. Xiao, Z. Wu, Q. Yao, J. Xie, *Aggregate* **2021**, *2*, 114–132.

Metal-Based Nanoclusters for Biomedical Applications

[92] N. Makarava, A. Parfenov, I. V. Baskakov, *Biophys. J.* **2005**, *89*, 572–580.

[93] S. I. Tanaka, J. Miyazaki, D. K. Tiwari, T. Jin, Y. Inouye, *Angew. Chemie* **2011**, *50*, 431–435.

[94] X. Huang, H. Ishitobi, Y. Inouye, *RSC Adv.* **2016**, *6*, 9709–9716.

[95] P. Wang, L. Lin, Z. Guo, J. Chen, H. Tian, X. Chen, H. Yang, *Macromol. Biosci.* **2016**, *16*, 160–167.

[96] J. Xu, L. Shang, *Fluoresc. Mater. Cell Imaging.* **2020**, 97–128.

[97] X. Zhang, F. G. Wu, P. Liu, H. Y. Wang, N. Gu, Z. Chen, *J. Colloid Interface Sci.* **2015**, *455*, 6–15.

[98] R. Khandelia, S. Bhandari, U. N. Pan, S. S. Ghosh, A. Chattopadhyay, *Small* **2015**, *11*, 4075–4081.

[99] T. T. Zhao, Q. Y. Chen, H. Yang, *Spectrochim. Acta - Part A.* **2015**, *137*, 66–69.

[100] L. Li, L. Zhang, T. Wang, X. Wu, H. Ren, C. Wang, Z. Su, *Small* **2015**, *11*, 3162.

[101] B. Chatterjee, A. Ghoshal, A. Chattopadhyay, S. S. Ghosh, *ACS Biomater. Sci. Eng.* **2018**, *4*, 1005–1012.

[102] F. Zhou, B. Feng, H. Yu, D. Wang, T. Wang, J. Liu, Q. Meng, S. Wang, P. Zhang, Z. Zhang, Y. Li, *Theranostics* **2016**, *6*, 679–687.

[103] H. Y. Chen, K. Albert, C. C. Wen, P. Y. Hsieh, S. Y. Chen, N. C. Huang, S. C. Lo, J. K. Chen, H. Y. Hsu, *Coll. Surf. B.* **2017**, *152*, 423–431.

[104] R. Liu, W. Xiao, C. Hu, R. Xie, H. Gao, *J. Control. Release.* **2018**, *278*, 127–139.

[105] Q. Li, Y. Pan, T. Chen, Y. Du, H. Ge, B. Zhang, J. Xie, H. Yu, M. Zhu, *Nanoscale* **2018**, *10*, 10166–10172.

[106] Y. Tao, Y. Zhang, E. Ju, H. Ren, J. Ren, *Nanoscale* **2015**, *7*, 12419–12426.

[107] Y. Tao, M. Li, J. Ren, X. Qu, *Chem. Soc. Rev.* **2015**, *44*, 8636–8663.

[108] Y. Wang, J. Chen, J. Irudayaraj, *ACS Nano.* **2011**, *5*, 9718–9725.

[109] H. Chen, B. Li, X. Ren, S. Li, Y. Ma, S. Cui, Y. Gu, *Biomaterials* **2012**, *33*, 8461–8476.

[110] L. V. Nair, S.S. Nazeer, R.S. Jayasree, A. Ajayaghosh, *ACS Nano.* **2015**, *9*, 5825–5832.

[111] P. Huang, J. Lin, S. Wang, Z. Zhou, Z. Li, Z. Wang, C. Zhang, X. Yue, G. Niu, M. Yang, D. Cui, X. Chen, *Biomaterials* **2013**, *34*, 4643–4654.

[112] H. Tian, Z. Guo, J. Chen, L. Lin, J. Xia, X. Dong, X. Chen, *Adv. Healthc. Mater.* **2012**, *1*, 337–341.

[113] Y. Tao, Z. Li, E. Ju, J. Ren, X. Qu, *Nanoscale* **2013**, *5*, 6154–6160.

[114] Y. Tao, E. Ju, Z. Li, J. Ren, X. Qu, *Adv. Funct. Mater.* **2014**, *24*, 1004–1010.

[115] Z. Lu, F.Y. Huang, R. Cao, L. Zhang, G.H. Tan, N. He, J. Huang, G. Wang, Z. Zhang, *Sci. Rep.* **2017**, *7*, 1–10.

[116] Y. Wang, T. Yang, H. Ke, A. Zhu, Y. Wang, J. Wang, J. Shen, G. Liu, C. Chen, Y. Zhao, H. Chen, *Adv. Mater.* **2015**, *27*, 3874–3882.

[117] W. Yang, W. Guo, W. Le, G. Lv, F. Zhang, L. Shi, X. Wang, J. Wang, S. Wang, J. Chang, B. Zhang, *ACS Nano.* **2016**, *10*, 10245–10257.

12 Radiometals in Molecular Imaging and Therapy

Izabela Cieszykowska, Wioletta Wojdowska,
Dariusz Pawlak, and Renata Mikołajczak*
National Centre for Nuclear Research
Radioisotope Centre POLATOM,
Andrzej Sołtan 7, PL-05-400 Otwock,Poland
Renata.Mikolajczak@polatom.pl

CONTENTS

1 Introduction 320
2 Properties of Radiometals 321
    2.1 The Types of Radioactive Decays 321
    2.2 Choice of Radiometal for Medical Application 323
3 Production Methods of Radiometals 326
    3.1 Nuclear Reactors 326
    3.2 Accelerators 327
    3.3 Radionuclide Generators 327
    3.4 Impact of Production Method on the Suitability of Radiometals
        for Medical Applications 328
4 Characteristics of Selected Radiometals Used in Radiopharmaceuticals 329
    4.1 Technetium-99m, Rhenium-186 and Rhenium-188 330
    4.2 Indium-111 331
    4.3 Gallium-68 331
    4.4 Copper-61, Copper-64, and Copper-67 332
    4.5 Scandium-43, Scandium-44, and Scandium-47 332
    4.6 Zirconium-89 333
    4.7 Yttrium-86 and Yttrium-90 333
    4.8 Lutetium-177 333
    4.9 Alpha-Emitting Radiometals 334
5 Chelators for Metal Complexation 335
6 Current Trends in Radiometals for Medical Application 337
7 General Conclusions 340
Acknowledgement 340
Abbreviations and Definitions 340
References 341

---

* Corresponding author

DOI: 10.1201/9781003272250-12

319

ABSTRACT

The radiometals are of particular interest for radiopharmaceutical development due to their wide range of nuclear properties such as half-life, type of radioactive decay, and rich coordination chemistry. In recent years, the number of novel target-specific radiotracers introduced to clinical practice is growing rapidly. This is not only due to the introduction of novel tumour targeting molecules but also due to the increasing availability of radionuclides, both for diagnostic imaging in PET and SPECT and for therapy. This chapter presents the radiometals which currently find application in nuclear medicine, their chemical and radiation characteristics, production methods and strategies allowing their incorporation into radiopharmaceuticals as well as future trends in the development of radiometals into medically useful tracers.

KEYWORDS

Radiopharmaceuticals; Targeting Molecules; Radiometals; Bifunctional Chelators; Diagnostic Imaging; Radionuclide Therapy

1 INTRODUCTION

The idea of using radiation to cure cancer originates from the times when Maria and Pierre Curie discovered the radioactive elements polonium and radium. The discovery of artificial radioactivity in 1934 by Frederic Joliot and Irene Curie was a major breakthrough in the field of nuclear sciences, paving the way to the synthesis of radioisotopes with better properties than the naturally occurring ones. At present, practically all radioisotopes used in nuclear medicine are artificially produced using man-made devices, invented in the 1930s and 1940s, i.e. nuclear reactors and accelerators of charged particles. The first use of beta-radiation emitter radiometal strontium-89 (^{89}Sr) in the treatment of metastatic bone cancer was reported in 1942 [1]. Since then several radiometals have been administered to patients in the form of medicinal products named radiopharmaceuticals and nuclear medicine is the medical speciality utilizing them in various diagnoses and treatments, especially for cancer [2, 3].

To date, with the deeper insight into targeting mechanisms, the development of novel, specific carrier molecules, and the broadening portfolio of radiometals, allowing to adjust their physical characteristics to the disease, the role of nuclear medicine techniques can't be overestimated [4]. In particular, molecular imaging which can be defined as the visualization, characterization and the measurement of biological processes at the molecular and cellular levels in humans and other living systems is the field in which novel radiopharmaceuticals provide superior spatial resolution and the advantage of visualizing the dynamics of these processes [5]. In addition, the same biological processes which govern the uptake of radiotracers *in vivo* for imaging can be used for delivering the therapeutic

Radiometals in Molecular Imaging and Therapy

radiation dose directly to the targeted organ or tissue [6]. This chapter presents the radiometals which currently find application in nuclear medicine, their chemical and radiation characteristics, methods allowing their incorporation into radiopharmaceuticals as well as future trends in the development of radiometals into medically useful tracers.

2 PROPERTIES OF RADIOMETALS

2.1 THE TYPES OF RADIOACTIVE DECAYS

Radioactive decay is the desired property of radiometals and determines their potential for application in nuclear medicine. It is the result of decay of unstable nuclei, which can differ in the form of emission, emitted energy and its penetrating range in tissue [7]. The types of radioactive decay comprise:

α **decay** – type of radioactive disintegration in which some unstable atomic nuclei lose excess energy by spontaneously ejecting an alpha particle (the nuclei of helium atom). Alpha radiation is much more ionizing than beta radiation. Typical energy of alpha particles is several MeV and the range in living tissues is in the order of tenths of a millimetres, usually not more than a few diameters of living cells. Additionally it can damage DNA irreversibly. These properties make alpha radioactive radionuclides very useful in the treatment of, in particular, neoplastic diseases [8].

β **decay** – type of radioactive decay, in which the atomic nucleus emits high-energy electrons (β^-) or positrons (anti-electrons, β^+). The β decay is usually accompanied by gamma-ray emission. The energies of the β particles are similar to gamma radiation and range from keV to several MeV, but β particles are more ionizing than gamma rays, which translates into the greater damage to living tissue and lower penetrating. The range of beta particles in tissues is up to several millimetres and depends on their energy. The β^- particles emitting radionuclides have found application in therapy [9]. In contrast to β^- radiation, the positron (β^+) emissions are used in imaging [10].

EC (electron capture) – a type of radioactive decay in which an electron from an electron shell is absorbed by a proton-rich nucleus [11]. The decay of the EC is accompanied by the emission of characteristic X-rays, Auger electrons and gamma rays. The energy of Auger electrons is low, on the order of several dozen eV. Due to their low kinetic energy, Auger electrons travel over a very short range: way less than the size of a single cell, on the order of less than a few hundred nanometres, which translates into the possibility of depositing very high energies in a single cell. This property can be used medicinally as Auger therapy [12].

IT (isomeric transition) – a type of radioactivity in which unstable atomic nuclei lose excess energy by emitting high-energy photons (gamma ray). The energy of the photons is different for each radionuclide and ranges from keV to several MeV. Gamma rays are penetrating and, for this reason, photon-emitting radiometals like technetium-99m (^{99m}Tc) are usually used in diagnostics [13].

The **fission** is a radioactive decay, induced by neutron capture, in which the nucleus splits into two nearly equal fragments and several free neutrons. A large amount of energy is also released. These neutrons may induce a nuclear fission chain reaction occurring in a nuclear reactor. The radiometal molybdenum-99 (Mo-99), a parent radionuclide used in radionuclide generators ^{99}Mo/^{99m}Tc, is the fission product of uranium-235 (U-235) [14]. Figure 1 illustrates the types of radioactive decay with the demonstration of the soft tissue penetration range [15].

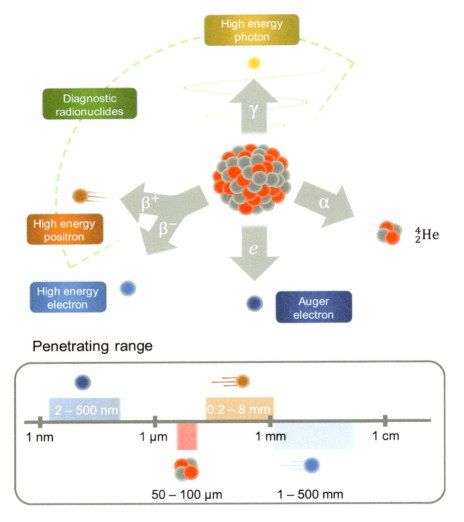

FIGURE 1 Types of radioactive decay with the demonstration of the soft tissue penetration range. (Reproduced by permission from Ref. [15]. Peltek, O.O., Muslimov, A.R., Zyuzin, M.V. et al. *J. Nanobiotechnol.* **17,** *90* (2019).)

Radiometals in Molecular Imaging and Therapy

2.2 Choice of Radiometal for Medical Application

The potential application of radionuclide is determined by its nature. In diagnostic applications, the emitted radiation is expected to leave the human body, it is then detected and converted into an image which demonstrates the localization of radioactivity in the diagnosed organism. The diagnostic radiometals are those characterized by gamma or positron emission, with a high enough energy to penetrate the body and to be detected externally by a camera and with no accompanying emission of particle (α or β^-) radiation. Gamma-emitting radionuclides (such as e.g. ^{99m}Tc) are used for diagnostic imaging by single photon emission tomography (SPECT). Radioisotopes that emit positrons are useful for imaging using positron emission tomography (PET). In a β^+ decay, the proton and electron annihilate, releasing two gamma rays of energy of 511 keV each, emitted in opposite directions. These gamma rays are called annihilation radiation. In the PET scanner, the annihilation radiation is detected simultaneously, which allows the location of the annihilation to be determined. Gallium-68 (Ga-68) is an example of a positron emitter that has played an important role in the development of novel PET tracers over the past two decades.

In therapy, the emitted corpuscular radiation (α, β^- or Auger electrons) is absorbed in the targeted tissue thus leading to its damage while sparing the adjacent tissues and organs. The action of radiation into matter can be described by linear energy transfer (LET) – the amount of energy that an ionizing particle transfers to the tissue per unit distance (keV/μm). Since the emitting particles vary in penetrating range and LET, the choice of radionuclide will depend on several factors, such as the type and size of targeted disease, density of the target and its heterogeneity. Alpha emitters characterized by high LET values deliver a very high energy in a very small volume and are therefore particularly useful in the case of micro-metastases and blood-borne cancer cells [16].

At present, β^- emitters play a dominant role in targeted therapy due to their well-known production methods and thus great availability [2, 3, 17]. The value of LET for β^- emitters is lower than for α emitters. Its penetration range in soft tissue is between a few micrometres to a few centimetres, proportionally to the energy of the particle. Thus, low to medium energy β^- particle-emitting radionuclides, e.g., lutetium-177 (^{177}Lu), are considered more effective for treating small tumor, while high-energy β^- particle-emitting radionuclides, e.g., ^{90}Y, are more appropriate for treatment of larger tumor [18]. Some β-emitting radionuclides also decay with γ-radiation, which provides the ability to visualize distribution of the radiopharmaceutical within the patient's body using SPECT (e.g. ^{177}Lu).

Regardless of the application, the "ideal" radiometals should present the adequate *in vivo* stability, suitable half-life, well-known chelation chemistry and ease of production.

Table 1 presents the radiometals discussed in this chapter, their physical properties and medical applications.

TABLE 1
Physical Characteristics of Radiometals for Molecular Imaging and Therapy, Production Methods and Medical Application

Radionuclide	$T_{1/2}$	E [keV] Particle/Photons per 100 Decay	Production Method	Medical Application
^{43}Sc	3.9 h	β^+ 1199 (70.9), 826 (17.2); γ 511 (176.2), 372 (22.5)	^{40}Ca(α,p)^{43}Sc ^{42}Ca(d,n)^{43}Sc ^{46}Ti(p,α)^{43}Sc ^{43}Ca(p,n)^{43}Sc	PET
^{44}Sc	3.97 h	β^+ 1474 (94.3); γ 511 (188), 1157 (99.8)	^{44}Ti$\rightarrow$^{44}Sc generator ^{nat}Ca(p,n)^{44}Sc	PET
^{47}Sc	3.35 d	β^- 441 (68.5), 601 (31.5); γ 159 (68.1)	^{47}Ti(n,p)^{47}Sc ^{46}Ca(n,γ)^{47}Ca$\rightarrow$^{47}Sc	Therapy
^{52}Mn	5.59 d	β^+ 575 (29.4); γ 511 (58.8), 744 (90.0), 935 (94.5), 1434(100)	^{52}Cr(p,n)^{52}Mn	PET
^{55}Co	17.5 h	β^+ 2535 (46), 2059 (25.6); γ 477 (26.9), 511 (151.8), 931 (100), 1408 (22.5)	^{58}Ni(p,α)^{55}Co	PET
^{61}Cu	3.4 h	β^+ 1215 (61.4); γ 282.9 (12.2), 511 (123.8), 656 (10.8)	^{61}Ni(p, n)^{61}Cu	PET
^{64}Cu	12.7 h	β^+ 653 (17.5); β^- 579 (38.5); γ 511 (35.0)	^{64}Ni(p,n)^{64}Cu ^{68}Zn(p,α)^{64}Cu	PET
^{67}Cu	2.7 d	β^- 562 (20), 468 (22), 377 (57); γ 93 (16.1), 185 (48.7)	^{67}Zn(n,p)^{67}Cu ^{64}Ni(α,p)^{67}Cu ^{70}Zn(p,α)^{67}Cu ^{68}Zn(γ,p)^{67}Cu	Therapy
^{68}Ga	67.8 m	β^+ 1899 (87.7); γ 511 (177.8), 1077 (3.2)	^{68}Ge $\rightarrow$^{68}Ga generator ^{68}Zn(p,n)^{68}Ga	PET
^{86}Y	14.7 h	β^+ 1545 (5.6), 1221 (11.9); γ 511 (63.8), 1076 (82.5), 1153 (30.5), 1921 (20.8)	^{86}Sr(p,n)^{86}Y ^{67}Zn(p,n)^{86}Y	PET
^{90}Y	2.7 d	β^- 2280 (100%);	^{235}U(n,f)^{90}Sr $\rightarrow$^{90}Y ^{89}Y(n,γ)^{90}Y	Therapy
^{89}Zr	78.4 h	β^+ 902 (22.8); γ 511 (45.4), 909 (99)	^{89}Y(p,n)^{89}Zr	PET
^{99}Mo	2.75 d	β^- 436 (16.4), 1214 (82.2) γ 739.5 (12.3),	^{235}U(n,f)^{99}Mo ^{98}Mo(n,γ)^{99}Mo	
^{99m}Tc	6.01 h	γ 140.5 (88.5)	^{99}Mo$\rightarrow$^{99m}Tc generator	SPECT
^{111}In	2.8 d	γ 17.3 (90.6), 245.4 (94.1)	^{111}Cd(p,n)^{111}In ^{112}Cd(p,2n)^{111}In	SPECT, Therapy Auger

(*Continued*)

TABLE 1 (*Continued*)
Physical Characteristics of Radiometals for Molecular Imaging and Therapy, Production Methods and Medical Application

Radionuclide	$T_{1/2}$	E [keV] Particle/Photons per 100 Decay	Production Method	Medical Application
[117m]Sn	13.6 d	γ 156 (86.4)	[nat]In(α,xn)[117m]Sn [nat]Cd(α,xn)[117m]Sn	Therapy Auger
[132]La	4.8 h	β^+ 3203 (14), 2636 (11); γ 464.5 (76), 511 (84.2)	[nat]Ba(p,xn)[132/135]La	PET
[135]La	19.5 h	γ 480.5 (1.5)	[nat]Ba(p,xn)[132/135]La	Therapy Auger
[153]Sm	1.93 d	β^- 641 (31.3), 694 (49.4); γ 103 (29.2)	[152]Sm(n,γ)[153]Sm	Therapy
[149]Tb	4.12 h	α 3967 (16.7); β^+ 1409 (4.6); γ 165 (31.6), 352 (35.3), 389 (22.0), 511 (9.2), 652 (19.5), 853 (18.6) [[149]Gd, [149]Em, [149]Sm, [145]Nd][a]	[181]Ta(p,spallation)[149]Tb	Therapy
[152]Tb	17.5 h	β^+ 2968 (8.0), 2624 (5.9); γ 344 (63.5), 511 (40.6)	[181]Ta(p,spallation)[152]Tb	PET
[155]Tb	5.32 d	γ 87 (32.0), 105 (25.1)	[155]Gd(p,n)[155]Tb [nat]Gd(p,xn)[155]Tb [nat]Gd(d,xn)[155]Tb [155]Dy decay	SPECT
[161]Tb	6.89 d	β^- 460 (25.7), 522 (65.0); γ 26 (23.2), 49 (17.0), 75 (10.2)	[160]Gd(n,γ)[161]Gd→[161]Tb	Therapy
[166]Ho	26.8 h	β^- 1773 (49.9), 1855 (48.8); γ 81 (6.6)	[nat]Dy(n,γ)[166]Dy →[166]Ho [165]Ho(n,γ)[166]Ho	Therapy
[169]Er	9.4 d	β^- 343 (45), 351 (55);	[168]Er(n,γ)[169]Er	Therapy
[177]Lu	6.65 d	β^- 177 (11.6), 498 (79.3); γ 113 (6.2), 208 (10.4)	[176]Lu(n,γ)[177]Lu [176]Yb(n,γ)[177]Yb→[177]Lu	Therapy
[186]Re	3.72 d	β^- 932 (21.5), 1069 (70.9); γ 137 (9.4)	[185]Re(n,γ)[186]Re [186]W(p,n)[186]Re [186]W(d,2n)[186]Re	Therapy
[188]Re	17.0 h	β^- 965 (25.6), 2120 (71.1); γ 155 (15.2)	[187]Re(n,γ)[188]Re [187]W(n,γ)[188]W→[188]Re generator	Therapy
[212]Pb	10.6 h	β^- 590 (11.9), 335 (83.1); γ 238.6 (43.6) [[212]Bi, [212]Po, [208]Tl][a]	[228]Th decay	Therapy
[213]Bi	45.6 m	α 5869 (1.9); β^- 983 (30.8), 1423 (66.2); γ 440.4 (26.1) [[213]Po, [209]Tl, [209]Pb][a]	[209]Bi(α,2n)[213]Bi [225]Ac→[213]Bi generator	Therapy

(*Continued*)

326   Mikołajczak et al.

TABLE 1 (*Continued*)
Physical Characteristics of Radiometals for Molecular Imaging and Therapy, Production Methods and Medical Application

Radionuclide	$T_{1/2}$	E [keV] Particle/Photons per 100 Decay	Production Method	Medical Application
^{223}Ra	11.4 d	α 5607 (25.8), 5716 (49.6), 5747 (10.0); γ 154 (5.8), 269 (14.2) [^{219}Rn, ^{215}Po, ^{215}At, ^{211}Pb, ^{211}Bi, ^{211}Po, ^{207}Tl][a]	^{235}U(n,f)^{223}Ra ^{226}Ra(n,γ)^{227}Ra$\rightarrow^{223}$Ra ^{227}Ac$\rightarrow^{223}$Ra	Therapy
^{225}Ac	10.0 d	α 5793 (18.9), 5830 (52.4); γ 99 (1.1) [^{221}Fr, ^{221}Ra, ^{217}At, ^{217}Rn, ^{213}Bi, ^{213}Po, ^{209}Tl, ^{209}Pb][a]	^{226}Ra(p,2n)^{225}Ac ^{233}U$\rightarrow^{229}$Th$\rightarrow^{225}$Ac ^{232}Th(p,spallation)^{225}Ac	Therapy
^{227}Th	18.7 d	α 6038 (24.2), 5978 (23.5), 5757 (20.4); γ 236 (12.9), 256 (7) [^{223}Ra, ^{219}Rn, ^{215}Po, ^{211}Pb, ^{211}Bi, ^{211}Po, ^{207}Tl][a]	^{227}Ac decay	Therapy

[a] Decay chain of main radionuclide.

3 PRODUCTION METHODS OF RADIOMETALS

There are four common methods of radionuclide production: fission and neutron activation in nuclear reactors, charged particle activation in accelerator and radionuclide generator.

3.1 NUCLEAR REACTORS

Nuclear reactors are the main source of neutrons of various energies (thermal, epithermal and fast) which can be utilized for irradiation of wide range target materials to produce radiometals. The direct neutron capture reaction (n,γ) results in carrier-added radioisotopes of relatively low specific activity, since the radionuclide cannot be chemically separated from the target of the same element. The higher the thermal neutron flux, cross section of the reaction and isotopic enrichment of the target, the higher the specific activity that can be achieved [19].

The presence of the carrier metal and rather low specific activity of radiometals produced by direct neutron irradiation may hamper their applications for radiolabelling of vector molecules, such as peptides, which can be administered to patients in a very limited mass. The indirect production route, utilizing neutron absorption reactions, leading to an intermediate product with β decay to the desired final product: (n,γ)$\rightarrow\beta^-$, or via reactions inducted by higher energy neutrons such as (n,p) or (n,α) would be preferred. In particular, the (n,p) nuclear reaction requires the irradiation in a fast neutron flux [19].

Radiometals in Molecular Imaging and Therapy

3.2 ACCELERATORS

The cyclotrons are the most often used accelerators for production of radiometals. This is typically accomplished by solid target irradiation with charged particles (protons, deuterons or alphas). Typically, radionuclides produced by cyclotrons yield a product of a different element than the target material, which can be chemically separated. Thus, most radionuclides produced via charged particle reactions have high specific activity (non-carrier-added, n.c.a.). The examples of radiometals produced in cyclotrons are ^{64}Cu, ^{89}Zr, ^{86}Y, and ^{111}In.

3.3 RADIONUCLIDE GENERATORS

Radionuclide generators play an important role as a source of diagnostic and therapeutic radionuclides for medical application [20, 21]. They operate on the principle that, while the long-lived parent radionuclide of one element decays to the shorter-lived daughter radionuclide of another element, this daughter radionuclide can be separated from the parent using chemical or physical methods. As a result, if the process is efficient, the isolated daughter radionuclide is of high radionuclide and radiochemical purity and is obtained in a n.c.a. form [22, 23]. The most commonly used radionuclide generator system is the one utilizing ^{99}Mo ($T_{1/2}=66$ h) as a parent radionuclide of ^{99m}Tc ($T_{1/2}=6$ h) [24]. The generators, as portable devices, can be delivered from manufacturing site to the remote users. Thanks to this, medical procedures can be performed at sites located far away from the reactors and accelerators. To this day, several radionuclide generator systems providing radiometals have been developed. Their brief characteristics are provided in Table 2.

TABLE 2
Examples of Radionuclide Generators of Radiometals for Medical Applications

Generator System	Parent Radionuclide		Daughter Radionuclide	
	$T_{1/2}$	Nuclear Reaction	$T_{1/2}$	Mode of Decay
^{99}Mo/^{99m}Tc	2.75 d	Fission, ^{98}Mo(n,γ)^{99}Mo	6.01 h	γ
^{68}Ge/^{68}Ga	270.8 d	^{69}Ga(p,2n)	1.36 h	β^+
^{82}Sr/^{82}Rb	25.6 d	^{85}Rb(p,4n)	75 s	β^+
^{44}Ti/^{44}Sc	60.3 a	^{45}Sc(p,2n)	3.93 h	β^+
^{90}Sr/^{90}Y	28.5 a	Fission	2.67 d	β^-
^{188}W/^{188}Re	69.4 d	^{186}W(n,γ)^{187}W ^{187}W(n,γ)^{188}W	16.98 h	β^-, γ
^{225}Ac/^{213}Bi	10.0 d	Decay chain of ^{233}U	45.6 min	β^-, α

3.4 Impact of Production Method on the Suitability of Radiometals for Medical Applications

The production of radiometals in sufficient radioactivity and quality is critically important for their use in nuclear medicine. The isotopically enriched target materials are necessary in order to increase the specific activity and to achieve high radionuclide and chemical purity of the product. The parameters of obtained radiometal will depend on the production route (target material, nuclear reaction, accompanying nuclear reactions, chemical processing, etc.). The final form of the radiometal to be used in radiopharmaceuticals is the solution for radiolabelling; it is thus of high chemical purity and concentrated into a small volume, typically in moderately acidic eluate. The separation and purification of desired radionuclide from macro-quantities of the irradiated target material along with other impurities are crucial steps. The employed separation technique should be efficient, relatively fast, especially in the case of short-lived radiometals, and possibly allowing an efficient target material recovery. A variety of techniques are used to isolate the desired radionuclide and to eliminate potential contaminants, including i.a. liquid-liquid (solvent) extraction (LLE), extraction chromatography, ion exchange, electrodeposition, precipitation and sublimation. They can be accomplished in one step or in a combination of multiple steps. The solid phase extraction (SPE) (chromatography) and LLE utilize the difference in affinity of the metals for either a stationary phase or an aqueous/organic phase. SPE, by ion exchange chromatography, is a prevalent chromatographic technique for radiometal separation and purification. Both cation- and anion-exchange resins can be used.

In the assessment of suitability of radiometals for medical applications, both the chemical and physical parameters are important. Radiometal identity is determined by assessing the physical characteristics of radionuclide emissions. The specific activity of radiometal is defined as radioactivity per unit mass of the product [25]. Several factors that could affect the specific activity of the produced radiometal include cross-sections, target impurities, secondary nuclear reactions, target burn-up, and post-irradiation processing [26]. An additional term used in this context is "effective specific activity" [25]. This addresses the chemically, biologically or pharmacologically "active" fraction of radioactive and non-radioactive materials. The term is often used to consider other (unknown) material present in a sample, competing with the labelled product in its chemical or biological reactions, such as the complexation process. For instance, the presence of metal cations of Zn, Cu or Fe in solutions of trivalent radiometals (^{68}Ga, ^{90}Y, ^{177}Lu, etc.) would compete with the radiometal in the chelator such as DOTA (2,2′,2″,2‴-(1,4,7,10-tetraazacyclododecane-1,4,7,10-tetrayl)tetraacetic acid, for the structure see Figure 4 in Section 4.10) coordination sphere [27–29]. Limits for individual metal impurities for radionuclides intended for radiopharmaceutical preparation are described in Ph. Eur. monographs [30–32].

Radionuclidic purity, defined as the ratio of the radioactivity of the desired radionuclide to the total radioactivity content of the sample, is usually assessed by gamma spectroscopy. When the radiolabelling process needs to be established, radiochemical purity is the measure of its yield. Radiochemical purity is defined as the fraction of the total radioactivity of the radionuclide in the sample, which is present as its desired chemical form. It is generally tested by radio-chromatographic methods, such as thin-layer chromatography (TLC) or high-performance liquid chromatography (HPLC) [26].

4 CHARACTERISTICS OF SELECTED RADIOMETALS USED IN RADIOPHARMACEUTICALS

The fate of a radiometal in the human body will depend on its affinity to certain tissues. Both ^{89}Sr and ^{223}Ra are present in the cationic form in the approved radiopharmaceuticals, since they are similar to calcium (Ca) in its biological behavior. When administered intravenously they are rapidly concentrated in the bones, mainly in osteoblastic areas [33]. Several radiometals produced in nuclear reactors have found their well-established place in nuclear medicine as colloidal suspensions for radio-synovectomy (^{90}Y, ^{186}Re, ^{169}Er) or resin/glass microspheres for catheter-directed embolization of hepatic malignancy and metastases (^{90}Y, ^{166}Ho, ^{188}Re) [34]. Also ^{153}Sm, ^{186}Re, ^{188}Re, ^{177}Lu can be targeted to bone by complexing the radionuclide to phosphonate chelators like EDTMP (lexidronam; ethyl enediaminetetra(methylenephosphonic acid; {ethane-1,2-diylbis[nitrilobis(methylene)]}tetrakis(phosphonic acid)) or HEDP (etidronate; (1-hydroxy-1,1-ethanediyl) bis(phosphonic acid)) and a few of them are approved for bone pain palliation in prostate cancer metastasized to bone [35, 36]. In these tracers, the relatively large mass of the injected substance is not affecting their biodistribution in the human body. However, this is not the case for the tracers used in molecular imaging, as excess mass of the vector molecule can cause saturation of the binding site in the biological target. For these vectors, radiolabelling with radiometals is based on the formation of chelated complexes with coordination bonds. Functional groups containing donor atoms with free electron pairs such as carboxylate, hydroxylate, amino or thiolate groups ($-COO^-$, $-O^-$, $-NH_2$, $-S^-$) are involved in binding the radiometal by the ligand molecule. The targeting vector is generally a biomolecule of interest (e.g. peptide, protein, small molecule, antibody, antibody fragment) that exhibits strong binding affinity for over-expressed tumour surface receptors; these are the vehicles that transport the radioactivity specifically to the tumour [37]. The principal design of a radiopharmaceutical composed of radiometal, linker, bifunctional chelating agent (BFC) and targeting vector to accumulate at a biological target is shown in Figure 2 [38].

The selection of a suitable molecule as a targeting vector rests on many factors. These include (i) biologic specificity and *in vivo* stability, (ii) the biologic mechanism(s) that bind it to target cells and the affinity of the carrier for these sites and (iii) the stability of the complex thus formed. Obviously, the chemical properties of the carrier molecule must enable the conjugation of a therapeutic/or diagnostic radionuclide without degradation of the intrinsic characteristics of the

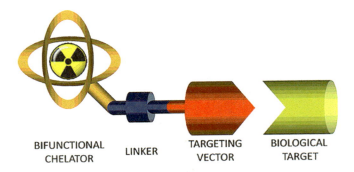

FIGURE 2 Principal design of a radiopharmaceutical composed of radiometal, linker, BFC and targeting vector to accumulate at a biological target. (Reproduced by permission from Ref [38]. Z. Baranyai, G. Tircsó, F. Rösch, *Eur. J. Inorg. Chem.* **2020**, *1*, 36–56.)

molecule. Finally, the physical half-life of the radionuclide must be at least equal to, and preferably much longer than, the biologic half-life of a carrier molecule [39, 40].

4.1 TECHNETIUM-99M, RHENIUM-186, AND RHENIUM-188

Technetium-99m, obtained from the generator, was first used clinically as early as in 1962 [41]. Since then, ^{99m}Tc has become the workhorse of nuclear medicine. Currently, nearly 80% of all radiopharmaceuticals used in clinical studies are based on ^{99m}Tc, due to its monoenergetic gamma line of 140 keV, ideal for SPECT imaging, easy availability (generator produced) and low cost [42]. Typically, the ^{99}Mo/^{99m}Tc generator consists of a chromatographic column filled with alumina. While the parent radionuclide Mo-99 as ^{99}MoO$_4^{2-}$ is absorbed on alumina, the daughter can be eluted with 0.9% (isotonic) saline solution as pertechnetate [^{99m}Tc]TcO$_4^-$.

The rich coordination chemistry and suitable physical characteristics of ^{99m}Tc along with its easy availability radionuclide generators ^{99}Mo/^{99m}Tc prompted the development of various ligands for ^{99m}Tc. In the pertechnetate ion ([^{99m}Tc]TcO$_4^-$) technetium is at the oxidation level of +7 and is practically inert chemically. Only after its reduction to the lower oxidation levels can it form coordination bonds with selected ligands. A few examples of ^{99m}Tc complexes at various oxidation levels which are used for diagnostic purposes in approved radiopharmaceuticals are presented in Figure 3.

The chemical similarity between technetium and rhenium has attracted the attention of researchers to design the therapeutic radiopharmaceuticals utilizing rhenium radionuclides [43–45]. There are two radioisotopes of rhenium with therapeutic potential: ^{186}Re and ^{188}Re. Both can be produced in nuclear reactors by irradiation of ^{185}Re and ^{187}Re, respectively. Their specific activity depends on the neutron flux and target material enrichment. ^{188}Re can be obtained with high radionuclide purity and specific activity (almost theoretical) as a daughter

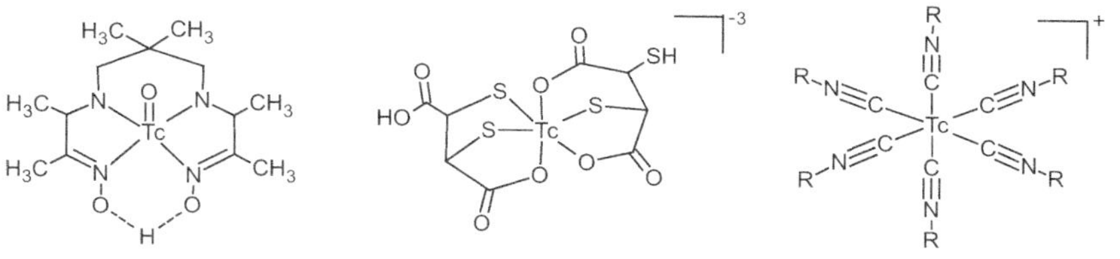

Radiometals in Molecular Imaging and Therapy

331

^{99m}Tc(V)-D,L-HMPAO ^{99m}Tc(III)-DMSA ^{99m}Tc(I)-MIBI [R=(CH$_2$-C(CH$_3$)$_2$OCH$_3$)]

FIGURE 3 Examples of ^{99m}Tc complexes used as radiopharmaceuticals. *Left*: [^{99m}Tc]-d,l–HMPAO (hexamethyl propylene amine oxime; 3,6,6,9-tetramethyl-4,8-diazaundecane-2,10-dione dioxime) indicated for imaging of central nervous system. *Middle*: [^{99m}Tc]-DMSA; 2,3 dimercaptosuccinic acid, renal imaging agent. *Right*: [^{99m}Tc](methoxy-isobutylisonitrile)$_6$]$^-$; hexakis(2-methoxy-2-methylpropyl-1-isonitrile-technetium(I), which is an approved myocardial perfusion agent.

product of the ^{188}W/^{188}Re radionuclide generator [46]. However, the high cost of parent radionuclide ^{188}W limits the availability of these generators.

The chemistry of perrhenate is similar to the well-described chemistry of pertechnetate [44, 45], but there are distinct differences, which include the requirement for stronger reducing conditions for the conversion of perrhenate [Re(VII)] to Re(V). In addition, care must be taken to avoid re-oxidation of Re(V) by the use of inert conditions and introduction of antioxidant agents during the radiolabelling procedures. These chemical challenges for facile introduction of Re into Re-targeting molecules result in under-utilization of ^{186}Re and ^{188}Re in medical applications [47].

4.2 INDIUM-111

Indium-111 (In-111) is another radiometal that has found use in medicine. It is produced in the cyclotron by proton irradiation of cadmium targets [48]. Due to its relatively long half-life and favourable radiation pattern, ^{111}In is used in biodistribution and pharmacokinetic studies of new radiopharmaceuticals. Indium, like gallium, has just one stable oxidation state in water: +3. Indium complexes incorporating chelators such as EDTA (ethylenediaminetetraacetic acid) and DTPA (diethylenetriaminepentaacetic acid) are highly thermodynamically stable. Several radiopharmaceuticals based on ^{111}In have been granted marketing authorization, among them ^{111}In-ProstaScint and ^{111}In-pentetreotide (Octreoscan) [49, 50]. Indium-111 is a source of gamma radiation for SPECT and also the source of low-energy Auger electrons, making it suitable for therapeutic applications [51].

4.3 GALLIUM-68

Gallium-68 (Ga-68) is a positron emitter produced in the ^{68}Ge/^{68}Ga generator and is used in PET diagnostics [52–54]. It can also be obtained by irradiating ^{68}Zn with protons with an energy of about 12 MeV. Due to the short half-life of ^{68}Ga, this method is applicable mostly in the clinics located near the cyclotrons [55, 56].

The chemistry of gallium-68 is similar to that of iron and is based on well-defined coordination complexes with macrocycle or chelates having strong binding properties, particularly suitable for linking peptides that allow resistance to *in vivo* transchelation of the metal ion [57]. Depending on the peptide to which it is attached, in ^{68}Ga-based radiopharmaceuticals, cyclic chelators such as DOTA ([^{68}Ga]Ga-DOTATATE, [^{68}Ga]Ga-DOTA-exendin-4) are used. An acyclic chelator HBED (*N,N'*-bis(2-hydroxybenzyl)ethylenediamine-*N,N'*-diacetic acid) has been proposed for coupling with PSMA (Prostate-Specific Membrane Antigen) inhibitor ([^{68}Ga]Ga-PSMA-11), where PSMA-11 is Glu-NH-CO-NH-Lys(Ahx)-HBED-CC [57].

4.4 COPPER-61, COPPER-64, AND COPPER-67

Among several copper isotopes, the ^{61}Cu and ^{64}Cu are positron emitters useful in PET diagnostics. In addition, ^{64}Cu emits β particles, which can be utilized for therapy. Cu-61 and Cu-64 are obtained in the cyclotron by proton irradiation of ^{61}Ni and ^{67}Ni, respectively [58–60]. Both positron emitters, ^{61}Cu and ^{64}Cu, have been widely used for the radiolabelling of peptides, antibodies and antibody fragments [60]. These radionuclides have also been suggested as diagnostic isotope pairs to the therapeutic ^{67}Cu. Copper-67 is a β-particle emitter with potential therapeutic application; it also emits photons with energy useful for imaging via planar imaging or SPECT. There are several production methods, such as irradiation with fast neutrons of ^{67}Zn, deuterons of ^{70}Zn, alpha particles of ^{64}Ni or protons of ^{68}Zn, but the efficiency of these reactions is not high, which significantly reduces the availability of ^{67}Cu [60, 61].

The chemistry of copper is dominated by two oxidation states: Cu^+ and Cu^{+2}, but Cu^{+2} is most common in Cu-radiopharmaceuticals. The stability of Cu^{+2} metal complexes with common macrocyclic ligands, such as DOTA and TETA was considered not satisfactory for biomedical applications [62, 63], but copper-attached to hexaazamacrobicyclic or bis (thiosemicarbazones) ligands possess excellent *in vitro* and *in vivo* stability [60].

4.5 SCANDIUM-43, SCANDIUM-44, AND SCANDIUM-47

The two scandium isotopes: ^{43}Sc and ^{44}Sc are positron emitters and are proposed for molecular imaging; ^{47}Sc is a β particle emitter useful for therapy. Scandium-43 can be obtained by proton irradiation with either ^{43}Ca or ^{46}Ti, deuteron irradiation of ^{42}Ca and α particles irradiation of ^{40}Ca [64, 65]. Scandium-44 can be obtained by proton irradiation of natural Ca or ^{44}Ca as well as from a ^{44}Ti/^{44}Sc radionuclide generator [64, 66, 67]. Scandium-47 can be produced by proton irradiation of ^{48}Ca or in nuclear reactors by neutron irradiation of ^{46}Ca [64, 66]. Both methods use expensive target material, which limits the availability of Sc-47. Scandium chemistry is intermediate between that of Al, Y, and the lanthanides [2]. Most of the ligands used to chelate Y or rare earth elements, such as DTPA or DOTA, can be used to bind scandium.

Radiometals in Molecular Imaging and Therapy 333

4.6 Zirconium-89

Zirconium-89 is a positron emitter produced in a cyclotron by irradiating yttrium targets with protons [68]. Zirconium occurs mainly in the +4 oxidation state. It is classic hard acceptor and prefers hard donors such as oxygen and nitrogen. Its maximum coordination number is 8. The optimal ligand for imaging applications of [89]Zr is polydentate with a denticity of 6–8 with oxygen or nitrogen donor atoms and a charge when deprotonated of 3$^-$ or 4$^-$ to minimize the overall charge on the complex [69]. However, to be utilized effectively in PET applications, it must be stably bound to a targeting ligand, and the most successfully used [89]Zr chelator is desferrioxamine B (DFO, N'-{5-[acetyl(hydroxy)amino]pentyl}-N-[5-({4-[(5-aminopentyl)(hydroxy)amino]-4-oxobutanoyl}amino)pentyl]-N-hydroxysuccinamide), which is commercially available as the iron chelator Desferal®. Despite the prevalence of DFO in [89]Zr-immuno-PET applications, the development of new ligands for this radiometal is an active area of research [70, 71]. The long half-life of [89]Zr ($T_{1/2}=3.27$ d), when compared to [68]Ga ($T_{1/2}=67.7$ min), makes it well suited for imaging of biological vectors with low circulation time in the bloodstream, such as antibodies and nanoparticles. Several studies have illustrated the utility of [89]Zr-labelled agents for PET imaging in both preclinical and clinical research [73–76].

4.7 Yttrium-86 and Yttrium-90

To date, two yttrium isotopes have been used in nuclear medicine: [86]Y and [90]Y. Ittrium-90 is a pure β$^-$ particle-emitting radionuclide. It is mainly produced in the ^{90}Sr/^{90}Y generator systems in high specific activity. The maximum range of β particles in soft tissues is 11 mm, which makes it suitable for the treatment of large-sized tumor [77–81]. Positron emitting [86]Y has been used as a substitute for PET imaging for therapeutic ^{90}Y radionuclide [82]. It is produced by protons or deuterons irradiation of [86]Sr [83, 84]. A significant limitation in the use of this isotope in PET diagnostics is the co-emission of high-energy gamma quanta, which contributes to the patient radiation dose [85].

The strong affinity of unchelated Y for bone and liver dominates the bio-inorganic chemistry of Y^{3+}, which necessitates the use of macrocycle chelators and emphasizes the importance of complex stability. Yttrium(III) has an ionic radius of 6–9 Å, giving the ability to achieve coordination numbers of 7 and 10 in its complexes. The octadentate lanthanide chelator DOTA is nearly a perfect match [83].

4.8 Lutetium-177

The lanthanide (rare earths) elements possess quite similar chemistries, with the most common oxidation state being +3 and a coordination number from 6 to 9. The predicted stability of lanthanide complexes increases on moving across the series from La to Lu, which follows the decrease in ionic radii and denticity required to result in a stable lanthanide complex *in vivo*. In aqueous media, the lanthanides are stabilized by chelation to multidentate ligands that provide "hard" donor atoms, such as oxygen or nitrogen [86].

Lutetium-177 is the most important representative of the rare earth elements used in nuclear medicine. It is an emitter of medium energy β particles. It is obtained by irradiating a target material enriched in ^{176}Lu or ^{176}Yb with neutrons. Using the latter it is possible to obtain ^{177}Lu with high specific activity and free from the long-lived ^{177m}Lu, which is co-produced in the process of neutron activation of ^{176}Lu. However, an effective process for separation of micro-quantities of ^{177}Lu from macro-quantities of ^{176}Yb is required [87].

Lutetium is the last member of the lanthanide series. The coordination number is usually 8 or 9, and the resultant complexes are thermodynamically very stable with both acyclic and cyclic polyaminopolycarboxylate-type ligands. Among the ligands, the macrocyclic DOTA ligand forms complexes of lanthanides with high thermodynamic stability and kinetic inertness [88, 89]. The use ^{177}Lu in therapeutic radiopharmaceuticals increased rapidly in recent years due to the success of peptide receptor radionuclide therapy (PRRT) of neuroendocrine tumor [90] and prostate cancer [91].

4.9 ALPHA-EMITTING RADIOMETALS

The characteristics of radioactive decay of α-emitting radiometals raised an increasing interest in the development of new radiopharmaceuticals. This is due to, i.a., high LET values, low range in living tissues and relatively easy binding of the radiometal to the biological vector. From the clinical point of view, the most important α emitters are: ^{223}Ra, ^{225}Ac, ^{213}Bi, ^{212}Pb and ^{227}Th, the parent radionuclide of ^{223}Ra. Alpha emitters can be produced by various methods: separation from the decay products of long-lived trans uranium elements (e.g. separation of daughter ^{212}Pb decaying from ^{228}Th), production as a result of high-energy proton spallation, e.g. ^{232}Th(p, spallation) ^{225}Ac, through irradiation with protons, deuterons, α particles or photons, e.g. ^{226}Ra(p,2n)^{225}Ac or from radionuclide generators (e.g. ^{225}Ac/^{213}Bi generator) [92–100]. Typically, the decay of α emitters results in the emission of several α particles per decay. For example, as a result of a single decay of ^{225}Ac, five α particles, three β particles as well as γ radiation are emitted.

Most α-emitting radiometals exist most stably in the +3 or +4 oxidation state and possess chemical properties that are similar to lanthanides. They form stable complexes with cyclic and linear aminopolycarboxylic ligands, so most of the ligands used to chelate rare earth elements, such as DTPA or DOTA can be used to bind them. The lack of suitable chelating agents to coordinate ^{223}Ra has limited the development of radioconjugates using this radionuclide. Recently, a biologically stable radiocomplex with the 18-membered macrocyclic chelator macropa (*N*,*N'*-bis[(6-carboxy-2pyridyl)methyl]-4,13-diaza-18-crown-6), [^{223}Ra][Ra(macropa)] has been reported [101]. Macropa (for the structure see Figure 4) has shown success for stable chelation of ^{225}Ac and ^{227}Th. On the other hand, ^{227}Th, with its +4 oxidation state, can be stably chelated by DOTA [102] and an

Radiometals in Molecular Imaging and Therapy

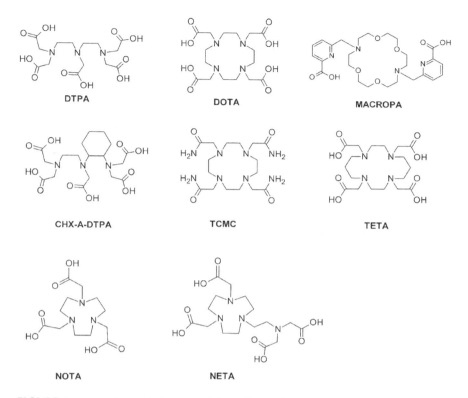

FIGURE 4 Examples of chelators used for radiometals.

octadentate chelator with 3-hydroxy-*N*-methyl-2-pyridinone coordinating moieties (Me-3,2-HOPO).

Therapy with α emitters holds the promise of effective tumour treatment. Thus, besides actinium-225 and bismuth-213, other new α emitters are under investigation [103]. Despite the recent success of novel radiotracers labelled with α-emitters for therapy, their use in nuclear medicine applications is still limited.

5 CHELATORS FOR METAL COMPLEXATION

Each radiometal ion has unique coordination chemistry properties; these must be properly attended to if these isotopes are to be safely harnessed for medical applications and use *in vivo* [104]. They are conjugated via a chelator that binds to the metal ion [105]. The ideal chelator is synthetically straightforward, allows rapid radiolabelling under mild conditions (neutral pH, low temperatures) with quantitative radiochemical yields at low concentration, can be conjugated to a range of vectors without disrupting the vector's function or pharmacokinetic profile and is thermodynamically and kinetically stable to prevent transchelation and hydrolysis. There is no "one-size-fits-all" chelator as the chemical properties of the metal, including size, charge, donor ligand preference and aqueous coordination chemistry directly influence the stability of the complex and linking group can influence the pharmacokinetic properties of the tracer [17, 19, 35, 106, 107].

To effectively radiolabel the peptides, nucleotides, antibodies or nanoparticles with radiometals the use of a bifunctional chelating agent (BFC) is mandatory. The BFC's contain in their structure donor atoms allowing binding of metallic cations and, at the other end, they contain functional groups which connect them stably to the biomolecule. Common bioconjugation techniques utilize functional groups such as carboxylic acids or activated esters (e.g. N-hydroxy-succinimide NHS-ester, tetrafluorophenyl TFP-ester) for amide couplings, isothiocyanates for thiourea couplings and maleimide for thiol couplings [105].

The choice of an appropriate BFC is based on the best fit of the radiometal governed by preferences in coordination chemistry and donor-ability of the ligand in order to form a stable and inert metal–chelate complex [37]. It is recommended that the ligand occupies the coordination sphere of metal cation. The chelators can be acyclic, e.g. DTPA or HYNIC (6-hydrazinonicotinamide), or macrocyclic (e.g. DOTA). The HYNIC core with N-hydroxysuccinimidyl hydrazinonicotinamide (NHS-HYNIC) has become one of the most popular BFCs for ^{99m}Tc labelling [108]. DTPA can form an octadentate coordination with three tertiary amine nitrogen donors and five oxygen donors from the carboxylic acid arms. CHX-A"-DTPA is a derivative of DTPA with improved stability, however still lower than DOTA. Macrocyclic chelators are more thermodynamically favourable than their acyclic counterparts and are more kinetically inert, with higher degrees of preorganization reducing entropic loss upon metal ion coordination [109], which can be problematic when radiolabelling chelators are appended to biological targeting vectors [110]. The most popular chelator used for labelling with radiometals is DOTA. DOTA chelates metals with four tertiary amine nitrogen donors and four oxygens from carboxylic acid, forming an octa-coordinate metal complex. TCMC (2,2',2'',2'''-(1,4,7,10-tetraazacyclododecane-1,4,7,10-tetrayl)tetraacetamide) is a derivative of DOTA with four primary amide pendant arms for stable chelation of ^{212}Pb. TETA is a selective chelator of $^{64/67}Cu$. NOTA (2,2',2''-(1,4,7-triazacyclononane-1,4,7-triyl)triacetic acid), and its derivative NETA (2,2'-((2-(4,7-bis(carboxymethyl))-1,4,7-triazonan-1-yl)ethyl)azanediyl) diacetic acid) is a hexadentate chelator that was utilized for radioisotopes such as ^{67}Ga and ^{90}Y, respectively. Structures of selected frequently used chelators are presented in Figure 4 [111].

The design of BFC depends upon a number of fundamental criteria. Foremost seems the metal complex stability followed by other coordination chemistry criteria such as charge, chelator, cavity size compatibility with the ionic radius of the radionuclide, chelate denticity and availability of donor binding groups of appropriate chemical character. Two additional properties are also critical to consider: the rate at which the metal complex forms and the rate of dissociation. All of these criteria are interrelated. Cavity size must accommodate the ionic radius of the radionuclide such that all of the required donor groups can be properly

Radiometals in Molecular Imaging and Therapy

aligned for optimal binding to the metal ion in such a way to adequately encapsulate the ion thereby providing high stability and limiting dissociation. The selection of BFC depends upon the oxidation state of the radiometal that makes it imperative to understand the coordination chemistry of chelators with any given radionuclide to be labelled. A BFC that forms a thermodynamically stable radiometal chelate with high kinetic inertness is considered as an ideal BFC [112].

The linker is used to connect the BFC to the targeting vector. The linker should be stable under physiological conditions and must not significantly compromise the binding affinity or specificity of the targeting vector or the metal-complexation performance of the chelator. The discovery process of PSMA-11 clearly emphasizes the complex characteristics of the PSMA binding site, requiring defined lipophilic interactions within the PSMA active-site, flanking funnel. It has been shown that aromatic moieties in the linker region of urea-based PSMA inhibitors can dramatically change the internalization properties and, accordingly, the tumour uptake [113]. As HBED-CC (*N,N'*-bis [2-hydroxy-5(carboxyethyl)benzyl]ethylenediamine-*N,N'*-diacetic acid) exhibits two aromatic moieties, it is introduced as a linker and chelator in the urea-based inhibitor. Hence, HBED-CC is simultaneously acting as a radiometal chelator for the incorporation of ^{68}Ga and as a functional moiety triggering internalization and tumour uptake [114].

6 CURRENT TRENDS IN RADIOMETALS FOR MEDICAL APPLICATION

Theranostics is a relatively new concept in nuclear medicine and refers to personalized patient management that involves targeted therapy and diagnostic imaging using a single or combination of radionuclide(s), with either therapeutic or diagnostic capabilities [116]. For the majority of the theranostics being developed in nuclear medicine, the chemical composition of the radiopharmaceuticals being used for diagnostic imaging and therapy are the exact same, with the exception of the isotope being swapped out. This ensures that the biodistribution remains the exact same throughout the imaging and therapy phases. For example, [^{68}Ga]Ga-PSMA-11 together with (DOTA)-functionalized PSMA ligand [^{177}Lu]Lu-DOTA-PSMA-617 (vipivotide tetraxetan) were considered a theranostic couple, which is very well suited for the diagnosis or treatment of prostate cancer as the ^{68}Ga/^{177}Lu-radiolabelled tracers show a very similar biological behavior [117].

Table 3 presents selected examples of biological targets, which were explored for radiotracer design. In recent years, the number of novel target-specific radiotracers introduced to clinical practice is growing rapidly. This is not only due to the introduction of novel tumor-targeting molecules but also due to the increasing availability of radionuclides, both for diagnostic imaging in PET and SPECT and for therapy [3, 118].

In this context, the use of ^{43}Sc/^{44}Sc for PET is regarded as advantageous when compared to the currently employed ^{68}Ga ($T_{1/2} = 68$ min): the almost

TABLE 3
Examples of Biological Targets and Their Targeting Radiotraces for Molecular Imaging and Therapy

Targets	Target Expression in Tumor	Radiopharmaceuticals
Somatostatin receptor subtype-2 (SST2)	Neuroendocrine tumor, carcinoids, pituitary, small cell lung cancer (SCLC)	[^{99m}Tc]Tc-HYNIC-TOC [^{68}Ga]Ga-DOTATATE [^{177}Lu]Lu-DOTATATE
Prostate-specific membrane antigen (PSMA)	Prostate carcinoma, breast cancer tumour cells and the endothelial cells of tumour vessels	[^{68}Ga]Ga-PSMA-11 [^{177}Lu]Lu-PSMA-617 [^{225}Ac]Ac-PSMA-617
Cholecystokinin-2 receptor (CCK2)	Medullary thyroid carcinoma, SCLC, astrocytoma, stromal ovarian cancer	[^{99m}Tc]Tc-Demogastrin [^{68}Ga]Ga-DOTA-MGS5
Bombesin receptor subtype-2 (BB2)	Breast, pancreas, prostate, SCLC	[^{64}Cu]Cu-NODAGA-BBN
Integrin $\alpha(v)\beta$	Ovarian, lung carcinoma, neuroblastomas	[^{68}Ga]Ga-DOTA-RGD [^{68}Ga]Ga-NOTA-RGD
Glucagon-like peptide-1 receptor (GLP1)	Insulinomas, gastrinomas	[^{68}Ga]Ga-DOTA-exendin-4, [^{99m}Tc]Tc-HYNIC-exendin-4
Carbonic anhydrase IX (CAIX)	Renal cell carcinoma	[^{89}Zr]Zr-DOTA-girentuximab

four-fold longer half-life of these scandium radionuclides could ensure the acquisition of late-time-point images, along with enabling shipment of ^{43}Sc/^{44}Sc-radiopharmaceuticals to distant PET centres. Another point of consideration is the stable coordination of Sc with (DOTA), allowing the subsequent application of the same targeting agents for therapeutic applications [2]. ^{43}Sc/^{44}Sc may, therefore, be employed for diagnosis, as well as for planning and monitoring of targeted radionuclide therapy with ^{177}Lu and ^{90}Y. The utilization of the exact matched therapeutic counterpart, ^{47}Sc, would be even more appealing as it can enable the concept of using chemically identical radiopharmaceuticals with the same kinetic properties for diagnosis and therapy [66]. Scandium and copper radioisotopes are particularly interesting in this respect, as they can provide true theranostic pairs allowing the use of radioactive isotopes of the same element for imaging ($^{43/44}$Sc, ^{64}Cu) and therapy (^{47}Sc, ^{67}Cu) [66]. Such pairs of radioisotopes are also named "matched pairs" [17].

The concept of using terbium-149 (Tb-149) for potential α-therapy and terbium-152 (Tb-152) for imaging/dosimetry was proposed by Beyer and Allen *et al.* already in the late 1990s [119, 120] and was further pursued by addressing the potential of terbium radioisotopes towards theranostics. The quadruplet of terbium radionuclides, i.e. ^{152}Tb ($T_{1/2} = 17.5$ h; PET) and ^{155}Tb ($T_{1/2} = 5.3$ d; SPECT) for imaging, while ^{149}Tb ($T_{1/2} = 4.1$ h; α-emitter) and ^{161}Tb ($T_{1/2} = 6.9$ d; β^--emitter) proposed as potentially effective for radionuclide therapy, are recommended

Radiometals in Molecular Imaging and Therapy

as true theranostic radiometals [121]. Chemistry of terbium is similar to that of yttrium and lutetium, with ^{90}Y and ^{177}Lu widely used in targeted radiotherapy. Terbium, as a trivalent lanthanide, forms stable complexes with many oxygen-containing bifunctional chelators, such as derivatives of DOTA, DTPA, which makes it possible to use standard methods for coordinating it to peptides or immunoconjugates [122]. In particular, ^{161}Tb is believed to be an alternative to the popular ^{177}Lu, due to its high quantity of Auger and conversion electrons with the potential to enhance the therapeutic effect [123, 124]. It can be obtained in high specific activity form through neutron irradiation of isotopically enriched ^{160}Gd target to produce ^{161}Gd which subsequently decays to ^{161}Tb. However, the availability of ^{149,152,155}Tb is still limited, needing highly specialized facilities such as an ISOL (Isotope Separation Online) system (ISOLDE-CERN). Therefore, at present, only few works have been reported related to preclinical and clinical studies with terbium radionuclides [125–128].

Lanthanum radiometals are also well positioned to serve as theranostic PET radiometals for targeted radionuclide therapy [129]. Although there are no radio-lanthanum isotopes with suitable decay properties for SPECT imaging, several radiolanthanum radionuclides: ^{132}La ($T_{1/2}$=4.6 h), ^{133}La ($T_{1/2}$=3.9 h) and a ^{134}Ce ($T_{1/2}$=3.2 d)/^{134}La ($T_{1/2}$=6.45 min) pair have shown significant potential to become PET imaging surrogates for ^{225}Ac. Another radiolanthanum radionuclide, ^{135}La ($T_{1/2}$=18.9 h), possesses Auger emissions and favourable decay characteristics, with potential for precise Auger electron therapy. These radionuclides have easily accessible production routes on medical cyclotrons, and there are established separation techniques to produce radiolanthanum of suitable purity for radiopharmaceutical applications. As lanthanum, cerium, and actinium possess 3+ cations with similar ionic radius, the chelation chemistry of radiolanthanum is robust with common chelators, such as DOTA, and especially well suited for chelators designed for ^{225}Ac, such as macropa and crown [130].

Commonly used β^+ emitters for PET imaging are usually short-lived (e.g. ^{15}O, ^{13}N, ^{11}C, and ^{18}F) and used to estimate the location of the disease and to quantitatively examine various biochemical and physiological processes. However, the interest in the application of long-lived β^+ emitters (^{89}Zr, ^{64}Cu and ^{52}Mn) has arisen, since they can be used to monitor the course of treatment for long periods of time (2–3 weeks). The use of positron emitters with longer half-life not only is expected to improve the diagnostic imaging but also may allow for improved dosimetry calculation for therapy [72].

Manganese-52 (Mn-52), due to its paramagnetic character, is considered for a multimodal imaging approach in which a mixture of ^{nat}Mn^{2+} and the PET radio-metal ^{52}Mn is used for dual PET/MRI application. ^{52}Mn can be readily produced in standard 16 MeV cyclotrons at low proton energies using pressed natural chromium targets [131]. ^{55}Co ($T_{1/2}$=17.5 h) offers slightly different chemistry and the potential for better *in vivo* stability than some of the radiocopper analogues [132, 133]. ^{55}Co has also been used for imaging in the form of a simple metal salt to study various disease processes [134], it has also been suggested as a theranostic isotope for the Auger emitter ^{58m}Co ($T_{1/2=}$9.10 h, 100% IC).

Relatively new approaches to production of radiometals are photoneutron (γ,n) and photoproton (γ,p) reactions using high-power electron linear accelerators (linacs) [115, 135]. In this process, a beam of electrons (typically in the energy range of 20–50 MeV) strikes a dense conversion target to produce high-energy photons which then strike the isotope production target producing appropriate radionuclide. Certain radioisotopes, e.g. ^{47}Sc, ^{44}Ti, ^{67}Cu, ^{117m}Sn, ^{169}Er, ^{195m}Pt or ^{225}Ac, with higher specific activity than with classical methods can be produced [113]. Non-carrier-added ^{186}Re can also be produced by proton or deuteron bombardment of ^{186}W using a cyclotron [136]. Another novel approach uses mass separation to produce certain radiometals and is expected to increase their availability. This novel approach is currently studied within the recently granted EU project (PRISMAP) [137].

7 GENERAL CONCLUSIONS

The radiometals are of particular interest for radiopharmaceutical development due to their wide range of nuclear properties such as half-life, type of radioactive decay, and rich coordination chemistry. This is of utmost importance nowadays, in the era of theranostics and precision medicine [138]. Further progress in the production process is needed to advance the availability of these new emerging radionuclides for clinical use. Finally, also the choice of the labelling method plays an important role for the overall performance of the radiopharmaceutical, and novel targeting vectors with improved pharmacokinetic profile are awaited [107].

ACKNOWLEDGEMENT

This work was supported with the funds awarded by CERAD project, financed under Smart Growth Operational Programme 2014–2020, Priority IV, Measure 4.2.

ABBREVIATIONS AND DEFINITIONS

BFC	bifunctional chelating agent
CHX-A''-DTPA	[(R)I-2-amino-3-(4-isothiocyanatophenyl)propyl]-trans-(S,S)-cyclohexane-1,2-diamine-pentaacetic acid
d	days
DFO	N'-{5-[acetyl(hydroxy)amino]pentyl}-N-[5-({4-[(5-amino-pentyl)(hydroxy)amino]-4-oxobutanoyl}amino)pentyl]-N-hydroxysuccinamide
DOTA	2,2′,2″,2‴-(1,4,7,10-tetraazacyclododecane-1,4,7,10-tetrayl)tetraacetic acid
DTPA	diethylenetriaminepentaacetic acid; 2,2′,2″,2‴-{[(carboxymethyl)azanediyl]bis(ethane-2,1-diylnitrilo)}tetraacetic acid
EC	electron capture

Radiometals in Molecular Imaging and Therapy

EDTA	ethylenediamine tetraacetic acid
eV	electronvolt
h	hours
HBED	*N,N'*-bis(2-hydroxybenzyl)ethylenediamine-*N,N'*-diacetic acid
HBED-CC	(*N,N'*-bis[2-hydroxy-5(carboxyethyl)benzyl]ethylenediamine-*N,N'*-diacetic acid)
LET	linear energy transfer
LLE	liquid-liquid (solvent) extraction
Macropa	*N,N'*-bis[(6-carboxy-2pyridyl)methyl]-4,13-diaza-18-crown-6
n.c.a.	non-carrier-added
NODA-GA	2,2'-(7-(1-carboxy-4-((2,5-dioxopyrrolidin-1-yl)oxy)-4-oxobutyl)-1,4,7-triazonane-1,4-diyl)diacetic acid
NOTA	2,2',2''-(1,4,7-triazacyclononane-1,4,7-triyl)triacetic acid
PET	positron emission tomography
PSMA	prostate-specific membrane antigen
PSMA-11	HBED-CC-PSMA, urea-based peptidomimetic that has a covalently bound chelator (HBED-CC). The peptide has the amino acid sequence Glu-NH-CO-NH-Lys(Ahx)-HBED-CC
PSMA-617	DOTA-functionalized PSMA ligand
SCLC	small cell lung cancer
SPE	solid phase extraction
SPECT	single photon emission computed tomography
$T_{1/2}$	half-life
TCMC	2,2',2'',2'''-(1,4,7,10-tetraazacyclododecane-1,4,7,10-tetrayl)tetra-acetamide
TETA	2,2',2'',2'''-(1,4,8,11-oxy)tetraazacyclotetradecane-1,4,8,11-tetrayl)tetraacetic acid

REFERENCES

[1] C. Pecher, *Biological Investigations with Radioactive Calcium and Strontium; Preliminary Report on the Use of Radioactive Strontium in the Treatment of Metastatic Bone Cancer*, University of California Press, Berkeley, Los Angeles, **1942**, pp. 117–149.

[2] C. S. Cutler, H. M. Hennkens, N. Sisay, S. Huclier-Markai, S. S. Jurisson, *Chem. Rev.* **2013**, *113*, 858–883.

[3] R. Mikołajczak, N. P. van der Meulen, S. E. Lapi, *J. Labelled Comp. Radiopharm.* **2019**, 62, 615–634.

[4] F. G. Blankenberg, H. W. Strauss, *J. Magn. Reson. Imaging* **2002**, 16, 352–361.

[5] D. A. Mankoff, *J. Nucl. Med.* **2007**, 48, 18N–21N.

[6] L. B. Solnes, R. A. Werner, K. M. Jones, M. S. Sadaghiani, C. R. Bailey, C. Lapa, M. G. Pomper, S. P. Rowe, *J. Nucl. Med.* **2020**, 61, 311–318.

[7] J. Konya, N. Nagy, in *Nuclear and Radiochemistry*, Elsevier, Amsterdam, **2012**, pp. 68–127.

[8] S. K. Imam, *Int. J. Radiat. Oncol. Biol. Phys.* **2001**, 51, 271–278.

[9] D. J. Kwekkeboom, W. W. de Herder, B. L. Kam, C. H. van Eijck, M. van Essen, P. Kooij, R. A. Feelders, M. O van Aken, E. P Krenning, *J. Clin. Oncol.* **2008**, 26, 2124–2130.

[10] J. J. Vaquero, P. Kinahan, *Annu. Rev. Biomed. Eng.* **2015**, 17, 385–414.

[11] IUPAC, *Compendium of Chemical Terminology*, 2nd ed. (the "Gold Book"), **1997**. Online corrected version: Auger effect, 2006.

[12] A. Kassis, *J. Nucl. Med.* **2003**, 44, 1479–1481.

[13] U. Mazzi, R. Schibli, H. J. Pietzsch, J. U. Kunsler, H. Spies, in *Technetium-99m Pharmaceuticals*, Eds I. Zolle, Springer, Berlin, Heidelberg, New York, **2007**, pp. 7–58.

[14] *Feasibility of Producing Molybdenum-99 on a Small Scale Using Fission of Low Enriched Uranium or Neutron Activation of Natural Molybdenum*, Technical Reports Series No. 478, IAEA, Vienna, Austria, **2015**.

[15] O. O. Peltek, A. R. Muslimov, M. V. Zyuzin, A. S. Timin, *J. Nanobiotechnol.* **2019**, 17, 1–34.

[16] R. Eychenne, M. Chérel, F. Haddad, F. Guérard, J. F. Gestin, *Pharmaceutics* **2021**, 13(6) 906.

[17] S. M. Qaim, J. Radioanal. *Nucl. Chem.* **2019**, 322, 1257–1266.

[18] M. de Jong, W. A. Breeman, R. Valkema, B. F. Bernard, E. P. Krenning, *J. Nucl. Med.* **2005**, 48 (suppl 1), 13S–7S.

[19] R. Mikołajczak, J. L. Parus, *World J. Nucl. Med.* **2005**, 4, 184–190.

[20] J. Pijarowska-Kruszyna, M. Pocięgiel, R. Mikołajczak, *Reference Module in Biomedical Sciences*, Elsevier, Amsterdam, **2021**.

[21] A. Dash, F. F. Knapp, M. R. A. Pillai, *RSC Adv.* **2013**, 3, 14890–14909.

[22] E. Lebowitz, P. Richards, *Semin. Nucl. Med.* **1974**, 4, 257–268.

[23] F. F. Knapp, S. Mirzadeh, *Eur. J. Nucl. Med.* **1994**, 21, 1151–1165.

[24] E. Segré, G. T. Seaborg, *Phys. Rev.* **1938**, 54, 772–772.

[25] H. H. Coenen, A. D. Gee, M. Adam, G. Antoni, C. S. Cutler, Y. Fujibayashi, J. M. Jeong, R.H. Mach, T. L. Mindt, V. W. Pike, A. D. Windhorst, *Nucl. Med. Biol.* **2017**, 55, v–xi.

[26] Z. Talip, Ch. Favaretto, S. Geistlich, N. P. van der Meulen, *Molecules* **2020**, 25(4), 966.

[27] M. Asti, M. Tegoni, D. Farioli, M. Iori, C. Guidotti, C. S. Cutler, P. Mayer, A. Versari, D. Salvo, *Nucl. Med. Biol.* **2012**, 39, 509–517.

[28] J. Šimeček, P. Hermann, H. Wester, J. Notni, *Chem.Med.Chem.* **2013**, 8, 95–103.

[29] E. Oehlke, S. Le Van, N. Lengkeek, P. Pellegrini, T. Jackson, I. Greguric, R. Weiner, *Appl. Radiat. Isot.* **2013**, 82, 232–238.

[30] EDQM. *Lutetium (^{177}Lu) Solution for Radiolabelling*, Monograph: 2798. in European Pharmacopeia; Council of Europe, Strasbourg, France, **2020**.

[31] EDQM. *Gallium-68 (^{68}Ga) Solution for Radiolabelling*, Monograph: 2464. in European Pharmacopeia, Council of Europe, Strasbourg, France, **2020**.

[32] EDQM, *Yttrium-90 (^{90}Y) Solution for Radiolabelling*, Monograph: 2803. in European Pharmacopeia, Council of Europe, Strasbourg, France, **2020**.

[33] https://www.ema.europa.eu/en/medicines/human/EPAR/xofigo

[34] V. Kyle, B. L. Hazleman, E. P. Wraight, *Ann. Rheum. Dis.* **1983**, 42, 132–137.

[35] https://radiologykey.com/targeted-therapy-for-bone-metastasis/#CR52

[36] H. Palmedo, S. Guhlke, H. Bender, J. Sartor, G. Schoeneich, J. Risse, F. Grünwald, F. F. Knapp Jr., H. J. Biersack, *Eur. J. Nucl. Med. Mol. Imaging* **2000**, 27, 123–130.

[37] C. F. Ramogida, C. Orvig, *Chem. Commun.* **2013**, 49, 4720–4739.

[38] Z. Baranyai, G. Tircsó, F. Rösch, *Eur. J. Inorg. Chem.* **2020**, 1, 36–56.

[39] D. L. Morse, R. J. Gillies, *Biochem. Pharmacol.* **2010**, 80, 731–738.

Radiometals in Molecular Imaging and Therapy   343

[40] M. J. Welch, C. S. Redvanly, *Handbook of Radiopharmaceuticals: Radiochemistry and Applications*, Wiley, UK, **2003**, pp. 1–862.

[41] P. V. Harper, G. Andros, K. Lathrop, Washington DC: US Atomic Energy Commission, **1962**, 77–88. Report ACRH-18.

[42] A. Boschi, L. Uccelli, P. Martini, *Appl. Sci.* **2019**, 9, 1–16.

[43] J. R. Dilworth, S. J. Parrot, *Chem. Soc. Rev.* **1998**, 27, 43–55.

[44] E. Deutsch, K. Libson, J. K. Vanderheyden, A. Ketring, H. R. Maxon, *Nucl. Med. Biol.* **1986**, 13, 465–477.

[45] P. J. Blower, S. Prakash, in *Perspectives on Bioinorganic Chemistry*, Vol. 4, Eds R. W. Hay, J. R. Dilworth, K. B. Nolan, JAI Press, **1999**, pp. 91–143.

[46] F. F. Knapp, *Int. J. Nucl. Med.* **2017**, Special Issue, 3–15.

[47] B. M. Zeglis, J. L. Houghton, M. J. Evans, N. Viola-Villegas, J. S. Lewis, *Inorg. Chem.* **2014**, 53, 1880–1899.

[48] S. Takács, F. Tárkányi, A. Hermanne, *Nucl. Instrum. Methods Phys. Res. B Nucl. Instrum. Meth. B.* **2005**, 240, 790–802.

[49] M. J. Manyak MJ, *Expert Rev. Anticancer. Ther.* **2008**, 8, 175–181.

[50] D. J. Kwekkeboom, E. P. Krenning, *Semin Nucl. Med.* **2002**, 32, 84–91.

[51] G. S. Limouris, A. Chatziioannou, D. Kontogeorgakos, D. Mourikis, M. Lyra, P. Dimitriou, A. Stavraka, A. Gouliamos, L. Vlahos, *Eur. J. Nucl. Med. Mol. Imaging* **2008**, 35, 1827–1837.

[52] G. I. Gleason, *Int. J. Appl. Radiat.* Isot. **1960**, 8, 90–94.

[53] N. P. van der Meulen, S. G. Dolley, G. F. Steyn, T. N. van der Walt, H. G. Raubenheimer, *Appl. Radiat. Isot.* **2011**, 69, 727–737.

[54] K. P. Zhernosekov, D. V. Filosofov, R. P. Baum, P. Aschoff, H. Bihl, A. A. Razbash, M. Jahn, M. Jennewein, F. Rösch, *J. Nucl. Med.* **2007**, 48, 1741–1748.

[55] F. Alves, V. H. Alves, A. B. C. Neves, S. J. C. do Carmo, B. Nactergal, V. Hellas, E. Kral, C. Gonçalves-Gameiro, A. J. Abrunhosa, "Cyclotron Production of Ga-68 for Human Use from Liquid Targets: From Theory to Practice," AIP Conference Proceedings, 2017.

[56] M. Jensen, J. Clark, "Direct Production of ^{68}Ga from Proton Bombardment of Concentrated Aqueous Solutions of [^{68}Zn] Zinc Chloride," Proceedings of the 13th International Workshop on Targetry and Target Chemistry, Danmark, 2011.

[57] C. Morgat, E. Hindié, A. K. Mishra, M. Allard, P. Fernandez, *Cancer Biother. Radiopharm.* **2013**, 28, 85–97.

[58] D. W. McCarthy, R. E. Shefer, R. E. Klinkowstein, L. A. Bass, W. H. Margeneau, C. S. Cutler, C. J. Anderson, M. J. Welch, *Nucl. Med. Biol.* **1997**, 24, 35–43.

[59] A. R. Jalilian, J. Osso Jr., *Iran. J. Nucl. Med.* **2017**, 25, 1–10.

[60] L. Mou, P. Martini, G. Pupillo, I. Cieszykowska, C. S. Cutler, R. Mikołajczak, *Molecules* **2022**, 27(5), 1570.

[61] S. Mirzadeh, L. F. Mausner, S. C. Srivastava, *Int. J. Rad. Appl. Instrum. A. Appl. Radiat. Isot.* **1986**, 37, 29–36.

[62] G. Hao, A. N. Singh, O. K. Oz, X. Sun, *Curr. Radiopharm.* **2011**, 4, 109–121.

[63] L. A. Bass, M. Wang, M. J. Welch, C. J. Anderson, *Bioconjug. Chem.* **2000**, 11, 527–532.

[64] R. Mikołajczak, S. Huclier-Markai, C. Alliot, F. Haddad, D. Szikra, V. Forgacs, P. Garnuszek, *EJNMMI Radiopharm. Chem.* **2021**, 6, 19.

[65] K. A. Domnanich, R. Eichler, C. Müller, S. Jordi, V. Yakusheva, S. Braccini, M. Behe, R. Schibli, A. Türler, N. P. van der Meulen, *EJNMMI Radiopharm. Chem.* **2017**, 2, 14.

[66] S. Huclier-Markai, C. Alliot, R. Kerdjoudj, M. Mougin-Degraef, N. Chouin, F. Haddad, *Cancer Biother. Radiopharm.* **2018**, 33, 316–329.

[67] E. Eppard, A. de la Fuente, M. Benešová, A. Khawar, R. A. Bundschuh, F. C. Gärtner, B. Kreppel, K. Kopka, M. Essler, F. Rösch, *Theranostics* **2017**, 7, 4359–4369.

[68] J. P. Holland, Y. Sheh, J. S. Lewis, *Nucl. Med. Biol.* **2009**, 36, 729–739.

[69] J. R. Dilworth, S. I. Pascu, *Chem. Soc. Rev.* **2018**, 47, 2554–2571.

[70] N. B. Bhatt, D. N. Pandya, T. J. Wadas, *Molecules* **2018**, 23 (3) 638.

[71] B. Klasen, D. Lemcke, T. L. Mindt, G. Gasser, F. Rösch, *Nucl. Med. Biol.* **2021**, 102–103, 12–23.

[72] S. A. Graves, R. Hernandez, J. Fonslet, C. G. England, H. F. Valdovinos, P. A. Ellison, T. E. Barnhart, D. R. Elema, C. P. Theuer, W. Cai, R. J. Nickles, G. W. Severin, *Bioconjug. Chem.* **2015**, 26, 2118–2124.

[73] B. N. McKnight, A. N. W. Kuda-Wedagedara, K. K. Sevak, D. Abdel-Atti, W. N. Wiesend, A. Ku, D. Selvakumar, S. D. Carlin, J. S. Lewis, N. T. Viola-Villegas. *Sci. Rep.* **2018**, 8, 9043.

[74] F. Dehdashti, N. Wu, R. Bose, M.J. Naughton, C. X. Ma, B. V. Marquez-Nostra, P. Diebolder, C. Mpoy, B.E. Rogers, S. E. Lapi, R. Laforest, B. A. Siegel, *Breast Cancer Res. Treat.* **2018**, 169, 523–530.

[75] F. Bensch, M. M. Smeenk, S. C. van Es, J. R. de Jong, C. P. Schroder, S. F. Oosting, M. N. Lub-de Hoog, C. W. Menke-van der Houven van Oordt, A. H. Brouwers, R. Boellaard, E. G. E. de Vries, *Theranostics* **2018**, 8, 4295–4304.

[76] G. Srimathveeravalli, D. Abdel-Atti, C. Perez-Medina, H. Takaki, S. B. Solomon, W. J. M. Mulder, T. Reiner, *Mol. Imaging* **2018**, 17, 1–9.

[77] D. Minarik, K. S. Gleisner, M. Ljungberg, Phys. Med. Biol. **2008**, 53, 5689–5703.

[78] S. J. Knox, M. L. Goris, K. Trisler, R. Negrin, T. Davis, T. M. Liles, A. Grillo-López, P. Chinn, C. Varns, S. C. Ning, S. Fowler, N. Deb, M. Becker, C. Marquez, R. Levy. *Clin. Cancer Res.* **1996**, 2, 457–470.

[79] J. E. Dancey, F. A. Shepherd, K. Paul, K. W. Sniderman, S. Houle, J. Gabrys, A. L. Hendler, J. E. Goin, *J. Nucl. Med.* **2000**, 41, 1673–1681.

[80] A. Otte, E. Jermann, M. Behe, M. Goetze, H. C. Bucher, H. W. Roser, A. Heppeler, J. Mueller-Brand, H. R. Maecke, *Eur. J. Nucl. Med.* **1997**, 24, 792–795.

[81] J. Kunikowska, L. Królicki, A. Hubalewska-Dydejczyk, R. Mikołajczak, A. Sowa-Staszczak, D. Pawlak, *Eur. J. Nucl. Med. Mol. Imaging* **2011**, 38, 1788–1797.

[82] N. Bandara, T. J. Stott Reynolds, R. Schehr, R. P. Bandari, P. J. Diebolder, S. Krieger, J. Xu, Y. Miao, B. E. Rogers, Ch. J. Smith, *Nucl. Med. Biol.* **2018**, 62–63, 71–77.

[83] F. Rösch, S. M. Qaim, G. Stöcklin, *Appl. Radiat. Isot.* **1993**, 44, 677–681.

[84] E. Aluicio-Sarduy, R. Hernandez, H. F. Valdovinos, C. J. Kutyreff, P. A. Ellison, T. E. Barnhart, R. J. Nickles, J. W. Engle, *Appl. Radiat. Isot.* **2018**, 142, 28–31.

[85] T. K. Nayak, M. W. Brechbiel, *Med. Chem.* **2011**, 7, 380–388.

[86] C. S. Cutler, C. J. Smith, G. J. Ehrhardt, T. T. Tyler, S. S. Jurisson, E. Deutsch, *Cancer Biother. Radiopharm.* **2000**, 15, 531–545.

[87] A. Dash, M. R. Pillai, F. F. Knapp Jr., Nucl. Med. Mol. Imaging. **2015**, 49, 85–107.

[88] J. L. Parus, D. Pawlak, R. Mikołajczak, A. Duatti, *Curr. Radiopharm.* **2015**, 8, 86–94.

[89] S. Banerjee, M. R. A. Pillai, F. F. Knapp, *Chem. Rev.* **2015**, 115, 2934–2974.

[90] B. L. Kam, J. J. Teunissen, E. P. Krenning, W. W. de Herder, S. Khan, E. I. van Vliet, D. J. Kwekkeboom, *Eur. J. Nucl. Med. Mol. Imaging* **2012**, 39(Suppl 1), S103–S112.

[91] G. Liu, T. Tang, X. P. Liu, Z. H. Zhou, F. J. Li, Medicine **2021**, 100, e25612.

[92] S. Poty, L. C. Francesconi, M. R. McDevitt, M. J. Morris, J. S. Lewis, *J. Nucl. Med.* **2018**, 59, 878–884.

Radiometals in Molecular Imaging and Therapy

[93] M. R. McDevitt, D. Ma, L. T. Lai, J. Simon, P. Borchardt, R. K. Frank, K. Wu, V. Pellegrini, M. J. Curcio, M. Miederer, N. H. Bander, D. A. Scheinberg, *Science* **2001**, 16, 1537–1540.

[94] C. Apostolidis, R. Molinet, G. Rasmussen, A. Morgenstern, *Anal. Chem.* **2005**, 77, 6288–6291.

[95] R. A. Boll, D. Malkemus, S. Mirzadeh, *Appl. Radiat. Isot.* **2005**, 62, 667–679.

[96] J. R. Griswold, D. G. Medvedev, J. W. Engle, R. Copping, J. M. Fitzsimmons, V. Radchenko, J. C. Cooley, M. E. Fassbender, D. L. Denton, K. E. Murphy, A. C. Owens, E. R. Birnbaum, K. D. John, F. M. Nortier, D. W. Stracener, L. H. Heilbronn, L. F. Mausner, S. Mirzadeh, *Appl. Radiat. Isot.* **2016**, 118, 366–374.

[97] G. Melville, H. Meriarty, P. Metcalfe, T. Knittel, B. J. Allen, *Appl. Radiat. Isot.* **2007**, 65, 1014–1022.

[98] N. A. Thiele, J. J. Wilson, *Cancer Biother. Radiopharm.* **2018**, 33, 336–348.

[99] P. I. Ivanov, S. M. Collins, E. M. van Es, M. Garcia-Miranda, S. M. Jeorme, B. C. Russell, *Appl. Radiat. Isotopes.* **2017**, 124, 100–105.

[100] G. Henriksen, P. Hoff, J. Alstad, R. H. Larsen, *Radiochim. Acta* **2001**, 89, 661–666.

[101] D. S. Abou, N. A. Thiele, N. T. Gutsche, A. Villmer, H. Zhang, J. J. Woods, K. E. Baidoo, F. E. Escorcia, J. J. Wilson, D. J. Thorek, *J. Chem. Sci.* **2021**, 12, 3733–3742.

[102] J. Dahle, J. Borrebaek, K. B. Melhus, O. S. Bruland, G. Salberg, D. R. Olsen, R. H Larsen, *Nucl. Med. Biol.* **2006**, 33, 271–279.

[103] B. J. B. Nelson, J. D. Andersson, F. Wuest, *Pharmaceutics* **2021**, 13, 49.

[104] E. W. Price, C. Orvig, *The Chemistry of Inorganic Nuclides ($^{86}Y,^{68}Ga,^{64}Cu,^{89}Zr,^{124}I$)* in *Chem. Mol. Imaging.* Eds N. J. Long, W. T. Wong., 1st ed., John Wiley & Sons, Inc., Hoboken, NJ, **2014**, pp. 105–135.

[105] E. W. Price, C. Orvig, *Chem. Soc. Rev.* **2014**, 43, 260–290.

[106] D. Sneddon, B. Cornelissen, *Curr. Opin. Chem. Biol.* **2021**, 63, 152–162.

[107] M. Fani, H. R. Maecke, *Eur. J. Nucl. Med. Mol. Imaging.* **2012**, 39(suppl 1), S11–S30.

[108] D. Krois, C. Riedel, H. Kalchhauser, H. Lehner, P. Angelberger, I. Virgolini, *Liebigs Ann.* **1996**, 1996, 1463–1469.

[109] K. P. Carter, G. J. P. Deblonde, T. D. Lohrey, A. T. Bailey, D. D. An, K. M. Shield, W. W. Lukens Jr., R. J. Aberge, *Commun. Chem.* **2020**, 3, 61.

[110] D. Sneddon, B. Cornelissen, *Curr. Opin. Chem. Biol.* **2021**, 63, 152–162.

[111] J. M. White, F. E. Escorcia, N. T. Viola, *Theranostics* **2021**, 11, 6293–6314.

[112] A. Ghai, N. Singh, S. Chopra, B. Singh, in *Dendrimers - Fundamentals and Applications*, Eds C. M. Simonescu, Intech Open, London, **2018**, pp. 47–63.

[113] D. Habs, U. Köster, *Appl. Phys. B.* **2011**, 103, 501–519.

[114] U. Hennrich, M. Eder, *Pharmaceuticals* **2021**, 14, 713.

[115] V. N. Starovoitova, L. Tchelidze, D. P. Wells, *Appl. Radiat. Isot.* **2014**, 85, 39–44.

[116] W. A. Weber, J. Czernin, C. J. Anderson, R. D. Badawi, H. Barthel, F. Bengel, L. Bodei, I. Buvat, M. DiCarli, M. M. Graham, J. Grimm, K. Herrmann, L. Kostakoglu, J. S. Lewis, D. A. Mankoff, T. E. Peterson, H. Schelbert, H. Schöder, B. A. Siegel, H. W. Strauss. *J. Nucl. Med.* **2020**, 61 (suppl 2), 263S–272S.

[117] M. Meisenheimer, Y. Saenko, E. Eppard, in *Medical Isotopes*, Eds S. A. R. Naqvi, M. B. Imrani, Intech Open, London, **2019**, pp. 1–21.

[118] L. Uccelli, P. Martini, C. Cittanti, A. Carnevale, L. Missiroli, M. Giganti, M. Bartolomei, A. Boschi, *Molecules* **2019**, 24, 640.

[119] G. J. Beyer, J. J. Čomor, M. Daković, D. Soloviev, C. Tamburella, E. Hagebo, B. Allan, S. N. Dmitriev, N. G. Zaitseva, *Radiochim. Acta.* **2002**, 90, 247–252.

[120] B. J. Allen, G. Goozee, S. Sarkar, G. Beyer, C. Morel, A. P. Byrne, *Appl. Radiat. Isot.* **2001**, 54, 53–58.

[121] C. Müller, K. Zhernosekov, U. Köster, K. Johnston, H. Dorrer, A. Hohn, N. T. van der Walt, A. Türler, R. Schibli, *J. Nucl. Med.* **2012**, 53, 1951–1959.

[122] A. G. Kazakov, R. A. Aliev, A. Y. Bodrov, A. B. Priselkova, S. N. Kalmykov, *Radiochim. Acta.* **2018**, 106, 135–140.

[123] C. Müller, K. A. Domnanich, C. A. Umbricht, N. P. van der Meulen, *Br. J. Radiol.* **2018**, 91, 20180074.

[124] R. P. Baum, A. Singh, H. R. Kulkarni, P. Bernhardt, T. Rydén, C. Schuchardt, N. Gracheva, P. V. Grundler, U. Köster, D. Müller, M. Pröhl, J. R. Zeevaart, R. Schibli, N. P. Van der Meulen, C. Müller, *J. Nucl. Med.* **2021**, 63, 6.

[125] C. Müller, J. Reber, S. Haller, H. Dorrer, U. Köster, K. Johnston, K. Zhernosekov, A. Türler, R. Schibli, *Pharmaceuticals* **2014**, 7, 353–365.

[126] R. P. Baum, A. Singh, M. Benešová, C. Vermeulen, S. Gnesin, U. Köster, K. Johnston, D. Müller, S. Senftleben, H. R. Kulkarni, A. Türler, R. Schibli, J. O. Prior, N. P. van der Meulen, C. Müller, *Dalton Trans.* **2017**, 46, 14638–14646.

[127] C. Müller, J. Reber, S. Haller, H. Dorrer, P. Bernhardt, K. Zhernosekov, A. Türler, R. Schibli, *Eur. J. Nucl. Med. Mol. Imaging* **2014**, 41, 476–485.

[128] S. Haller, G. Pellegrini, C. Vermeulen, N. P. van der Meulen, U. Köster, P. Bernhardt, R. Schibli, C. Müller, *EJNMMI Res.* **2016**, 6, 13.

[129] B. J. B. Nelson, J. D. Andersson, F. Wuest, *Nucl. Med. Biol.* **2022**. In press.

[130] D. Filosofov, E. Kurakina, V. Radchenko, *Nucl. Med. Biol.* **2021**, 94–95, 1–19.

[131] E. Aluicio-Sarduy, P. A. Ellison, T. E. Barnhart, W. Cai, R. J. Nickles, *J. Label. Com. Radiopharm.* **2018**, 61, 636–651.

[132] T. Mastren, B. V. Marquez, D. E. Sultan, E. Bollinger, P. Eisenbeis, T. Voller, S. E. Lapi, *Mol. Imaging.* **2015**, 14, 526–532.

[133] J. H. Dam, B. B. Olsen, C. Baun, P. F. Hoilund-Carlsen, H. Thisgaard, *Mol. Imaging. Biol.* **2017**, 19, 915–922.

[134] J. De Reuck, P. Santens, K. Strijckmans, I. Lemahieu, *J. Neurol. Sci.* **2001**, 193, 1–6.

[135] D. J. Schlyer, T. J. Ruth, in *Industrial Accelerators and Their Applications*, Eds R. W. Hamm, M. E. Hamm, R & M Technical Enterprises, California, USA, **2012**, pp. 139–181.

[136] M. E. Moustapha, G. J. Ehrhardt, J. Smith, L. Szajek, W. Eckelman, S. Jurisson, *Nucl. Med. Biol.* **2006**, 33, 81–89.

[137] PRISMAP—Building a European Network for Medical Radionuclides. Available online: https://www.arronax-nantes.fr/en/radionuclide-production/news/prismap-building-a-european-network-for-medical-radionuclides/ (accessed on July 10, 2022).

[138] T. Langbein, W. A. Weber, M. Eiber, *J. Nucl. Med.* **2019**, 60 (suppl 2), 13S–19S.

Index

Abiraterone, 54
Absorption, distribution, metabolism, excretion (ADME), 46, 49
Absorption window, 92
Acac *see* Acetylacetonate
Acacen, 112, 139, 147, 149, 150; *see also* Bis(acetylacetone) ethylenediamine
Accelerator, 272, 320, 326, 327, 340
ACE-2 *see* Angiotensin-converting enzyme, 2
Acetylacetonate (acac), 199, 200, 228
Acetyl-CoA, 74
N-Acetylcysteine, 129
N-Acetylglucosamine, 166
N-Acetylmuramic acid, 166
Acinetobacter baumannii, 178
Acquired immunodeficiency syndrome (AIDS), 107, 108, 125, 126, 182
Actinic keratosis, 44
Actinium-225 (Ac-225), 325–327, 334, 335, 338–340
Activation by reduction, 2, 3, 5, 7, 8, 17, 18, 21, 23, 31
Active site, 82, 123, 128, 129, 183, 229, 272, 273
Acute myeloid leukaemia, 181
Acyclovir, 121
Acyl enzyme, 183
Adenosine monophosphate (AMP), 299, 300, 302, 303
Adenosine triphosphate (ATP), 21, 67, 68, 72, 75, 78, 79, 81, 88, 90, 94, 95, 259
    ATPase, 68, 81, 150
    depletion, 88
    synthase, 76
    synthesis, 78, 79, 90
Adenoviruses, 111, 113, 121
ADME *see* Absorption, distribution, metabolism, excretion
Ado-Cbl *see* 5'-Deoxyadenosyl-cobalamin
Aerobic glycolysis, 6, 72, 79
Aggregation, 227, 297, 299, 308
AIDS *see* Acquired immunodeficiency syndrome
AIF *see* Apoptosis-inducing factor
5-ALA *see* 5-Aminolevulinic acid
Albumin, 6, 11, 12–14, 22, 85, 205, 274, 295
    albumin/paclitaxel nanoformulation Abraxane®, 12
    albumin-based nanosystem, 22
    albumin-coated Pt(IV)-IDOi, 12, 13
    chlorin e6-conjugated albumin, 22
Alkoxy radical, 252, 253

Alkylphosphine, 84
Alkynyl, 84, 127, 295
Alpha-emitting radiometals/alpha emitters, 333, 334
Alpha particle, 321, 332
Alpha radiation, 321
α-tocopherol succinate (α-toc), 80
Alphaviruses, 122
Alpidem, 81
Alumina (aluminium oxide), 330
Alzheimer's disease, 71, 272
Amantadine, 114
Amino acids *see individual names*
Aminoacrylate, 55
Aminoglycoside, 166, 171, 182
5-Aminolevulinic acid (5-ALA; Lexulan), 44, 57
3-Aminopyridine-2-carboxaldehyde thiosemicarbazone (Triapine), 90
Ammonium trichloro(dioxoethylene-*O,O'*) tellurate (AS-101), 181, 182
AMP *see* Adenosine monophosphate
Ampicillin, 172
Amyl nitrite, 221, 223
Amyotrophic lateral sclerosis, 71
Androgen-independent PCa cells, 78
Angiogenesis, 90, 276
Angiotensin-converting enzyme 2 (ACE-2), 110, 112, 120–122, 127–131, 140, 145, 146, 148, 152, 154, 155
Annihilation radiation, 323
Anthracene, 251, 253
Anthraquinone, 94
Anti-apoptotic proteins, 72, 77
Antibacterial
    activity, 149, 166, 169–172, 174, 176–179, 181–183, 185
    agents/drugs, 119, 142, 153, 164, 166, 168–170, 172–174, 176, 177, 178, 180, 184
        copper-based, 169–173
        gallium-based, 178–180
        gold-based, 176–178
        silver-based, 174–176
        tellurium-based, 180–182
    compounds, 164, 170, 171, 173–176, 178, 179, 181–183, 186
    properties, 121, 148, 168, 169, 174, 180
Anti-biofilm activity, 177, 180
Antibiotics
    anti-pseudomonal, 180
    β-lactam, 167

347

Antibiotics (*cont.*)
  metal-based, 168, 172
  overview of conventional, 166
Antibody, 26, 28, 122, 123, 306, 329, 332
  antibody-conjugated photocatalyst, 51
  antibody-directed enzyme prodrug therapy, 28
  antibody drug conjugate, 55
Anti-chemokine receptor antibody (anti-CXCR4-Ab), 306
Anti-COVID-19, 140, 147
  agents/drugs, 139, 140, 147
    Auranofin, 148
    bismuth compounds, 150–152
    $[Co(acacen)(NH_3)_2]Cl$, 149–150
    silver sulfadiazine, 148–149
Anti-CXCR4-Ab *see* Anti-chemokine receptor antibody
Anti-cyanide compounds, 220
Antidote kits *see* Cyanide antidote kits
Antidotes metal/metallo antidotes, 216, 220, 221, 223, 225, 227, 228, 230, 231, 232; *see also* Cyanide antidots
Antifungal
  activity, 174
  agents, 199
Antimicrobial
  activity, 170, 171, 174, 176–179
  agents, 129, 164, 166, 168, 178, 185, 279
  drugs, 278
  resistance, 164–166
Antimonials, 196, 197
Antimony(III) potassium tartrate (tartar emetic), 197
Anti-MRSA activities, 172
Antiparasitic, 178, 197–200, 209
  activity, 198–200
  agents/compounds, 178, 194, 197–199
Antiretroviral therapy (HAART), 108
Antirheumatic drugs, 125, 178
Antirhinovirus activity, 118
Anti-SARS-Cov-2
  activity, 278
  agents, 152–155
Antitrypanosomal
  agents, 206
  drugs, 208
Antitumor
  activity, 9, 10, 12, 13, 24, 26, 58
  agents, 82, 106
  immunity, 48, 73
  resistance, 73
Antiviral
  activity, 109–111, 113–119, 121, 122, 124, 125, 128, 149, 154, 155

  agents, 106, 107, 109, 111, 112–115, 119, 121, 122, 124–126, 129, 130, 147, 152, 154
  drugs, 106, 107, 126, 129, 154
  drug targets of relevance for metal-based compounds, 108
  metal complexes, 106, 109, 119, 122
AP5346 *see* ProLindac™
Apoptogenic proteins, 70
Apoptosis
  pathways of apoptosis, 69
  resistance to apoptosis, 72, 98
Apoptosis-inducing factor (AIF), 70, 269
Aptamer, 309
Argyosis, 175
Argyria, 175, 281
Arsenic (As)/metalloid As, 29, 142, 276
  As(III), 143
  As-based drugs/prodrugs, 29, 141, 142, 143, 269, 276
  As compounds/arsenicals, 141, 142
  arsenic trioxide, 4, 29, 269, 276
  organoarsenic compounds
    4-(*N*-(*S*-glutathionylacetyl)amino) phenylarsonous acid, 29, 276
    4-(*N*-(*S*-penicillaminyl)-amino) phenylarsonous acid, 29, 276
    arsenic-biotin conjugate, 276
    darinaparsin (*S*-dimethylarsion-glutathione, ZIO-101), 29, 276, 277, 278
    salvarsan, 168
Arsenic-binding proteins, 270, 276–278
Arsenical probes, 270, 271, 276, 277
Artesunate, 89
AS-101 *see* Ammonium trichloro(dioxoethylene-*O,O*') tellurate
Ascorbate, 8, 78
Atomic absorption spectroscopy, 74
Atomic emission spectroscopy, 240
ATP *see* Adenosine triphosphate (ATP)
Auger electron, 241, 321, 323, 331, 339
Auranofin *see* Gold complexes
Aurothioglucose *see* Gold complexes
Aurothiomalate *see* Gold complexes
Autoimmune inflammatory diseases, 71
Autophagic cell death, 69
Autophagosomes, 70
Autophagy, 14, 70, 84, 170
Autosis, 70
A/WSN/33 virus, 114
Axial ligand/axial position, 8, 9, 10, 11, 57, 79–81, 112, 225, 227, 228
Azobenzene, 22, 23, 55, 56

B16F10 melanoma, 85
Bacillus calmette-guerin, 44
Background fluorescence, 248, 249
Bacteria
    antibiotic-resistant, 166, 169, 171, 172, 176, 179, 180
    with copper-resistant mechanisms, 173
    drug-resistant, 163, 166, 169, 186
    gram-negative, 166, 172, 177–179, 181, 183, 281
    gram-positive, 167, 169, 170, 172, 176–179, 182
    MBL-producing, 182–184
    resistant, 163, 164, 166
Bacterial
    infection, 165, 166, 169, 183, 184, 281
    pathogen, 165, 166, 186
    pathogenicity, 181
    strains, 166, 174, 184
Bactericidal
    activity, 170, 171, 173, 177, 282
    effects, 176
Bacterioferritin, 57
Barrett's esophagus, 44
Basal respiration, 75, 79, 81
Bax, 70, 75, 80, 85, 91
BBB *see* Blood brain barrier
BCA *see* Bis(2-chloroethyl)amine
BCE *see* N,N′-Bis(2-chloroethyl) ethylenediamine
BCG Refractory/Intolerant Non-Muscle Invasive Bladder Cancer (NMIBC), 44
Bcl-2 protein, 70, 86
Bcl-xL-Bax interaction, 80
BenzIm *see* Benzimidazole
Benzimidazole (BenzIm), 225
Benznidazole, 195
β-oxidation of fatty acids, 68
β-particles, 321, 332–334
β-radiation, 320
Bifunctional chelating agent (BFC), 329, 336
Biguanidine ligand, 113
Biliary excretion, 173
(4Z,15Z)-Bilirubin, 41
Bioavailability, 22, 46, 118, 174, 175, 198, 218, 220, 221, 229–231
Biocompatibility, 229, 290, 297, 304, 305, 307
Bioenergetics, 68, 71, 97
Biofilm, 165, 175, 177, 180
    biofilm-living bacteria, 180
    biofilm-producing bacteria, 180
Bioimaging, 290, 291, 293, 304, 305, 306, 307
Bioinformatics, 273, 282
Biolabeling, 290, 291, 304, 306, 307
Biological reducing agents, 78

Biomedical applications, 122, 253, 289, 292, 293, 295, 297, 312, 332
Biosensors, 297
Biosynthetic pathways, 57
Biotin, 11, 80, 274, 276
    biotinilated compounds, 11, 51, 80, 276, 277
2,2′-Bipyridine (bipy), 53, 172, 256
2,2′-Biquinoline (biq), 53
[2,2′-Biquinoline]-4,4′-dicarboxylic acid, 54
1,1′-Bis(diphenylphosphino)ferrocene (dppf), 204, 207–209
Bis(2-chloroethyl)amine (BCA), 19
Bis(acetylacetone)ethylenediamine (acacen), 112, 139, 147, 149, 150
N,N′-Bis[(6-carboxy-2pyridyl)methyl]-4,13-diaza-18-crown-6 (Macropa), 334
N,N-Bis(2-chloroethyl)ethylenediamine (DCE), 20
Bis(cyclopentadienyl) titanium complexes, 109
N,N′-Bis(2-hydroxybenzyl)ethylenediamine-N,N′-diacetic acid (HBED), 332
Bis(phosphine), 83, 84
Bismuth (Bi)
    Bi-213, 325–327, 334, 335
    Bi(III), 170, 272
    Bi-based drugs, 152, 157, 170, 278, 279
        bismuth subsalicylate, 152, 170, 278
        colloidal bismuth subcitrate (CBS), 152, 170, 278, 280
        complexes with citrate, 143, 150, 152, 170, 278
        complexes with porphine derivatives, 151
        ranitidine bismuth citrate (RBC), 150, 152, 170, 278
    bismuth compounds, 140, 141, 147, 150, 278
Blood brain barrier (BBB), 46, 231
BODIPY *see* Difluoro-boraindacene
Bond dissociation, 62
    heterolytic, 62
    homolytic, 62
Bovine viral diarrhoea virus (BVDV), 111
2,2′-Bpy *see* 2,2′-Bipyridine
BRC-ABL fusion of break point cluster (Bcr) and Abelson (Abl) tyrosine kinase protein (Bcr-Able), 59
Brc-Abl fusion protein, 56
Brd2, Brd 4 *see* Bromodomain-containing protein
Bromodomain-containing protein, 2, 4, 56
Breast cancer cells, 55, 81, 86, 275, 276, 308, 309
    MCF-7, 11, 15, 16, 55, 81, 89, 95, 97, 251, 275, 276, 309
    MDA-MB-468 cells, 55
    MDA-MB-468 cells (EGFR+), 55
Burn wounds, 174

350   Index

Buthionine sulfoximine, 125
BVDV *see* Bovine viral diarrhoea virus

Cadmium (Cd), 122, 291, 298, 331
   cadmium acetate, 122
   cadmium complexes, 106, 121, 122
CA-4 *see* Combretastatin A-4
Calcium (Ca), 329
   Ca isotopes, 332
   calcium phosphate, 308
   homeostasis, 68
CA-MRSA *see* Methicillin-resistant *S. aureus*
Cancer
   bladder, 14, 44, 58, 92
   bone, 320
   brain, 74
   breast, 11, 15, 55, 81, 86, 90, 95, 251, 275,
      276, 308, 309
   cell immortality, 68
   colorectal, 22, 25, 26, 141
   esophageal, 41, 44
   head and neck, 81
   lung, 10, 17, 41, 44, 95, 97, 338
   ovarian, 25, 79–82, 243, 244, 338
   prostate, 9, 44, 329, 334, 337
   stem cells, 86
   therapy, 3, 4, 23, 41, 44, 73, 197, 293, 310
Cancer cell immortality, 68
Cancer-specific stimuli, 1, 30
Cancer therapy, 3, 4, 23, 41, 44, 73, 197, 293, 310
Candida parapsilosis (*C. parapsilosis*)
      biofilms, 175
Capcid proteins, 113
Capillary electrophoresis (CE), 267
Carbapenem, 183
Carbazole, 258
Carbon dioxide, 6, 293
Carbon dots, 305
Carbon monoxide, 217, 257, 259
   poisoning, 217
   releasing molecules (CORMs), 58, 258, 259
Carboplatin, 3, 9, 25, 28, 76, 124, 141; *see also*
      Platinum(II) drugs
Carboxyhemoglobin, 223
Cardiolipin, 68
Cardiovascular disease, 71
Carrier, 9, 11, 12, 14, 23–26, 79, 80, 81, 171,
      320, 326, 329, 330
   nanocarrier, 4, 6, 11, 12, 14, 17, 26, 76,
      309, 311
CasIIgly *see* Casiopeinas®
Casiopeinas® *see* Copper complexes
Caspase, 71, 75, 86, 88, 89, 94
Catalysis, 50, 51, 94, 229, 293
Catalyst, 92, 229, 266, 302; *see also* Additional
      items at Photocatalysts

Cathepsin B, 28, 54, 145
Cbi *see* Cobinamide
Cbl *see* Cobalamin
CBS *see* Colloidal bismuth subcitrate
CcO *see* Cytochrome c oxidase
CcO-cyanide complex, 222
CD *see* Circular discroism
CE *see* Capillary electrophoresis
Cells
   bacterial, 176, 180, 268
   cycle, 8, 10, 69, 74, 79, 80, 94, 171, 269
   death pathways, 69, 74, 125
   death programs, 67, 73
   death signaling, 68, 69
   division, 71, 167, 274
   epithelial, 11, 168, 208, 274
   immune, 71, 269
   lysis, 166
   organelle dyes, 256
   organelles, 68–70, 75, 94, 108, 171,
      240, 243
   wall, 121, 165–167, 183
Cellular
   energy metabolism, 68
   imaging, 95
   morphology, 243
   stress response, 172
   stressors, 69, 97
   thermal shift assay (CETSA), 267
   uptake, 11, 16, 84–86, 90, 308, 309, 311
Cellulitis *see* Infections
Cerium (Ce), 339
Cervical carcinoma HeLa cells, 88
CETSA *see* Cellular thermal shift assay
Carboxyfluoresceindiacetate (CFDA), 274
CF *see* Cystic fibrosis
CFDA *see* Carboxyfluoresceindiacetate
CFDA-cisplatin, 274
Channel proteins, 95, 114
Charged particle activation, 326
Chelate, 84, 113, 115, 150, 224, 329, 332, 334,
      336, 337
Chemical stability, 169, 307
Chemoresistance, 73
Chemosensitization, 73
Chemosensitizer, 79
Chemotherapy-induced bone marrow toxicity, 182
Chikungunya virus (CHIKV), 121
Chloramphenicol, 177
Cholesterol, 68
Chromatin, 70
Chromophore, 54, 241, 247–250, 252–256,
      258, 260
Chryseobacterium indologenes, 183
3-Chymotrypsin-like protease (3CLpro),
      111, 118, 119, 123, 130, 149, 154

Index

351

Ciprofloxacin (CipA), 172, 173
CipA *see* Ciprofloxacin
Circular dichroism (CD), 267
Cisplatin, 3, 5, 9, 10, 11, 12, 16, 23, 24, 26, 30,
53, 76, 77, 78, 79, 80, 81, 82, 84,
85, 86, 89, 91, 94, 95, 97, 106, 124,
141, 154, 243, 244, 246, 269, 270,
274, 308, 309; *see also* Platinum(II)
drugs
    cisplatin-resistant cells, 9, 78, 79, 81, 82, 85,
86, 89, 91, 94, 95, 97, 243
    cisplatin-selective fluorescent sensor, 76
Chelator, 17, 25, 90, 170, 182–185, 320, 328,
329, 331–337
Chromium, 131, 339
Citrate, 78
    citrate-based complexes, 117, 143, 150, 152,
170, 179, 278, 280, 282
Citric acid cycle, 68, 74
Clindamycin, 168
Clinical trials, 9, 13, 14, 18, 21, 25, 29, 43–45,
47, 59, 90, 92, 110, 130, 148, 152,
179, 180, 182, 197, 274
    INDYGO, 58
    Phase I 9, 12, 13, 17, 18, 25, 29, 43, 44, 82,
90, 179, 182
    Phase II 9, 13, 14, 18, 21, 25, 29, 30, 43, 44,
45, 82, 113, 125, 130, 179, 180, 182
    Phase III 9, 11, 12, 18, 182
    Phase I/IIa randomised, double-blind,
multicentre study, 179
    Phase Ib non-randomised, 179
    Phase II multicentre, randomised, placebo-
controlled study, 179
CLint *see* Intrinsic clearance
Clotrimazole (CTZ), 170, 199, 206
3CLpro *see* 3-Chymotrypsin-like protease
(3C-like protease)
Cobalamin (Cbl), 217, 224–227, 230–232
    $[Cbl(CN)_2]^-$, 226
    5'-deoxyadenosyl-cobalamin (Ado-Cbl), 225
    cyanocobalamin, 224, 225
    hydroxocobalamin, 221, 225, 226
Cobalt (Co), 106, 112, 216, 217, 221, 224,
225, 291
    Co(II), 221
    Co(III), 112, 149, 221
        hypoxia-responsive Co complexes,
19–21
    cobalt(II) compounds, 112, 113, 130, 147,
149, 224, 225, 228
    hypoxia-responsive cobalt(III) complexes
with BCA, BCE and DCE nitrogen
mustards, 19, 20
        with erlotinib analogs Co(III)-EGFR,
20, 21

        with ponatinib analogs Co(III)-FGFR,
20, 21
    selected cobalt complexes
        $[Co(acacen)(2-methylimidazole)_2]^+$
(CTC-96), 110, 112, 113, 130
        $[Co(acacen)(imidazole)_2]^+$
(CTC-82), 110
        antiviral cobalt(III) CTC complexes
$[Co(acacen)(NH_3)_2]Cl$, 110, 112, 147,
149, 150
        cobalt(II) and (III) cyano complexes
$[Co(CN)_6]^{3-/4-}$, 224
        cobalt(II) complexes
$[Co_2(EDTA)(H_2O)_4]$, 221,
224, 230
Cobinamide (Cbi), 224–227, 230, 231
Cofactor, 44, 57, 70, 117, 225, 266, 281
    mimics, 57
Co-ligands, 172, 194, 195, 198–201,
203–206, 209
    bioactive, 205, 206
    non-active, 199
Colloidal particle, 290, 293, 297
Co-localization, 245, 246, 260
Colorectal adenocarcinoma, 88
Combretastatin A-4 (CA-4), 55
Computed tomography (CT), 308
Conductance channel, 69
Confocal microscopy, 75, 97, 247, 249, 251
    fluorescence microscopy, 74
    laser scanning microscopy, 253, 256–259
Conjugation, 5, 12, 17, 28, 76, 86, 167, 270,
308, 329, 336
Contrast-enhancing group, 245
Copper (Cu)
    Cu isotopes, 324, 332
    Cu(I), 18, 21, 90, 171
    Cu(I) complexes, 18
    Cu(II), 8, 17, 18, 19, 21, 90, 150, 169, 171,
172, 173, 272, 299
    Cu(II) complexes, 17, 18, 21, 114, 115
Copper complexes, 18, 68, 105, 114–116, 130,
171–173
    as antibacterial agents, 169–173
    as anticancer agents, 17, 18, 21, 90
    as antiviral agents, 114
    hypoxia-responsive, 21
    redox-responsive, 17
    selected copper complexes containing,
1,10-phenanthroline, 18
        $[Cu(II)(4,4'-dimethyl-2,2'-bipyridine)$
$(acetylacetonato)]NO_3$ (Casiopeina
CasIII-ia), 17
        Casiopeinas® [Cu(glycinate)
(4,7-dimethyl-1,10-phenanthroline)]
NO_3 (CasIIgly), 90

352 Index

Copper complexes (*cont.*)
   containing a-*N*-heterocyclic
      thiosemicarbazones Cu-diacetyl-
      bis(N4-methylthiosemicarbazone
      (Cu-ATSM), 21
   containing mustard derivative of
      1,4,7, 10-tetraazacyclododecane
      (Cu-TAD), 21
   containing quinoline Cu(II)-
      Triapine®, 18
   Cu chaperone, 76
   Cu(II)-phthalocyanine, 300
Copper-dependent protein, 173
CORMs *see* Carbon monoxide
Coronavirus, 107, 108, 144–147, 153
Coumarin, 52, 258, 271, 277
Coumarin-4-ylmethyl groups, 52
COVID-19, 106, 108, 126, 140, 144–148, 152,
   156, 157
COX17, 76
Coxsackie virus type B4, 109
Cp *see* Cyclopentadienyl
CRGD (cyclic RGD peptide), 13, 26, 27
Cross-linking, 166, 167, 183
   domain of penicillin-binding proteins, 167
CryoEM *see* Cryogenic electron microscopy
Cryogenic electron microscopy (CryoEM), 267
Cryo-preservation, 242
CT *see* Computed tomography
CTC complexes *see* Acacen-chelated Co(III)
   antiviral complexes
CTZ *see* Clotrimazole
Curcumin, 97
Cyanide (CN⁻), 216, 222, 226
   administration routes of, 218
   antagonist, 225, 226
   binding, 222–224, 226
   concentrations *in vivo*, 217–218
   detoxification, 229
   detoxifying inorganic compounds, 217, 221
      cobalt-based complexes, 224–228, 231
      MetHb former salts, 221–224
      molybdenum-based complexes,
      228, 231
      sulfur donor salts, 217
   detoxifying organic compounds, 220
   elimination routes of, 219
   exposure routes of, 217
   neurotoxic effects of, 219
   poisoning, 215–217, 219, 221, 222, 224, 232
   tissue uptake and distribution of, 218–220
   transport routes of, 217
Cyanide antidote kits, 221, 223
   Cyanide Antidote Kit (CAK™), 223
   Cyanokit™, 221, 223, 224, 225, 226
   4-DMAP, 221

Kelocyanor™, 221, 224, 225
Nithiodote™, 221
Thiosulfate, 221
Cyanide-based compounds/ions, 216, 217, 218
   hydrogen cyanide, 216, 217
   thiocyanate anion, 216, 219, 220, 223, 227,
      229, 232
cyanMetHb *see* Cyanmethemoglobin
Cyanmethemoglobin (CyanMetHb),
   222, 223, 224
Cyanokit® 221, 224, 225; *see also* Cyanide
   antidote kits
(L-Cyclohexyl alanine-D-arginine), 76
Cyclometalating ligands, 79, 84, 86, 92
Cyclometallated Pt(II), 249, 250
Cyclopentadienyl (Cp), 109, 120
Cyclotron, 327, 331–333, 339, 340
H6-p-Cymene, 199, 200
CYP17A1 inhibitor, 54
CYP1B1, 54
CYP3A4, 54
CYP450 *see* Cytochrome P450
Cysteine (Cys)
   protease, 53, 127, 128, 145, 181
   residue, 29, 82, 115, 123, 124, 127, 128, 149,
      155, 185
Cystic fibrosis (CF), 179
Cytochrome c, 8, 70, 75, 91
Cytochrome c oxidase (CcO), 216, 220,
   222, 230
Cytochrome P450 (CYP450), 17, 46
Cytokines, 126, 127
Cytomembrane, 257
Cytoplasm, 8, 80, 174, 185, 250, 257
Cytosolic TrxR1, 73
Cytosolic-free Ca level, 220
Cytotoxins, 53, 78, 81, 90

Daptomycin, 168
Database for annotation, visualization, and
   integrated discovery (DAVID), 273
DAVID *see* Database for annotation,
   visualization, and integrated
   discovery
DBET1 PROTAC, 52
DCA *see* Dichloroacetate
DCE *see* *N*,*N*-Bis(2-chloroethyl)
   ethylenediamine
Death-receptor-mediated pathway, 69
Death-signaling cascade, 70
Degenerative disorders, 71, 72
Demethylases, 90
Dendrimer, 290, 292, 293, 295, 303
Density functional theory (DFT), 256
5′-Deoxyadenosyl-cobalamin (Ado-Cbl), 225
Deoxyguanosine 5′-triphosphate (dGTP), 309

Index

Deoxynucleotides, 79, 311
Deoxyribonucleic acid (DNA)
  damage, 8, 14, 53, 69, 70, 73, 76, 77, 79, 81, 88, 93, 94, 97, 228
  damage response, 76, 79
  mutations, 71, 72
  platination, 95
  polymerase, 108, 116, 124
  repair, 172, 243
  replication, 82, 88, 172, 176, 185
Deoxyribonucleotides, 73
Depolarization, 78, 81, 84, 88
Dequalinium, 76
Desferal® see Desferrioxamine B
Desferrioxamine B (Desferal® or DFO), 281, 333
Detector technology advancement, 241
Deuteron, 327, 332–334, 340
DFO see Desferrioxamine B
DFT see Density functional theory
DGTP see Deoxyguanosine 5'-triphosphate
Diagnosis, 26, 301, 310, 337, 338
Diagnostics, 290, 291, 293, 309, 312, 321, 331–333
Diarrhoea, 111, 167, 173, 175
Diazines, 53
Dichloroacetate (DCA), 79
Diethylenetriaminepentaacetic acid (DTPA), 331
Difluoro-boraindacene, 95–97, 271
Difluoro-boraindacene dyes (BODIPY dyes), 95–97
4-Dimethylaminophenol (4-DMAP), 221
1-[(3-Dimethylamino)-propyl]-3-ethylcarbodiimide hydrochloride (EDC), 306
4,4'-Dimethyl bipyridine (dimethylbipy), 207
6,6'-Dimethyl-2,2'-bipyridine (dmbpy), 54
Dimethyltrisulfide, 220
Dinuclear, 79, 85, 88, 150, 250, 251
Dipyridophenazine, 86, 172
Disulfide bond, 128, 176, 185
Dithiocarbamate, 8, 127
Dithiocarbazate Schiff base, 90
4-DMAP see 4-Dimethylaminophenol
Dmbpy see 6,6'-Dimethyl-2,2'-bipyridine
2D monolayer cell models, 246
DNA see Deoxyribonucleic acid (DNA)
Dopamine, 52, 220, 298, 303
Dosimetry, 45, 58, 338, 339
DOTA see 2,2',2'',2'''-(1,4,7,10-Tetraazacyclododecane-1,4,7,10-tetrayl)tetraacetic acid
DOTA-(Tyr3)-octreotate (DOTATATE), 332, 338
DOTATATE see DOTA-(Tyr3)-octreotate

DOX see Doxorubicin
Doxorubicin (DOX), 308
Doxovir™ see CTC-96 cobalt complex
Doxycycline, 172
Dppf see 1,1'-Bis(diphenylphosphino)ferrocene
Drp1, 91
Drug/prodrug activation, 4, 5, 6, 28, 42, 57, 80
  by biological (enzymatic) triggers, 5
  by hypoxia, 18, 19, 21, 22, 23
  by reduced pH, 5–6
  by reduction, 2, 3, 5, 7, 8, 17, 21, 23, 31
Drug delivery, 55, 289, 290, 291, 307, 308, 312
Drug-resistant strain HTLVIIIB (HIV-1), 111
Drug-resistant bacterial pathogens, 166
3D tissue culture models 246
DTPA see Diethylenetriaminepentaacetic acid
Duocarmycin, 55
Dynamin-protein 1, 71
Dysplasia, 41, 44

ECAR see Extracellular acidification rate
EDC see 1-[(3-Dimethylamino)-propyl]-3-ethylcarbodiimide hydrochloride
EDT see Ethanedithiol
EDTA see Ethylenediaminetetraacetic acid
Effective PDT dose (EPDTD), 47, 48
EGFR see Epidermal growth factor receptor
Electron linear accelerators, 340
Electron microscopy, 68
Electron transport chain (ETC), 68
Element-specific energy, 241
Elizabethkingia meningoseptica (E. meningoseptica), 183
Emitter, 320, 323, 331, 332, 333, 334, 338, 339
En see Ethylenediamine
Encephalopathy, 219
Endogenous biosynthetic pathways, 57
Endonuclease G, 70
Endoperoxide, 251, 253
Endoplasmic reticulum (ER), 14, 70, 95, 274
  ER proteases, 95
  ER stress, 14, 274
Energy dispersive X-ray spectroscopy, 74
Energy transfer, 42, 54, 92, 323
Enhanced permeability and retention (EPR), 6
Enterobacter cloacae (E. cloacae), 178, 181, 182
Enterococcus faecalis (E. faecalis), 170, 177
Enterococcus faecium (E. faecium), 177
Enveloped virus, 112, 113
Enzyme
  enzyme-activatable metal-based drugs, 28–30

Enzyme (*cont.*)
enzyme-activatable nanomaterials releasing metal drugs, 30
enzyme-activatable nanomaterials sPLA2 sensitive liposomal cisplatin formulation (LiPlaCis®), 30
enzyme-activatable prodrugs, 28–29
enzyme inhibition, 52, 53, 54, 121
EPDTD *see* Effective PDT dose
Epidermal growth factor receptor (EGFR), 21, 26, 55
Epigenetic, 14, 72, 90
Epithelial herpetic keratitis, 112
EPR *see* Enhanced permeability and retention
Equilibrium constant, 222, 226
Equine arteritis virus (EAV), 118
ER *see* Endoplasmic reticulum
Erbium-169 (Er-169), 325
ERK1/2 inhibitoe, 52
Escherichia coli (*E. coli*), 170, 171, 178, 182, 281
ESKAPE pathogens (*Enterococcus faecium, Staphylococcus aureus, Klebsiella pneumoniae, Acinetobacter baumannii, Pseudomonas aeruginosa,* and Enterobacter Pathogens), 166, 180, 186
gram negative ESKAPE pathogens, 166
Estrogen receptor antagonist, 55
ETC *see* Electron transport chain
Et3P *see* Triethylphosphine, 83
Etchenique, R., 53, 54
Ethanedithiol (EDT), 270, 271, 283
Ethylenediamine (en), 9, 199
Ethylenediaminetetraacetic acid (EDTA), 115, 118, 221, 224, 230, 231, 270, 272, 331
7-Ethyl-10-hydroxycamptothecin (SN-38), 55
Etidronate *see* 1-Hydroxy-1,1-ethanediyl) bis(phosphonic acid)
Etomidate, 53
Eudragit RL100, 252
Europium (Eu), 256
Excitation, 53, 241, 242, 254, 256; *see also* Two-photon excitation
Excitation wavelength, 47, 48
Extracellular acidification rate (ECAR), 75
Extracellular signal-regulated kinase (ERK), 52
Extrinsic pathway of programmed cell death, 69

FAD *see* Flavin adenine dinucleotide
FDA *see* Food and Drug Administration
Fenton catalyst, 92
Fenton reaction, 70, 91

Fermi wavelength, 295, 312
Ferric reductases, 179
Ferroptosis, 69, 70, 88, 89, 278
Ferroptotic cell death, 90
FGFR *see* Fibroblast growth factor receptor
Fibroblast growth factor receptor (FGFR), 21
Fission, 68–71, 91, 95, 322, 326, 327
Flavin adenine dinucleotide (FAD), 57
Flavin adenine mononucleotide (FMN), 57
Flavin-conjugated prodrugs, 57
Flavoproteins, 57
Flow cytometry, 75, 269
Fluorescence lifetime spectrometer, 247
Fluorescent, 17, 75, 76, 91, 269–272, 274, 276, 277, 279, 281, 292, 295, 298–302, 304–311; probes, 270, 281, 305
Fluorophore, 247, 254, 270, 274, 277, 304, 306
Fluoroquinolone, 166, 172, 182
FMN *see* Flavin adenine mononucleotide
Folic acid, 302, 303, 308, 310
Food and drug administration (FDA), 174, 274
Förster (Fluorescence) Resonance Energy Transfer (FRET), 54
Fosfomycin, 177
Freeze-drying, 242
FRET *see* Förster (Fluorescence) Resonance Energy Transfer
Fumarate, 72, 207, 208
Fusidic acid, 177
Fusion, 29, 56, 68, 71, 95, 108, 112, 116, 117
Fusion proteins, 17, 122

Gadolinium (Gd), 245, 292, 311, 325, 339
Gd-160, 325, 339
Gd-161, 325, 339
oxide nanostructures (Gd_2O_3), 311
Galleria mellonella larvae (*G. mellonella* larvae), 173
Gallium (Ga), 169, 178
Ga-68, 321, 324, 327, 328, 331–333, 337, 338
[68Ga] Ga-PSMA-11, 332
[68Ga]Ga-DOTA-exendin-4, 332
Ga-68-based radiopharmaceuticals [68Ga]Ga-DOTATATE, 332
Ga(III), 179, 180, 185, 272, 281
gallium-based antibacterial agents, 179, 180, 281
Gallium complexes
Ga-based fluorescent probes Ga(III)-TRACER, 281
Ga-IMAC, 281
gallium citrate, 179
gallium DFO, 281
gallium maltolate, 179

Index

gallium nitrate, 179, 180
gallium porphyrins, 180, 279
gallium-based antibacterial drugs
Ganite®, 180
Ga-loaded carboxymethyl cellulose
(Ga-CMC), 281
γ-H2AX, 81
Gamma rays, 321, 323, 331
Gamma spectroscopy, 329
Ganite®, 180
Gasotransmitter, 53, 58
Gastric ulcer, 171
Gastrointestinal tract, 167
GE *see* Gel electrophoresis
Gel electrophoresis (GE), 267
Gene ontology (GO), 273
Gene therapy, 311
Genome, 69, 71, 108, 117, 196, 278, 282
Genomics, 266, 268, 273
Genotoxicity, 73, 171
Glioblastoma, 49, 58, 81
Glioma cells, 81
Glucose, 11, 96, 180, 224, 298, 301–303
Glucose oxidation, 74, 88, 94, 302
Glucose-modified terpyridine Pt(II)
complex, 77
Glutathione (GSH), 5, 8, 14–17, 29, 70, 71,
78, 85, 88, 89, 125, 176, 205, 297,
300, 307
Glutathione peroxidase, 4 (GPX4), 70
Glycolysis, 6, 72–74, 79, 80, 85, 88, 94, 276,
281, 282
Glycolytic pathway, 75
Glycoprotein, 116, 123, 124, 145, 146
GO *see* Gene ontology
Gold (Au)
as anticancer agents
Au(I/III) complexes with NHC-based
ligands, 83, 84, 85
Au(III) porphyrin complexes, 83, 85
Auranofin, 82–84
bis(phosphine)-Au(I) complexes, 83, 84
chloro(triethylphosphine)gold(I)
(Et₃PAuCl), 83
PTA-Au(I) complex, 83, 84
triethylphosphine-based Au(I)
complexes, 22, 83
as antimicrobial agents sodium
tetrachloroaurate (Na[AuCl₄]), 176
Au(I)-phosphine, 176
Auranofin, 177, 178
NHC-Au(I) complex, 177, 178
potassium dicyanidooaurate(I)
(K[Au(CN)₂]), 176
Au(I), 22, 82, 83, 85, 176, 178
Au(III), 82, 85, 176, 178, 292

hypoxia-responsive Au complexes,
21–22
Au(I) complexes, 82, 84, 124, 125, 126,
130, 143, 148, 157
Au(III) complexes, 82, 83, 84, 85, 86, 125,
126, 127, 128, 130, 176, 274
gold-NHC probe, 274
selected Au complexes as antiviral agents
Auranofin, 124, 125, 126
aurothioglucose, 124, 125,
128, 130
aurothiomalate, 83, 124, 125, 127, 128,
155, 156
bis(thioglucose)gold(I), 124
bis(thiosemicarbazonate) gold(III), 125
chloro(triethylphosphine)gold(I), 143
dicyanogold(I), 125
gold(I) phosphine complexes, 126
gold(III) dithiocarbamate complexes,
84, 127
gold(III) porphyrin complex, 126
NHC-based gold complexes, 127
Golgi apparatus, 257
GPX4, 4; *see also* Glutathione peroxidase
G-quadruplex, 52, 178
G-quadruplex DNA, 52
GSH *see* Glutathione

HAART *see* Antiretroviral therapy
HA-MRSA *see* Methicillin-resistant *S. aureus*
HAT *see* Human African tripanosomiasis
Hb *see* Hemoglobin
HBED *see* N,N'-Bis(2-hydroxybenzyl)
ethylenediamine-N,N'-diacetic
acid
HBED-CC (*N,N'*-bis[2-hydroxy-
5(carboxyethyl)benzyl]
ethylenediamine-*N,N'*-diacetic
acid), 332
HCMV *see* Human cytomegalovirus
HCV *see* Hepatitis C virus
HDAC7, 89
Head and neck squamous carcinoma cell
lines, 81
Heat-shock protein 60, 86
HEDP *see* 1-Hydroxy-1,1-ethanediyl)
bis(phosphonic acid)
HeLa *see* Human cervical cancer cells
Heme, 41, 50, 57, 68, 222, 275, 302
Hemoglobin (Hb), 221–224, 231
Hep G2, 46
Hepatitis C virus (HCV), 115, 117
Hepatotoxicity, 46, 141
Heptamethine cyanine dye, 97
Heptaplatin, 3
Herceptin, 310

356   Index

Herpes, 107, 108, 113, 121, 124, 149
  herpes simplex encephalitis, 107
  herpes simplex labialis, 113
  herpex simplex virus (HSV)/HSV-1, HSV-
    2, 107, 109, 111, 113, 116, 121, 124
Heterodinuclear Ir(III)-Pt(II) complexes, 79
Heterodinuclear Pt(II)-Gd(III) complex, 245
HSV see Herpes
Hexokinase, 73, 81, 276; inhibitors, 73
Histidine, 112, 114, 149, 150, 270, 279, 303
Histone, 71, 90
Histone deacetylase (HDAC), 10, 11, 23, 89,
    277, 278
High-performance liquid chromatography
    (HPLC), 329
HIV see Human immunodeficiency virus
Hmpo see Pyridine-2-thiol N-oxide
Holmium (Ho)-166, 325
Homeostasis, 2, 7, 17, 68, 70, 73, 82, 90, 97,
    173, 178, 224, 266, 278, 279
Hospital-acquired infection, 169
HPLC see High-performance liquid
    chromatography
HPV see Human papilloma virus
HRV see Human rhinovirus
Hsp60, 86, 274, 277, 278
Human African tripanosomiasis (HAT,
    sleeping sickness), 195, 196
Human lung adenocarcinoma cells, 50
  A549, 10–12, 21, 24, 49, 50, 78, 86, 89,
    94–97, 245, 251, 253
  A549R cells, 11, 94, 95
Human immunodeficiency virus (HIV)/HIV-1,
    HIV-2, 107–130, 148, 149, 160, 195
  envelope glycoproteins gp-120 and
    gp-41, 123
  HIV-1 integrase, 111
  HIV-1 reverse transcriptase, 111
  integrase, 119
  protease, 114, 115, 130
  replication, 116, 125
Human ovarian cancer cells
  human cervical cancer cells (HeLa), 12, 79,
    88, 92, 94, 96, 97, 246, 257, 258,
    306, 307, 309
  human ovarian, 2008 cells, 243, 244
  human ovarian adenocarcinoma (IGROV1)
    cells, 243
  human ovarian cancer cells (A2780), 9, 11,
    78, 80, 243, 244
Huntington's disease, 71
6-Hydrazinonicotinamide (HYNIC), 336
Hydrazones, 201
Hydrogen peroxide, 258, 299
Hydrogen sulfide, 56, 58, 222
Hydrogeneration process, 293

Hydrolysis, 8, 15, 23, 30, 55, 181, 183, 205,
    226, 336
Hydroxocobalamin see Cyanokit®
4-Hydroxycyclofen, 55
1-Hydroxy-1,1-ethanediyl)bis(phosphonic acid)
    (HEDP; Etidronate), 329
2-Hydroxyglutarate, 72
Hydroxyl, 92, 270, 271, 329
Hydroxypropylmethacrylamide copolymer, 25
8-Hydroxyquinoline (8HQ), 184, 202
HYNIC see 6-Hydrazinonicotinamide
Hyperbaric oxygen therapy, 223
Hypercalcaemia, 180
Hyperproliferative diseases, 72
Hypochlorous acid, 257
Hypoxia/hypoxic, 3, 5, 6, 8, 18, 19, 20, 21, 22,
    23, 50, 51, 54, 56, 58, 73, 94, 95,
    144, 251, 252
Hypoxia-responsive metal-based prodrugs,
    18–23

ICP-MS see Inductively coupled plasma-mass
    spectrometry
IDOi see Indolamine-2, 3-dioxygenase
    inhibitor
IMAC see Immobilized metal affinity
    chromatography
Imatinib, 54
Imidazole, 26, 53, 95, 149
IMM see Inner mitochondrial membrane
Immobilized metal affinity chromatography
    (IMAC), 272
Immune response, 72, 116, 125, 173, 174, 184
  innate immune repsonse, 173
Immune system
  evasion, 167
  suppression, 167
Immunomodulation, 74
  immunomodulatory effect, 109, 118
Immunotherapy, 12, 311
Impetigo see Infections
IMS see Intermembrane space
Indenoisoquinoline, 86–88
Indium (In) In-111, 324, 327, 331
  ^{111}In-pentetreotide (Octreoscan), 331
  ^{111}In-ProstaScint, 331
Indolamine-2,3-dioxygenase inhibitor
    (IDOi), 12
Inductively coupled plasma-mass spectrometry
    (ICP-MS), 74, 267–270, 279
  time resolved analysis mode of ICP-MS
    (TR-ICP-MS), 268–269
INDYGO clinical trial, 58
Infections
  bacterial, 164–169, 171, 179, 180, 183,
    184, 186

Index

nosocomial, 168
skin infection, 167; *see also individual words (e.g.,* impetigo, cellulitis, wound infection)
systemic, 167; *see also individual words (e.g.,* pneumonia, sinusitis, osteomyelitis)
Infectious diseases, 106, 112, 114, 124
Inflammation, 30, 126, 128, 130, 148, 167
Influenza viruses, 109, 111, 113, 114, 122
Inhalation injuries, 215–219, 223, 226, 227
Inhaled formulation, 179
Inhibiting/inhibitory, 11, 21, 52, 73, 79, 80, 82, 88, 90, 113, 116–118, 127, 129, 149, 150, 154, 155, 169, 185, 197, 199, 207, 208, 243, 261, 274, 281
Inner mitochondrial membrane (IMM), 68
Integrin, 13, 26, 86, 181, 338
Intermembrane space (IMS), 68
Intersystem crossing (ISC), 92
Intrauterine devices, 173
Intrinsic clearance (CLint), 46
Intrinsic pathway of programmed cell death, 69
Iridium (Ir)
 Ir(III), 79, 86, 87, 92, 93, 94, 95, 170, 251, 253
 Ir(III) complexes, 79, 86, 92, 93, 95, 170, 251, 253
  anthracene Ir(III) prodrug, 251, 253
  endoperoxide Ir(III) prodrug, 251, 253
  Ir(III)-based PS/PDT complexes, 93, 94, 97
  Ir(III)polypyridyl, 87, 92, 93
Iron (Fe)
 Fe(II), 221, 222, 223, 230, 299
 Fe(III), 19, 22, 179, 221, 222, 223, 230, 299
 Fe(III) complexes with hydroxamic acids, 22
 Fe homeostasis, 90, 224
 Fe/S clusters, 68
 hypoxia-responsive Fe complexes, 21–22
 iron complexes
  as antiviral agents, 111, 112
 iron uptake, 179
 iron-dependent enzymes, 179, 185
Irradiation, 23, 26, 48, 50, 52–58, 79, 92, 94, 95, 96, 119, 246, 251, 253, 256, 272, 274, 310, 311, 326, 327, 328, 330–334, 339
 light, 26, 52, 251, 310
 laser, 311
 NIR, 92, 311
ISC *see* Intersystem crossing
Ischemia-reperfusion injury, 71
ISOL *see* Isotope separation online system
Isomeric transition (IT), 321

Isotope separation online system (ISOL), 339
Isothermal titration calorimetry (ITC), 267
IT *see* Isomeric transition
ITC *see* Isothermal titration calorimetry

J aggregates, 75
JC-1, 252

KDAC, 52
Kelocyanor™ antidote kit, 221, 224–225; *see also* Cyanide antidote kits
Keratoconjunctivitis, 113
Keratosis, 44, 57
Kerr cell, 247
Kinase inhibitor, 19, 31, 54, 73, 278
Klebsiella pneumoniae (K. pneumoniae), 178, 183
K-lines, 241
Krebs cycle, 225

β-lactam, 166, 182–184, 278
β-lactam antibiotics, 182, 183
β-lactamase enzyme, 167
Lactic acid, 81, 219
Lactic acidosis, 219
Lactoferrin, 111
Lanthanides, 44, 122, 269, 332, 333, 334, 339
Lanthanum (La), 106, 122, 339
 radiolanthanum radionuclides, 339
Laser pyrolysis method, 293
Laser, 4, 44, 252, 253, 254, 255, 256, 257, 258, 259, 272, 293, 311
LC *see* Liquid chromatography
Lead (Pb), 153, 293, 299, 325, 326, 334, 336
 Pb-212, 325, 334, 336
Leishmania–HIV co-infection, 195
Leishmaniasis, 194, 195, 197, 200
 leishmaniasis drugs, 197, 200
LET *see* Linear energy transfer
Leukocytes, 168
Lexulan *see* 5-Aminolevulinic acid
Lifetime sensors, 250
Ligand exchange, 83, 112, 124, 198, 225, 226, 227, 230, 249
Ligand-to-metal charge transfer (LMCT), 296
Ligand-to-metal-metal charge transfer, 296
Light therapy, 41
Linear energy transfer (LET), 323, 334
Linezolid, 177
Linkage photoisomerism, 56
Lipids, 5, 11, 70, 72
 lipid peroxidation, 89, 278
 lipid peroxides, 70
Lipinski's rule of 5, 45, 46
LiPlaCis® *see* Enzyme activable nanomaterials
Lipophilic cationic fluorescent dye, 75

Liquid chromatography (LC), 267, 274, 283, 329
LLC solid tumor, 92
L-lines, 241
LMCT *see* Ligand-to-metal charge transfer
LMMCT *see* Ligand-to-metal-metal charge transfer
Lobaplatin, 3
Localized surface plasmon resonance (LSPR), 294
Lonidamine, 81
Lowest unoccupied molecular orbital (LUMO), 54, 294
LSPR *see* Localized surface plasmon resonance
Luminescence
    lifetime, 240, 241, 247, 248, 249, 250, 251, 252, 253, 256, 260
    lifetime imaging microscopy, 247–250, 260
    lifetime spectrometer, 247
Luminescent
    luminescent two-photon chromophores, 260
    metal complexes as luminescent lifetime sensors, 250–251
Luminophores, 247, 249, 259
LUMO *see* Lowest unoccupied molecular orbital
Lung cancer cells, 17, 49, 96, 97
    A549, 10, 11, 12, 21, 24, 49, 50, 78, 86, 94, 95, 96, 97, 245, 251, 253, 277
Lung inflammation, 128, 148
Lung injury, 127
Lupus, 41
Lutetium (Lu), 44, 323, 334, 329
    Lu-177, 323, 325, 328, 329, 334, 337, 338, 339
LUZ111, 44
Lymphocytic leukemia, 82
Lymphoid cells, 181
Lymphokines, 181
Lymphopoiesis, 181
Lysine deacetylase *see* KDAC

M2 ion channel, 114, 130
MAA *see* Mercaptoacetic acid
Macropa *see* N,N'-Bis[(6-carboxy-2pyridyl)methyl]-4,13-diaza-18-crown-6
Macrophage, 108, 171, 173, 180, 196, 207
Magnetic nanoparticles (MNPs), 293
Major histocompatibility complex (MHC) Class II, 167
MAL *see* Methyl 5-aminolevulinate
MALDI-TOF-MS, 82, 274
Maloplatin-B, 96
Manganese (Mn), 111, 113, 170, 266, 339
    Mn-52, 324, 339

Mn complexes with antiviral activity, 111, 112
Mass cytometry imaging (MCI), 269, 270
Mass imaging cytometry (IMC), 269
Mass spectrometry (MS), 74, 82, 84, 240, 267, 268, 274
Matrix Assisted Laser Desorption/Ionization Time-of-Flight Mass Spectrometry (MALDI-TOF-MS) *see* MALDI-TOF-MS
Matrix metalloproteinase (MMP), 19, 22, 30, 304
MBL *see* Metallo-β-lactamases
MBL-producing bacteria *see* Bacteria
MCCNN *see* Multichannel convolutional neural network
MCI *see* Mass cytometry imaging
Meca, 167
Membrane integrity, 171
Membrane-permeable fluorescent probes, 270
MeNCs *see* Metal nanoclusters
Mercaptoacetic acid, 306
Mercaptopyruvate (sulfanegen), 220, 227
Mercury (Hg) complexes, 129, 256, 276, 141
    as anti viral agents, 129
    mercury chloride, 129
    with N-acetylcysteine, 129
    organomercury derivatives
        thiomersal, 129
        merbromin, 129
        methylmercury, 129
        phenylmercuric acetate, 129
Meropenem, 183
Mesoporous silica nanoparticle (MSN), 17, 86
MERS-CoV *see* Middle East Respiratory Syndrome Coronavirus
Mesocates, 95
Metabolic pathway(s), 14, 165, 166, 171, 217, 220, 276
Metabolic processes, 178
Metabolomics, 266, 281
    metabolomic studies, 279, 281
Metal-to-ligand charge transfer (MLCT), 54
Metals *see individual names*
Metal-based antiviral agents, 105–138
    Period 4 metal-based antiviral agents, 109–119
    Period 5 metal-based antiviral agents, 119–122
    Period 6 and 7 metal-based antiviral agents, 122–129
Metal-based photosensitizers, 68, 92–97
Metal-binding
    affinity, 270
    capability, 266

Index

domain, 115
protein, 272
sites, 266, 272, 273
Metallic nanoparticles, 293
Metallic nanostructures, 290, 294
Metallo-drug targets, 273, 275
Metallohelicates, 95
Metallome, 266
Metallomics, 266–267
Metalloprotein, 221, 222, 267, 270, 272, 282
Metalloproteinase, 19, 181, 304
Metalloproteome, 266, 272
microbial, 282
Metalloproteomics, 266–268
methodology, 267
implementation on biomedical studies
anticancer drugs, 274–278
antimicrobial drugs, 278–282
Metallo-β-lactamases (MBL), 278, 182
Metal nanoclusters (MeNCs), 290–312
Ag-based NCs (AgNCs), 295, 296, 297, 298, 299, 302, 303, 304, 306, 308, 309
Au-based NCs (AuNCs), 292, 294, 295, 296, 297, 298, 299, 300, 301, 302, 303, 304, 307, 308, 309, 310, 311
bimetallic Au/Ag NCs, 302, 303, 306
biomedical applications, 297–311
Cu-based NCs (CuNCs), 299, 302, 304, 306
glutathione-directed AuNCs, 297, 300
Ni-based NCs (NiNCs), 295
optical characteristics, 295–297
Pt-based NCs (PtNCs), 306
self-assembled NCs, 293
structural characteristics, 294–295
Thiol-protected NCs, 292
Metastases, 323, 329
Metastasis, 90, 275, 309
MetHb see Methemoglobin
Methemoglobin (MetHb), 216, 217, 221, 222, 223
Methicillin, 167
Methicillin-resistant *S. aureus* (MRSA), 167–168, 170, 172, 174, 175, 176, 177, 178, 180, 182
MRSA infections
community-acquired (CA) infection (CA-MRSA), 168
healthcare-acquired (HA) infection (HA-MRSA), 168
MRSA treatment, 168
Methionine, 84, 181, 185, 303
Methyl 5-aminolevulinate (MAL, Metvix), 44, 57
Methylation, 21, 90
N7-Methyltransferase, 128, 129

Metvix *see* Methyl 5-aminolevulinate
Metyrapone, 53
MHC *see* Major histocompatibility complex (MHC) Class II
MIBI *see* Multiplexed ion beam imaging
Microsomal stability, 46
Microtubule, 54, 55
polymerization, 55
targeting agent, 54
Middle East Respiratory Syndrome Coronavirus (MERS-CoV), 146, 147
Mitaplatin, 9, 79
Mitocan(s), 73–74
Mitochondria
and cancer, 72
as drug targets, 72–74
mitochondria-directing entities, 68, 86
mitochondria-directing ligands, 76
mitochondria-mediated pathway, 69
mitochondria-penetrating peptide, 76, 78, 91
mitochondria-targeting, 67, 68, 74, 76, 77, 85, 86, 87, 89, 91, 92, 94, 96, 97, 98, 257
mitochondria-targeting metal-based cancer drugs
copper-based, 90–92
gold-based, 82–86
iridium-based, 88
platinum-based, 76–82
rhenium-based, 88–90
ruthenium-based, 86–88
Mitochondrial
biogenesis, 71
deoxynucleotide carrier, 79
depolarization, 81, 88
diabetes, 71
diseases, 71–72
DNA (mtDNA), 69, 71, 73, 74, 75, 76, 77, 78, 79, 80, 81, 87, 88, 93, 94, 95
dynamics, 71, 91
dysfunction, 71, 72, 75, 81, 82, 84, 85, 86, 88, 92, 94, 95, 97
fission, 70, 91, 95
matrix, 68
membrane, 9, 68, 70, 73, 74, 75, 76, 81, 82, 86, 91
membrane density, 91
membrane permeabilization, 70, 73
membrane potential, 9, 76, 81, 82, 86
metabolism, 68, 71, 88, 90, 97
morphology, 80, 88
outer membrane permeabilization (MOMP), 70, 72
oxidative phosphorylation, 176

360 Index

Mitochondrial (*cont.*)
  permeability transition (MPT), 69, 72, 76, 92, 95
  respiration, 71, 72, 85, 88, 90, 94, 95, 178
  ROS, 81, 85, 90, 91, 94
  superoxide levels, 79
  topoisomerase I (TOP1MT), 87, 88
  transition pore, 79
  transmembrane potential, 69
  TrxR2, 73, 81
Mitophagosomes, 82
Mitophagy, 70, 71, 72, 81, 82, 88
MitoTam, 74
MitoTracker Orange, 85
MLCT *see* Metal-to-ligand charge transfer
MM *see* Mitochondria
MMP *see* Matrix metalloproteinase
MNPs *see* Magnetic nanoparticles
Molar extinction coefficient (ε), 47
Molecular imaging, 319, 320, 324, 325, 326, 329, 332, 338
Molecular oxygen, 41, 42
Molybdenum (Mo), 216, 217, 221, 228, 229
  Mo-99, 322, 324, 327, 330
MOMP *see* Mitochondria
Monobactam, 166, 182
Monocarboxylate transporter, 81
Monoclonal anti-EGFR antibody, 55
Morpholine, 94
Morphological damage, 75, 81
Morphology, 68, 79, 80, 88, 243, 290, 293, 307
Motexafin lutetium, 44
MPT *see* Mitochondria
MRC-5 cells, 80
MRNA, 148, 165, 166
MS *see* Mass spectrometry
MSN *see* Mesoporous silica nanoparticle
MtDNA *see* Mitchondria
Multichannel convolutional neural network (MCCNN), 273
Multi-drug resistance *see* Resistance
Multiplexed ion beam imaging (MIBI), 269
Mupirocin, 177
Murine thigh infection model, 175, 176
Mutation(s), 71, 72, 114, 117, 144, 185, 273, 304
Mycobacterial clinical isolates, 179
Mycobacterium tuberculosis (*M. tuberculosis*), 170, 176, 177
Myelopoiesis, 181
Myoglobin, 57, 150
Myopathy, 71

NAD *see* Nicotinamide adenine dinucleotide radical
NAD⁺, 94

NADH cytochrome b5 reductase, 222
NADH fumarate reductase, 207, 208
NADH kinase Pos5, 82
NADH *see* Nicotinamide adenine dinucleotide
Nalidixic acid, 172
Nanocarrier(s), 4, 6, 11, 12, 23, 26, 76, 309
Nanoclusters (NCs), 289–312
Nanomedicine, 53, 58, 269, 312
NCs *see* Nanoclusters
Nicotinamide adenine dinucleotide (NADH), 57, 68, 94, 207
Nicotinamide adenine dinucleotide radical (NAD), 50
Nitrogen mustard, 19, 21
Nanoparticles (NPs), 10, 11, 12, 13, 17, 22, 25, 26, 27, 30, 78, 86, 107, 121, 149, 181, 250, 269, 289, 290, 291, 293, 294, 296, 297, 299, 300, 302, 304, 305, 307, 308, 309, 312, 333, 336
  magnetic (MNPs), 293
Nanostructures, 290, 291, 293, 294, 301, 304, 311, 312
  "hybrid" assemblies, 291
  inorganic-based, 290
  organic-based, 290
Naphthalimide, 17, 77
NBPs *see* Nitrogen-containing bisphosphonates
NCT00001006, 182
NCT01555112, 182
Necroptosis, 69, 71, 84, 88
Necrosis, 5, 71, 84, 168
Nedaplatin, 3
Neglected tropical diseases (NTDs), 193–196, 205
  Buruli ulcer, 194
  Chagas disease (American trypanosomiasis), 194–195
  cysticercosis, 194–195
  dengue fever, 194
  dracunculiasis, 194
  equinococcosis, 194
  fascioliasis, 194
  helminthiasis (soil-transmitted), 194
    ascaris, 194
    hookworm, 194
    whipworm, 194
  human African trypanosomiasis (HAT), 194–195
  leishmaniasis, 194, 195
    cutaneous leishmaniasis, 195
    mucocutaneous leishmaniasis, 195
    visceral leishmaniasis, 195
  leprosy, 180, 194
  lymphatic filariasis, 194
  mycetoma, 194

Index

onchocerciasis, 194
rabies, 194
schistosomiasis, 194–195
trachoma, 194
toxoplasmosis, 206
Neomycin, 172
Nephrotoxicity, 11, 84, 141
NETA *see* 2,2'-((2-(4,7-Bis(carboxymethyl))-1,4,7-triazonan-1-yl)ethyl)azanediyl) diacetic acid (NETA)
Neurodegenerative disorders, 71
Neuroendocrine tumor, 334, 338
Neuromodulator agents, 52
Neuropathy, 71
Neurosphere(s), 251, 252
Neurotoxin, 219
Neurotoxic effect, 219
Neurotransmitter(s), 53, 219, 303
Neutron, 322, 326, 330, 332, 334, 339
  activation, 326, 334
  capture, 322, 326
  flux, 326, 330
  irradiation, 326, 332, 339
Neutrophil, 168, 173, 180, 278
New Delhi MBL, 183
N-heterocyclic carbene (NHC), 15, 16, 83, 85, 122, 127, 174, 175, 176, 177, 178, 274, 275
NHC *see* N-heterocyclic carbene
NAMPT *see* Nicotinamide phosphoribosyltransferase (NAMPT)
Nanoliquid chromatography coupled to electrospray linear ion trap tandem mass spectrometry (nHPLC-ESI-LTQ-FT-MS/MS), 274
nDNA *see* Nuclear DNA
NHPLC-ESI-LTQ-FT-MS/MS *see* Nanoliquid chromatography coupled to electrospray linear ion trap tandem mass spectrometry
Nickel (Ni), 113, 198, 256, 270, 279, 291, 295
  nickel complexes as antiviral agents, 113
Nicotinamide phosphoribosyltransferase (NAMPT), 54
Nifurtimox, 195, 196, 203, 207, 208
Nifurtimox-eflornithine combination therapy, 196
NIR (near-infrared), 50, 92, 296, 305, 307, 310, 311
Nithiodote™ antidote kit, 221
Nitric oxide, 58, 219, 258
  releasing molecules (NORMs), 58
Nitriles, 53
Nitrilotriacetic acid (NTA), 270–271
Nitrite antidote, 223

Nitrites, 223–224
Nitrogen-containing bisphosphonates (NBPs), 206
  alendronate (ale), 206
  pamidronate (pam), 206
Nitrogen radical species, 51
Nitroreductase, 50
Nitroxoline, 184
NK-lysin, 73
NMIBC *see* BCG Refractory/Intolerant Non-Muscle Invasive Bladder Cancer
Non-apoptotic cell death, 70
Non-radiative decay, 254
Normoxia, 50, 54
NORMs *see* Nitric oxide releasing molecules
NOTA *see* 2,2',2''-(1,4,7-Triazacyclononane-1,4,7-triyl)triacetic acid
NOX4, 71
NPs *see* Nanoparticles
NTA-probes, 270–271
NTDs *see* Neglected tropical diseases
Nuclear DNA (nDNA), 73, 76, 79, 80, 81, 88, 94, 95, 97
Nuclear magnetic imaging, 245
Nuclear magnetic resonance (NMR) spectroscopy, 14, 267
Nuclear medicine, 119, 320, 321, 328, 329, 330, 333, 334, 335, 337
Nuclear reactor(s), 320, 322, 326, 329, 330, 332
Nucleic acid(s), 52, 58, 145, 171, 174, 249, 290, 298, 303, 304
Nucleotide excision repair, 71
Nucleotides, 68, 72, 78, 292, 293, 336

OCR *see* O$_2$ consumption rate
Octreoscan *see* Indium
Oligonucleotide, 298, 309
Oncogenesis, 68
One-photon excitation, 241, 254
Optical fluorescence microscopy, 242
Optical imaging-guided cancer therapy, 310
Optical transitions, 241
Oral administration, 78, 114, 128
Organic photocages, 51, 52, 55
Organic photoswitches, 55
Organometallic, 195, 203, 207, 209
  complexes, 27, 75, 84, 126, 127, 84, 126, 127, 177, 200, 203, 207, 209, 225, 228
Organophotoredox catalysis, 50
Organotellurium compounds, 181
Osmium (Os), 43, 44, 56, 58, 75, 95, 198, 247
  Os(II), 44, 75, 95
  Os(III), 95
  Os-arene complexes, 247

Oseltamivir, 122, 124
Osteomyelitis *see* Infections
Osteosarcoma cells, 52
O_2 consumption rate (OCR), 75, 88, 92, 94
Ovarian cancer cells, 79, 80, 81, 82, 243
Ovarian carcinoma, 9, 78, 94
Oxaliplatin, 3, 8, 9, 11, 13, 22, 24, 25, 26, 28, 76, 79, 141
Oxidative phosphorylation (OXPHOS), 67, 68, 72, 73, 75, 78, 79, 80, 176, 217
Oxidative stress, 71, 81, 82, 84, 88, 92, 95, 125, 176, 242, 276, 277, 279, 281
Oxoglutarate, 90
OXPHOS *see* Oxidative phosphorylation
Oxygen sensor(s), 250, 252

P388 murine leukemia, 82
P450 inhibitor, 53–54
P53, 70, 86, 91, 243, 278
PAA *see* Polyacrylic acid
Paclitaxel, 9, 12, 309
Padeliporfin, 44
Palladium (Pd), 44, 121, 153, 170, 198, 203, 204, 206, 207, 208, 209, 249, 258, 259, 274, 289, 291, 293, 295
    Pd(II), 203, 206, 207, 209, 249, 258, 259, 274
    Pd complexes containing thiosemicarbazone, 121, 203
    acyclovir, 121
Pam *see* Nitrogen-containing bisphosphonates
Pancreatic cancer cells, 90–91
Panitumumab, 25, 26, 55
Papain, 53, 303
Papain-like protease (PLpro), 109, 119, 127, 148, 152, 154
Parainfluenza virus type 3, 109
Paraptosis, 69, 70, 88, 98
Parasites, 194, 195, 196, 198, 200, 203, 206
    apicomplexan parasites, 206
        Toxoplasma gondii, 206
        Plasmodium falciparum, 206
    kinetoplastid pathogens, 195
    trypanosomatid parasites/trypanosomatids, 194, 195, 196, 203, 206, 207
    trypanosomaid leishmania, 196
        Trypanosoma cruzi (*T. cruzi*), 195, 196, 199, 200, 201, 202, 203, 204, 205, 206, 207, 208, 209
        Trypanosoma brucei (*T. brucei*), 196, 206, 209
        Trypanosoma brucei rhodesiense, 206
    Leishmania sp (Leishmania species), 195, 196
        Leishmania major (*L. major*), 200
        Leishmania donovani, 206

Parkinson's disease, 71, 282
Pathogenic viruses, 105, 106, 107
Pathogens, 164, 165, 166, 171, 175, 179, 181, 186, 195, 196, 279
Pathological trigger, 69
PBP *see* Penicillin
PDC-E1, 71
PDK *see* Pyruvate dehydrogenase kinase
PDT *see* Photodynamic therapy
PDT window, 46
PEG *see* Polyethylene glycol
Penicillin(s), 142, 166, 167, 169, 176, 183
    penicillin-binding protein 2a (PBP2a), 167
    penicillin-binding proteins (PBP), 167, 183
    penicillin-resistant bacteria, 167
Peptide receptor radionuclide therapy (PRRT), 334
Peptides, 11, 12, 13, 17, 26, 76, 78, 168, 268, 279, 290, 292, 293, 296, 301, 307, 326, 332, 336, 339
Peroxidation, 70, 89, 278
Peroxide(s), 70, 92, 219, 220, 258, 299, 301
Peroxiredoxin prx3, 82
Peroxisomes, 95
Pertechnetate [^{99}mTc]TcO$_4^-$, 330–331
PET *see* Positron emission tomography
Phagocytic activity, 173
Phagosome, 70, 82, 171
Pharmacokinetic(s), 46, 84, 196, 205, 227, 331, 335, 336, 340
Pharmacophore(s), 166, 202, 203, 205
Phen *see* 1,10-Phenanthroline
Phenanthrene, 172
1,10-Phenanthroline (phen), 17, 18, 90, 122, 170, 172, 173, 192, 201, 206, 207, 208
Phenol soluble modulin (PSM) cytolysin, 168
4-Phenylbutyrate, 80
Phosphate glycerin mutase 5, 71
Phosphatidylinositol 3-kinase (PI3K), 52
Phosphine, 83–86, 126, 176–178, 203, 204, 295
Phosphorescence, 89, 247, 248, 254
Photoacid, 94–95
Photoactivated chemotherapy (PACT), 43, 44, 47, 50, 51, 53, 86
Photoactivators, 40
Photoactivity index, 52
PI3K *see* Phosphatidylinositol 3-kinase
Photoaffinity chemical probes, 267, 270
    fluorescein arsenical hairpin binder-ethanedithiol (FlAsH-EDT2), 270
    NTA-based probes, 270
    organic arsenic EDT-containing probes, 270, 271
Photoallergic, 53
Photobiological properties, 41, 44

Index

363

Photocages, 50, 51, 52, 53, 54, 55
  inorganic, 53–55
  organic, 51–53, 55
Photocatalyst(s), 41, 42, 50, 51, 79
Photochemical, 40, 41, 42, 43, 50, 53, 56, 95
  isomerization, 41
Photochemotherapy (PCT), 50, 53
Photocontrol, 52, 53
Photodamage, 94, 95, 254
Photodynamic effect, 41
Photodynamic therapy (PDT), 4, 14, 22, 26, 41,
    43, 44, 45, 46, 47, 48, 49, 50, 57, 58,
    92, 93, 94, 95, 96, 97, 310, 311
  highlights of successful PDT
    drugs, 44–45
  ongoing challenges and missed
    opportunities, 45
Photoelectron, 241
Photoexcitation, 42
Photogeneration, 50
Photo-inactivation, 119
Photoluminescence (pl), 50, 290, 294, 295, 296,
    297, 299, 300, 302, 303, 304, 305,
    306, 312
Photon flux density, 253
Photoneutron, 340
Photooxidation, 41
Photopharmacology, 52
Photophysical, 40, 41, 42, 44, 46, 47, 48, 50, 53,
    55, 94, 95, 124, 241, 247, 249, 250,
    253, 256, 258, 304
Photoproducts, 53, 93
Photoproton, 340
Photoredox catalysis, 50
Photosensitivity, 41
Photosensitizer (PS), 22, 40, 41, 42, 44, 45, 46,
    50, 51, 55, 57, 68, 92, 93, 94, 96, 97,
    310, 311
  organic versus metal-containing PS, 50–51
Photostability, 44, 88, 290, 297, 304, 312
Photosubstitution, 48, 54
Photoswitchable, 55, 56
Photoswitches, 52, 55, 56, 57
  inorganic, 56–57
  organic, 55–56
Phototherapeutic index, 94
Phototherapy, 40, 41, 43, 45, 46, 48, 59, 310
Photothermal therapy (PTT), 311
Phototoxic, 53
Phototoxicity index (PI), 50, 52, 54, 55
Photo-uncaging, 55
pH-responsive complexes/prodrugs
    pH-responsive Pt(II) complexes,
    23–24
  bis-(0-ethyldithiocarbonato)Pt(II)
    (thioplatin), 23

bis(2-aminoethanol)dichloroplatinum(II), 23
bis[(R)-(-)-2-aminobutanol)]
    dichloroplatinum(II), 23
1,3-dihydroxyacetoneoximatoplatinum(II)
    complexes, 24
pH-responsive Pt nanomaterials, 24–26
pH-responsive Ru drugs and nanomaterials,
    26–28
  cRGD-containing ruthenium(II)-
    bipyridyl complex, 27
  MSN-conjugated ruthenium(II)-arene
    complex with a pH-sensitive
    hydrazone linker, 27
pH-responsive metal-based prodrugs, 23–28
Physicochemical properties, 28, 45, 198,
    199, 203
PI3K *see* Phototoxicity index
PK11195, 81
PL lifetime, 296, 304, 306
PL *see* Photoluminescence
Plaque formation, 112
Plasmonic feature, 296–297
Platin-M, 78
Platinum (Pt), 3, 43, 44, 58, 68, 76, 106, 121,
    122, 124, 141, 142, 154, 170, 197,
    198, 204, 205, 243, 256, 266, 274,
    289, 291
  with active targeting carriers (*e.g.*, peptides,
    vitamins, sugars, or lipids)
    biotin as a carrier, 11, 80
  with bioactive ligands
    aspirin, 9
    dichloroacetate, 9, 79
    gemcitabine, 9
    paclitaxel, 9
    valproic acid/valproate, 10, 11
  glycosylated Pt(IV) derivatives, 11
    albumin as nanocarrier, 11, 12, 13,
    22, 295
  with passive targeting carriers, 9, 25
  with non-bioactive ligands
    Iproplatin, 9, 10
    LA-12, 9, 10
    Satraplatin, 9, 10
    Tetraplatin, 9, 10
  Pt(II), 3, 7, 8, 15, 23, 24, 25, 28, 52, 57, 77,
    78, 79, 80, 81, 95, 96, 203, 205, 207,
    209, 243, 244, 245, 246, 249, 250,
    252, 274
  Pt(IV), 7–14, 17, 23, 57, 77, 78, 79, 80, 81,
    97, 205, 245
Pt-based nanomaterials, 12, 24
Pt(IV) complexes incorporated into
    polysilsesquioxane nanoparticles, 13
Pt-Gd complex, 245
Pt-195m, 340

364 Index

Platinum (*cont.*)
   platinum(II) drugs *see individual names,*
      e.g., cisplatin, carboplatin,
      oxaliplatin, nedaplatin, lobaplatin,
      heptaplatin
   platinum(II) complexes *see also*
      Platinum(II) drugs
      cisplatin-nucleotide conjugate, 124
      cyclometallated platinum(II), 124
   Pt(IV) complexes/prodrugs
      dihydroxido oxaliplatin(IV), 11
      oxoplatin, 10
      with axial maleimide moieties, 12
Plpro *see* Papain-like protease
PMS2, 86
Pneumonia *see* Infections
Poliovirus, 119, 121
Polyacrylic acid (PAA), 299, 308
Polyamine, 84
Polyelectrolyte(s), 295, 300, 306, 307, 311
Polyethylene glycol (PEG), 10, 12, 308,
   309, 311
Polymerase, 75, 79, 90, 108, 111, 116, 118, 124,
   145, 278, 281
Polyoxometalates (POMs), 119, 140, 153,
   154, 155
Polypyridine, 44, 250, 251, 256, 257
Polypyridyl (moiety/ligand/derivative), 14, 26,
   44, 86, 87, 92, 93, 119, 201, 206,
   208, 209
POMs *see* Polyoxometalates, 41, 42, 44, 47, 48,
   49, 50
Porphyria, 41
Porphyrin(s), 41, 44, 47, 50, 57, 84, 85, 86,
   111, 126, 150, 180, 222, 227, 228,
   249, 250
Positron, 21, 321, 323, 331, 332, 333, 339
Precursor(s), 23, 41, 44, 58, 72, 118, 292, 295
Pro-apoptotic proteins, 72, 77, 84
Pro-apoptotic signal, 69, 70
Proliferation, 5, 7, 72, 73, 74, 89, 125, 176, 181,
   206, 269, 276
ProLindac™ (AP5346), 25
Prolymphocytic lymphoma, 82
Prophylactic, 128, 172
Positron emission tomography (PET), 21, 323
Protease inhibitors, 53, 129, 130
Proteasome, 18, 70
Protein crystallography, 267
Protein disulfide isomerase, 274
Protein kinase c, 126
Protein separation, 268, 270, 282
Protein:protein interactions, 52
PROteolysis TArgeting Chimera (PROTAC),
   52, 55, 56
Proteome(s), 265, 266, 269, 276

Proteomic analysis, 172, 278
Proteomics, 85, 266, 268, 273, 275, 276,
   278, 279
Proteostasis, 70
Proton spallation, 325, 326, 334
Protoporphyrin IX, 57, 279, 310
PRRT *see* Peptide receptor radionuclide
   therapy
PS *see* Photosensitizer
Pseudomonas aeruginosa (*P. aeruginosa*),
   170, 178, 179, 180, 181, 182, 281
PSMA-11 (Glu-NH-CO-NH-Lys(Ahx)-
   HBED-CC), 332, 337, 338
Psoralens, 40
Psoriatic arthritis, 125
PTA *see* 1,3,5-Triaza-7-phosphaadamantane
PTT *see* Photothermal therapy
PVL *see* Toxins
PYGL, 71
Pyridine, 53, 78, 88, 95, 243
Pyridine-2-thiol N-oxide (Hmpo), 208
Pyridyl, 86, 93, 94
Pyriplatin, 78, 95
Pyruvate, 9, 73, 74, 81, 220, 225
Pyruvate dehydrogenase kinase (PDK), 9, 73,
   74, 79, 88

QCE *see* Quantum confinement effect
QPCR *see* Quantitative polymerase chain
   reaction
Quantitative polymerase chain reaction
   (qPCR), 75, 94
Quantum confinement effect (QCE),
   295, 296, 297
Quantum yield (QY), 47, 48, 88, 96, 124, 295,
   307, 308, 312
Quenching, 297, 299, 300, 302, 304
Quinolones, 172
QY *see* Quantum yield

Radar plot, 48
Radiation therapy, 45
Radical(s), 50, 51, 56, 92, 94, 198, 207, 208,
   252, 253
Radioactive decay, 320, 321, 322, 334, 340
   α decay, 321
   β decay, 321, 323, 326
   electron capture (EC), 321
   fission, 68, 69, 70, 71, 91, 95, 322,
      326, 327
   isomeric transition (IT), 321
Radioactivity, 320, 321, 323, 328, 329
Radiochemical purity, 327, 329
Radioimmunotherapy, 122
Radioisotopes, 119, 320, 323, 326, 330, 336,
   338, 340

Index

365

Radiolabelling, 326, 328, 329, 331, 332, 335–336
Radiometals, 319–340
   characteristics of selected radiometals used in radiopharmaceuticals, 329–335
   current trends for medical application, 337–340
   medical applications, 323–326, 337–340
   production methods, 326–329
   properties, 321–323
Radionuclide
   daughter radionuclide, 327
   generator, 332, 326–327, 330, 331, 332, 334
   parent radionuclide, 322, 327, 330–331, 334
   therapy, 320, 334, 338, 339
Radiopharmaceutical(s), 21, 178, 320–321, 323, 328–332, 334, 337, 338, 339
Radio-synovectomy, 329
Radiotracer(s), 320, 335, 337
Radium (Ra), 320, 334
   Ra-223, 326, 329, 334
Ranitidine bismuth citrate, 150, 152, 170, 278
RAPTA see Ruthenium(arene) "piano stool" complexes
RBC see Ranitidine bismuth citrate
RBD see Receptor binding domain
RdRp see RNA-dependent RNA polymerase
Reactive oxygen species (ROS), 5, 14, 15, 17, 25, 29, 34, 42, 58, 69, 71–78, 80, 81, 84–86, 88, 90–92, 94–97, 111, 126, 171, 174, 185, 198, 203, 219, 229
Receptor binding domain (RBD), 145, 154
Redox homeostasis, 2, 7, 68, 73, 82, 97, 178
Redox potential, 8, 18, 21, 90
Redox-responsive metal-based prodrugs, 7–18
Reducing agent, 5, 8, 17, 78, 115, 292, 294
Reductive environment of cancer cells, 5
Relaxation pathways, 42
Resistance
   gene, 165, 167, 185
   mechanisms, 30, 67, 73, 97, 165, 166, 169, 181, 182, 197, 198, 243
   multi-drug, 85, 92, 166
Respiration, 68, 71, 72, 75, 78, 79, 81, 85, 86, 88, 90, 94, 95, 174, 178, 217, 223
Respiratory syncytial virus (RSV), 118, 122
Respiratory virus, 117, 118, 130
Retrovirus, 108, 109
Reverse transcriptase (RT)
Reverse transcription-qPCR, 75
Rhenium (Re), 68, 86, 123, 170, 330
   perrhenate anion, 331
   Re(I), 88–90, 245–246
   Re(V), 331
   Re(VII), 331
   Re-186, 325, 329, 330, 331, 340

Re-188, 123, 325, 327, 329, 330, 331
   Re-188 labelled antibody, 123
   Re(I) tricarbonyl complexes, 123, 206
Rhesus macaques (monkey AIDS model), 125
Rheumatoid arthritis, 82, 124, 148, 176
Rhodamine, 75, 76, 77, 79
Rhodanese, 217, 218, 219, 221, 229, 230
Rhodaplatin 2, 79
Rhodium (Rh), 119, 120, 130, 153, 171, 198, 289, 291
   cyclopentadienyl derivatives, 120
Ribonucleotide reductase, 73
Ribonucleotides, 73
Ribosome, 141, 166
RIPK3, 71
RNA, 18, 86, 90, 108–109, 111, 115–119, 122, 145, 150, 266, 279, 281–282
RNA-dependent RNA polymerase (RdRp), 111, 118, 130
RNA virus, 108, 111, 116, 145
ROS see Reactive oxygen species
Rosacea, 41
Rotavirus, 111
Rotaxane, 52
RSV see Respiratory syncytial virus
RT, 108, 109, 111, 116, 117, 119, 122, 124, 126, 130; see also Reverse transcriptase
Ruthenium (Ru), 3, 43, 44, 53, 68, 119–121, 130, 142, 154, 171, 203, 256, 274, 275, 276, 289, 291
   pH-responsive Ru drugs and nanomaterials, 26–28
   redox-responsive Ru complexes, 13–16
   redox-responsive nanomaterials of Ru compounds, 17
   Ru(II), 13–16, 26–27, 44, 51, 53–58, 86–87, 92–93, 119, 171, 203, 207, 250, 251, 256, 257
   Ru(III), 8, 13–14, 17, 56, 119, 121, 203
   Ru(arene) "piano stool" complexes
      (NHC)-containing Ru(II)-arene complex, 15
      arene-Ru–CTZ complexes, 200
      NHC-17α-ethynyl testosterone ruthenium(II)-arene complex, 16
      phenylazopyridine-containing ruthenium(II)-arene complex, 15
      plecstatin (ruthenium(arene) pyridinecarbothioamide), 276
      RAPTA, 275–276
   Ru-polypyridyl complexes, 14, 26, 44, 86, 87, 92, 93, 119, 208, 209
      KP-1019, 14
      NAMI-A, 13–14, 121, 274
      NKP1339 (BOLD-100), 13–15
      TLD1433, 14, 44–48, 50, 58

Ruthenium (*cont.*)
  ruthenium complexes (clinically studied)
    see individual names, e.g.,
    NAMI-A, KP-1029, NKP1339
    (BOLD-100), (TLD1433)

SAHA *see* Suberoylanilide hydroxamic acid
Salophen, 228
Salvarsan, 141, 143, 168
Samarium (Sm)
  Sm-153, 325, 329
SARS-CoV *see* Severe acute respiratory
    syndrome
SARS-CoV-2 main protease, 128, 149
Saxitoxin, 52
Scandium (Sc), 109, 332, 338
  Sc-43, 324, 332, 337, 338
  Sc-44, 324, 327, 332, 337, 338
  Sc-47, 324, 340, 332, 338
SCCmec *see* Staphylococcal cassette
    chromosome mec
Schiff bases, 19, 90, 91, 112, 170, 201
SDS PAGE *see* Sodium dodecyl sulfate–
    polyacrylamide gel electrophoresis
Seahorse assay, 75
Secretory phospholipase A2 (sPLA2), 30
Selection rules, 241
Selective excitation, 241, 254
Selectivity index, 119, 121, 126, 128
Selenium (Se), 81, 82
Selenocysteine, 73, 81, 82, 84
Self-immolating linkers, 55
Semicarbazones, 201
Semliki forest virus (SFV), 109, 117
Sensor(s), 76, 250, 252, 258, 259, 290, 297–304
Serine, 145, 183
Serotonin, 52, 298, 303
Serum albumin, 12, 22, 85, 205, 295
Severe acute respiratory syndrome (SARS-
    CoV), 107, 144, 146, 278, 105–113,
    115, 117–130, 140, 144–157
SFV *see* Semliki forest virus
SHIV *see* Simian-human
    immunodeficiency virus
Shock-freezing, 242
SH-SY5Y neuroblastoma cells, 78
Siderophore, 179, 281
Signal-to-noise ratio, 257
Silver (Ag), 121, 122, 126, 130, 147, 148, 149,
    153, 155, 168, 169, 174–176, 185,
    256, 281, 282, 289, 290, 291, 293,
    295–299, 302–306, 308–209
  Ag(I), 174–176, 304
  Ag complexes as antiviral agents, 121–122
  Ag complexes as antibacterial agents,
    174–176

Ag nanomaterials, 281
Ag-impregnated glutaraldehyde hydrogel
    ethylmafenide, 121
  mafenide, 121
  colloidal silver, 175
Simian-human immunodeficiency virus
    (SHIV), 116
Sindbis virus (SINV), 109, 113, 119
Single photon emission computed tomography
    (SPECT), 320, 323, 324, 325, 330,
    331, 332, 337, 338, 339
Singlet oxygen, 22, 23, 42, 55, 251, 253
Singlet state, 42, 247–248, 254
Sinusitis *see* Infections
SINV *see* Sindbis virus
Skin keratinocyte (HaCaT) cells, 95
Small lymphocytic lymphoma, 82
Smoke inhalation, 219, 223
SN-38 *see* 7-Ethyl-10-hydroxycamptothecin
SOD *see* Superoxide dismutas
Sodium dodecyl sulfate–polyacrylamide gel
    electrophoresis (SDS PAGE), 281
Sodium stibogluconate, 143, 196
Sodium thiosulfate, 223, 227
SPECT *see* Single photon emission computed
    tomography
Spheroids, 20, 84, 92, 246, 247
Spike protein (S protein), 110, 122, 127, 128,
    148, 152, 154
Spin-orbit coupling, 42
SPLA2 *see* Secretory phospholipase A
S protein *see* Spike protein
SR-XRF *see* Synchrotron radiation X-ray
    fluorescence
SSSS *see* Staphylococcal scalded skin syndrom
Stabilizing agent, 292, 293
Staphylococcal cassette chromosome mec
    (SCCmec), 168
Staphylococcal scalded skin syndrome
    (SSSS), 157
Staphylococcus aureus (*S. aureus*), 167
Staphylococcus epidermidis, 177
Stenotrophomonas maltophilia
    (*S. maltophilia*), 183
Steroidogenesis, 74
Stimuli-responsive, 5, 12, 17, 18
  Pt(IV) nanomaterials, 12
  Ru nanomaterials, 17
Stokes shifted emission, 308
Stokes shifts, 88
Streptomycin, 172
STRING database, 273
Strontium (Sr)
  Sr-89, 320
Suberoylanilide hydroxamic acid (SAHA), 89
Sub-micro sized particle, 290

Index

367

Succinate, 72, 80
Sulfamethoxazole, 166
Sulfanegen *see* Mercaptopyruvate
Sulfhydryl group, 174, 185
Sulfitocyanocobinamide, 227
Sulfitohydroxocobinamide, 227
Sulfonamide, 121, 166, 182
Sulfoxide, 56
Sulfur dioxide, 258
Sulfur (S), 14, 23, 56, 57, 81, 84, 217, 220, 221, 223, 226, 232
 disulfide linker, 12, 13
 hydrogen sulfide, H2S, 56, 58, 222
 sulfur monoxide, SO, 222
Sulfur transferase enzymes, 216, 220
Superoxide, 42, 56, 58, 79, 92
Superoxide dismutase (SOD), 5, 220
Synchrotron, 74, 241, 242, 272
 X-ray fluorescence nanoprobe, 74
 X-ray radiation, 241
Synergistic effect, 80, 121, 169
Syphilis, 141, 169
Szeto-Schiller peptides, 76

T cells, 12, 108, 125, 167
Talaporfin, 44
Tartar emetic *see* Antimony(III) potassium tartrate
TAR-TAT complexes, 119
TAT (virus-encoded transactivator protein), 119
TB *see* Tuberculosis
TCMC *see* 2,2',2'',2'''-(1,4,7,10-Tetraazacyclododecane-1,4,7,10-tetrayl)tetraacetamide
Technetium (Tc), 119, 333
 pertechnetate anion [^{99m}Tc]TcO$_4$$^-$, 330
 Tc-99m, 330
 Tc-99m complexes, 330
Tellurium (Te), 142, 169, 180, 181
 organotellurium compounds telluro-cysteine, 181, 185
 telluro-methionine, 181
 Te(IV), 181, 182
 Te-based compounds, 180–182, 185
TEM *see* Transmission electron microscopy
Template-assisted preparation, 292
Terbium (Tb), 256, 338, 339
 Tb-149, 338
 Tb-152, 338
2,2',2'',2'''-(1,4,8,11-Tetraazacyclotetradecane-1,4,8,11-tetrayl)tetraacetic acid (TETA), 332, 336

Terpy *see* Terpyridine
Terpyridine (terpy), 54, 77, 79, 81, 91
2,2';6',2''-Terpyridine, 54, 79, 81
Testis-specific TrxR3, 73
TETA *see* 2,2',2'',2'''-(1,4,8,11-Tetraazacyclotetradecane-1,4,8,11-tetrayl)tetraacetic acid
Tetraarylporphyrins, 85
2,2',2'',2'''-(1,4,7,10-Tetraazacyclododecane-1,4,7,10-tetrayl)tetraacetic acid (DOTA), 184, 337, 338
Tetracycline, 166, 172, 174
Tetramethylpyridineporhyrin (TMPyP), 224, 227, 228, 231
Tetrapeptides, 76, 86
Texaphyrins, 44
Thallium (Tl)
 Tl(III), 275
Theranostic agents, 42
Theranostics, 40, 243, 309, 337, 338, 340
 heterobimetallic, 243
 involving targeted therapy and diagnostic imaging, 337
Therapeutic dose, 59, 169
Thin-layer chromatography (TLC), 204, 329
Thiocyanate anion, 216, 219, 220, 223, 227, 229, 232
Thioethers, 53, 55
Thiol redox modulators, 73
Thioredoxin (Trx), 73
Thioredoxin reductase (TrxR), 73, 74, 81–86
Thiosulfate, 220, 221, 223, 226, 227, 229, 232
 kit, 221
Thiosemicarbazones, 18, 22, 90, 203, 204, 332
 5-nitro-2-furaldehyde thiosemicarbazones, 203
 5-nitrofuryl containing thiosemicarbazones, 203, 204
Thorium (Th)
 Th-227, 326
Time-resolved emission spectroscopy, 256
Tin (Sn)
 Sn-117, 325
 tin porphyrinoid catalyst, 51
Tissue penetration, 47, 53, 92, 254, 255, 322
Titanium (Ti), 109, 142, 155
 Ti-46, 324, 332
 Ti-sapphire laser, 253
Titanocene dichloride, 109, 110, 143, 154, 155
TKI *see* Tyrosine kinase inhibitor
TLC *see* Thin-layer chromatography
TLD-1433, 14, 44–48, 50, 58
TMPyP *see* Tetramethylpyridineporhyrin
TOOKAD® soluble (Padeliporfin), 44
TOP1 *see* Topoisomerase I
TOP1MT-mtDNA, 88

Index

368

TOP1-nDNA, 88
Topoisomerase I (TOP1), 87
Topoisomerase-DNA complex, 87
Topoisomerases, 87
Toxicology, 164, 173, 175, 178, 180, 182, 183
Toxins α-toxin, 168
 exfoliative toxin, 167
 enterotoxin, 167
 panton-valentine leukocidin toxin (PVL), 168
 toxic shock syndrome toxin-1 (TSST-1), 167
TPP *see* Triphenylphosphonium
Trace element, 19, 111, 112, 173
TRACER ("metal-tunable" fluorescent probe),
 270, 279–281
Tracer, 270, 279–281, 323, 329, 336, 337
Tracking, 75, 241, 243, 310
Trans activation response (TAR) region (within
 HIV-1 RNA), 119
Trans uranium elements, 334
Transcription, 72, 73, 75–77, 86–88, 94, 112,
 116, 119, 122, 125, 145, 178, 276,
 278, 279, 281
Translation, 44, 57–59, 97, 166, 243, 279, 281
Translocase proteins, 95
Translocator protein 18 kDa (TSPO), 93
Transmission electron microscopy (TEM), 75
Transpeptidation, 166
Treponema pallidum, 169
Triapine® *see* 3-Aminopyridine-2-
 carboxaldehyde thiosemicarbazone
2,2′,2″,2‴-(1,4,7,10-Tetraazacyclododecane-
 1,4,7,10-tetrayl)tetraacetamide
 (TCMC), 336
2,2′,2″-(1,4,7-Triazacyclononane-1,4,7-triyl)
 triacetic acid (NOTA), 336, 338
1,3,5-Triaza-7-phosphaadamantane (PTA), 84,
 203, 204, 205, 275
Tricarboxylic acid cycle, 73
Triethylphosphine (Et3P), 22, 83, 148
Trifluoroacetate, 175
Trimethoprim, 166
Tripeptide integrin-recognizing tripeptide, 86
Triphenylphosphine (PPh3), 84, 155, 204, 257
Triphenylphosphonium (TPP), 76, 257
Triphenylsulfonium, 94
Triplet excited state, 42, 247, 248, 254, 256
Triplet metal-to-ligand charge transfer state
 (3MLCT), 256
TriTrypDB, 196
Trx *see* Thioredoxin
TrxR *see* Thioredoxin reductase
Trypanosomiasis, 178, 194, 195
TSPO protein, 92
TSST-1 *see* Toxins
Tuberculosis (TB), 171
Tumor ablation, 311

Tumor necrosis factor, 73, 278
Tumor progression, 68
Tumor spheroids, 84
Tumorigenesis, 72
Tungsten (W), 327
 W-186, 325, 327, 340
 W-188, 325, 327, 331
Two-photon
 absorption, 241, 255, 256
 excitation, 240, 251, 252, 254–260
 excitation microscopy, 240–241, 252–253,
 256–259
 excited chromophores, 255
 excited luminophores, 259
 excited sensors, 258
 fluorescence microscope, 253
Type I photoprocess, 92
Type II photoprocess, 92
L-Tyrosine ester, 172
Tyrosine kinase inhibitor (TKI), 19, 54

Ubiquinone, 90
Uganda S virus, 122
Ultraviolet (UV)-vis spectroscopy, 267
United States Environmental Protection
 Agency, 169
Uranium-235, 322, 324, 326
Uroporphyrinogen III synthase, 41
Uroporphyrins, 41
UV light, 52, 53, 56

Vaccinia virus, 109, 111, 121, 126
Vanadium (V), 110, 111, 200, 201, 202
 vanadium/oxovanadium complexes with
 antiviral activity
 with activity against neglected tropical
 diseases, 201
 oxidovanadium (IV) and (V)
 compounds, 201
 oxidovanadium compounds with
 porphyrins as ligands, 110, 111
 VO-based heteroleptic complexes with
 different bioactive ligands, 202
 VO-based homoleptic complexes with
 8HQ derivatives, 202
Vancomycin, 166, 168, 170, 172, 177, 180
Varicella-zoster virus (VZV), 112
Vector, 195, 196, 326, 329, 330,
 333–337, 340
Venetoclax, 74
Verteporfin (visudyne), 44
Vesicular stomatitis virus (VSV), 109, 111
Vibrational relaxation, 247
Viral infection, 108, 109, 124, 147, 155
Viral life cycles of HIV, 108, 109
 of SARS-CoV-2, 108, 109

Index

369

Viral replication, 108, 109, 111, 114, 117, 121, 122, 128, 130, 153–155
Viruses
  herpes simplex virus (HSV), 107, 109, 111, 113, 116, 121, 124 (*see also* Herpes)
  human cytomegalovirus (HCMV), 129
  human papilloma virus (HPV), 117, 130
  human rhinovirus (HRV), 118
Visudyne *see* Verteporfin
Vitamin B12, 19, 225–227
Vitamin E, 80
VSV *see* Vesicular stomatitis virus
VZV *see* Varicella-zoster virus

Warburg effect, 6, 72, 79
West Nile virus, 122
Western blots, 75
WHO *see* World Health Organization
World Health Organization (WHO), 144, 194
Wound infection, 167, 174; *see also* Infections

XAS *see* X-ray absorption spectrometry
X-ray, 74, 128, 240, 272, 295, 321
  synchrotron radiation X-ray fluorescence (SR-XRF), 272
  3D X-ray imaging, 272
  X-ray radiation, 241, 242, 272
X-ray fluorescence, 240–242
  imaging (XRF imaging), 240, 242 (*see also* X-ray fluorescence imaging)
  microscopy, 241–247, 259
  photon, 241

  radiation, 241
  tomography, 242
X-ray absorption spectrometry (XAS), 272
XRF imaging *see* X-ray

Yttrium (Y), 119, 333, 339
  Y-86, 333
  Y-90, 333

Zinc (Zn)
  Zn-68, 324, 331, 332
  Zn-lantanoides, 292
  Zn(II), 117, 118, 127, 173, 185
  zinc-binding domain of Plpro, 127, 155
  zinc complexes as antibacterial agents, 182–185
    complexes with zinc chelators, 169, 182–185, 169, 182
    complexes with zinc chelators combined with β-lactams, 183, 184
  zinc-finger enzyme PARP-1, 178
  zinc finger proteins, 112, 113
  zinc salts/complexes as antiviral agents, 115–118, 130
    zinc salts (acetate, chloride, nitrate, sulfate), 115–118
    zinc citrate (CIZAR®), 117
    zinc gluconate, 119
Zirconium (Zr), 333
  Zr-89, 324, 327, 333, 338, 339
  Zr-89 labelled agent, 333

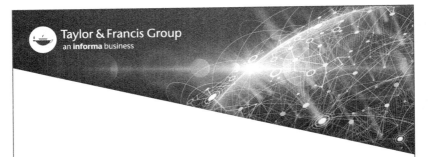